INTERNATIONAL
Trauma Life Support

for Emergency
Care Providers

eighth edition

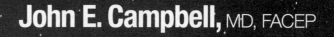

John E. Campbell, MD, FACEP

Roy L. Alson, PhD, MD, FACEP, FAAEM

and Alabama Chapter,
American College of Emergency Physicians

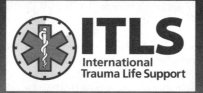

ITLS
**International
Trauma Life Support**

PEARSON

Boston   Columbus   Indianapolis   New York   San Francisco   Hoboken   Amsterdam
Cape Town   Dubai   London   Madrid   Milan   Munich   Paris   Montréal   Toronto
Delhi   Mexico City   São Paulo   Sydney   Hong Kong   Seoul   Singapore   Taipei   Tokyo

Publisher: Julie Levin Alexander
Publisher's Assistant: Sarah Henrich
Acquisitions Editor: Sladjana Repic Bruno
Program Manager: Monica Moosang
Development Editor: Jo Cepeda
Editorial Assistant: Lisa Narine
Project Management Lead: Cynthia Zonneveld
Project Manager: Julie Boddorf
Full-Service Project Manager: Peggy Kellar, iEnergizer Aptara®, Ltd.
Director of Marketing: David Gesell
Marketing Manager: Brian Hoehl
Marketing Specialist: Michael Sirinides
Marketing Assistant: Amy Pfund
Manufacturing Buyer: Mary Ann Gloriande
Interior and Cover Art Director: Diane Ernsberger
Interior Designer: Studio Montage
Cover Designer: Mary Siener
Cover Photos: Fuse/Getty Images; Blend Images - ERproductions Ltd/
 Getty Images; Steve Debenport/Getty Images
Composition: iEnergizer Aptara®, Ltd.
Printing and Binding: R.R. Donnelley
Cover Printer: Lehigh/Phoenix

Credits and acknowledgments for content borrowed from other sources and reproduced, with permission, in this textbook appear on the appropriate page within text.

Library of Congress Cataloging-in-Publication Data
International trauma life support for emergency care providers / [edited by] John Campbell.—8th edition.
 p. ; cm.
Includes bibliographical references and index.
ISBN 978-0-13-413079-8—ISBN 0-13-413079-0
I. Campbell, John E., 1943- , editor. [DNLM: 1. Emergency Medical Services. 2. Emergency Treatment—methods. 3. Life Support Care—methods. 4. Wounds and Injuries—therapy. WX 215]
 RA975.5.T83]
 362.18—dc23

 2015022267

Notice on Care Procedures

It is the intent of the authors and publisher that this textbook be used as part of an education program taught by qualified instructors and supervised by a licensed physician, in compliance with rules and regulations of the jurisdiction where the course is being offered. The procedures described in this textbook are based upon consultation with emergency care providers including EMTs, paramedics, nurses, and physicians, who are actively involved in prehospital care. As a field, prehospital medicine is constantly evolving. The authors and publisher have taken care to make certain that these procedures reflect currently accepted clinical practice; however, the procedures cannot be considered absolute recommendations, nor do they supersede applicable local laws or rules and the medical supervision of the prehospital provider.

The material in this textbook contains the most current information available at the time of publication. However, international, national, federal, state, provincial, and local guidelines concerning clinical practices, including, without limitation, those governing infection control and universal precautions, change rapidly. The reader should note, therefore, that new regulations may require changes in some procedures.

The references to products in this text do not represent an official endorsement by ITLS. Efforts have been made to include multiple types of devices, for illustrative purposes, when possible. It is impossible to include in this text an example of every type of device. As in other areas of medicine, there is ongoing development of equipment for use in the care of the prehospital trauma patient, which the authors and editors believe is good. It remains the responsibility of the ITLS provider in conjunction with local medical direction to determine which specific devices are applicable in their specific practice setting.

It is the responsibility of the reader to familiarize himself or herself with the policies and procedures set by federal, state, provincial, and local agencies as well as the institution or agency where the reader is employed. The authors and the publisher of this textbook and the supplements written to accompany it disclaim any liability, loss, or risk resulting directly or indirectly from the suggested procedures and theory, from any undetected errors, or from the reader's misunderstanding of the text. It is the reader's responsibility to stay informed of any new changes or recommendations made by any national, federal, state, provincial, and local agency as well as by his or her employing institution or agency.

Notice on Gender Usage

The English language has historically given preference to the male gender. Among many words, the pronouns, he and his are commonly used to describe both genders. Society evolves faster than language, and the male pronouns still predominate our speech. The authors have made great effort to treat the two genders equally, recognizing that a significant percentage of EMS providers are female. However, in some instances, male pronouns may be used to describe both males and females solely for the purpose of brevity. This is not intended to offend any readers of the female gender.

Notice on Prehospital Personnel Designation

Around the world, the credentialing and training of personnel who provide prehospital care vary greatly. In some jurisdictions, physicians and nurses respond as part of the EMS crew, whereas in other areas, those responding may only be trained to a basic life support (BLS) level. As the principles of care of the multiple trauma patient are the same regardless of the level of training of the persons providing care, the authors and publisher have attempted to describe those care providers in generic terms throughout the book. Common terms in English such as *medic* or *emergency medical responder* are, in some jurisdictions, actual certification levels of personnel. The term *emergency care provider* is used in this text to describe all levels of personnel who provide care in the prehospital setting. When other common terms are used to refer to persons providing care, it is intended to represent all persons who provide prehospital care and not to exclude or offend any care provider.

10 9 8 7 6 5 4 3

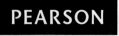

ISBN-10: 0-13-413079-0
ISBN-13: 978-0-13-413079-8

Dedication

The best way to find yourself is to lose yourself in the service of others.

– Mohandas K. Gandhi

This eighth edition of the ITLS textbook is dedicated to the men and women who each day answer the call for help. Every hour of every day they stand watch keeping our fellow citizens, our friends, and our families safe. When crises arise, they are there, providing care and comfort, often at great risk to themselves. And each year, all over the world, some of our colleagues make the ultimate sacrifice. We honor them and their families in our resolve to continue to "answer the call." We can think of no one who better epitomizes that dedication better than our friend and colleague Vickey G. Lewis, RN, BSN.

Vickey has been a first responder, ED RN, EMS and Nurse educator, and a fixture in ITLS for 30 years. She was certified in the first BTLS course taught in North Carolina in the early 1980s, served as the first chapter coordinator for North Carolina BTLS (now ITLS), establishing a training program that continues to grow. Furthermore, she has shared her knowledge and experience with others, all across the globe as they sought to bring the program to their communities. She taught hundreds of providers how to care for trauma patients as well as established educational programs for providers and citizens to deal with cardiac arrest. She has served as the speaker of the ITLS annual delegate meeting for over 10 years, "herding the cats" with both knowledge and humor. Over her long career, she consistently gives credit to others for what is accomplished. As an organization and as individual providers and educators, we have greatly benefited from her wisdom, experience, and dedication. For that we are truly grateful.

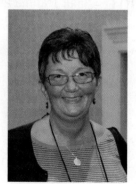

Vickey G. Lewis, RN, BSN

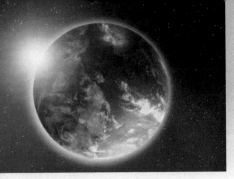

Table of Contents

About the Editors

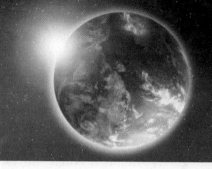

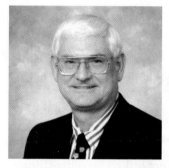

John E. Campbell, MD, FACEP

Dr. Campbell received his BS degree in pharmacy from Auburn University in 1966 and his medical degree from the University of Alabama at Birmingham in 1970. He has been in the practice of Emergency Medicine for 40 years, practicing in Alabama, Georgia, New Mexico, and Texas. He became interested in prehospital care in 1972 when he was asked to teach a basic EMT course to members of the Clay County Rescue Squad. He is still an honorary member of that outstanding group. Since then, he has served as medical director of many EMT and paramedic training programs. He recently retired as the Medical Director for EMS and Trauma for the State of Alabama.

From the original basic trauma life support course developed an international organization of teachers of trauma care called "International Trauma Life Support, Inc.," or ITLS. Dr. Campbell has served as its president since the inception of the organization.

Dr. Campbell is the author of the first edition of the *Basic Trauma Life Support* textbook and has continued to be the editor through to this new edition, now entitled *International Trauma Life Support for Emergency Care Providers*. He also is the coauthor of *Homeland Security and Emergency Medical Response* and *Tactical Emergency Medical Essentials*.

He was a member of the first faculty of Emergency Medicine at the School of Medicine, University of Alabama at Birmingham. In 1991 he was the first recipient of the American College of Emergency Medicine's EMS Award for outstanding achievement of national significance in the area of EMS. In 2001 he received the Ronald D. Stewart Lifetime Achievement Award from the National Association of EMS Physicians. He is currently retired from clinical practice and resides in Montgomery, Alabama.

Roy L. Alson, PhD, MD, FACEP, FAAEM

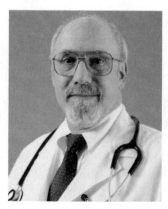

Dr. Roy L. Alson is an Associate Professor of Emergency Medicine at the Wake Forest University School of Medicine and Director of the Office of Prehospital and Disaster Medicine at Wake Forest. He is also an Associate Professor at the Childress Institute for Pediatric Trauma at Wake Forest University. He received his bachelor's degree from the University of Virginia in 1974 and both his PhD and MD from the Bowman Gray School of Medicine of Wake Forest University (1982, 1985). He completed his residency in emergency medicine at Allegheny General Hospital in Pittsburgh, Pennsylvania, and is board certified in both emergency medicine and emergency medical services by the American Board of Emergency Medicine.

His EMS career began in the early 1970s as an EMT in New York City. As a graduate student, Dr. Alson became a member of the Winston-Salem Rescue Squad and began working for the Forsyth County EMS as an EMT. Upon completion of his residency, Dr. Alson returned to Wake Forest University and the Forsyth County EMS system, serving as Assistant Medical Director for 14 years and Medical Director for the last 12 years. He remains actively involved in the education of EMS personnel.

Dr. Alson's involvement with ITLS dates to the 1980s. He served as the North Carolina Chapter Medical Director for 15 years. Since the 1990s he has been a member of the editorial board for ITLS as well as a contributing author. With this edition, he joins Dr. Campbell as co-editor in chief.

Along with EMS, disaster medicine is an area of interest. Dr. Alson serves as the Medical Director for the North Carolina State Medical Response System (NC SMAT) program. He has served as the Chairman of the Disaster Preparedness and Response Committee for American College of Emergency Physicians, as well as a member of the EMS Committee for the American Academy of Emergency Physicians. He is the Chairman for the NAEMSP Disaster Preparedness Committee for 2014-16.

He has served with the National Disaster Medical System (NDMS) for 20 years and is currently a member of the International Medical Surgical Response Team East (IMSURT–E). He previously served as the Commander and Deputy Commander for the North Carolina Disaster Medical Assistance Team (NC-DMAT-1).

Dr. Alson has responded to numerous nationally declared disasters. He continues to teach about the delivery of care in austere and surge-type conditions and has lectured nationally and internationally on prehospital trauma care and disaster medicine.

He and his wife, Rebecca, reside in Winston-Salem.

About the Authors

ITLS for Emergency Care Providers, 8th Edition

Roy L. Alson, PhD, MD, FACEP, FAAEM

Associate Professor of Emergency Medicine and Director, Office of Prehospital and Disaster Medicine, Wake Forest University School of Medicine, Winston-Salem, NC; Medical Director, Forsyth County EMS, Winston-Salem, NC; Medical Advisor, Disaster Services, NC Office of EMS, Raleigh, NC

James J. Augustine, MD

Director of Clinical Operations, EMP Ltd, Canton, OH; Assistant Clinical Professor, Department of Emergency Medicine, Wright State University, Dayton, OH; Chair, ASTM Task Group E54.02.01, Standards for Hospital Preparedness Under Committee E54 on Homeland Security Applications; former Medical Director, Atlanta Fire Rescue Department and the District of Columbia Fire and EMS Department.

Jere Baldwin, MD, FACEP, FAAFP

Chief, Department of Emergency Medicine and Ambulatory Services, Mercy Hospital, Port Huron, MI

Graciela M. Bauza, MD

Assistant Professor of Surgery, University of Pittsburgh, Pittsburgh, PA

Russell Bieniek, MD, FACEP

Director of Emergency Preparedness, UPMC Hamot, Erie, PA

William Bozeman, MD, FACEP, FAAEM

Professor, Department of Emergency Medicine, and Associate Research Director, Wake Forest University School of Medicine, Winston-Salem, NC; Lead Physician, Tactical Operations, Forsyth County EMS, Winston-Salem, NC

Walter J. Bradley, MD, MBA, FACEP

Medical Director, Illinois State Police; SWAT Team Physician, Moline Police Department; Physician Advisor, Trinity Medical Center, Moline, IL

Sabina A. Braithwaite, MD, MPH, FACEP, NREMTP

Clinical Associate Professor of Emergency Medicine, University of Kansas Medical Center, Kansas City; Clinical Associate Professor of Preventive Medicine and Public Health, University of Kansas Medical Center, Wichita; Associate Medical Director, Medical Control Board, EMS System for Metropolitan Oklahoma City and Tulsa; Vice Chair, Board of Directors, International Trauma Life Support

Jeremy J. Brywczynski, MD

Assistant Professor, Emergency Medicine, Vanderbilt University Medical Center, Nashville, TN; Medical Director, Vanderbilt LifeFlight; Medical Director, Vanderbilt FlightComm; Assistant Medical Director, Nashville (TN) Fire Department

John E. Campbell, MD, FACEP

Medical Director, EMS and Trauma, State of Alabama, Retired

Alexandra Charpentier, EMT-P

EMS Director, Heart of Texas Healthcare System EMS, Brady, TX

Leon Charpentier, EMT-P

Harker Heights (TX) Fire Chief, Retired

James H. Creel, Jr. MD, FACEP

Clinical Associate Professor and Program Director, Department of Emergency Medicine, University of Tennessee College of Medicine (UTCOM); Chief of Emergency Medicine, Erlanger Health System, Chattanooga, TN

Ann M. Dietrich, MD, FAAP, FACEP

Professor of Pediatrics, Ohio State University; Director of Risk Management, Section of Emergency Medicine, Columbus (OH) Children's Hospital; Pediatric Medical Advisor, Medflight of Ohio

Ray Fowler, MD, FACEP, DBAEMS

Professor and Chief, Division of Emergency Medical Services, The University of Texas, Southwestern Medical Center; Attending Emergency Medicine Faculty, Parkland Memorial Hospital, Dallas, TX

Pam Gersch, RN, CLNC
Program Director, AirMed Team, Rocky Mountain Helicopters, Redding, CA

Martin Greenberg, MD, FAAOS, FACS
Chief of Hand Surgery, Advocate Illinois Masonic Medical Center; Chief of Orthopedic Surgery, Our Lady of the Resurrection Medical Center, Chicago, IL; Reserve Police Officer, Village of Tinley Park, IL; Tactical Physician, South Suburban Emergency Response Team; ITOA Co-Chair, TEMS Committee

Kyee H. Han, MBBS, FRCS, FCEM
Consultant in Accident and Emergency Medicine; Medical Director, North East Ambulance Service NHS Trust; Honorary Clinical Senior Lecturer, The James Cook University Hospital, Middlesbrough, UK

Donna Hastings, MA, EMT-P, CPCC
Chair, ITLS Editorial Board; CEO, Heart and Stroke Foundation of Alberta, NWT and Nunavut, Calgary, Canada

Leah J. Heimbach, JD, RN, EMT-P
Principal, Healthcare Management Solutions, LLC, White Hall, WV

Eduardo Romero Hicks, MD, EMT
Director, Sistema de Urgencias del Estado de Guanajuato, Guanajuato State Emergency System, México; Associate Professor, University of Guanajuato Nursing School, Guanajuato, México; Medical Director, ITLS Guanajuato México Chapter

Ahamed H. Idris, MD
Professor of Surgery and Medicine and Director, DFW Center for Resuscitation Research, UT Southwestern Medical Center at Dallas, TX

David Maatman, NRP/IC

Kirk Magee MD, MSc, FRCPC
Associate Professor, Dalhousie Department of Emergency Medicine, Halifax, Nova Scotia

Patrick J. Maloney, MD
Staff Physician, Denver (CO) Health Medical Center and Denver Emergency, Center for Children; Clinical Instructor, University of Colorado School of Medicine, Denver, CO

David Manthey, MD, FACEP, FAAEM
Professor of Emergency Medicine and Vice Chair of Education, Wake Forest University School of Medicine, Winston-Salem, NC

Leslie K. Mihalov, MD
Chief, Emergency Medicine, and Medical Director, Emergency Services, Nationwide Children's Hospital; Associate Professor of Pediatrics at The Ohio State University College of Medicine

Richard N. Nelson, MD, FACEP
Professor and Vice Chair, Department of Emergency Medicine, The Ohio State University College of Medicine

Jonathan Newman, MD, MMM, FACEP
Assistant Medical Director, United Hospital Center, Bridgeport, WV

Bob Page, MEd, NRP, CCP, NCEE
Edutainment Consulting and Seminars, LLC

Wm. Bruce Patterson, Platoon Chief/EMT-P
Strathcona County Emergency Services

Andrew B. Peitzman, MD

Mark M. Ravitch
Professor and Executive Vice-Chairman, Department of Surgery, and Chief, Division of General Surgery, University of Pittsburgh

Paul E. Pepe, MD, MPH
Professor of Emergency Medicine, Internal Medicine, Pediatrics, Public Health and Riggs Family Chair in Emergency Medicine, University of Texas Southwestern Medical Center and Parkland Emergency-Trauma Center; Director, City of Dallas Medical Emergency Services for Public Safety, Public Health and Homeland Security, Dallas, TX

William F. Pfeifer, MD, FACS
Professor of Surgery, Department of Specialty Medicine, Rocky Vista University College of Osteopathic Medicine; Mile High Surgical Specialists, Littleton, CO; Colonel MC USAR (ret)

Art Proust, MD, FACEP
Associate Medical Director, SFVEMSS, Geneva, IL

Mario Luis Ramirez, MD, MPP
Tactical and Prehospital EMS Fellow and Clinical Instructor in Emergency Medicine, Department of Emergency Medicine, Vanderbilt University Medical Center, Nashville, TN

Jonathan M. Rubin, MD, FAAEM
Associate Professor of Emergency Medicine, Medical College of Wisconsin

S. Robert Seitz, MEd, RN, NRP
Assistant Professor, School of Health and Rehabilitation Sciences, Emergency Medicine Program, University of Pittsburgh; Assistant Program Director, Office of Education and International Emergency Medicine, University of Pittsburgh Center for Emergency Medicine; Continuing Education Editor, *Journal of Emergency Medical Services*; Editorial Board, International Trauma Life Support

Corey M. Slovis, MD, FACP, FACEP, FAAEM
Professor of Emergency Medicine and Medicine and Chairman, Department of Emergency Medicine, Vanderbilt University Medical Center, Nashville, TN; Medical Director, Metro Nashville Fire Department and International Airport

J. T. Stevens, NRP (ret.)
Sun City, SC

Ronald D. Stewart, OC, ONS, ECNS, BA, BSc, MD, FACEP, DSc, LLD
Professor Emeritus, Medical Education, and Professor of Emergency Medicine and Anaesthesia, Dalhousie University, Halifax, Nova Scotia, Canada

Shin Tsuruoka, MD
Vice director and Chief of Neurosurgical Department, JA Toride Medical Center, Toride, Japan; ITLS Japan Chapter Medical Director

Arlo Weltge, MD, MPH, FACEP
Clinical Associate Professor of Emergency Medicine, University of Texas, Houston Medical School; Medical Director, Program in EMS, Houston Community College

Howard A. Werman, MD, FACEP
Professor of Clinical Emergency Medicine, The Ohio State University; Medical Director, MedFlight of Ohio

Katherine West, BSN, MSEd, CIC
Infection Control Consultant, Manassas, VA; Member JEMS Editorial Board

Melissa White, MD, MPH
Assistant Professor, Assistant Residency Director, and Medical Director, John's Creek Fire Department; Medical Director, Emory Emergency Medical Services; Associate Medical Director, Emory Flight/Air Methods, GA; Department of Emergency Medicine, Emory University School of Medicine, Atlanta, GA

Janet M. Williams, MD
Professor of Emergency Medicine, University of Rochester (NY) Medical Center

E. John Wipfler, III, MD, FACEP
Attending Emergency Physician, OSF Saint Francis Medical Center Residency Program; Medical Director, STATT TacMed Unit, Tactical Medicine; Sheriff's Physician, Peoria County (IL) Sheriff's Office; Clinical Associate Professor of Surgery, University of Illinois College of Medicine, Peoria, IL

Arthur H. Yancey II, MD, MPH, FACEP
Deputy Director of Health for EMS, Fulton County Department of Health and Wellness, Atlanta, GA; Associate Professor, Department of Emergency Medicine, Emory University School of Medicine, Atlanta, GA

What's New in This Edition

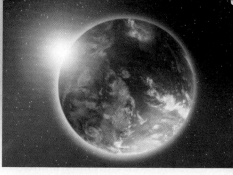

The eighth edition of the ITLS textbook, *International Trauma Life Support for Emergency Care Providers*, has been updated to provide the emergency care provider with information on the latest and most effective approaches to the care of the trauma patient. The science of trauma is constantly evolving, and the research working group at ITLS has worked to bring to the authors and the text information that is pertinent to the initial care of the trauma patient.

One of the biggest changes in this edition is that Dr. Roy Alson has joined Dr. John Campbell as co-editor in chief. Dr. Alson is a board-certified EM and EMS physician with extensive experience in EMS care and education and has been a contributor to the ITLS text and course for over 25 years.

The text again conforms to the latest AHA/ILCOR guidelines for artificial ventilation and CPR. The case presentations used in many of the chapters draw upon a single scenario as an effort to have the illustrative cases used reflect a more realistic situation. Although trauma can result in single-system injuries, major trauma victims often have multiple organ systems or body areas involved, and these must all be assessed and stabilized.

The text continues the presentation of Key Terms and updates of photos and drawings as needed. There is now also a new student and instructor resource Web site, which provides additional information beyond the core material of ITLS.

Some of the chapter-by-chapter changes and key components are listed here:

- In the Introduction it is explained what the concept of the "Golden Period" is and why it remains important to what we do.
- In Chapter 1, the emphasis on scene safety continues to be a central component, as is the concept that trauma care is a team effort involving many disciplines. There is a discussion of the changes in response put forth by the Hartford Consensus.
- In Chapter 2, minor changes have been made in the assessment sequence based on feedback from ITLS instructors and providers. The importance of identifying and controlling at the start of the assessment is reinforced. As the leader performs the assessment, he or she will delegate responses to abnormalities found in the initial assessment. This is to reinforce the rule that the leader must not interrupt the assessment to deal with

problems but must delegate the needed actions to team members. That emphasizes the team concept and keeps on scene time at a minimum. The order of presentation of the three assessments (ITLS Primary Survey, ITLS Ongoing Exam, and ITLS Secondary Survey) has been changed. The ITLS Ongoing Exam is performed before the ITLS Secondary Survey, a more common situation, and may replace it. The use of finger-stick serum lactate levels and prehospital abdominal ultrasound exams are mentioned as areas of current study to better identify patients who may be in early shock.

- Chapter 3 reflects the changes in Chapter 2.
- In Chapter 4, capnography is stressed as the standard for confirming and monitoring the position of the endotracheal tube as well as the best way to assess for hyperventilation or hypoventilation. The volume of air delivered with each ventilation now emphasizes the response of the patient (rise and fall of the chest) rather than a fixed volume amount.
- In Chapter 5, fiberoptic and video intubation are discussed as evolving technologies. Drug-assisted intubation is now included in this chapter, rather than in the appendix, because it is more commonly used. The key role of blind insertion airway devices (BIADs) in basic airway management is reinforced.
- In Chapter 6, a discussion of the indications for decompressing pericardial tamponade has been added, when such a procedure is in the emergency care provider's scope of practice. Also discussed is the use of ultrasound to identify such injuries and also to identify a pneumothorax.
- In Chapter 7, there is a revised discussion of needle decompression of the chest for a tension pneumothorax reflecting challenges faced by tactical EMS providers.
- In Chapter 8, the discussion of hemorrhagic shock has again been updated to reflect the latest experience of the military during the recent conflicts. A discussion of the role of tranexamic acid (TXA) in the management of hemorrhage has been added.
- Chapters 11 and 12 now reflect current science and published guidelines. There has been a complete revision of when to apply spinal motion restriction. In addition, the transport of a patient on a backboard is now discouraged. Included also is how to remove the patient from the backboard once placed on a transport stretcher. The standing backboard procedure has been eliminated.

- In Chapter 13, the use of finger-stick serum lactate levels and the use of prehospital abdominal ultrasound exams are mentioned.
- In Chapter 14, the discussion of management of bleeding from extremity injuries has been expanded, including discussion of hemostatic agents.
- In Chapter 15, procedures for use of a tourniquet and use of hemostatic agents have been expanded as well as discussion of pelvic binders for pelvic fractures.
- In Chapter 16, the use of Ringer's lactate as a resuscitation fluid in major burns is emphasized.
- Chapter 21 discusses the indications for termination of resuscitation for the trauma patient in the prehospital setting.
- Chapter 22 has been updated with the latest recommendations for postexposure prophylaxis and an expanded section on emerging infections that pose challenges to emergency care providers.

What's New on Student Resource Page

Student Resources can be found at *pearsonhighered.com/bradyresources*. Students can access additional skills and information for more practice and review.

- In "Additional Skills," the use of the new FastResponder™ sternal IO has been added.
- In "Role of the Medical Helicopter," the data has been updated.
- In "Trauma Scoring in the Prehospital Care Setting," the CDC Trauma Triage Scheme is included.
- In "Tactical EMS," the bibliography has been revised to reflect current thinking within the Hartford Consensus.

Acknowledgments

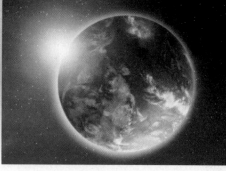

The creation of a text and course is a major undertaking and could not be done without a team effort. For many of those involved this is a true labor of love. We want to give special thanks to the following friends of ITLS who provided invaluable assistance with ideas, reviews, and corrections of the text. This was such a big job, and there were so many people who contributed, that we are sure we have left someone out. Please accept our apologies in advance.

We wish to thank the EMS professionals who reviewed material especially for this 8th Edition of *International Trauma Life Support for Emergency Care Providers*. Their assistance is appreciated:

Gary Bonewald, M.Ed., LP, Program Director / Coordinator, Wharton County Junior College, Emergency Medical Services Program

Scott Craig, CCEMT-P, I/C, Associate Professor of EMS, Johnson County Community College, Overland Park, KS

Ronald Feller, MBA, NRP, Director, Emergency Medical Services, Oklahoma City Community College, OKC, OK

Jerry Findley, Licensed Paramedic, BS Health Admin, MA Organizational Leadership EMS Program Director, South Plains College, Lubbock, Texas

Scott Jones, EMT-P, MBAEMS Professor, Victor Valley College, Regional Public Safety Training Center, Apple Valley, CA

Richard Main, M.Ed., NRP, Engelstad School of Health Sciences, College of Southern Nevada, Las Vegas, NV

Reylon Meeks, RN, BSN, MS, MSN, EMT, PhD Clinical Nurse Specialist, Blank Children's Hospital - Des Moines, IA

Christoper Mierek - CPT, MC,4th MEB Surgeon, Dauntless Clinic OIC

Brandon Poteet – EMS Program Director, Grayson College, Denison, TX

Roy Ramos, NRP, Pre/CEO Heart EMTS LL., Pueblo, CO

Rintha Simpson, BS, NRP, NCEE

Robert Vroman, M.Ed., BS NRP Associate Professor of EMS, Red Rocks Community College, Lakewood, CO

We wish to thank Jo Cepeda, our development editor, for her patience and for keeping us on track.

Thanks to the management and staff of AMR-Las Vegas for their assistance with photographs. Their hospitality and cooperation is greatly appreciated:

Carla Murreu
Jake Fan

Jason Blakley
Christi Cservenyak

Nathen Van Wingerden
Eric Dievendorf

Another special thanks goes to the following photographers who donated their work to help illustrate the text:

Roy Alson, MD, FACEP
Sabina Braithwaite, MD, FACEP
James Broselow, MD
Brant Burden, EMT-P
Anthony Cellitti, NRP
Alexandra Charpentier, EM-P
Leon Charpentier, EMT-P
Stanley Cooper, EMT-P
Delphi Medical
Pamela Drexel, Brain Trauma Foundation

David Effron, MD, FACEP
Ferno Washington, Inc.
Peter Gianas, MD
Peter Goth, MD
KING Airway Systems
Kyee H. Han, MD, FRCS, FFAEM
Michal Heron
Eduardo Romero Hicks, MD
Jeff Hinshaw, MS, PA-C, NRP
Kelly Kirk, EMT-P

Masimo Corporation
Lewis B. Mallory, MBA, REMT-P
Bonnie Meneely, EMT-P
Nonin Medical, Inc.
North American Rescue
Bob Page, MEd, NRP, CCP, NCEE
William Pfeifer, MD, FACS
Robert S. Porter
Don Resch
SAM Splints

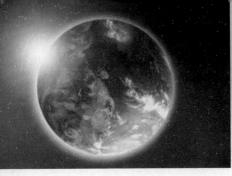

Introduction to the ITLS Course

Trauma, the medical term for *injury*, has become the most expensive health problem in the United States and most other countries. In the United States, trauma is the fourth-leading cause of death for all ages and the leading cause of death for children and adults under the age of 45 years. Trauma causes 73% of all deaths in the 15- to 24-year-old age group. For every fatality, there are 10 more patients admitted to hospitals and hundreds more treated in emergency departments. The price of trauma, in both physical and fiscal resources, mandates that all emergency medical services (EMS) personnel learn more about this disease to treat its effects and decrease its incidence.

Because the survival of trauma patients is often determined by how quickly they get definitive care in the operating room, it is crucial that you know how to assess and manage the critical trauma patient in the most efficient way. The purpose of the ITLS course is to teach you the most rapid and practical method to assess and manage critical trauma patients. The course is a combination of written chapters to give you the "why" and the "how" and practical exercises to practice your knowledge and skills on simulated patients so that at the end of the course you feel confident in your ability to provide rapid life-saving trauma care.

Philosophy of Assessment and Management of the Trauma Patient

Severe trauma, along with acute coronary syndrome and stroke, is a time-dependent disease. The direct relationship between the timing of definitive (surgical) treatment and the survival of trauma patients was first described by Dr. R Adams Cowley of the famous Shock-Trauma Center in Baltimore, Maryland. He discovered that when patients with serious multiple injuries were able to gain access to the operating room within an hour of the time of injury, the highest survival rate was achieved. He referred to this as the "Golden Hour." Over the years we have found that some patients (such as penetrating trauma to trunk) do not have a golden "hour" but rather a shorter period of minutes, whereas many patients with blunt trauma may have a golden period longer than an hour. It has been suggested that we now call the prehospital period the "Golden Period" because it may be longer or shorter than an hour.

The Golden Period begins at the moment the patient is injured, not at the time you arrive at the scene. Much of this period has already passed when you begin your assessment, so you must be well organized in what you do. In the prehospital setting it is better to think of the Golden Period for on scene care as being 10 minutes. In those 10 minutes, you must identify live patients, make treatment decisions, and begin to move patients to the appropriate medical facility. This means that every action must have a life-saving purpose. Any action that increases scene time but is not potentially life saving must be omitted. Not only must you reduce evaluation and resuscitation to the most efficient and critical steps, but you also must develop the habit of assessing and treating every trauma patient in a planned logical and sequential manner so you do not forget critical actions.

When performing patient assessment, it is best to proceed in a "head-to-toe" manner so that nothing is missed. If you jump around during your assessment, you will inevitably forget to evaluate something crucial. Working as a team with your partner is also important because many actions must be done at the same time.

It has been said that medicine is a profession that was created for obsessive-compulsive people. Nowhere is this truer than in the care of the trauma patient. Often the patient's life depends on how well you manage the details. It is very important to remember that many of the details necessary to save the patient occur before you even arrive at the scene of the injury.

You or a member of your team must:

- Know how to maintain your ambulance or rescue vehicle so that it is serviced and ready to respond when needed.
- Know the quickest way to the scene of an injury. Use of global positioning satellite (GPS) navigation has been shown to decrease not only the time to respond but also the time of transport.
- Know how to size up a scene to recognize dangers and identify mechanisms of injury.
- Know which scenes are safe and, if not safe, what to do about them.
- Know when you can handle a situation and when to call for help.
- Work effectively as a team so the care provided is appropriate and effective.

- Know when to approach the patient and when to leave with the patient.
- Know your equipment, and maintain it in working order.
- Know the most appropriate hospital and the fastest way to get there. (Organized trauma systems and transfer/bypass guidelines can shorten the time it takes to get a trauma patient to definitive care.)

As if all that were not enough, you also have to:

- Know where to put your hands, which questions to ask, what interventions to perform, when to perform them, and how to perform critical procedures quickly and correctly.

If you think the details are not important, then leave the profession now. Our job is saving lives, a most ancient and honorable profession. If we have a bad day, someone will pay for our mistakes with suffering or even death. Since the early beginnings of emergency medical services (EMS), patients and even rescuers have lost their lives because attention was not paid to the details listed here. Many of us can recall patients that we might have saved if we had been a little smarter, a little faster, or a little better organized.

Make no mistake, there is no "high" like saving a life, but we carry the scars of our failures all our lives.

Your mind-set and attitude are very important. You must be concerned but not emotional, alert but not excited, quick but not hasty. Above all, you must continuously strive for what is best for your patient. When your training has not prepared you for a situation, always fall back on the question: *What is best for my patient?* When you no longer care, burnout has set in, and your effectiveness is severely limited. When this happens, seek help. (Yes, all of us need help when the stress overcomes us.) Or seek an alternative profession.

Since 1982, the International Trauma Life Support (ITLS, formerly BTLS) organization has been identifying the best methods to get the most out of those few minutes that prehospital EMS providers have to save the patient's life. Not all patients can be saved, but our goal is never to lose a life that could have been saved. The knowledge in this book can help you make a difference. Learn it well.

John E. Campbell, MD, FACEP
Editor

About ITLS

International Trauma Life Support is a global not-for-profit organization dedicated to preventing death and disability from trauma through education and emergency trauma care.

The Smart Choice for Trauma Training

Train with the best. Train with ITLS. Together, we are improving trauma care worldwide. International Trauma Life Support—a not-for-profit organization dedicated to excellence in trauma education and response—coordinates ITLS education and training worldwide. Founded in 1985 as Basic Trauma Life Support, ITLS adopted a new name in 2005 to better reflect its global role and impact. Today, ITLS has more than 80 chapters and training centers around the world. Through ITLS, hundreds of thousands of trauma care professionals have learned proven techniques endorsed by the American College of Emergency Physicians.

ITLS is the smart choice for your trauma training, because it is

- *Practical.* ITLS trains you in a realistic, hands-on approach proven to work in the field—from scene to surgery.
- *Dynamic.* ITLS content is current, relevant, and responsive to the latest thinking in trauma management.

- *Flexible.* ITLS courses are taught through a strong network of chapters and training centers that customize content to reflect local needs and priorities.
- *Team centered.* ITLS emphasizes a cohesive team approach that works in the real world and recognizes the importance of your role.
- *Grounded in emergency medicine.* Practicing emergency physicians—medicine's frontline responders—lead ITLS efforts to deliver stimulating content based on solid emergency medicine.
- *Challenging.* ITLS course content raises the bar on performance in the field by integrating classroom knowledge with practical application of skills.

Focused Content That Delivers

ITLS empowers you with the knowledge and skill to provide optimal care in the prehospital setting. It offers a variety of training options for all levels and backgrounds of emergency personnel around the world. ITLS courses combine classroom learning, hands-on skills stations, and assessment stations that put your learning to work in simulated trauma situations. Not only are courses taught as a continuing education option, but they are also used as essential curricula in many Paramedic, EMT, and first responder training programs.

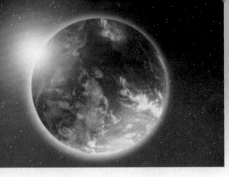

International Trauma Life Support Courses

ITLS Basic

ITLS Basic is designed for the Emergency Medical Technician (EMT-Basic) and the emergency care responder. This hands-on training course offers basic EMS providers complete training in the skills necessary for rapid assessment, resuscitation, stabilization and transportation of the trauma patient. The course provides education in the initial evaluation and stabilization of the trauma patient.

ITLS Advanced

ITLS Advanced is a comprehensive course covering the skills necessary for rapid assessment, resuscitation, stabilization, and transportation of the trauma patient for advanced EMTs, Paramedics, and Trauma Nurses. The course teaches the correct sequence of evaluation and the techniques of critical intervention, resuscitation, and packaging of a patient.

ITLS Combined

Many ITLS courses choose to train both Advanced and Basic level providers. In the **ITLS Combined** courses, the Basic level providers partake of all didactic sessions and observe the advanced skill stations.

ITLS Military

The ITLS Military Provider course combines the fundamentals of ITLS trauma assessment and treatment with recent military innovations utilized in the world's current war zones. The course adapts proven techniques taught in the civilian ITLS course to the military environment, where limited resources are the rule, not the exception.

eTrauma

ITLS eTrauma covers the eight hours of ITLS Provider classroom instruction providing online training on the core principles of rapid assessment, resuscitation, stabilization, and transportation of trauma patients. ITLS eTrauma is offered at both the Basic and Advanced levels. At the completion of eTrauma, the learner receives eight hours of CEU from CECBEMS and is qualified to take the ITLS Completer course that will lead to ITLS certification.

Completer Course

The ITLS Completer course is for the learner who has successfully completed eTrauma and wishes to become ITLS certified. The Completer course covers eight hours of skills learning and assessment as well as the ITLS written post course exam.

Provider Recertification

This course provides continuing education in ITLS for the experienced provider who has already completed the Basic or Advanced Course. Sample course agendas are available in the 8th edition ITLS Coordinator and Instructor Guide or from the International Office.

ITLS Instructor Bridge Course

The ITLS Instructor Bridge Course is designed for the instructor who has successfully completed an ATLS or PHTLS instructor course and wishes to transition to the ITLS program. The course typically runs eight hours, and a sample course agenda is available in the 8th edition ITLS Coordinator and Instructor Guide or from the International Office. Following completion of an ITLS Bridge course, a candidate must be monitored teaching an ITLS provider course to complete the steps to become an ITLS instructor.

ITLS Provider Bridge Course

The ITLS Provider Bridge Course is designed for the provider who has successfully completed a PHTLS, ATT, or TNCC course and wishes to transition to the ITLS program. The course typically runs eight hours. A sample course agenda is available in the 8th edition ITLS Coordinator and Instructor Guide or from the International Office.

ITLS Access

This ITLS Access course provides EMS crews and first responders with training to utilize the tools commonly carried on an ambulance or first responder unit to reach entrapped patients and begin stabilization and extrication.

ITLS Pediatric

Pediatric ITLS concentrates on the care of injured children. The course is designed to train EMS and nursing personnel in the proper assessment, stabilization, and packaging of a pediatric trauma patient. The course also covers communication techniques with pediatric patients and parents.

ITLS Instructor Courses

ITLS instructor courses are offered for both ITLS Advanced and ITLS Basic courses. Other methods of achieving instructor status are used for Pediatric ITLS and ITLS Access courses. To become an instructor, students must have successfully completed the provider level course with specific requirements on both the written and practical exams and be monitored teaching the lecture, skills, and testing portions of the Provider course.

Enrolling in an ITLS Course

ITLS provides its courses through chapters and training centers. The ITLS Course Management System makes it easy to find a course in your area. Log on to cms.itrauma.org to search for courses and contact the course administrator to register.

If you need information about your local chapter or training center, check our list at itrauma.org or call ITLS headquarters at 888-495-ITLS or +1-630-495-6442 (for international callers). We will put you in touch with your local organization—or help you start the program in your area.

International Trauma Life Support
3000 Woodcreek Drive, Suite 200
Downers Grove, Illinois 60515
Phone: 888-495-ITLS
+1-630-495-6442 (International)
Fax: 630-495-6404
Web: www.itrauma.org
E-mail: info@itrauma.org

ITLS Leadership
Board of Directors

John E. Campbell, MD, FACEP (USA)
Neil Christen, MD, FACEP (USA)
Tony Connelly, EMT-P, BHSc, PGCEd (Canada)
Jonathan L. Epstein, MEMS, NRP (USA)
Peter Macintyre, ACP (Canada)
Russell Bieniek, MD, FACEP (USA)

Gianluca Ghiselli, MD (Italy)
Peter Gianas, MD (USA)
John S. Holloway, Sr., MBA, FF/NRP (USA)
Wilhelmina Elsabe Nel, MD (Canada)
Eric Roy, MBA-HCM, BMaSc, CD OSJ Canada)
Chen Zhi, MD (Peoples Republic of China)

ITLS Leadership
Editorial Board

Chair: Donna Hastings, MA, EMT-P, CPCC (Canada)
Chair Emeritus: John E. Campbell, MD, FACEP, Editor*
  (USA)

Members

Roy Alson, MD, PhD, FACEP (USA) –Co-Editor
Sabina Braithwaite, MD, MPH, FACEP, NRP (USA)
Darby Copeland, EdD, RN, NRP (USA)
Ann Marie Dietrich, MD, FACEP, FAAP (USA)

Kyee Han, MBBS, FRCS, FFAEM (UK)
Tim Hillier, ACP (Canada)
David Maatman, NRP/IC (USA)
Bob Page, MEd, NRP, CCP, NCEE (USA)
William Pfeifer III, MD, FACS (USA)
Antonio Requena Lopez, MD (Spain)
S. Robert Seitz, MEd, RN, NRP (USA)

ITLS Editorial Teams
Research Team

Kyee Han, MBBS, FRCS, FFAEM, Team Leader
  (United Kingdom)
Liz Cloughessy, RN, MHM, FAEN
  (Australia)

Howard Mell, MD, FACEP (USA)
Art Proust, MD, FACEP (USA)
Eduardo Romero Hicks, MD (Mexico)
Hiroyuki Tanaka, MD (Japan)

Skills Team (Skills Chapters)

S. Robert Seitz, MEd, RN, NRP, Team Leader (USA)
J. David Barrick, EMT-P (USA)
Dale Bayliss, EMT-P (Canada)
Ron Kowalik, ACP (Canada)
William Oakley, CCEMT-P (USA)

Visual Team (Photos, Illustrations, Video, PPT)

Darby Copeland, EdD, RN, NRP, Team Leader (USA)
Jake Carroll, ThD, MBA, NRP, TN-I/C (USA)
Anthony Cellitti, CCEMTP, NRP, ATF (USA)
Youta Kanesaki, EMT-P (Japan)
David Maatman, NRP/IC (USA)
Bob Page, MEd, NRP, CCP, NCEE (USA)

Instructor Preparation Team (Instructor Guide)

Tony Connelly, EMT-P, BHSc, PGCEd, Team Leader (Canada)
Jake Carroll, ThD, MBA, NRP, TN-I/C (USA)
Darby Copeland, EdD, RN, NRP (USA)
Bob Page, MEd, NRP, CCP, NCEE (USA)
Brock Snedeker, MEd, NRP (USA)

Instructor Update Team

Sabina Braithwaite, MD, MPH, FACEP, NRP, Team Leader (USA)
Dale Bayliss, ACP (Canada)
Tim Hillier, ACP (Canada)
David Maatman, NRP/IC (Canada)
Bob Page, MEd, NRP, CCP, NCEE (USA)

Exam Team

S. Robert Seitz, MEd, RN, NRP, Team Leader (USA)
Marian Hands, BEd (Canada)
Tim Hillier, EMT-P (Canada)
David Maatman, NRP/IC (USA)
Roberto Rivera, RN (Puerto Rico)

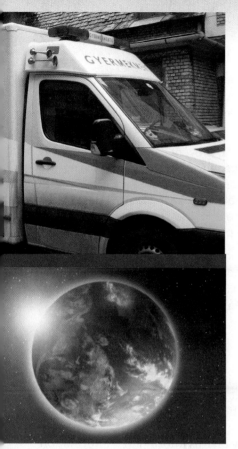

1

Scene Size-up

James H. Creel, Jr., MD, FACEP

Valoración de la Escena   Ocena miejsca zdarzenia   Procjena mjesta događaja

Ocena prizorišča   Valutazione della Scena   Taille-haute de scène

Beurteilung der Einsatzstelle   مسح الموقع   mesto nesreće

Helyszinfelmérés

Key Terms

Objectives

Upon successful completion of this chapter, you should be able to:

1. Discuss the steps of the scene size-up.
2. List the two basic mechanisms of motion injury.
3. Identify the three collisions associated with a motor-vehicle collision (MVC), and relate potential patient injuries to deformity of the vehicle, interior structures, and body structures.
4. Name the five common forms of MVCs.
5. Describe potential injuries associated with proper and improper use of seat restraints, headrests, and air bags in a head-on collision.
6. Describe potential injuries from rear-end collisions.
7. Describe the three assessment criteria for falls, and relate them to anticipated injuries.
8. Identify the two most common forms of penetrating injuries, and discuss associated mechanisms and extent of injuries.
9. Relate five injury mechanisms involved in blast injuries and how they relate to scene size-up and patient assessment.

scene size-up: observations made and actions taken at a trauma scene before actually approaching the patient. It is the initial step in the ITLS Primary Survey.

ITLS Primary Survey: a brief exam to find immediately life-threatening conditions. It is made up of the scene size-up, initial assessment, and either the rapid trauma survey or the focused exam.

standard precautions: steps each health-care worker takes to protect themselves and their patient from exposure to infectious agents; includes treating each patient and himself as if they were infectious. This always entails wearing gloves, frequently requires a face shield, and occasionally requires a protective gown.

Chapter Overview

Scene size-up is the first step in the **ITLS Primary Survey** (Table 1-1). It is a critical part of trauma assessment and begins before you approach the patient. If you fail to perform the preliminary steps of scene size-up, you may jeopardize your life as well as the life of your patient.

Scene size-up includes taking **standard precautions** to prevent exposure to blood and other potentially infective material, evaluating the scene for dangers, determining the total number of patients, determining essential equipment needed for the particular scene, and identifying the mechanisms of injuries (Table 1-2). Each step will be covered in detail in this chapter, with special emphasis on how to use your knowledge of the mechanisms of injury to predict occult injuries to the patient.

Motion (mechanical) injuries are by and large responsible for the majority of deaths from trauma in most countries. This chapter reviews the most common mechanisms of motion injuries and stresses the injuries that may be associated with those mechanisms.

Scene Size-up

Scene size-up begins at dispatch, when you anticipate what you will find at the scene. At that time, you should think about what equipment you may need and whether other resources (more units, special extrication equipment, multiple-casualty incident [MCI] protocols) may be needed. Although information from dispatch is useful to begin to think about a plan, do not overrely on this information. Information given to the dispatcher is often exaggerated or even completely wrong. Be prepared to change your plan depending on your own scene size-up.

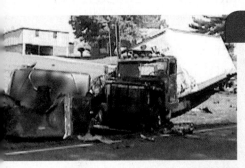

Courtesy of Roy Alson, PhD, MD, FACEP, FAAEM

Case Presentation

An Advanced Life Support (ALS) ambulance is dispatched along with the fire service to the scene of a truck rollover. Dispatch advises responding personnel that bystanders report fluid leaking from the truck. Upon arrival, the fire department establishes command and orders the ambulance to stage approximately one-half mile (800 meters) upwind of the incident. Two minutes later, Incident Command (IC) advises medical personnel that the minor petroleum spill is controlled and that there may be more than one patient: the truck driver, who is out of his truck, alert, and walking around, and the drivers of an auto and motorcycle, which were damaged in the collision. Command tells them they should proceed to the site.

As you arrive with the ambulance, you observe fire personnel containing the spill.

You smell diesel fuel. You see a four-door sedan damaged in the front and left fender with a starred front windshield. Some 30 feet (9 meters) behind it, you see a man on the ground near a heavily damaged motorbike, not moving. What are the first steps and decisions you need to make?

Before proceeding, consider these questions: Is the scene safe? Are responders and/or victims in potential danger? What protective clothing is required? Other than the spill, are there other potential hazards? How many patients do you have? What additional equipment may be required?

Keep these questions in mind as you read through the chapter. Then, at the end of the chapter, find out how the emergency care providers managed this emergency.

Table 1-1: ITLS Patient Assessment

ITLS Primary Survey	Perform a scene size-up
	Perform initial assessment
	Perform a rapid trauma survey or focused exam
	Make critical interventions and transport decision
	Contact medical direction
ITLS Secondary Survey	Repeat initial assessment
	Repeat vital signs and consider monitors
	Perform a neurological exam
	Perform a detailed (head-to-toe) exam
ITLS Ongoing Exam	Repeat initial assessment
	Repeat vital signs and check monitors
	Reassess the abdomen
	Check injuries and interventions

Standard Precautions

Trauma scenes are among the most likely to subject the emergency care provider to contamination by blood or other potentially infectious material (**OPIM**). The subject of OPIM will be covered in more detail in Chapter 22. Not only are trauma patients often bloody, but they also frequently require airway management under adverse conditions. **Personal protective equipment (PPE)** is necessary at trauma scenes. Protective gloves are always needed, and many situations will require eye protection. It is wise for the emergency care provider in charge of airway management to don a face shield or eye protection and mask. In highly contaminated situations, impervious gowns with mask or face shield may be needed as well. In a toxic environment, chemical suits and gas masks may be needed. Remember to protect your patient from body fluid contamination by changing your gloves between patients.

OPIM: short for *other potentially infectious material* to which an emergency care provider may be exposed (other than blood).

personal protective equipment (PPE): equipment that an emergency care provider dons for protection from various dangers that may be present at a trauma scene. At a minimum that entails wearing protective gloves. At a maximum it is a chemical suit and self-contained breathing apparatus.

Scene Safety

Begin sizing up the scene for hazards as you approach it in your vehicle. Your first decision is to determine the nearest safe place to park the ambulance or rescue vehicle. You would like the vehicle as close to the scene as possible, and yet it must be far enough away for you to be safe while you are performing the scene size-up. In some situations you should not enter the scene until it has been cleared by fire personnel, law enforcement, or hazmat technicians. Try to park facing away from the scene, so

Table 1-2: Steps of the Scene Size-up

1. Standard precautions (personal protective equipment)

2. Scene safety

3. Initial triage (total number of patients)

4. Need for more help or equipment

5. Mechanism of injury

if dangers arise, you can load the patient and leave quickly. Next, determine if it is safe to approach the patient. Perform a "windshield survey" before leaving your response vehicle. Consider the following:

- *Crash/rescue scenes.* Is there danger from fire or toxic substances? Is there danger of electrocution? Are unstable surfaces or structures present such as ice, water, a slope, or buildings in danger of collapse? Areas with potential for low oxygen levels or toxic chemical levels (sewers, ship holds, silos, and so on) should never be entered until you have the proper protective equipment and breathing apparatus. You should never enter such areas without proper training, safety equipment, and appropriate backup support.

- *Farms.* Silos are confined spaces and should not be entered without proper equipment and training. Livestock also can pose hazards to emergency care providers. Be aware of the machinery present as well as manure pits or ponds.

- *Crime scenes.* Danger may exist even after a crime has been committed. Be alert for persons fleeing the scene, for persons attempting to conceal themselves, and for persons who are armed or who make threatening statements or gestures. Do not approach a known crime scene if law enforcement personnel are not present. Wait for law enforcement, not only for your own safety and the safety of victims, but also to help preserve evidence. Do not approach the scene if you see that law enforcement personnel are in defensive positions or have their weapons drawn.

- *Bystanders.* You and the victims may be in danger from bystanders. Are bystanders talking in loud, angry voices? Are people fighting? Are weapons present? Is there evidence of the use of alcohol or illegal drugs? Is this a domestic-violence scene? You may not be recognized as an emergency care provider, but as a symbol of authority and thus attacked. Are dangerous animals present? Request law enforcement personnel at any sign of danger from violence.

- *Mass-Shooting Events.* Unfortunately, mass-shooting events have become too common worldwide. Classic instructions for emergency care providers have been not to enter the scene until law enforcement has "secured" it, which could take a very long time. Based on the analysis of a number of events, the Hartford Consensus document recommends that EMS responders enter the scene with law enforcement protection, when an area with victims has been rendered "safe," meaning there are no immediate threats in the area in which EMS personnel are operating. Then control any life-threatening hemorrhage in victims found, and rapidly evacuate them to a safer area for further assessment and treatment.

Another type of hazardous scene is the *blast scene.* Explosions usually are associated with industrial accidents, but because the threat of terrorist activity is both common and worldwide, it should be considered when approaching the scene of an explosion. In addition, in some countries the proliferation of illegal methamphetamine labs has been associated with an increased incidence of chemical explosions.

Whatever the cause of an explosion, if possible, law enforcement personnel, along with a bomb technician and a hazmat technician, should first evaluate the blast scene to make sure it is safe to enter and that no chemical, biological, or radiological hazards exist. If possible, park your vehicle outside the blast zone (the area where glass is broken). If you are not sure of scene safety, call for ambulatory victims to leave the scene by following a designated emergency responder to a safe area for triage and decontamination.

If it is necessary to enter the blast zone to save lives, try to do so in protective clothing using respiratory protection (which may include a chemical suit and gas mask). Identify those who are still alive prior to entry if possible. Rapidly rescue patients who are too injured to walk using "load-and-go" tactics with expedient spinal motion-restriction techniques. If the scene could be dangerous, the best policy is not to provide treatment on scene but rather to immediately remove all living patients. Take the patients directly to the casualty collection point, and begin patient assessment and treatment there or in the ambulance. If resources are available, those patients should be taken directly from the scene to the appropriate hospital. Leave the dead in place.

The proper management of blast scenes is beyond the scope of this course, which is focused mainly on assessment and management of the injured patient. Other courses are available for more in-depth knowledge of this subject.

Consider whether or not the scene poses a continued threat to the patient. If there is danger of fire, water, structure collapse, toxic exposure, and so on, the patient may have to be moved immediately. This does not mean that you should expose yourself or your partners to unnecessary danger. You may need to call for special equipment and proper backup from law enforcement, fire services, or the power company. If the scene is unsafe, you should make it safe or try to remove the patients from the scene without putting yourself in danger. Sometimes there is no clearly good way to do this. Use good judgment. You are there to save lives, not give up your own.

Total Number of Patients

Next, determine the total number of patients. If there are more patients than your team can effectively handle, call for additional resources. Based on dispatch information and additional information received en route, you may need to do this while still responding to the incident. Remember that you usually need one ambulance for each seriously injured patient. If there are many patients, establish medical command and initiate multiple-casualty incident (MCI) protocols.

When determining the total number of patients, consider this question: Are all patients accounted for? If a patient is unconscious, and there are no witnesses to the incident, look for clues that other patients might be present (schoolbooks or diaper bag, passenger list in a commercial vehicle). Carefully evaluate the scene for patients. As you do so, not only look toward the vehicle or the center of the scene, but also look outward to see if there are victims behind you. This is especially important at night or if there is poor visibility.

Essential Equipment and Additional Resources

If possible, carry all **essential equipment** to the scene. This prevents loss of time returning to the vehicle. Remember to change gloves between patients. The following equipment is always needed for trauma patients.

- Personal protection equipment
- Patient transport device (stretcher, long spine board, and so on) with effective strapping and head motion-restriction device
- Rigid cervical extrication collar of an appropriate size
- Oxygen and airway equipment, which should include suction equipment and a bag-valve mask (BVM)
- Trauma box (bandage material, hemostatic agent, tourniquet, blood pressure cuff, stethoscope)

If special extrication equipment, more ambulances, or additional personnel are needed, call now. You are less likely to call for help when involved in patient care. Be sure to tell additional responders exactly where to respond and of any dangers present. In larger events, a staging area for ambulances and other responding units may be established. Use of designated radio channels, if available, helps in effective communications.

Mechanism of Injury

Once you determine that it is safe to approach the patient, begin to assess for the **mechanism of injury (MOI)**. This may be apparent from the scene itself, but it may require questioning the patient or bystanders. Injuries are caused by the transfer of

PEARLS
Equipment

It is wise to invest in a high-intensity tactical flashlight. It is small enough to carry in your shirt pocket, but it is many times brighter than regular flashlights.

essential equipment: equipment that is worn or carried when the team approaches the trauma patient. It includes personal protective equipment, long backboard and strapping, rigid cervical extrication collar, oxygen and airway equipment, and trauma box.

mechanism of injury (MOI): the means by which the patient was injured, such as a fall, motor-vehicle collision, or explosion.

energy. Kinetic energy is equal to the mass (M) of the object in motion multiplied by the square of the velocity (V) divided by two.

$$\textbf{Kinetic Energy} = \tfrac{1}{2}\,(\textbf{M} \times \textbf{V}^2)$$

high-energy event: a mechanism of injury in which it is likely that there was a large release of uncontrolled kinetic energy transmitted to the patient, thus increasing the chances for serious injury.

You are not expected to calculate how much energy was transferred in a traumatic event but rather to estimate whether the collision was a low-energy event (such as an auto that backed into another in a parking lot) or **high-energy event** (such as an auto that hit a tree at a speed of 40 miles [64 kilometers] per hour). The formula is shown only to stress that speed (velocity) has a much larger effect on energy than does mass. A small increase in speed causes a large increase in energy transferred. Energy transmission follows the laws of physics; therefore, injuries present in predictable patterns (Table 1-3). Knowledge and appreciation of the mechanism of injury is very helpful in your evaluation of the patient for occult injuries. By performing a careful patient assessment, guided in part by the MOI, you should be able to identify the majority of injuries the patient has sustained. Missed or overlooked injuries may be catastrophic, especially when they become known only after the compensatory mechanisms of the body are exhausted.

Remember that patients who are involved in a high-energy event are at risk for severe injury. Despite normal vital signs and no apparent anatomic injury upon the initial assessment, 5% to 15% of those patients will later exhibit severe injuries that

Table 1-3: Mechanisms of Injury and Potential Injury Patterns

Mechanisms of Injury	Potential Injury Patterns
Frontal impact 　Deformed steering wheel 　Dashboard knee imprints 　Spider-web deformity of windscreen	• Cervical-spine fracture • Flail chest • Myocardial contusion • Pneumothorax • Aortic disruption • Spleen or liver laceration • Posterior hip dislocation • Knee dislocation
Lateral impact (T-bone)	• Contralateral neck sprain • Cervical-spine fracture • Lateral flail chest • Pneumothorax • Aortic disruption • Diaphragmatic rupture • Laceration of spleen, liver, kidney • Pelvic fracture
Rear impact	• Cervical-spine injury
Ejection	• Exposure to all mechanisms and mortality increased
Pedestrian vs. car	• Head injury • Aortic disruption • Abdominal visceral injuries • Fracture lower extremities and pelvis

are discovered on repeat examinations. Therefore, a high-energy event signifies a large release of uncontrolled energy. Consider the patient injured until you have proven otherwise.

It is important to be aware of whether the mechanism of injury is generalized or focused. Generalized mechanisms include motor-vehicle collisions, falls from a height, and so on. Focused mechanisms cause injuries to discrete areas of the body, such as a stab wound of the abdomen or an amputation of a foot. Generalized mechanisms require a **rapid trauma survey** of the whole body, whereas focused mechanisms may only require a **focused exam**, which is a limited exam of the affected areas or systems.

rapid trauma survey: a brief exam from head to toe performed to identify life-threatening injuries.

focused exam: an exam used when there is a focused (localized) mechanism of injury or an isolated injury. The exam is limited to the area of injury.

Factors to be considered are direction and speed of impact, patient kinetics and physical size, and the signs of energy release (such as major vehicle damage). A strong correlation exists between injury severity and automobile velocity changes, as measured by the amount of vehicle damage. So, it is important that you consider these two questions: What happened? How was the patient injured?

The mechanism of injury is an important triage tool. It provides information you should report to the emergency physician or trauma surgeon. Severity of vehicle damage has been suggested as a nonphysiologic sign of injury. Taking a few brief photos with a digital camera of the vehicle's damage can be helpful for emergency department personnel to recognize the severity of forces involved. It is essential to develop an awareness of mechanisms of injury and thus have a high **index of suspicion** for occult injuries. Always consider the potential injury to be present until it is ruled out in a hospital setting.

index of suspicion: the medical provider's estimate of a disease or injury being present in a patient. A high index of suspicion means there is a high probability the injury is present. A low index of suspicion means there is a low risk of the injury.

Mechanisms of Motion Injury

Motion injuries are by and large responsible for the majority of the mortality from trauma in the world. The most common are discussed in the sections that follow. The important concept to appreciate is that energy is neither created nor destroyed but is only changed in form (law of conservation of energy). Thus the kinetic energy of motion must be absorbed. It is this absorption of energy that is the major component in producing injury.

The two basic mechanisms of motion injury are blunt and penetrating (Table 1-4), although patients can have injuries from both at the same time. In the United States, penetrating injury is a major cause of young minority males needing trauma care. For the nonurban areas of the United States and for most of the world (outside of combat zones), blunt force trauma remains the major cause.

Motor-Vehicle Collisions

The patterns of injuries from collisions with automobiles, motorcycles, all-terrain vehicles (ATVs), personal watercraft, and tractors are varied. Therefore, you should keep in mind that all MVCs occur as three separate events (Figure 1-1):

- Machine collision
- Body collision
- Organ collision resulting in rupture, shearing, or bruising

Table 1-4: Basic Mechanisms of Motion Injury	
Blunt Injuries	**Penetrating Injuries**
• Rapid forward deceleration (collisions) • Rapid vertical deceleration (falls) • Energy transfer from blunt instruments (baseball bat, blackjack)	• Projectiles • Knives • Falls on fixed objects

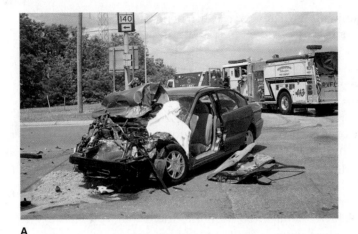

A

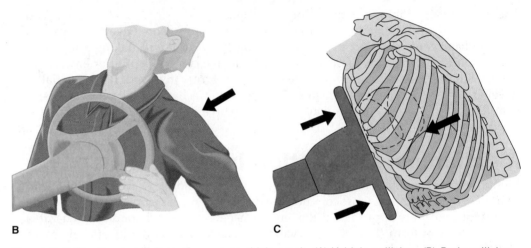

B   C

Figure 1-1 The three collisions of a motor-vehicle crash. (A) Vehicle collision. (B) Body collision. (C) Organ collision. *(Photo copyright Mark C. Ide)*

For example, consider approaching an MVC in which an automobile has hit a tree head-on at 40 miles (64 kilometers) per hour. The tree brings the auto to an immediate stop by transferring the energy into damage to the tree and the automobile. The person inside the auto is still traveling at 40 miles (64 kilometers) per hour until he strikes something that stops him (such as seat belts, steering wheel, windshield, or dashboard). At that point, energy transfers into damage to the person and to the surface struck. The organs inside the person are also traveling at 40 miles (64 kilometers) per hour until they are stopped by striking a stationary object (such as inside of skull, sternum, steering wheel, dashboard) or by their ligamentous attachments (such as the aorta by ligamentum arteriosum). In this auto-versus-tree example, appreciation of the rapid forward decelerating mechanism (high-energy event) coupled with a high index of suspicion should make you concerned that the victim may have possible head injury, cervical-spine injury, myocardial contusion, any of the "deadly dozen" chest injuries (described in Chapter 6), intra-abdominal injuries, and musculoskeletal injuries (especially fracture or dislocation of the hip).

To explain the forces involved, consider Sir Isaac Newton's first law of motion: A body in motion remains in motion in a straight line unless acted on by an outside force. Motion is created by force (energy exchange), and therefore force will stop motion. If this energy exchange occurs within the body, tissue damage occurs. This law is well exemplified in the automobile crash. The kinetic energy of the vehicle's forward motion is absorbed as each part of the vehicle is brought to a sudden halt by

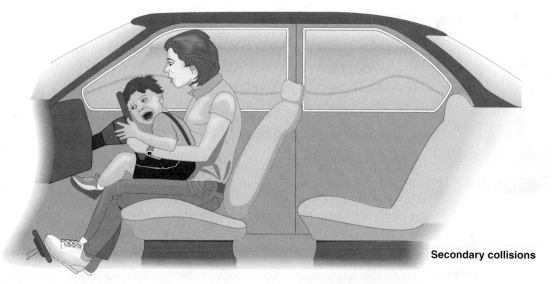

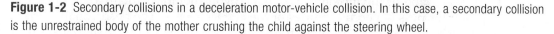

Secondary collisions

Figure 1-2 Secondary collisions in a deceleration motor-vehicle collision. In this case, a secondary collision is the unrestrained body of the mother crushing the child against the steering wheel.

the impact. Remember that the body of the occupant is also traveling at 40 miles (64 kilometers) per hour until impacted by some structure within the car. With awareness of this mechanism, one can see the multitude of injuries that could occur. Be aware of the following clues:

- Deformity of the vehicle (indication of forces involved—energy exchange)
- Deformity of interior structures (indication of where the patient impacted—energy exchange)
- Deformity or injury patterns of the patient (indication of what parts of the body may have been impacted)

Additional collisions other than the three already mentioned may occur. Objects inside the automobile (books, bags, luggage, and other persons) will become missiles traveling at the original speed of the auto and may strike persons in front of them. These are called *secondary collisions*. A good example occurs when an unrestrained parent is holding a child in her lap and crushes the child between her and the dashboard in a deceleration collision (Figure 1-2).

In rear-impact auto collisions, multiple impacts may occur if the auto strikes another auto in the rear and is then in turn struck from behind by another auto following. Also, vehicles frequently deflect from hitting one object and then collide with a second or even third vehicle or stationary object. They are similar to what occurs in a rollover collision: the persons inside the vehicle are subjected to energy transfer from multiple directions. It is often more difficult to predict injuries in these cases. You must quickly but carefully look for clues inside the vehicle. Remember that in multiple-impact collisions, the airbag only works for the first one.

MVCs occur in several forms, and each form is associated with certain patterns of injury. The five common forms of MVCs are the following:

- Frontal-impact or head-on collision
- Lateral-impact or T-bone collision
- Rear-impact collision
- Rollover collision
- Rotational collision

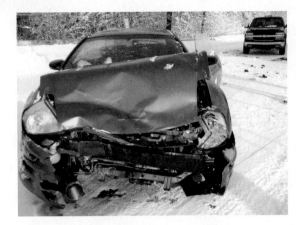

Figure 1-3 In a head-on collision, most injuries are inflicted by the windshield, steering wheel, and dashboard. *(Photo courtesy of Maria Dryfhout, Shutterstock)*

Frontal-Impact Collision (Head-on)

In an MVC involving a frontal-impact collision, an unrestrained body is brought to a sudden halt. The energy transfer is capable of producing multiple injuries.

Windshield injuries occur in the rapid forward-decelerating type of event, in which the unrestrained occupant impacts the windshield forcefully (Figure 1-3). The possibility for injuries is great under those conditions. Of utmost concern is the potential for serious airway and cervical-spine injury.

Remembering the three separate collision events, note the following:

- *Machine collision*—deformed front end
- *Body collision*—spider-web pattern of windshield
- *Organ collision*—coup/contracoup brain, soft-tissue injury (scalp, face, neck), hyperextension/flexion of the cervical spine

From the spider-web appearance of the windshield and an appreciation of the mechanism of injury, you should maintain a high index of suspicion for possible occult injuries of the cervical spine. The head usually strikes the windshield, resulting in direct trauma to the face and head. External signs of trauma include cuts, abrasions, and contusions. They may be quite dramatic in appearance. However, the key concern is airway maintenance with motion restriction of the cervical spine and evaluation of level of consciousness.

Steering-wheel injuries most often occur to an unrestrained driver of a vehicle in a head-on collision. The driver may subsequently impact with the windshield. The steering wheel is the vehicle's most lethal weapon for the unrestrained driver, and any degree of steering-wheel deformity (check under collapsed airbags) must be treated with a high index of suspicion for face, neck, thoracic, or abdominal injury. The two components of this weapon are the ring and column (Figure 1-4). The ring is a semirigid, plastic-covered metal circle attached to a fixed inflexible post, which essentially is a battering ram.

Utilizing the three-collision concept, check for the presence of the following:

- *Machine collision:* Look for front-end deformity of the vehicle.
- *Body collision:* Check the steering wheel for ring fracture and deformity and the column for any displacement.
- *Organ collision:* Look for traumatic tattooing of patient's skin.

The head-on collision is entirely dependent on the area of the body that impacts with the steering wheel, dashboard, or other portion of the vehicle's interior. Signs may be readily visible, with direct trauma such as lacerations of mouth and chin, contusion/bruises of the anterior neck, traumatic tattoos of the chest wall, and bruising of the abdomen. These external signs may be subtle or dramatic in appearance, but more important, they may represent only the tip of the iceberg. Deeper structures and organs may harbor occult injuries due to shearing forces, compression forces, and displacement of kinetic energy.

Organs that are susceptible to shearing injuries due to their ligamentous attachments are the aortic arch, liver, spleen, kidneys, and bowel. With the exception of small-bowel tears, those injuries are sources for occult bleeds and hemorrhagic shock. Compression injuries are common for the lungs, heart, diaphragm, and urinary bladder. An important sign is respiratory distress, which may be due to pulmonary contusions, pneumothorax, diaphragmatic hernia (bowel sounds in chest), or flail chest. Consider a bruised chest wall as a myocardial contusion that requires monitoring of cardiac rhythm and, if available, a 12-lead ECG. In short, the steering wheel is a lethal weapon capable of producing devastating injuries,

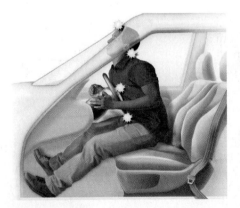

Figure 1-4 Steering wheel injuries.

DASHBOARD INJURIES

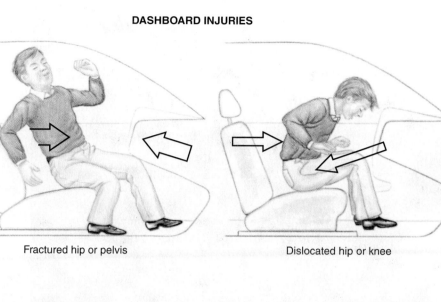

Fractured hip or pelvis

Dislocated hip or knee

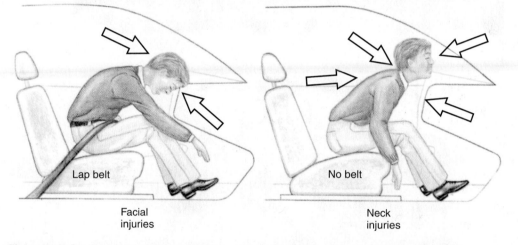

Lap belt

Facial
injuries

No belt

Neck
injuries

Figure 1-5 Dashboard injuries.

many of which are occult. Steering wheel deformity is a cause for alarm and must heighten your index of suspicion. You also must relay this information to the receiving physician.

Dashboard injuries occur most often to an unrestrained passenger. The dashboard has the capability of producing a variety of injuries, depending on the area of the body that strikes the dashboard. Most frequently, injuries involve the face and knees. However, many types of injuries have been described (Figure 1-5). Applying the three-event concept of collision, you will note the following:

- *Machine collision:* Look for deformity of the vehicle.
- *Body collision:* Check the dash for fracture and deformity.
- *Organ collision:* Look for facial trauma, coup/contracoup brain, hyperextension/flexion of the cervical spine, pelvis, hip, and knee trauma.

Facial, brain, and cervical-spine injuries have already been mentioned. These are more likely if the crash forces send the victim up over the dash into the windshield. Like chest contusion, knee trauma may represent only the tip of the iceberg. Knees commonly impact with the dashboard, especially if the patient is thrown down under it. Knee trauma may range from a simple contusion to a severe compound fracture of the patella. Frank dislocation of the knees also can occur, along with fractures of the

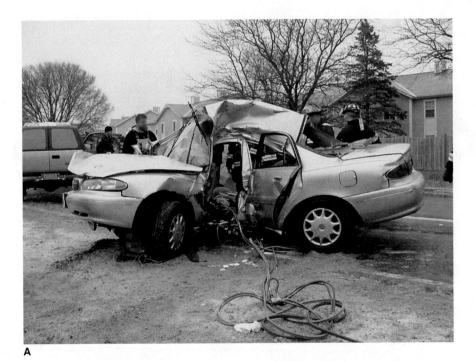

A

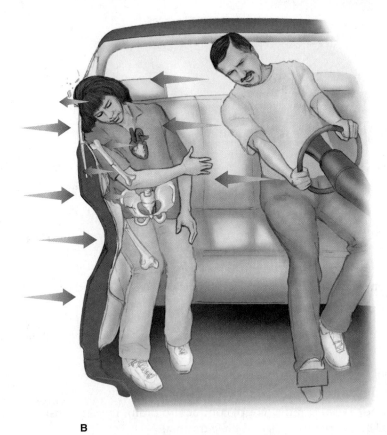

B

Figure 1-6 In a lateral-impact collision, most injuries are inflicted by intrusion of the door, armrest, side window, or door post. *(Photo courtesy of Anthony Cellitti, NREMT-P)*

proximal tibia (tibial plateau fracture). In addition, kinetic energy may be transmitted proximally and result in fracture of the femur or fractured/dislocated hip. On occasion, the pelvis can impact with the dash, resulting in acetabulum and pelvic fractures. Such pelvic injuries are often associated with hemorrhage that may lead to shock. Maintain a high index of suspicion, and always palpate the femurs, gently squeeze the pelvis, and palpate the symphysis pubis.

Deceleration collisions are most commonly associated with secondary collisions with people or loose objects in the vehicle, which can become missiles causing deadly injuries.

Lateral-Impact or T-Bone Collision

The mechanism of the lateral-impact collision is similar to that of the frontal-impact collision, with the addition of lateral energy displacement (Figure 1-6). Applying the three-collision concept to the lateral-impact collision, look for the presence of the following:

- *Machine collision:* Look for primary deformity of the vehicle, being sure to check the impact side (driver or passenger).
- *Body collision:* Determine the degree of door deformity (for example, armrest bent, outward or inward bowing of door).
- *Organ collision:* This cannot be predicted by external exam alone. Instead, consider organs beneath areas of external injury.

Look for the following common injuries:

- *Head.* Coup/contracoup is due to lateral displacement.
- *Neck.* Lateral displacement injuries range from cervical-muscle strain to fracture or subluxation with neurologic deficit.
- *Upper arm and shoulder.* Injuries appear on the side of the impact and are common, as are injuries to the lower extremities.
- *Thorax/abdomen.* Injury is due to direct force either from inward bowing of the door on the side of the impact or from an unrestrained passenger being propelled across the seat. Injuries vary from soft-tissue injuries to flail chest, lung contusion, pneumothorax, hemothorax, or possible traumatic aortic dissection. Abdominal injuries include those to solid and hollow organs.
- *Pelvis/legs.* Occupants on the side of the impact are likely to have pelvic, hip, or femur fractures. Pelvic injuries may also include dislocation, bladder rupture, and urethral injuries.

Emergency care providers do need to be aware that many new vehicles are equipped with side airbags and air curtains (Figure 1-7). They pose a hazard to responders, if those safety devices did not activate in the collision.

Rear-Impact Collision

In the most common form of rear-impact collision, a stationary car is struck from the rear by a moving vehicle (Figure 1-8). Or a slower-moving car may be impacted

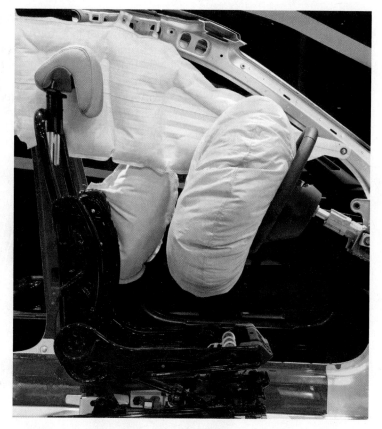

Figure 1-7 Side airbags and air curtains pose a hazard to responders, if the devices did not activate in the collision. *Note:* See the *Access: First on Scene—Rapid Vehicle Entry Provider Manual* from ITLS for more information about rendering nondeployed airbags safe. *(testing. Shutterstock)*

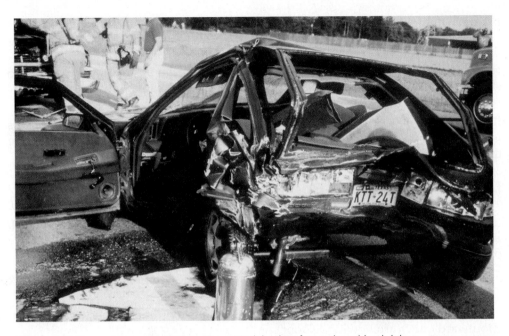

Figure 1-8 In a rear-impact collision, the potential exists for neck and back injury. *(Photo courtesy of Bonnie Mcneely, EMT-P)*

from the rear by a faster-moving car. The sudden increase in acceleration produces posterior displacement of the occupants and possible hyperextension of the cervical spine if the headrest is not properly adjusted. If the seat back breaks and falls backward into the rear seat, there is greater chance of lumbar-spine injury. Rapid forward deceleration may also occur if the car suddenly strikes something in the front or if the driver applies the brakes suddenly. Note deformity of the auto anterior and posterior as well as interior deformity and headrest position. The potential for cervical-spine injuries is great (Figure 1-9). Be alert for associated deceleration injuries as well.

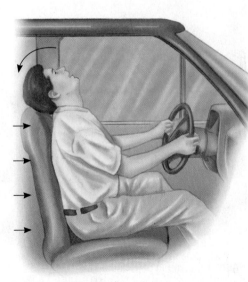

A Victim moves ahead while head remains stationary. Head rotates backward. Neck extends.

B Head snaps forward. Head rotates forward. Neck flexes.

Figure 1-9 Mechanism of cervical-spine injury in a rear-impact collision.

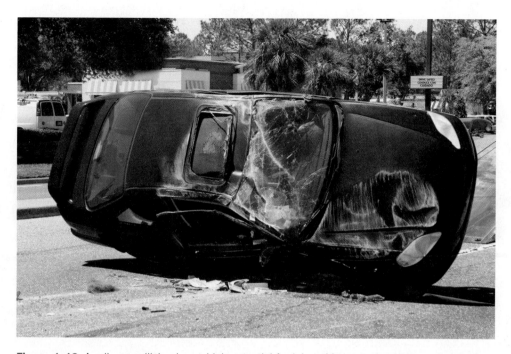

Figure 1-10 A rollover collision has a high potential for injury. Many mechanisms are involved, and unrestrained victims are frequently ejected. *(Rob Wilson. Shutterstock)*

Rollover Collision

During a vehicle rollover, the body may be impacted from any direction. Thus, the potential for injuries is great (Figure 1-10). The chance for axial-loading injuries of the spine is increased in this form of MVC. Emergency care providers must be alert for clues that suggest the car turned over (such as roof dents, scratches, debris, and deformity of roof posts). Lethal injuries often occur in this form of collision because of the greater likelihood of occupants being ejected. Occupants ejected from the car are three times as likely to be killed or have serious injuries.

Rotational Collision

A rotational mechanism is best described as what occurs when one part of the vehicle stops and the rest of the vehicle remains in motion. A rotational collision usually occurs when a vehicle is struck in the front or rear lateral area. This converts forward motion to a spinning motion. The results are a combination of the frontal-impact and the lateral-impact mechanisms with the same possibilities of injuries of both mechanisms.

Occupant Restraint Systems

Restrained occupants are more likely to survive a collision, because they are protected by **occupant restraint systems** from much of the impact inside the auto and are unlikely to be ejected from the auto. Those occupants are, however, still susceptible to certain injuries.

A lap belt is intended to go across the pelvis (iliac crests), not the abdomen. If the lap belt is in place and the victim is subjected to a frontal deceleration crash, the body tends to fold together like a clasp knife (Figure 1-11). The head may be thrown forward into the steering wheel or dashboard. Facial, head, or neck injuries are common. Abdominal injuries also occur if the lap belt is positioned improperly. The compression forces that are produced when a body is suddenly folded at the waist may injure the abdomen or the lumbar spine.

occupant restraint systems: systems built into a vehicle to prevent the driver and passengers from being thrown about the interior of the vehicle or from being ejected from the vehicle in the event of a collision.

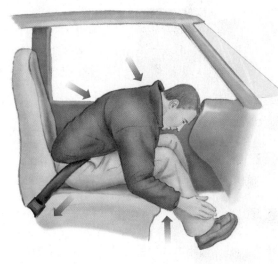

Figure 1-11 Clasp-knife effect.

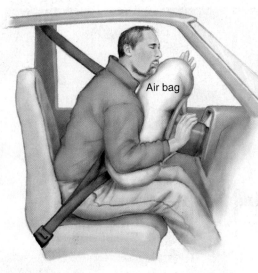

Air bag and three-point restraint
prevents collisions 2 and 3.

Figure 1-12 Air bag and three-point restraint.

The three-point restraint or cross-chest lap belt (Figure 1-12) secures the body much better than a lap belt alone. The chest and pelvis are restrained, so life-threatening injuries are much less common. The head is not restrained, and therefore the neck is still subjected to stresses that may cause fractures, dislocations, or spinal-cord injuries. Clavicle fractures (at the point where the chest strap crosses) are common, as are chest-wall injuries. Internal organ damage may still occur due to organ movement inside the body.

Like belt restraints, air bags (passive restraints) will reduce injuries in victims of MVCs in most but not all situations. Air bags are designed to inflate from the center of the steering wheel and the dashboard to protect the front-seat occupants in case of a frontal deceleration crash. If functioning properly, they cushion the head and chest at the instant of impact, thus effectively decreasing injury to the face, neck, and chest. Be sure to stabilize the neck, however, until it has been adequately examined. Air bags deflate immediately, so they protect against only one impact. The driver whose car hits more than one object is unprotected after the initial collision. Air bags also do not prevent "down and under" movement, so drivers who are extended (tall drivers and drivers of small, low-slung autos) may still impact the dash with their legs and suffer leg, pelvis, or abdominal injuries. It is important for occupants to wear chest and lap belts even when the car is equipped with air bags.

Researchers have recently shown that some drivers who appear uninjured after deceleration crashes have been later found to have serious internal injuries. A clue to possible internal injuries to the driver is the condition of the steering wheel. A deformed steering wheel is just as important a clue in an auto equipped with an air bag as in those that are not. This clue may be missed because the deflated air bag covers the steering wheel. Thus, a quick "lift and look" under the air bag should be part of the routine examination of the steering wheel (Figure 1-13).

Cars manufactured in the last few years now also include side airbags. They may be built into the body, seat, or headrest. Just like frontal airbags, they only protect the driver during the initial collision. Some vehicles have air bags that come down from the roof to protect the head, and at least one make of auto has air bags under the dash to protect the legs. They obviously give much-needed extra protection.

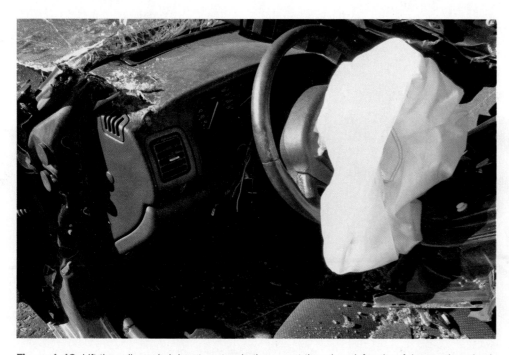

Figure 1-13 Lift the collapsed air bag to note whether or not there is a deformity of the steering wheel.

(Photo courtesy of Olivier Le Queinec, Shutterstock.com)

Certain dangers are associated with air bags. Small drivers who bring the seat up close to the steering wheel may sustain serious injuries when the bag inflates. Infants in car seats placed in the front seat, especially front-facing car seats, may be seriously injured by deployment of the air bag. The smoke seen with airbag deployment is really powder (talc or cornstarch) that is used to "lubricate" the nylon bag so it slides smoothly during inflation. Abrasions from the nylon bag, corneal abrasions, and superficial burns on arms in the vicinity of the airbag vents have been reported.

In summary, when at the scene of an MVC, note the type of collision and the clues (such as deformities of the vehicle) that imply high kinetic energy has been spent. Maintain a high index of suspicion for occult injuries, and thus keep scene time to a minimum. In addition, knowledge of anatomy and physiology is essential. Focus on what injuries can be predicted, and appreciate that age and environment may suggest the probability of other injuries. Last, comorbidities (for example, diabetes, cardiovascular disease, chronic obstructive pulmonary disease) and medications (for example, anticoagulants) can make the case more complex and demanding. Those observations and clues are essential to quality patient care and must be relayed to medical direction and the receiving physician.

Tractor Accidents

Another large motorized vehicle with which you must be familiar is the farm tractor. Worldwide about 50% of all farm-accident fatalities are from tractor overturns. Each year over 200 people in the United States and Canada and hundreds more worldwide die from tractor accidents. Although safety features such as rollover protection systems (ROPS) are present on newer tractors, many older tractors lack this feature.

The two basic types of tractors are the two-wheel drive and the four-wheel drive. In both, the vehicle's center of gravity is high, and thus the tractors can easily turn over (Figure 1-14). The majority of fatal accidents are due to the tractor turning over and crushing the driver. Most overturns (85%) are to the side, which are less likely to pin the driver, who has a chance to jump or be thrown clear. Rear overturns, although less frequent, are more likely to entrap and crush the driver because there is almost no opportunity to jump free.

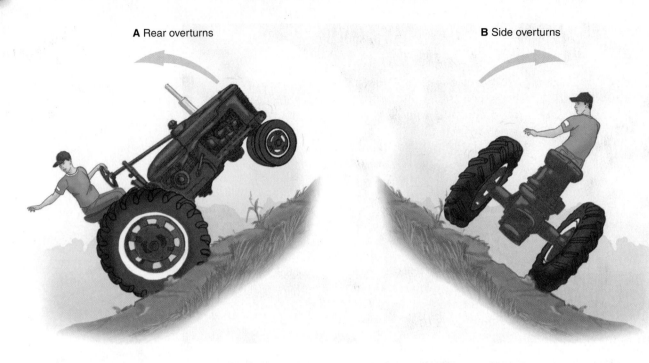

A Rear overturns   **B** Side overturns

Figure 1-14 Tractor accidents.

The primary mechanism of injury in a tractor accident is the crush injury. Severity depends on the part of the anatomy involved. Additional mechanisms are chemical burns from gasoline, diesel fuel, hydraulic fluid, or even battery acid. Thermal burns from hot engine parts or ignited fuel are also common. Last, the injured driver may not be found for an extended period if he or she is working alone.

Emergency management of the patient's injuries consists of scene stabilization followed quickly by the primary survey and resuscitation. The following questions are used as a checklist in scene stabilization:

- Is the engine off?
- Are the rear wheels locked?
- Have the fuel situation and fire hazard been addressed?
- Are there hydraulic fluid leaks or radiator leaks?

While you are assessing the patient, other emergency responders must stabilize the tractor. The center of gravity must be identified before any attempt is made to lift the tractor. The center of gravity of the two-wheel-drive tractor is located approximately 10 inches (25 cm) above and 24 inches (61 cm) in front of the rear axle. The center of gravity of a four-wheel-drive tractor is closer to the midline of the machine.

Because tractors usually overturn on soft ground and their centers of gravity are tricky to determine, great care must be taken during lifting to avoid a second crush injury. Because of the tractor weight and the usually prolonged length of time the driver is pinned, anticipate serious injuries. Often, the patient will go into profound shock as the compressing weight of the tractor is removed and blood rushes to the formerly compressed tissue. Just as with any other crush injury, large-bore IV access with fluid infusion prior to removing the compressing object may decrease hypotension post extrication. If the patient has been entrapped for a long period, be aware that he or she may develop crush syndrome.

Rapid, safe management of tractor accidents requires special expertise in lifting heavy machinery as well as good trauma management.

Small-Vehicle Crashes

Other small vehicles that fall into the motion-injury category include the motorcycle, all-terrain vehicle (ATV), personal watercraft (PWC), and the snowmobile. The operators of those machines are not encased within them and, of course, wear no restraining devices. When the operator is subjected to the classic head-on, lateral-impact, rear-end, or rollover collision, the only forms of protection are evasive maneuvering, protective clothing (such as helmets, leathers, and boots), and the use of the vehicle to absorb kinetic energy (such as a bike slide).

Motorcycles It is extremely important for motorcycle riders to wear helmets. Helmets help prevent head injury, which causes 75% of motorcycle deaths, but give no protection to the spine, especially the neck. The operator of a motorcycle involved in a crash is much like an ejected automobile occupant, and severe injuries are common. Injuries depend on the part of the anatomy subjected to kinetic energy. The lack of protective encasement leads to a higher frequency of head, neck, and extremity injuries. Important clues to injury include deformity of the motorcycle, distance of skid, distance the rider was thrown, and deformity of stationary objects or cars. Often the rider is thrown onto the other vehicle in the collision and then sustains another impact when he or she lands on the roadway.

All-Terrain Vehicles The all-terrain vehicle (ATV) was designed as a vehicle to traverse rough terrain. The ATV was used initially by ranchers, hunters, and farmers. Unfortunately, some people view it as a fast toy. Carelessness and misuse have resulted in an ever-increasing morbidity and mortality from ATV accidents—sadly and frequently, among the very young. Often alcohol consumption is a contributing factor to the accidents. The two basic designs of ATVs are three-wheeled (no longer made and, so, rare) and four-wheeled. The four-wheel design affords reasonable stability and handling, but the three-wheeled ATV has a high center of gravity and is prone to roll over when turned sharply. Listed here are the most common mechanisms of injury:

- Vehicle rollover
- Fall-off of rider or passenger
- Forward deceleration of rider from vehicle impact with stationary object
- Impact to rider or passenger's head or extremities when passing too close to stationary objects (trees)
- "Clothesline" type injuries of the neck with resulting airway compromise

The injuries produced depend on the mechanism and the part of the anatomy impacted. The most frequent injuries are fractures, about half of which are above and half below the diaphragm. The major bony injuries involve the clavicles, sternum, and ribs. Be very suspicious for head or spine injury.

Personal Watercraft The use of personal watercraft (PWC), such as the Jet Ski®, Sea-Doo®, or WaveRunner®, has become a popular water recreational activity. Over a million PWCs are in operation in the United States. The U.S. Coast Guard reported in 2006 that 24% of all boating accidents involved one or more PWCs. In the United States, California reports that PWCs represent 16% of all registered vessels but account for 55% of all injuries. The rate of emergency department–treated injuries related to PWCs is about 8.5 times higher than the rate of that of motorboats.

In the United States, the total number of accidents, deaths, and injuries is higher for open motorboats. However, the rate of deaths and injuries is higher with PWCs because they have a higher percentage of accidents relative to the number of vessels registered. (This is similar to the situation when comparing injury rates between cars and motorcycles.) Consumption of alcohol while boating greatly increases the risk of accidents and deaths.

The PWC is designed to be operated by a driver who is in a sitting, standing, or kneeling position, with one or more passengers located behind the driver in tandem. PWCs are able to obtain high speeds quickly, but have no braking mechanism. Like motorcycles, PWCs offer no protection to the driver or passengers. Most injuries are caused by PWC collisions, either with other watercraft or with fixed objects such as docks or tree stumps. Most are due to driver inattention, inexperience, and error.

PWCs are unique in that they are steered by the flow of water through the motor so that when the motor is shut off, the craft cannot be steered. The usual response when approaching an obstruction (tree stump, dock) is to slow down and turn to avoid it. However, with a PWC, when you slow the engine, you lose the ability to steer and often hit the object.

PWC collisions produce injury patterns similar to those encountered with motorcycle–auto collisions. Rectal and vaginal trauma may occur when rear-seat passengers or the driver fall off backward, impacting the water (buttocks first) at high speeds. The likelihood of drowning (even with the use of personal flotation devices) is always a danger. Remember, water is not soft when a body impacts with it at high speeds. Therefore, you must assess and practice the same index of suspicion as with any high-energy event. Because these events occur in water, there is also the possibility of submersion injury.

Snowmobiles Snowmobiles are used both as recreational and utility vehicles. The snowmobile has a low clearance and a low center of gravity. The injuries common to this vehicle are similar to those that occur with ATVs. Turnovers are somewhat more common, and because the vehicle is usually heavier than an ATV, crush injuries are seen more frequently. Again, the injury pattern depends on the part of the anatomy that is directly involved. Be alert for possible coexisting hypothermia. A common injury with the snowmobile is the "hangman" or "clothesline" injury that results from running under wire fences. Be alert for occult cervical-spine injuries and potential airway compromise.

Pedestrian Injuries

A pedestrian struck by a car almost always suffers severe internal injuries as well as fractures. This is true even if the vehicle is traveling at low speed. The mass of the auto is so large that high speed is not necessary to impart high-energy transfer. When high speed is involved, the results are disastrous.

There are two associated mechanisms of injury. The first is when the bumper of the auto strikes the body, and the second is when the body, accelerated by the transfer of forces, strikes the ground or some other object. An adult usually has bilateral lower leg or knee fractures plus whatever secondary injuries occur when the body strikes the hood of the car and then later the ground. Children are shorter, so the bumper is more likely to hit them in the pelvis or torso. They usually land on their heads in the secondary impact. The classic pattern is referred to as Waddell's Triad, in which the bumper causes a femur or pelvis fracture. The child is struck in the chest by the fender or car body and sustains a head injury when striking the pavement. A similar pattern would be seen in adults, but the site of injury varies with the height of the victim. When answering a call to an auto–pedestrian accident, be prepared for broken bones, internal injuries, and head injuries.

Falls

The mechanism of injury for falls is vertical deceleration. The types of injuries sustained depend on the following three factors, which you must identify and relay to medical direction:

- Distance of fall
- Anatomic area impacted
- Surface struck

The primary groups involved in vertical falls are adults and children under the age of 5. In children, the falls most commonly involve boys and occur mostly in the summer months in urban high-rise, multiple-occupant dwellings. Predisposing factors include poor supervision, defective railings, and the curiosity associated with that age group. Head injuries are common in falls by children because the head is the heaviest part of the body and thus impacts first.

Adult falls are generally occupational or due to the influence of alcohol or drugs. It is not uncommon for falls to occur during attempts to escape from fire or criminal activity. Teenagers, predominantly males also are at risk because they attempt to be "daredevils." Generally, adults attempt to land on their feet; thus their falls are more controlled. In this landing form, the victim usually impacts initially on the feet and then falls backward, landing on the buttocks and outstretched hands. Classically, this "lover's leap" fall may result in the following injuries (Figure 1-15):

- Fractures of the feet or legs
- Hip and/or pelvic injuries
- Axial loading to the lumbar and cervical spine
- Vertical deceleration forces to the organs
- Colles fractures of the wrists

The greater the height, the greater is the potential for injury. However, serious injury can occur in a short-distance fall. Surface density (concrete versus sawdust) and irregularity (gym floor versus staircase) also influence the severity of injury. Relay information about distance fallen and surface struck with other pertinent information to medical direction. One must also be aware that even a seemingly trivial fall, such as a fall from a standing position, can produce a hip fracture in older adults. Pain control is an important part of their care.

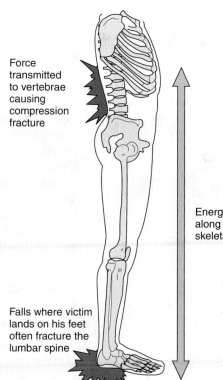

Force transmitted to vertebrae causing compression fracture

Energy transmitted along the skeletal system

Falls where victim lands on his feet often fracture the lumbar spine

Figure 1-15 Axial loading.

Penetrating Injuries

Numerous objects are capable of producing penetrating injuries. They range from the industrial saw blade that breaks off at an extremely high rate of speed to the foreign body hurled by a lawn mower. Most high-velocity objects are capable of penetrating the thorax or abdomen. Common forms of penetrating wounds come from the knife and gun.

The severity of a knife wound depends on the anatomic area penetrated, length of the blade, and angle of penetration (Figure 1-16). Knife wounds are low-energy injuries, and tissue damage is confined to the direct path of the blade. Remember, an upper abdominal stab wound may cause intrathoracic organ injury, and stab wounds below the fourth intercostal space may have penetrated the abdomen. Arrow wounds usually penetrate deeper than a knife due to higher velocity and thus energy. The golden rule with any impaled object is to stabilize it in place. It will be removed at the hospital. Impaled objects in the cheek of the face and those blocking the airway are exceptions to this rule.

Most penetrating wounds inflicted by firearms are due to handguns, rifles, and shotguns. In combat situations or terrorist events, penetrating wounds can result from shrapnel. (See *ITLS Military* for more information about dealing with combat casualty care.) Important factors to obtain, if possible, are the type of weapon, its caliber (size of bullet), and the distance from which the weapon was fired. However, *remember that you must treat the patient and the wound, not the weapon.*

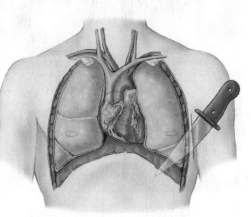

Stab wounds at nipple level or below frequently penetrate the abdomen.

Figure 1-16 Stab wounds.

Wound Ballistics

As was stated earlier in the chapter, injury to tissue results from the transfer of kinetic energy to the tissue. Because the kinetic energy produced by a projectile is mostly dependent on velocity, weapons are classified as either high or low velocity. Weapons with projectile velocities less than 2,000 feet (610 meters) per second are considered low velocity and include essentially all handguns and some rifles. Injuries from these weapons are much less destructive than those sustained from high-velocity weapons, such as a military or hunting rifle. Low-velocity weapons are certainly capable of lethal injuries, depending on the body area struck. More civilians are killed by low-velocity bullets because they are more often shot by low-velocity weapons. All wounds inflicted by high-velocity weapons carry the additional factor of hydrostatic pressure and resulting cavitation. This factor alone can increase the injury because tissues are torn or displaced beyond those directly damaged as the bullet passes through. Useful terminology associated with these weapons include the following:

- *Caliber.* Referring to the internal diameter of the barrel, caliber corresponds to the ammunition used for the particular weapon.
- *Rifling.* The series of spiral grooves in the interior surface of the barrel of some weapons is called rifling.
- *Ammunition.* The term *ammunition* refers to the case, primer, powder, and bullet, which is the projectile fired from the gun.
- *Bullet construction.* Bullets are usually made of solid lead alloy and may have a full or partial copper or steel jacket. The shape of the nose of the bullet may be rounded, flat, conical, or pointed. The bullet nose may also be soft or hollow (for expansion or fragmentation), which can result in greater injury.

Bullet factors that contribute to tissue damage include the following:

- *Missile size.* The larger the bullet, the more resistance and the larger the permanent tract.
- *Missile deformity.* Hollow point and soft nose flatten out on impact, resulting in the involvement of a larger surface and thus more tissue damage.
  - *Semijacket.* The jacket expands and adds to surface area.
  - *Tumbling.* Tumbling of the missile causes a wider path of destruction.
  - *Yaw.* The missile can oscillate vertically and horizontally (wobble) about its axis, resulting in a larger surface area presenting to the tissue.

The wounds caused by bullets consist of the following three parts:

- *Entry wound.* Usually smaller than the exit wound, it may have darkened, burned edges if the bullet is fired from very close range (Figure 1-17).
- *Exit wound.* Not all gunshot victims will have exit wounds, and on occasion there may be multiple exits due to fragmentation of bone and missile. Generally, the exit wound is larger and has ragged edges. (*Note:* It is less important to identify entrance and exit wounds in the field than it is to determine the total number of wounds present.)

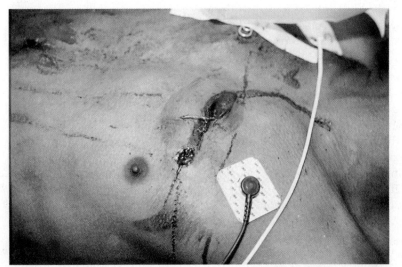

Figure 1-17 Example of entrance (lateral) and exit (medial) wounds. Because EMS personnel are not forensic experts, wounds should not be labeled as entrance and exit in the report. Note location and number of wounds.
(Photo © Edward T. Dickinson, MD)

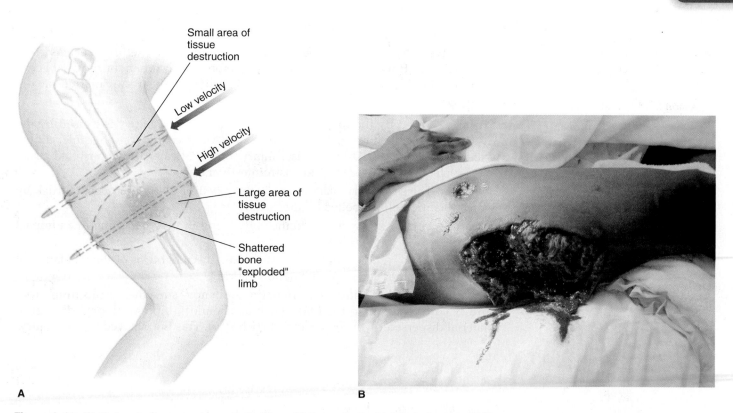

Figure 1-18 (A) High-velocity versus low-velocity injury. (B) Example of a high-velocity wound of leg. *(Photo courtesy of Roy Alson, MD)*

- *Internal wound.* Low-velocity projectiles inflict damage primarily by damaging tissue by way of direct contact. High-velocity projectiles inflict damage by tissue contact and transfer of kinetic energy to surrounding tissues (Figure 1-18). Damage is related to the following:
  —Shock waves
  —Temporary cavity, which is 30 to 40 times the bullet's diameter and creates immense tissue pressures
  —Pulsation of the temporary cavity, which creates pressure changes in the adjacent tissue

Generally, damage done is proportional to tissue density. Highly dense organs such as bone, muscle, and the liver sustain more damage than less dense organs such as the lungs. Bone damaged by a gunshot can fragment and damage surrounding tissues. A key factor to remember is that once a bullet enters a body, its trajectory will not always be in a straight line. Any patient with a missile penetration of the head, thorax, or abdomen should be transported immediately because many will require emergent surgery. Patients who have wounds far from the spine do not usually need spinal motion restriction (SMR), and delaying transport to perform SMR actually can increase the death rate because of prolonged scene time. Personnel who have been shot while wearing ballistic armor should be managed with caution. Be alert for possible cardiac and other organ contusions because those organs have sustained blunt trauma.

In shotgun wounds, injury is determined by kinetic energy at impact, which is influenced by powder charge, size of pellets, choke of muzzle, and distance to target. For shotguns, velocity and kinetic energy dissipate rapidly as distance is traveled. At 40 yards (37 meters), the velocity is one-half the initial muzzle velocity. Remember that at close range (<15 yards or <14 meters) shotgun wounds are high energy because the pellets are still tightly grouped and act like a massive single bullet.

Blast Injuries

blast injuries: injuries commonly produced by the different mechanisms associated with an explosion (air blast, shrapnel, burns, and so on).

Blast injuries in North America occur primarily in industrial settings such as grain elevator and gas fume explosions but may also be from criminal or terrorist activity. The mechanism of injury by blast or explosion is the result of five factors (Figure 1-19):

- *Primary.* Caused by the initial air blast, a primary blast injury is caused by the direct effect of blast overpressure on tissue. Air is easily compressible, unlike water. As a result, the primary blast injury almost always affects air-filled structures such as the lungs, ears, and gastrointestinal tract.
- *Secondary.* The secondary blast injury is the result of the patient being struck by material (shrapnel) propelled by the blast force.
- *Tertiary.* A tertiary injury is due to the body being thrown, resulting in an impact with the ground or other object.
- *Quaternary.* As a result of the explosion fireball, thermal burns or the inhalation of toxic dust or fumes can cause inhalation injuries.
- *Quinary.* The quinary injury is the hyperinflammatory state that results from exposure to contaminants in the blast, such as chemical, biological, or radiological material dispersed by the explosion (dirty bomb). This is a delayed type of injury.

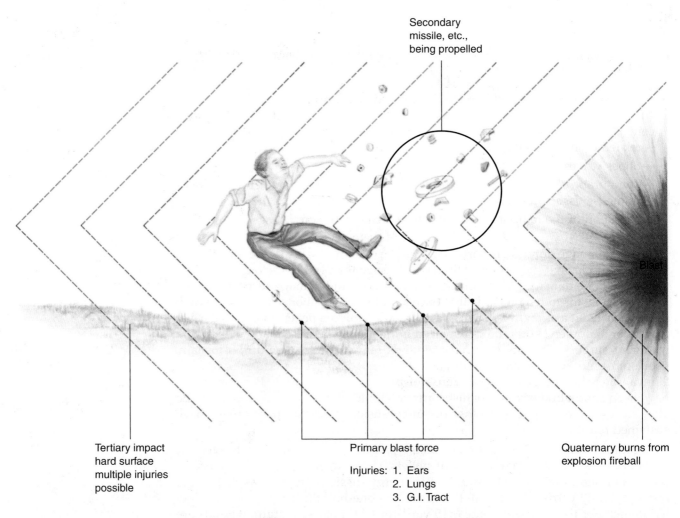

Secondary missile, etc., being propelled

Tertiary impact hard surface multiple injuries possible

Primary blast force

Injuries: 1. Ears
2. Lungs
3. G.I. Tract

Quaternary burns from explosion fireball

Figure 1-19 Explosions can cause injury with the initial blast, when the victim is struck by debris, or by the victim being thrown against the ground or other fixed objects by the blast.

Primary blast injury is less common in the civilian setting than in combat. Injuries due to the primary air blast are almost exclusive to the air-containing organs. The auditory system often involves ruptured tympanic membranes. Once thought of as a marker of exposure to blasts sufficient to cause primary injury, recent data suggests that this is not a good triage tool. Lung injuries resulting from primary blast injury can include pneumothorax, parenchymal hemorrhage, and especially alveolar rupture. Alveolar rupture may cause air embolus that may be manifested by bizarre central nervous system symptoms. Gastrointestinal tract injuries may vary from mild intestinal and stomach contusions to frank rupture. Always suspect lung injuries in a blast victim.

Injuries caused by the secondary factors may be penetrating or blunt. Fragments of shrapnel from an explosion may attain velocities of 14,000 feet (4,270 meters) per second. This is over four times the velocity of the most powerful high-velocity rifle bullets. A piece of shrapnel traveling at this velocity would impart more than 16 times the energy of a similarly sized high-velocity rifle bullet. Any shrapnel wound should be considered serious.

Tertiary injuries are much the same as when a person is ejected from an automobile or has fallen from a height. The blast wave may propel the person at a high velocity for a varying distance. The injuries will depend on what the person impacts (solid object versus water or soft ground, for example).

Quaternary injuries are seen when there is a large fireball associated with the explosion or when toxic fumes or dust are produced by the explosion. They are more common when the victim is in an enclosed space or has previous lung disease such as asthma or emphysema.

Quinary injuries are relatively new and reflect a terrorist's attempts to make bombs more deadly by using the explosion to disperse toxic chemicals, biological agents, or radiological agents. Such bombs are called "dirty bombs" for that reason.

Case Presentation (continued)

As you pull up, your windshield survey reveals a possible multiple patient scene with hazards. Incident Command assures you that the spill is under control, and that other than a slight fuel odor, there is no fire danger or other hazardous materials (hazmat) threat. He also says that the truck driver seems uninjured, but there are two passengers awake, "stunned," but alert in the car, and that "at least the guy from the bike is breathing."

Having donned gloves, you head toward the car. The truck driver assures you he does not need emergency medical attention, that his neck is "just a little stiff," and that he swerved in order to avoid the motorcyclist who ran into the car "pretty much head-on."

At the car, the EMS crew finds an elderly couple. The husband is in the driver's seat. He is alert, talking normally, and complaining of left arm and left ankle pain. "He just swerved into me," he says, "just flew over the hood right into the windshield in front of me. Ripped my side mirror off as he fell past me!"

The passenger, his wife, says, "I'm okay. Just take care of my husband and our granddaughter." You then discover an upside-down car seat, which has been thrown onto the car floor. As you carefully lift it up, the baby buckled in it begins to cry.

The emergency care provider in charge advises the Incident Commander to request two more ambulances and to have fire personnel check on the other patients, He then proceeds with the trauma kit to the cyclist. Because the nearest trauma center is a considerable distance from the scene, the emergency care provider considers requesting air medical transport (a helicopter).

Summary

Trauma is the most serious disease affecting young people. Being an emergency care provider is among the most important professions but requires great dedication and continuous training. Saving patients who have sustained severe trauma requires attention to detail and careful management of time. Teamwork is essential because many actions must occur at the same time.

At the scene of an injury, there are certain important steps to perform before you begin care of the patient. Failure to perform a scene size-up will subject you and your patient to danger and may cause you to fail to anticipate serious injuries your patient may have sustained. Take standard precautions and assess the scene for dangers first. Then determine the total number of patients and the need for additional emergency care providers or special equipment. If there are more patients than your team can manage, report to dispatch and initiate multiple-casualty incident protocols.

Identify the mechanism of injury and consider it as part of the overall management of the trauma patient. Ask yourself: What happened? What type of energy was applied? How much energy was transmitted? What part of the body was affected? If there is a motor-vehicle collision involved, consider the form of the crash, and survey the vehicle's interior and exterior for damage.

Note that tractor accidents require careful stabilization of the machine to prevent a second injury to the patient. Falls require identification of distance fallen, surface struck, and position of the patient upon impact. Stab wounds require knowledge of the length of the instrument as well as the angle at which it entered the body. When evaluating a shooting victim, you need to know the weapon, caliber, and distance from which it was fired.

Information about the high-energy event (for example, a fall, a vehicle collision) is also important to the emergency physician. Be sure not only to record your findings but also to give a verbal report to the emergency department physician or trauma surgeon when you arrive. With this knowledge and a high index of suspicion, you can give your patient the greatest chance of survival.

Bibliography

Almogy, G., Y. Mintz, G. Zamir, T. Bdolah-Abram, R. Elazary, L. Dotan, M. Faruga, and A.I. Rivkind. "Suicide Bombing Attacks: Can External Signs Predict Internal Injuries?" *Annals of Surgery* 243, no. 4 (April 2006): 541–46.

Alson, R.L., and W. B. Patterson. *Access: First on Scene—Rapid Vehicle Entry Provider Manual*, 2nd ed. Downers Grove, IL: ITLS, 2006.

American Academy of Pediatrics, Committee on Injury and Poison Prevention. "Personal Watercraft Use by Children and Adolescents." *Pediatrics* 105, no. 2 (February 1, 2000): 452–53.

Brinsfield, K., et al. *Bombings: Injury Patterns and Care Curriculum*. Course offered by the American College of Emergency Physicians (ACEP) and the Centers for Disease Control and Prevention (CDC). Information page accessed December 27, 2014, at http://www.acep.org/blastinjury/

Campbell, J.E., W. Pfeifer, and A. Kagel. *ITLS Military*, 2nd ed. Downers Grove, IL: ITLS, 2014.

Campbell, J.E., and J. Smith. "Incendiaries and Explosives." In *Homeland Security and Emergency Medical Response*, 117–39. New York: McGraw-Hill, 2008.

De Haven, H. "Mechanical Analysis of Survival in Falls from Heights of Fifty to One Hundred and Fifty Feet." *Injury Prevention* 6, no. 1 (March 2000): 62–68.

Jacobs, L., and K. J. Burns. "The Hartford Consensus to Improve Survivability in Mass Casualty Events: Process to Policy," *American Journal of Disaster Medicine* 9, no. 1 (Winter, 2014): 67–71.

Newgard, C.D., K.A. Martens, and E.M. Lyons. "Crash Scene Photography in Motor Vehicle Crashes Without Air Bag Deployment." *Academic Emergency Medicine* 9, no. 9 (September 2002): 924–29.

Sochor M., S. Althoff, D. Bose, R. Maio, and P. Deflorio. "Glass Intact Assures Safe Cervical Spine Protocol." *Journal of Emergency Medicine* 44, no. 3 (March 2013): 631-36.

Wightman, J.M., and S.L. Gladish. "Explosions and Blast Injuries." *Annals of Emergency Medicine* 37, no. 6 (June 2001): 664–78.

Get more information about this course by calling
ITLS International at 888-495-4875
(outside the United States call +1-630-495-6442) or visit

www.itrauma.org

2

Trauma Assessment and Management

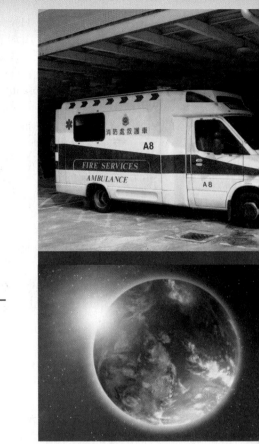

John E. Campbell, MD, FACEP
John T. Stevens, NREMT-P
Leon Charpentier, EMT-P
Alexandra Charpentier, NREMT-P

Reconocimiento Primario   Badanie wstępne   Primarni pregled

Primarni Pregled   Valutazione Primaria   Enquête Primaire

Schnelle Traumauntersuchung   التقييم الأولي   primarni pregled

Első áttekintés

Kate Blackwelder

Key Terms

Objectives

Upon successful completion of this chapter, you should be able to:

1. Outline the steps in trauma assessment and management.
2. Describe the ITLS Primary Survey.
3. Explain the initial assessment and how it relates to the rapid trauma survey and the focused exam.
4. Describe when the initial assessment can be interrupted.
5. Describe when critical interventions should be made and where to make them.
6. Identify which patients have critical conditions and how they should be managed.
7. Describe the ITLS Ongoing Exam.
8. Describe the ITLS Secondary Survey.

Chapter Overview

ITLS **patient assessment** is made up of the **ITLS Primary Survey**, the ITLS Secondary Survey, and the ITLS Ongoing Exam. The ITLS Primary Survey is made up of the scene size-up, **initial assessment**, and a **rapid trauma survey** or **focused exam**. The purpose of the ITLS Primary Survey is to determine if immediately life-threatening conditions exist and to identify those patients who should have immediate transport to the hospital. The **ITLS Ongoing Exam** is meant to identify changes in the patient's condition, and the **ITLS Secondary Survey** is an evaluation for all injuries, not just life-threatening ones.

The scene size-up will set the stage for how you will perform the rest of the ITLS Primary Survey. If a dangerous generalized mechanism of injury exists (such as an auto crash or fall from a height) or if the patient is unconscious and the mechanism of injury is unknown, you should extend the ITLS Primary Survey to include a rapid examination of the head, neck, chest, abdomen, pelvis, extremities, and back. You would then perform critical interventions and transport. The ITLS Ongoing Exam and possibly an ITLS Secondary Survey would be performed en route to the hospital.

If there is a dangerous localized mechanism of injury suggesting an isolated injury (such as a stab or bullet wound of the thigh or amputation of the hand), you would perform the initial assessment, but the focused exam would be limited to the area affected by the injury. The full rapid trauma survey is not required. You would then perform critical interventions and transport. The ITLS Ongoing Exam and possibly an ITLS Secondary Survey would be performed en route.

If there is no significant life threat in the mechanism of injury (such as an amputation of the great toe) you would do the initial assessment and, if normal, go directly to a focused exam based on the patient's chief complaint. The ITLS Secondary Survey would not be necessary in this situation.

To make the most efficient use of time, ITLS prehospital assessment and management of the trauma patient is divided into three assessments (ITLS Primary Survey, ITLS Ongoing Exam, and ITLS Secondary Survey), and each assessment is made up of certain steps (Figure 2-1). Those assessments are the foundation on which prehospital trauma care is built.

patient assessment: the process by which the emergency care provider evaluates a trauma patient to determine injuries sustained and the patient's physiologic status; made up of the ITLS Primary Survey, ITLS Ongoing Exam, and ITLS Secondary Survey.

ITLS Primary Survey: a brief exam to find immediately life-threatening conditions; made up of the scene size-up, initial assessment, and either the rapid trauma survey or the focused exam.

initial assessment: a rapid assessment of airway, breathing, and circulation to prioritize the patient and identify immediately life-threatening conditions; part of the ITLS Primary Survey.

rapid trauma survey: a brief exam from head to toe performed to identify life-threatening injuries.

Case Presentation

Your ambulance has responded to a motor-vehicle collision involving an overturned truck, a sedan, and a motorcycle. The fire service has contained the hazards. As part of the scene size-up, you identify a total of five victims.

Basic life support (BLS) personnel assess the minor patients at your instructions, and you have called for additional EMS units due to the number of patients. As the senior emergency care provider on the scene, you approach the motorcyclist, who is lying on his left side at the side of the road approximately 35 feet (10 meters) from the car he struck. The victim is apparently unaware of your arrival, gasping for air,

and lying in an expanding pool of blood under his right knee.

Before proceeding, consider these questions: As you approach the patient, what should you be looking for? What does the mechanism of injury suggest? What is your first priority? What type of injuries is the motorcyclist likely to have? How can you immediately identify those that are life threatening? What type of assessment should be performed? Is this a load-and-go situation? Keep these questions in mind as you read through the chapter. Then, at the end of the chapter, find out how the emergency care providers managed this patient.

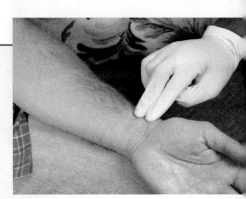

Figure 2-1 Steps in the assessment of the trauma patient.

focused exam: an exam used when there is a focused (localized) mechanism of injury or an isolated injury; an exam that is limited to the area of injury.

ITLS Ongoing Exam: an abbreviated exam to determine changes in the patient's condition.

ITLS Secondary Survey: a comprehensive head-to-toe exam to find additional injuries that may have been missed in the ITLS Primary Survey.

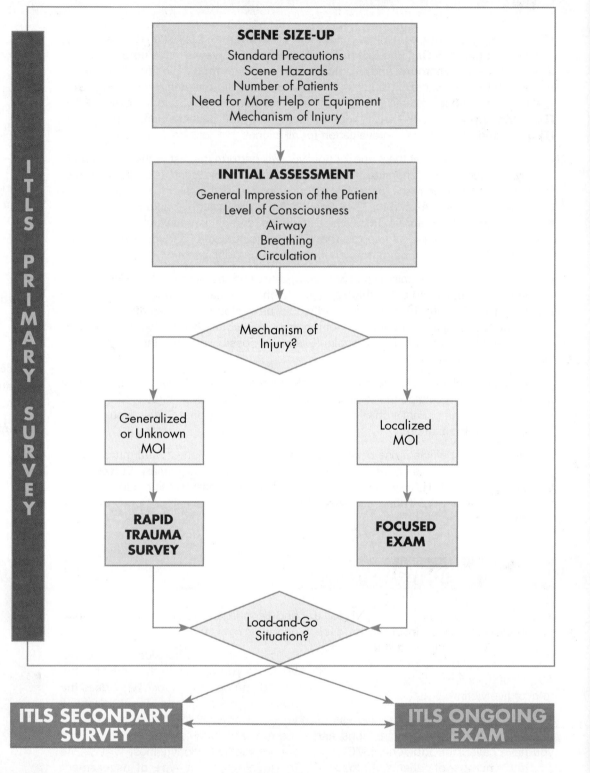

ITLS Patient Assessment

ITLS PRIMARY SURVEY

SCENE SIZE-UP
Standard Precautions
Scene Hazards
Number of Patients
Need for More Help or Equipment
Mechanism of Injury

INITIAL ASSESSMENT
General Impression of the Patient
Level of Consciousness
Airway
Breathing
Circulation

Mechanism of Injury?

Generalized or Unknown MOI

Localized MOI

RAPID TRAUMA SURVEY

FOCUSED EXAM

Load-and-Go Situation?

ITLS SECONDARY SURVEY

ITLS ONGOING EXAM

ITLS Primary Survey

The ITLS Primary Survey includes an evaluation of the scene and preparation for patient assessment and management. It begins with the scene size-up and then, if the scene is safe to enter, moves on to the initial assessment and a rapid trauma survey or focused exam (Figures 2-2 and 2-3).

ITLS PRIMARY SURVEY

SCENE SIZE-UP
Standard Precautions
Hazards, Number of Patients, Need for additional resources,
Mechanism of Injury

↓

INITIAL ASSESSMENT
GENERAL IMPRESSION
Age, Sex, Weight, General Appearance, Position,
Purposeful Movement, Obvious Injuries, Skin Color
Life-threatening Bleeding (CABC)
|
LOC
(A-V-P-U)
Chief Complaint/Symptoms
|
AIRWAY
(CONSIDER C-SPINE CONTROL)
(Snoring, Gurgling, Stridor; Silence)
|
BREATHING
(Present? Rate, Depth, Effort)
|
CIRCULATION
(Radial/Carotid Present? Rate, Rhythm, Quality)
Skin Color, Temperature, Moisture; Capillary Refill
Has bleeding been controlled?

↓

RAPID TRAUMA SURVEY
HEAD AND NECK
Neck Vein Distention?
Tracheal Deviation?
|
CHEST
Asymmetry; (w/Paradoxical Motion?), Contusions, Penetrations,
Tenderness, Instability, Crepitation
Breath Sounds
(Present? Equal? If unequal: percussion)
Heart Tones
|
ABDOMEN
(Contusions, Penetration/evisceration; **Tenderness, Rigidity, Distention)**
|
PELVIS
Tenderness, Instability, Crepitation
|
LOWER/UPPER EXTREMITIES
Obvious Swelling, Deformity
Motor and Sensory
|
POSTERIOR
Penetrations, Obvious Deformity
|

If critical patient - transfer to ambulance to complete exam

If radial pulse present:
VITAL SIGNS
Measured Pulse, Breathing, Blood Pressure
|
If altered mental status:
PUPILS
Size? Reactive? **Equal?**
|
GLASGOW COMA SCALE
Eyes, Voice, Motor

Figure 2-2 The ITLS Primary Survey including the rapid trauma survey.

ITLS PRIMARY SURVEY

SCENE SIZE-UP
Standard Precautions
Hazards, Number of Patients, Need for additional resources,
Mechanism of Injury

- ↓ -

INITIAL ASSESSMENT
GENERAL IMPRESSION
Age, Sex, Weight, General Appearance, Position,
Purposeful Movement, Obvious Injuries, Skin Color
Life-threatening Bleeding
|
LOC
A-V-P-U
Chief Complaint/Symptoms
|
AIRWAY
(WITH C-SPINE CONTROL)
Snoring, Gurgling, Stridor; Silence
|
BREATHING
Present? Rate, Depth, Effort
|
CIRCULATION
Radial/Carotid Present? Rate, Rhythm, Quality
Skin Color, Temperature, Moisture; Capillary Refill
Has bleeding been controlled?

- ↓ -

FOCUSED EXAM
Focused exam of the identified injury
Also evaluate the spine if distracting injury and any possibility of spinal injury
|
If radial pulse present:
VITAL SIGNS
Measured Pulse, Breathing, Blood Pressure
|
If altered mental status: Brief Neurologic exam
PUPILS
Size? Reactive? **Equal?**
|
GLASGOW COMA SCALE
Eyes, Voice, Motor

Figure 2-3 The ITLS Primary Survey including the focused exam.

Scene Size-up

On-scene trauma assessment begins with certain actions that are performed before you approach the patient. It cannot be stressed enough that the failure to perform preliminary actions can jeopardize your life as well as the patient's life. Perform the scene size-up as described in Chapter 1.

Once you begin your assessment of the critical patient, you may not have time to return to the vehicle for needed equipment. For this reason, always carry essential medical equipment with you to the patient's side. Anticipate that the following equipment may be needed for trauma patients, depending on your level of practice:

- Personal
  —Portable radio
  —Small, high-intensity light

  —Personal protective equipment (gloves, goggles)

  —Spring-loaded punch for window entry

  —EMS scissors

  —Stethoscope

  —Pen and pad; felt-tip pen (initial triage marker)

- Trauma Kit (carried by the team leader)

  —Airway equipment: suction device, blind insertion airway device (BIAD), endotracheal (ET) intubation kit (including surgical mask/goggles), cricothyroidotomy set

  —Bag-valve-mask device

  —Age-appropriate pediatric airway supplies

  —Oxygen (D-tank), nonrebreather mask

  —One- and two-inch tape, 10-pack sterile 4 × 4s, four-inch roller-gauze bandage, four-inch elastic bandage, one each sterile 5 × 9 and 8 × 10 inch dressings

  —Commercial combat-style tourniquet, hemostatic dressing (examples include Combat Gauze™, HemCon™ dressing, ChitoSam 100™ dressing™)

  —Seal for sucking chest wound (examples include Asherman™ Chest Seal, Bolin™ Chest Seal, Halo™ vent, SAM™ Chest Seal, or Vaseline™ Gauze)

  —Device for chest decompression (examples include Cook™ Emergency Pneumothorax Set, Turkel™ Safety Needle, or 14-gauge 3.25 inch [8 cm] angiocath)

  —Rescue or warming blanket (may be contained with stretcher)

- Spinal motion restriction (SMR) package (carried by second emergency care provider)

  —Long backboard or scoop stretcher

  —Three to four straps

  —Cervical immobilization device (CID) or sheet rolls + two-inch tape

  —Adjustable cervical collar

- Other equipment (brought by a third emergency care provider or first responder, based on dispatch information)

  —Stretcher or Stokes basket

  —Burn sheets/irrigation fluids

  —Spinal extrication device

  —Monitor/defibrillator

  —Additional heavy dressings

Once the scene is safe to enter, as team leader, you must focus your attention on the rapid assessment of your patient. All decisions on treatment require that you have identified life-threatening conditions. Remember, once you begin patient assessment in the ITLS Primary Survey, only four things should cause you to interrupt completion of the assessment. You may interrupt the assessment sequence only if (1) the scene becomes unsafe, (2) you must treat exsanguinating hemorrhage, (3) you must treat an airway obstruction, or (4) you must treat cardiac arrest. (Respiratory arrest, dyspnea, or bleeding management should be delegated to other team members while you continue assessment of the patient.)

For critical patients, the goal should be to complete the ITLS Primary Survey in less than two minutes and to have on-scene times of five minutes or less. Internal bleeding can usually be stopped only in the operating room, so all on-scene interventions should be life saving. Other interventions in the critical patient should be delayed until the patient is in the ambulance on the way to the hospital.

Experience has shown that injuries are missed or treatment errors occur because the team leader stops the initial assessment to perform an intervention and forgets to

PEARLS
Interruptions
The team leader should delegate any intervention required during the ITLS Primary Survey and should not interrupt the completion of the survey except for airway obstruction, cardiac arrest, exsanguinating hemorrhage, or scene danger.

perform part of the assessment. To prevent this, when immediate interventions are needed, delegate them to your team members while you continue the assessment. This is an important concept that immediately addresses problems encountered and yet does not interrupt the assessment sequence and does not increase scene time. Teamwork is essential to good patient outcomes.

As you perform your assessment, you will identify critical interventions that need to be performed immediately. You should instruct the other members of the emergency medical team to carry out these interventions. For example, as you check the airway, another team member can apply a nonrebreather mask at 15 LPM, or prepare to maintain the airway with a BVM or BIAD. When you check the neck, other team members should be applying a cervical collar.

Initial Assessment

The purpose of the initial assessment is to prioritize the patient and to identify immediately life-threatening conditions. The information gathered is used to make decisions about critical interventions and time of transport. Once you determine that the patient may be safely approached, assessment should proceed quickly and smoothly. The next steps in the ITLS Primary Survey (initial assessment and rapid trauma survey) should take less than two minutes. As you begin, you will place the trauma bag beside the patient and direct another emergency medical responder to stabilize the patient's neck (if needed) and to assume responsibility for the airway. Emergency care provider 3 will place the backboard or scoop beside the patient and address any major bleeding while you are proceeding with your exam. This team approach makes the most efficient use of time and allows you to rapidly perform the initial assessment without becoming distracted by performing the necessary interventions yourself, which can interrupt your thought process.

The initial assessment is made up of your general impression on approaching the patient; an evaluation of the patient's level of consciousness (LOC); manual spinal motion restriction (if needed); and an assessment of the patient's airway, breathing, and circulation (ABCs).

Form a General Impression of the Patient on Approach

You have already sized up the scene, determined the total number of patients, and initiated multiple-casualty incident (MCI) protocols if there are more patients than your team can effectively handle. (See Chapter 1.) Try to approach a patient from the front so he does not turn his head to look at you. As you approach, note the patient's approximate age, sex, weight, and general appearance. The elderly and the very young are at increased risk. Female patients may be pregnant. Observe the position of the patient, both body position and position in relation to surroundings. Note the patient's activity. (Is the patient aware of surroundings, moving purposefully, anxious, obviously in distress, and so on?) Does the patient have any obvious major injuries or major bleeding? (If so, this changes the priority to C-A-B-C.) The first C stands for control life-threatening bleeding. (Do not confuse this with the American Heart Association/ILCOR's "CAB" for cardiac arrest, where the C stands for compressions.) If your patient has major external bleeding, you must immediately direct another team member to control it. As team leader, you may need to initially control the bleeding if no other emergency care provider is immediately available.

Your observation of the patient in relation to the scene and the mechanism of injury will help you prioritize the patient. If there are multiple patients, rapidly triage them. Triage will be different for a small group than for a mass-casualty event in which the number of patients exceeds the care available. When there are only a limited number of patients, the main decision is which patient will be treated and transported first. When there are mass casualties, the emergency care provider must decide who will receive care and who will not.

Evaluate Initial Level of Consciousness While Obtaining Cervical-Spine Stabilization

Assessment begins immediately, even if the patient has to be extricated. If there is a mechanism of injury that suggests spine injury, emergency care provider 2 immediately and gently but firmly stabilizes the head and neck in a neutral position. Holding the head (with hands or knees), rather than holding the neck, keeps the hands from being in the way when another team member applies a cervical collar later. As team leader, you may need to initially stabilize the neck if there is not a second emergency care provider immediately available. If you elect to do this, you should immediately turn this responsibility over to the first emergency care provider arriving to help you. (You cannot stabilize the neck and perform an adequate assessment at the same time.) If the head or neck is held in an angulated position and the patient complains of pain on any attempt to achieve a neutral position, you should stabilize the neck in the position found. The same is true of the unconscious patient whose neck is held to one side and does not move when you gently attempt to align it in neutral position. The emergency care provider stabilizing the neck must not release the neck until he or she is relieved or until a suitable motion-restriction device is applied.

As you approach the patient, identify yourself: "My name is _____. We are here to help you. Can you tell me what happened?" The patient's reply gives immediate information about both the status of the airway and the LOC. If the patient responds appropriately to questioning, it indicates the airway is open and the LOC is normal. If the response is not appropriate (the patient is unconscious or awake but confused), make a mental note of the LOC using the **AVPU** scale (Table 2-1). Anything below "A" (alert) should trigger a systematic search for the causes of the altered mental status during the rapid trauma survey. Loss or decrease in LOC can be caused by many things, including obstructed airway, respiratory failure, shock, and increased intracranial pressure, as well as drugs or metabolic disorders. The rapid trauma survey leads you in a systematic, organized way to look for the causes of the altered LOC.

AVPU: an abbreviated description of the patient's level of consciousness. AVPU stands for alert, responds to verbal stimuli, responds to pain, and unresponsive.

Assess the Airway

If the patient cannot speak or is unconscious, further evaluation of the airway should follow. Look, listen, and feel for movement of air. Emergency care provider 2 should position the airway as needed. Because of the ever-present danger of spine injury, avoid extending the neck to open the airway of a trauma patient. If the airway is obstructed (apnea, snoring, gurgling, stridor), use an appropriate method (reposition, sweep, suction) to open it immediately (Figure 2-4). Failure to quickly provide an open airway is one of the four reasons to interrupt the patient assessment part of the ITLS Primary Survey. If simple positioning and suctioning fail to provide an adequate airway, or if the patient has stridor, advanced airway techniques may be necessary immediately.

Assess Breathing

Look, listen, and feel for movement of air. If the patient is unconscious, place your ear over the patient's mouth so you can judge both the depth (tidal volume; see

Table 2-1: Levels of Mental Status (AVPU)
A—Alert (awake, oriented, and obeys commands)
V— Responds to Verbal stimuli (awake but confused, or unconscious but responds in some way to verbal stimuli)
P—Responds to Pain (unconscious but responds in some way to touch or painful stimuli)
U—Unresponsive (no gag or cough reflex)

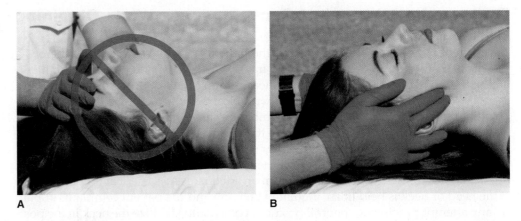

A   **B**

Figure 2-4 Opening the airway using the modified jaw thrust. (A) Do not extend the neck. (B) Maintain in-line stabilization while pushing up on the angles of the jaw.

Chapter 4) and rate of ventilations. Look at the movement of the chest (or abdomen), listen to the sound of air movement, and feel both the movement of air on your cheek and the movement of the chest wall with your hand. If the chest is moving but you do not feel air at the mouth or nose, the patient is *not* breathing adequately. Notice if the patient uses accessory muscles to breathe. If ventilation is inadequate (Table 2-2), emergency care provider 2 should begin to assist ventilation immediately using his or her knees to restrict movement of the patient's neck, which will free his hands to apply oxygen or use a bag-valve mask to assist ventilation (Figure 2-5). When assisting or providing ventilation, be sure that the patient gets an adequate ventilatory rate (one breath every six to eight seconds) and an adequate volume, as evidenced by an adequate chest rise (about 500 mL for an adult or 10 mL/kg for a child). Emergency care providers tend to ventilate too fast when using a bag-valve mask.

Later, when you are able, monitor ventilation with capnography (recommended). You should maintain the end-tidal CO_2 (ETCO$_2$) at about 35–45 mm Hg. All patients who are breathing too fast should receive supplemental high-flow oxygen. As a general rule, all patients with multiple-system trauma should receive supplemental high-flow oxygen. Several recent studies suggest that too much oxygen may be harmful, so it would be prudent to try to keep the pulse oximeter reading around 95% rather than 100%.

Assess Circulation

Has the external bleeding been controlled? Most bleeding can be stopped by direct pressure or pressure dressings. Tourniquets have been discouraged in the past, but recent military experience has found that for bleeding not adequately controlled with pressure, an appropriate tourniquet should be used immediately. If a dressing becomes blood soaked, remove the dressing and redress once to be sure direct pressure is being placed on the bleeding area. Hemostatic dressings such as QuikClot™ Combat Gauze (kaolin based) should be used in this situation. Use of elevation and pressure points is now discouraged due to lack of evidence that they are effective. It

Table 2-2: Normal and Abnormal Respiratory Rates		
	Normal	**Abnormal**
Adult	10–20	<8 and >24
Small child	15–30	<15 and >35
Infant	25–50	<25 and >60

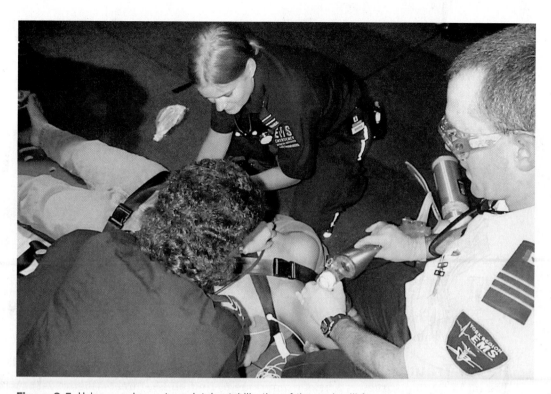

Figure 2-5 Using your knees to maintain stabilization of the neck will free your hands to assist ventilation. *(Photo courtesy of ITLS Ontario, Steve McNenly, Jennifer Lundren, and Sheryl Jackson)*

is important to report excessive bleeding to the receiving physician. Do not blindly clamp inside the wound to stop bleeders; this can cause injuries to other structures. (Nerves are present alongside arteries.)

Now note the rate and quality of the pulses at the radial artery (brachial in the infant). Decide whether the rate is too slow (< 60 in an adult) or too fast (> 120). For pediatric patients, the limits vary with age. (See Table 17-2, p. 337.) Also note its quality (thready, bounding, weak, or irregular). While at the wrist, note skin color, temperature, and condition (and capillary refill in an infant or small child). Pale, cool, clammy skin, thready radial pulse, and decreased LOC are all early assessments of decreased perfusion (shock). If the pulse is not palpable at the wrist, check for the presence of a carotid pulse. If pulses are absent at the neck, immediately start CPR unless there is massive blunt trauma or other nonsurvivable injury. (See Chapter 21.) Address the treatable causes of traumatic cardiac arrest. This is also one of the four reasons to interrupt assessment during the ITLS Primary Survey.

Rapid Trauma Survey or Focused Exam

The choice between the rapid trauma survey and the focused exam depends on both the mechanism of injury and the results of the initial assessment. If there is a dangerous generalized mechanism of injury (such as an auto crash or fall from a height), you should perform a rapid trauma survey (Figure 2-2). You also should perform a rapid trauma survey if the patient is unconscious and you do not know the mechanism of injury. If there is a dangerous focused mechanism of injury suggesting an isolated injury (bullet wound of the thigh or amputation of the hand, for example), you may perform the focused exam (Figure 2-3), which is limited to the area affected by the injury. As a practical matter, remember that where there appears to be only one isolated injury (stab or bullet wound), there may be others of which the patient is not aware. You should have a low threshold for doing a rapid trauma survey rather than a focused exam. Finally, if there is no significant mechanism of injury (such as a dropped a rock on a toe) and the initial assessment is normal (alert with no loss of consciousness, normal breathing, radial pulse less than 120, and no complaint of dyspnea, chest, abdominal, or pelvic pain), you may move directly to the focused exam based on the patient's chief complaint.

If you identify a priority (high-risk) patient, you need to find the cause of the abnormal findings to determine if this is a load-and-go patient.

You have identified a priority patient if you find any of the following:

- Dangerous mechanism of injury
- High-risk group (very young, very old, chronically ill)
- Initial assessment reveals
  —Altered mental status
  —Abnormal breathing
  —Abnormal circulation (shock or uncontrolled bleeding)
- History that reveals
  —Loss of consciousness
  —Difficulty breathing
  —Severe pain of head, neck, or torso

Rapid Trauma Survey

The rapid trauma survey is a brief exam done to find all life threats (Figure 2-2). A more thorough assessment—the ITLS Secondary Survey—will follow later if time permits. Having completed the initial assessment, begin obtaining a brief, targeted history (What happened? Where do you hurt?). Quickly assess (look and feel) head and neck for obvious wounds.

Evaluate neck veins, which, if engorged, indicate positive pressure in the chest (possible tension pneumothorax or cardiac tamponade). If they are distended, look and palpate at the sternal notch for tracheal deviation. A rigid cervical extrication collar may be applied at this time.

Expose and examine the chest. Look to see if it is moving symmetrically. If not, is there paradoxical motion? Are there contusions or abrasions? Are there penetrations or sucking wounds? Briefly palpate for tenderness, instability, or crepitation. Then listen to see if breath sounds are present and equal bilaterally. Listen with the stethoscope over the lateral chest about the fourth intercostal space in the midaxillary line on both sides. If breath sounds are not equal (decreased or absent on one side), percuss the chest to determine whether the patient is just splinting from pain or if a pneumothorax (hyperresonant) or a hemothorax (dull) is present. If abnormalities are found during the chest exam (open chest wound, flail chest, tension pneumothorax, hemothorax), treat them as you discover them. Delegate the appropriate intervention (seal an open wound, hand stabilize flail chest) to another team member. If a tension pneumothorax is identified, and the patient has altered mental status, cyanosis, and signs of shock, prepare to decompress immediately. Before moving to the abdominal exam, very briefly notice heart sounds so you will have a baseline for changes, such as development of muffled heart sounds.

Briefly examine the abdomen, looking for bruises, penetrating wounds, or impaled objects. Palpate briefly for tenderness, rigidity, or distention. Be aware that an unconscious patient or one with a cervical-spine injury may have a false-negative exam.

Briefly palpate the pelvic girdle for tenderness, instability, or crepitation by gently pressing down on the symphysis and gently squeezing in on the anterior iliac crests. Note that tenderness is not the same thing as being unstable. The pelvis may be tender and yet stable. If the pelvis is unstable, you can feel the pelvic ring collapse as you apply pressure. If the pelvis is unstable, direct another team member to get the

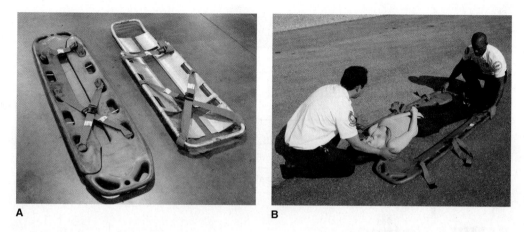

A   B

Figure 2-6 Scoop stretchers may be used to transfer patients onto a stretcher.

scoop stretcher and possibly the pelvic compression belt or a sheet. If the pelvis is unstable, do *not* check again.

Very quickly, examine the lower and upper extremities for gross deformity or swelling. An unstable pelvis and bilateral femur fractures indicate an unstable patient at risk for shock. Before moving such patients, check to make sure they can feel and move their feet and hands.

At this point, log roll the patient onto a long backboard, and transfer him to the ambulance stretcher. Remember to check the posterior of the patient as you do this. If the patient has an unstable pelvis or bilateral femur fractures, to prevent further injuries, use a scoop stretcher (Figure 2-6) to transfer the patient to the ambulance stretcher. Research has shown that a scoop stretcher (Ferno™) provides stabilization equal or superior to a rigid backboard, and it is acceptable to use instead of a backboard. Remember that if you use a scoop stretcher, you are still responsible to do your best to evaluate the posterior side of the patient. Transfer your patient to the ambulance as soon as you have secured him or her to the stretcher (or backboard, if clinically indicated).

If a critical situation is present, transport now and obtain the vital signs during transport. Otherwise, you should now obtain baseline vital signs (blood pressure, pulse, and respiratory rate) and the rest of the **SAMPLE history**. (See the following section.)

If the patient has an altered mental status, do a brief neurologic exam to identify possible increased intracranial pressure (ICP). It is critical to identify this condition (see Chapter 10) because it will have important implications with respect to the rate at which you provide ventilation, your aggressiveness in treating shock, and also the destination of the patient. This exam should include the pupils, Glasgow Coma Scale (GCS) score, and signs of cerebral herniation. (See Chapter 10.) Head injury, shock, and hypoxia are not the only things that cause altered mental status; also think about nontraumatic causes such as hypoglycemia and drug or alcohol overdose. All patients with altered mental status should have a finger-stick glucose performed as soon as they are placed in the ambulance.

During the rapid trauma survey, if encountered, you should note the presence of any medical identification tags, giving information about the patient's existing medical conditions. Also, if the emergency care provider finds a medical patch, such as a nitroglycerin or nicotine or analgesic patch, these should be removed and their presence noted and reported at the hospital. Finally, note the presence of implanted medical devices, such as a pacemaker or insulin pump or vascular access catheters for dialysis or chemotherapy. Emergency care providers should not access these indwelling catheters without direct medical orders and only if trained to do so.

SAMPLE history: the minimum amount of information needed for a trauma patient; the letters in SAMPLE stand for symptoms, allergies, medications, past medical history, last oral intake, and events preceding the incident.

Table 2-3: SAMPLE History
S —Symptoms
A —Allergies
M —Medications
P —Past medical history (Other illnesses?)
L —Last oral intake (When was the last time there was any solid or liquid intake?)
E —Events preceding the incident (Why did it happen?)

SAMPLE History

At the same time as you are performing the patient assessment part of the ITLS Primary Survey (initial assessment and rapid trauma survey or focused exam), you or one of the other emergency care providers should obtain a SAMPLE history (Table 2-3). This is especially important if you must gather information from bystanders because they will not be going with you when you transport the patient.

Remember, prehospital providers are the only ones who get to see the scene and also may be the only ones who get to take a history because many patients who are initially alert lose consciousness before arriving at the hospital. You are not only making interventions to deliver a living patient to the hospital, but you also must be the detective who figures out what happened and why. Pay special attention to the patient's complaints (symptoms) and events prior to the incident (the S and E of the SAMPLE history). A more detailed history may be taken later during the ITLS Secondary Survey. The patient's symptoms can suggest other injuries, and this will affect further examination. It is important to know as much about the mechanism of injury as possible. (Was she restrained? How far did she fall? What caused her to fall?) Look for clues to serious injury such as a history of loss of consciousness, shortness of breath, or pain in the neck, back, chest, abdomen, or pelvis.

Critical Interventions and Transport Decision

When you have completed the initial assessment and rapid trauma survey or focused exam, enough information is available to decide if a critical situation is present. Patients with critical trauma situations are transported immediately. Most treatment interventions will be done during transport.

If your patient has any of the following critical injuries or conditions, transport immediately.

- *Initial assessment reveals:*
  —Altered mental status
  —Abnormal breathing
  —Abnormal circulation (shock or uncontrolled bleeding)
- *Signs discovered during the rapid trauma survey of conditions that can rapidly lead to shock:*
  —Penetrating wounds of the torso
  —Abnormal chest exam (flail chest, open wound, tension pneumothorax, hemothorax)
  —Tender, distended abdomen
  —Pelvic instability
  —Bilateral femur fractures

PEARLS
On-Scene Time

Survival of many trauma patients is time-dependent. Critical trauma patients often need definitive care in the operating room. Delegate interventions that must be done on scene. If possible, do interventions during transport.

- *Significant mechanism of injury and/or poor general health of patient.* Even though the patient appears to be stable, if there is a dangerous mechanism or other dangers (such as age, poor general health, death of another passenger in the same auto), consider early transport. "Stable" patients can become unstable quite rapidly.

If the patient has one of the critical conditions listed, after the rapid trauma survey or focused exam, immediately load the patient into an ambulance and transport rapidly to the nearest appropriate emergency facility. When in doubt, transport early.

The following procedures are done at the scene, and most of them can be delegated to team members to perform while you continue the ITLS Primary Survey: control major external bleeding, open and maintain a patent airway (position, sweep, suction; intubate if indicated and necessary), ventilate, apply oxygen, CP, seal sucking chest wounds, stabilize flail segments, decompress tension pneumothorax when indicated, stabilize penetrating objects, and maintain SMR if indicated.

Procedures that are not life saving, such as splinting, bandaging, insertion of IV lines, or even elective endotracheal intubation, must not hold up transport of the critical patient. At this point, the ITLS Primary Survey is over, and the team leader may help the other emergency care providers with patient care.

Contacting Medical Direction

When you have a critical patient, it is extremely important to contact medical direction as early as possible. It takes time to get the necessary resources such as the appropriate surgeon and the operating room team in place, and the critical patient may have no time to wait after arrival at the hospital. Always notify the receiving facility of your estimated time of arrival (ETA), the condition of the patient, and any special needs on arrival.

ITLS Ongoing Exam

Ongoing assessment and management includes the critical procedures performed on scene and during transport and communication with medical direction. The ITLS Ongoing Exam is an abbreviated exam to assess for changes in the patient's condition. In contrast to the ITLS Secondary Survey, which is performed only once, the ITLS Ongoing Exam may be performed multiple times during a long transport. In critical cases with short transport times, there may not be time to perform an ITLS Secondary Survey. The ITLS Ongoing Exam may take its place. It should be performed and recorded no less than every five minutes for critical patients and every 15 minutes for stable patients. The ITLS Ongoing Exam also should be performed as follows:

- Each time the patient is moved
- Each time an intervention is performed
- Any time the patient's condition worsens

This exam is meant to find any changes in the patient's condition, so concentrate on reassessing only those things that may change. For example, if you have applied a traction splint, reassess the limb for decreased pain and for the presence of distal pulses, motor function, and sensation (PMS). In contrast, if you decompress a chest, you must reassess almost everything in the initial assessment and rapid trauma survey down through the abdominal exam.

Having moved the patient to the ambulance and completed the ITLS Primary Survey and vital signs (including a brief neurologic exam if the patient is not alert), transport the patient and begin the ITLS Ongoing Exam, completing exposure of the patient if he or she is unstable. In the critical, multiple-trauma patient, the first ITLS Ongoing Exam may essentially be a repeat of the ITLS Primary Survey, including the initial assessment and rapid trauma survey.

Procedure

Performing an ITLS Ongoing Exam

The ITLS Ongoing Exam should be performed in the following order (Figure 2-7):

1. Ask the patient if there have been any changes in how he or she feels. Complete the SAMPLE history if not already done.

2. Reassess mental status (LOC and pupils). If the patient has an altered mental status, check a finger-stick glucose and recheck the GCS.

Figure 2-7 ITLS Ongoing Exam.

ITLS ONGOING EXAM
|
PATIENT HISTORY
Complete S.A.M.P.L.E. History if not already done
|
LOC
A-V/P-U
Pupils
|
If altered mental status:
Finger-stick Glucose
GLASCOW COMA SCALE
Eyes, Voice, Movement
|
VITAL SIGNS
Measured Pulse, Respiratory Rate, Blood Pressure
Pulse Oximeter, Cardiac Monitor, CO_2 Monitor, Temperature
|
AIRWAY
Patency? If burn patient assess for signs of inhalation injury
|
BREATHING
Present? Rate, Depth, Effort
|
CIRCULATION
Skin Color, Temperature, Moisture; Capillary Refill
|
BLEEDING STILL CONTROLLED?
|
Examine Neck
Obvious Wounds, Tenderness, Swelling
Neck Vein Distention? Tracheal Deviation?
|
Examine CHEST
Asymmetry (Paradoxical Motion?), Contusions, Penetrations,
Tenderness, Instability, Crepitation
|
BREATH SOUNDS
Present? Equal? (If unequal: **Percussion**)
Heart Tones
|
Examine ABDOMEN
Contusions, Penetration/evisceration; Tenderness, Rigidity, Distention
|
Recheck Identified INJURIES
|
Check INTERVENTIONS
ET tube, Oxygen, IVs, seals on chest wounds, decompression needle,
splints & dressings, impaled objects, position of pregnant patients
|
Recheck MONITORS
Cardiac, Capnograph, Pulse Oximeter

3. Reassess the ABCs.
   a. Reassess the airway.
      (1) Recheck patency.
      (2) If this is a burn patient, assess for signs of inhalation injury.
   b. Reassess breathing and circulation.
      (1) Recheck vital signs.
      (2) Note skin color, condition, and temperature.
      (3) Check the neck for jugular venous distention (JVD) and tracheal deviation. (If a cervical collar has been applied, remove the front to examine the neck.)
      (4) Recheck the chest. Notice the quality of breath sounds. If breath sounds are unequal, evaluate for splinting, pneumothorax, and hemothorax. Listen to the heart to see if the sounds have become muffled.
4. Reassess the abdomen, if mechanism suggests possible injury. Note the development of tenderness, rigidity, or distention.
5. Check each of the identified injuries (lacerations for bleeding, PMS distal to all injured extremi-ties, flails, pneumothorax, open chest wounds, and so on).
6. Check interventions.
   a. Check ET tube for patency and position.
   b. Check oxygen for flow rate.
   c. Check IVs for patency and rate of fluid.
   d. Check seals on sucking chest wounds.
   e. Check patency of tension pneumothorax decompression needle.
   f. Check splints and dressings.
   g. Check impaled objects to be sure they are well stabilized.
   h. Check body position of pregnant patients.
   i. Check cardiac monitor, capnograph, and pulse oximeter.

Accurately record what you see and what you do. Record changes in the patient's condition during transport. Record the time that you perform each intervention. Extenuating circumstances or significant details should be recorded in the comments or remarks section of the written report.

ITLS Secondary Survey

The ITLS Secondary Survey is a more comprehensive exam meant to pick up additional injuries that might have been missed in the brief ITLS Primary Survey. This assessment also establishes the baseline from which treatment decisions will eventually be made. It is important to record the information discovered in this assessment. Whether or not to perform an ITLS Secondary Survey as well as when to perform one depends on the situation:

- Critical patients should have this assessment done during transport rather than on scene.
- If there is a short transport and you must perform interventions, you may not have time to do the ITLS Secondary Survey.
- If the ITLS Primary Survey does not reveal a critical condition, the ITLS Secondary Survey may be performed on scene. Stable patients with no dangerous mechanism of injury (such as a dropped rock on a toe) do not require an ITLS Secondary Survey.

When you perform the ITLS Secondary Survey, you should always begin by quickly repeating the initial assessment. You can do this as another team member is checking the vital signs.

You should have obtained the SAMPLE history during the ITLS Primary Survey and ITLS Ongoing Exam, but now you can obtain further information if needed. Perform your ITLS Secondary Survey while you are obtaining the rest of the history (if the patient is conscious).

Procedure

Performing an ITLS Secondary Survey

The exam should contain the following elements (Figure 2-8).

1. Repeat the initial assessment.
2. Consider using monitors (cardiac, pulse oximeter, CO_2). These are usually applied during transport.
3. Record vital signs again. Record pulse rate, respiratory rate, and blood pressure. Remember, the pulse pressure is as important as the systolic pressure. Many people now consider the pulse oximetry and capnography readings as part of the vital signs. These are useful tools, but you must know their limitations. (See Chapters 4 and 5.)
4. Do a brief neurologic exam. It gives important baseline information that is used in later treatment decisions. This exam should include the following:
   a. *Level of consciousness.* If the patient is conscious, describe his or her orientation, emotional status, and whether he or she follows commands. If the patient has an altered mental status, record the level of coma (for Glasgow Coma Scale score, see Table 2-4). If there is altered mental status, check fingerstick blood glucose (if not already done) and check the oxygen saturation level. If there is any chance of narcotic overdose, administer

Naloxone (IV or IN). For elderly or other special-needs patients, try to determine from a caretaker if the patient is at the usual baseline level of alertness and responsiveness.
   b. *Pupils.* Note the size of the pupils and whether they are equal or unequal. Do they respond to light?
   c. *Motor.* Can the patient move fingers and toes?
   d. *Sensation.* Can the patient feel you when you touch his or her fingers and toes? Does the unconscious patient respond when you pinch fingers and toes?
5. Perform a detailed (head-to-toe) exam. Pay particular attention to the patient's complaints and also recheck the injuries that you found previously. The exam should consist of inspection, auscultation, palpation, and sometimes percussion. Last, look for and note the presence of medical identification tags, medication patches (remove them), and implanted medical devices, if not done previously.
   a. Begin at the head examining for deformities, contusions, abrasions, penetrations, burns, lacerations, and swelling (**DCAP-BLS**), and palpating for tenderness, instability, and crepitus (**TIC**). Also check for raccoon eyes, Battle's sign, and drainage of blood or fluid from the ears or nose. Assess the mouth. Assess the airway again. (*Continued on page 46.*)

Table 2-4: Glasgow Coma Scale

Eye Opening	Points	Verbal Response	Points	Motor Response	Points
Spontaneous	4	Oriented	5	Obeys commands	6
To voice	3	Confused	4	Localizes pain	5
To pain	2	Inappropriate words	3	Withdraws	4
None	1	Incomprehensible sounds	2	Abnormal flexion	3*
		Silent	1	Abnormal extension	2**
				No movement	1

* *Decorticate posturing to pain.*

** *Decerebrate posturing to pain.*

ITLS SECONDARY SURVEY

|

INITIAL ASSESSMENT

|

GENERAL IMPRESSION

Does the patient appear better, worse, or unchanged?

|

LOC

A-V/P-U

|

AIRWAY

(WITH C-SPINE CONTROL)

Snoring, Gurgling, Stridor, etc.; Silence

|

BREATHING

Present? Rate, Depth, Effort

|

RADIAL PULSE – CAROTID if no radial

Present? Rate, Rhythm, Quality

Skin Color, Temperature, Moisture; Capillary Refill

|

BLEEDING STILL CONTROLLED?

- -

DETAILED EXAM

PATIENT HISTORY

Complete S.A.M.P.L.E. History if not already done

|

VITAL SIGNS

Measured Pulse, Respiratory Rate, Blood Pressure

Consider Pulse Oximeter, Cardiac Monitor, CO_2 Monitor, Blood Sugar, Temperature, prn

GLASCOW COMA SCALE

(Eyes, Voice, Movement); Emotional State

Examine Head

DCAP-BLS, TIC

(Pupils, Battles Sign, Raccoon Eyes, Drainage from ears or nose

|

Examine Neck

DCAP-BLS, TIC Neck Vein Distention? Tracheal Deviation?

|

Examine CHEST

Asymmetry, Paradoxical motion, DCAP-BLS, TIC

BREATH SOUNDS

Present? Equal? (If unequal: **Percussion**) Abnormal Breath Sounds?

Heart Tones

Examine ABDOMEN

Contusions, Penetration/evisceration; Tenderness, Rigidity, Distention

|

Examine PELVIS

DCAP-BLS, TIC

|

Examine LOWER/UPPER EXTREMITIES

DCAP-BLS, TIC, Distal PMS

POSTERIOR

Examine only if not done in Primary Survey

DCAP-BLS, TIC

Figure 2-8 ITLS Secondary Survey.

DCAP-BLS: short for deformities, contusions, abrasions, penetrations, burns, lacerations, and swelling.

TIC: short for tenderness, instability, and crepitus.

Procedure (*continued*)

b. Check the neck for DCAP-BLS, TIC, distended neck veins, and deviated trachea.

c. Check the chest for DCAP-BLS and TIC. Also check for paradoxical movement of the chest wall. Be sure that breath sounds are present and equal on each side (check all four fields). Note rales, wheezing, or "noisy" breath sounds. Notice if heart sounds are as loud as before. (A noticeable decrease in heart sounds may be an early sign of cardiac tamponade.) Recheck seals over open wounds. Be sure flails are well stabilized. If you detect decreased breath sounds, percuss to determine whether the patient has a pneumothorax or hemothorax.

d. Perform an abdominal exam. Look for signs of blunt or penetrating trauma. Feel all four quadrants for tenderness or rigidity. Do not waste time listening for bowel sounds; it provides the emergency care provider with no useful information. If the abdomen is painful to gentle pressure during examination, you can expect the patient to be bleeding internally. If the abdomen is both distended and painful, you can expect hemorrhagic shock to occur very quickly. Assess perineum for bleeding or hematoma.

e. Assess pelvis and extremities. (The unstable pelvis noted in the rapid trauma survey is not rechecked.) Examine for DCAP-BLS and feel for TIC. Be sure to check and record pulse, motor function, and sensation (PMS) on all fractures. Do this before and after straightening any fracture. Angulated fractures of the upper extremities can be splinted as found. Most fractures of the lower extremities are gently straightened and then stabilized using traction splints or air splints. Critical patients have all splints applied during transport.

Transport immediately if the ITLS Secondary Survey reveals the development of any of the critical trauma situations. After you finish the ITLS Secondary Survey, you should finish bandaging and splinting.

Adjuncts for Trauma Patient Assessment

One of the decisions to be made when assessing a trauma patient is determining the level of trauma center to which to take the patient. Patients with unstable vital signs and those with serious anatomic injuries are usually taken to trauma centers, but the decision can be more difficult for patients with normal vital signs and a normal level of consciousness who also have a significant mechanism of injury.

Ideally, you should take the most severely injured patients to the appropriate trauma center as quickly as possible because this has been shown to have the best patient outcomes. However, avoid taking every injured patient to a trauma center, which would overload this resource with patients who do not have critical injuries. Better tools are needed to distinguish between patients who have injuries that are either not severe or not time critical and will remain stable, and those who appear stable initially and then decompensate later, requiring emergent transfer to a trauma center. There are at least two adjuncts for trauma triage that may prove to be helpful in that situation by distinguishing between the two patient groups: serum lactate and ultrasound.

Serum lactate is a marker for tissue hypoxia and has been used in the hospital setting to monitor critical patients. In the field it appears to be useful to predict which patients with normal vital signs are having occult internal bleeding and will soon develop hemorrhagic shock. Multiple services have been using prehospital finger-stick serum lactate levels to predict who will develop shock. If further studies confirm its predictive value, it will be very useful.

Portable ultrasound can be used to assess for intra-abdominal hemorrhage, pneumo-thoraces, and cardiac tamponade, among other things. Abdominal trauma sonography is very commonly used in the initial assessment of trauma patients in the emergency department and is called the FAST exam (focused assessment with sonography in trauma). It is noninvasive and only takes from one to three minutes to perform. In many emergency departments FAST has replaced the diagnostic peritoneal lavage in the initial assessment for blood in the abdomen after blunt trauma. Because it is portable and not difficult to learn to use for simple exams, FAST is being used in the field by some ground and air services (especially in Europe), and the information obtained is being used to determine which patients are transported directly to a trauma center and which are transported to a community hospital instead. Initial studies are reporting that it has a very high (90% and higher) predictive value for intra-abdominal bleeding. Studies of its use in moving ambulances and helicopters have been mixed, and as with most procedures, success depends on the skill and training of the operator.

Hopefully, those and other assessment adjuncts will prove to give emergency care providers more options to improve patient care and health-care resource utilization.

Case Presentation (continued)

The emergency care providers are at the scene of a multiple-casualty incident involving an overturned truck, a sedan, and a motorcycle. The fire service has contained hazards, and the scene is safe to enter. As the ambulance crew approaches the motorcyclist, they look for any hazards that might endanger themselves or the patient. Finding none, they note the motorcyclist is not wearing a helmet, is lacking awareness, and is in obvious respiratory distress. With the mechanism of injury in mind, they ask the Incident Commander (IC) to have one of his crew bring an orthopedic (scoop) stretcher or a long spine board, straps, and a C-collar from the ambulance. If the unit does not have a scoop stretcher, a long spine board should be used.

Seeing the obvious major bleeding from behind the left knee, the first priority is to stop the bleeding. While providing spinal motion restriction, they gently turn the patient onto his back, the second crew member applies direct pressure to the laceration behind the knee and prepares to apply a pressure dressing. As they roll the patient to a supine position, they quickly assess the back for major injury.

The lead emergency care provider takes a position at the head of the patient, maintains in-line spinal motion restriction, and speaks to the patient, who opens his eyes briefly and moans. In the absence of snoring, gurgling, or stridor, the responder carefully listens and feels for air movement at the nose and mouth. Finding very poor movement with rapid respiratory efforts, the responder then feels for and finds a rapid carotid pulse.

The third emergency care provider arrives with the equipment, places it beside the patient, and then takes over manual in-line spinal motion restriction after placing a high-flow oxygen mask on the patient. The lead emergency care provider notes generally pale, clammy skin, but is able to palpate a rapid, thready radial pulse. His partner reports that he is unable to stem the hemorrhage and is going to place a tourniquet on the upper left leg.

The lead emergency care provider declares a "load-and-go" situation, and due to the mechanism and the decreased level of consciousness of the victim, decides to perform a rapid trauma survey. He sees a large hematoma over the right eye, a contusion at the front of the neck, notes flat neck veins and a midline trachea. He instructs his team member to apply the C-collar. Upon cutting away the biker's body shirt, he sees a large contusion over the right anterior chest wall, asymmetrical movement with the right side not moving at all, but no open or puncture wounds. He then listens bilaterally and finds breath sounds diminished on the right. He hears faint heart sounds. He quickly inspects the abdomen finding obvious bruising, and palpates for tenderness, rigidity, or distention, and quickly palpates the pelvic girdle for tenderness, instability, or crepitus. Finding the pelvis stable, he quickly checks the lower extremities, notes control of the hemorrhage with the tourniquet, and notes swelling and deformity of the right thigh. He notes no reaction to pain when pinching the feet, but the patient withdraws both arms when his thumb is pinched. While maneuvering the patient onto the scoop stretcher, he notes only numerous abrasions to the middle and lower back.

With packaging complete, the patient is transferred to the ambulance, and the third member of the team is assigned to drive the ambulance. The lead emergency care provider asks the IC to have one of his crew monitor the remaining patients for any apparent changes in condition, pending arrival of additional ambulance personnel. (Given the critical nature of the cyclist's injuries and the apparent stability of other patients, it is appropriate to leave them in the care of BLS responders still on the scene until arrival of additional ambulances.)

Before leaving for the trauma center, a brief set of initial vital signs is obtained while the lead emergency care provider performs a neurologic exam, discovering large (8 mm) sluggish but equal pupils, and a patient whose GCS is now 1+1+4: withdraws to pain induced by pinching the left thumbnail. (There is no reaction or movement in the lower extremities.)

While en route, the lead emergency care provider contacts the trauma center to identify themselves, report the situation, the life-threatening injuries discovered and suspected, including the life-threatening external hemorrhage now controlled, findings of the exam indicating possible head, chest, and abdominal injuries, concern for possible spine injury occasioned by lack of movement in the lower extremities, the treatment performed and to be performed, including SMR, supplemental oxygen, fluid administration, and their ETA.

While his partner establishes IV lines, the lead emergency care provider prepares to reassess the patient. While team member 2 attaches a cardiac monitor and a pulse oximeter, the leader checks the wound again to confirm that bleeding is still controlled and then calls the emergency department at the trauma center to advise them of their ETA and the status of the patient.

If there is time during transport, the leader will conduct a thorough ITLS Secondary Survey in search of any additional injuries.

Summary

Patient assessment is key to trauma care. The interventions required are not difficult, but their timing often is critical. If you know what questions to ask and how to perform the exam, you will know when to perform the life-saving interventions without unnecessarily prolonging time on scene. This chapter has described a rapid, orderly, and thorough examination of the trauma patient with examination and treatment priorities always in mind. The continuous practice of approaching the patient in the way described will allow you to concentrate on the patient, rather than on what to do next. Optimum speed is achieved by teamwork. Teamwork is achieved by practice. You should plan regular exercises in patient evaluation to perfect each team member's role. Current research may provide future assessment adjuncts to help us make better decisions about the level of care our patients may need.

Bibliography

Alam, H. B., D. Burris, J. A. DaCorta, and P. Rhee. "Hemorrhage Control in the Battlefield: Role of New Hemostatic Agents." *Military Medicine* 170, no. 1 (January 2005): 63–69.

Brooke, M., J. Walton, and D. Scutt. "Paramedic Application of Ultrasound in the Management of Patients in the Prehospital Setting: A Review of the Literature." *Emergency Medicine Journal* 27, no. 9 (September 2010): 702–7.

Jansen, T. C., J. van Bommel, P. G. Mulder, J. H. Rommes, S. J. Schieveld, and J. Bakker. "The Prognostic Value of Blood Lactate Levels Relative to That of Vital Signs in the Prehospital Setting: A Pilot Study." *Critical Care* 12, no. 6 (2008): 160–66.

Korner, M., M. M. Krotz, C. Degenhart, K. J. Pfeifer, M. F. Reiser, and U. Linsenmaier. "Current Role of Emergency Ultrasound in Patients with Major Trauma." *Radiographics* 28, no. 1 (January-February 2008): 225–42.

Krell, J. M., M. S. McCoy, P. J. Sparto, G. L. Fisher, W. A. Stoy, and D. P. Hostler. "Comparison of the Ferno Scoop Stretcher with the Long Backboard for Spinal Immobilization." *Prehospital Emergency Care* 10, no. 1 (January-March 2006): 46–51.

MacKenzie, E. J., F. P. Rivara, G. J. Jurkovich, A. B. Nathens, K. P. Frey, B. L. Egleston, D. S. Salkever, and D. O. Scharfstein. "A National Evaluation of the Effect of Trauma-Center Care on Mortality." *New England Journal of Medicine* 354, no. 4 (January 26, 2006): 366–78.

Sasser S. M., R. C. Hunt, M. Faul, D. Sugerman, W. S. Pearson, T. Dulski, M. M. Wald, G. J. Jurkovich, C. D. Newgard, E. B. Lerner, et al. "Guidelines for Field Triage of Injured Patients: Recommendations of the National Expert Panel on Field Triage, 2011." *Morbidity and Mortality Weekly Report* 61 (RR01) (January 13, 2012). Available on the Centers for Disease Control and Prevention website, last reviewed/updated January 13, 2012. Accessed January 8, 2015, at http://www.cdc.gov/mmwr/preview/mmwrhtml/rr6101a1.htm

Sochor, M., S. Althoff, D. Bose, R. Maio, and P. Deflorio. "Glass Intact Assures Safe Cervical Spine Protocol." *Journal of Emergency Medicine* 44, no. 3 (March 2013): 631-36.

van Beest, P. A., P. J. Mulder, S. B. Oetomo, B. van den Broek, M. A. Kuiper, and P. E. Spronk. "Measurement of Lactate in a Prehospital Setting Is Related to Outcome." *European Journal of Emergency Medicine* 16, no. 6 (December 2009): 318–22.

Get more information about this course by calling
ITLS International at 888-495-4875
(outside the United States call +1-630-495-6442) or visit

www.itrauma.org

3

Assessment Skills

S. Robert Seitz, M.Ed., RN, NRP
Eduardo Romero Hicks, MD

Evaluación del Paciente   Ocena stanu chorego   Pregled ozljeđenika

Ocena stanja pacienta   Valutazione del paziente   D'évaluation des Patients

Patientenbeurteilung   تقييم حالة المصاب   procena pacijenta

Sérültvizsgálat

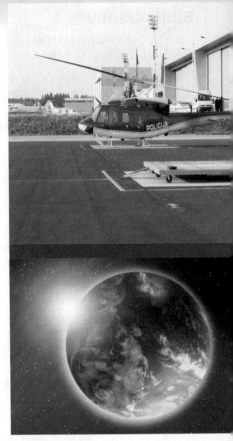

Kate Blackwelder

Objectives

Upon successful completion of this chapter, you should be able to:

1. ITLS Primary Survey
   a. Correctly perform the ITLS Primary Survey.
   b. Identify within two minutes which patients require load and go.
   c. Describe when to perform critical interventions.
2. ITLS Ongoing Exam and ITLS Secondary Survey
   a. Correctly perform the ITLS Ongoing (reassessment) Exam.
   b. Correctly perform the ITLS Secondary Survey.
   c. Describe when to perform critical interventions.
   d. Demonstrate proper communications with medical direction.
3. Assessment and Management of the Trauma Patient
   a. Demonstrate the proper sequence of rapid assessment and the management of the multiple-trauma patient.

Procedure

ITLS Primary Survey

During the ITLS class, short written scenarios will be used along with a model to simulate the patient. You will divide into teams to practice conducting an initial assessment, performing critical interventions, and making a transport decision. Each member of the team must practice being team leader at least once. The critical information represents the answers you should be seeking at each step of the survey. The Treatment Decision Tree (Table 3-1) represents the actions that should be taken (personally or delegated) in response to your assessment.

Table 3-1: Trauma Assessment—Treatment Decision Tree

Assessment	Action
SCENE SIZE-UP	
Safety	Put on gloves, protective clothing. Remove hazards or patient from hazards.
Number of patients	Call for help, if needed.
Extrication/rescue needed	Call for special equipment, if needed.
Mechanisms of injury	Suspect appropriate injuries (e.g., cervical spine).
GENERAL IMPRESSION	Begin to establish priorities.
Age, sex, weight	
Position (in surroundings, body position/posture)	
Activity	
Obvious major injuries	
Major bleeding	Direct pressure, tourniquet, hemostatic agent, as needed.
LEVEL OF CONSCIOUSNESS	
Alert/responsive to voice	Initiate cervical-spine motion restriction, *if indicated by dangerous mechanism of injury.*
Unresponsive to voice	Establish cervical-spine motion restriction.
AIRWAY	*You must fix any airway problems when you find them.*
Snoring	Modified jaw thrust.
Gurgling	Suction.
Stridor	Intubate, confirm tube placement, and apply waveform capnography, if available.
Silence	Attempt to ventilate. If unsuccessful:
	– Reposition; initiate rapid extrication.
	– Visualize.
	– Suction.
	– Consider foreign body removal or decompression of tension pneumothorax.
	– Initiate bag-mask ventilation, and consider BIAD or intubation, confirm tube placement, and apply waveform capnography, if available.
	– Consider translaryngeal jet ventilation or crycothyroidotomy.
BREATHING	*If ventilation is inadequate,* assist ventilations.
Absent	Ventilate twice (check pulse before continuing ventilation at 8–10 breaths per minute with oxygen).
< 8	Assist ventilation at 8–10 breaths per minute with oxygen.
Low tidal volume	Assist ventilation at 8–10 breaths per minute with oxygen.
Labored	Oxygen by nonrebreather at 15 liters/minute.
Normal or rapid	Consider oxygen.

(continued)

Procedure (*continued*)

Table 3-1: Trauma Assessment–Treatment Decision Tree (*continued*)

Assessment	Action
CIRCULATION	
RADIAL PULSE	
Absent	Check carotid pulse (see below). Note late shock.
Present	Note rate and quality.
Bradycardia	Consider spinal shock, head injury.
Tachycardia	Consider hypovolemic shock.
	Consider need for pain management.
	Consider cardiac monitor.
CAROTID PULSE	Check, if no radial pulse.
Absent	Initiate CPR and ventilation with oxygen, consider immediate intervention, transport, or terminate resuscitation.
Present	Note rate and quality.
Bradycardia	Consider spinal shock, head injury.
Tachycardia	Consider late shock.
SKIN COLOR AND CONDITION	
Pale, cool, clammy	Consider hypovolemic shock.
Cyanosis	Reassess ventilatory assistance and consider intubation.
MAJOR BLEEDING	Direct pressure, tourniquet, and/or hemostatic agent.
HEAD	
Major facial injuries	Consider intubation.
NECK	
Swelling, bruising, retracting	Consider intubation.
Neck vein distention	Consider tamponade, tension pneumothorax.
Tracheal deviation	Consider tension pneumothorax.
Tenderness, deformity, or altered mental status	Apply cervical collar.
CHEST	Inspect and palpate.
Symmetrical, stable	Continue exam.
Bruises, crepitation	Consider early cardiac monitoring.
Penetrating wounds	Occlusive dressing.
Paradoxical motion	Stabilize flail. Consider early intubation.
BREATH SOUNDS	
Present and equal	Continue exam.
Unequal	Percuss chest to determine pneumothorax versus hemothorax.
	If indicated, initiate needle decompression.
HEART TONES	Note for comparison later.
Muffled with JVD and bilateral breath sounds	Consider pericardial tamponade.
ABDOMEN, PELVIS, UPPER LEGS	
If tender abdomen, unstable pelvis, or bilateral femur fractures	Anticipate development of shock.

Table 3-1: (continued)

Assessment	Action
MOVEMENT/SENSATION IN EXTREMITIES	
Present	Record.
Decreased or absent.	Suspect spine injury.
POSTERIOR	
Injuries identified.	Appropriately manage identified injuries.
	Transfer to backboard.
	TRANSPORT IMMEDIATELY IF CRITICAL TRAUMA SITUATION PRESENT.
SAMPLE HISTORY	Obtain and record.
VITAL SIGNS	Measure and record level of consciousness, respirations, pulse, blood pressure, pulse oximetry, core temperature, and level of discomfort.
Systolic < 90 with signs of shock	Consider IV fluid therapy en route to hospital.
Systolic < 80	IV fluid therapy en route to hospital
Systolic < 60	*Treat decompensated shock. Consider CPR.*
Increasing systolic blood pressure and decreasing heart rate	Consider increased intracerebral pressure. Maintain systolic blood pressure of 110–120 mm Hg. Consider adjustment of ventilations to maintain an $ETCO_2$ of 30–35 mm Hg.
PUPILS	
Unequal	Suspect head injury unless patient is alert, then suspect eye injury.
Unequal or dilated and fixed with GCS < 8	Give 100% oxygen. Do not let patient get hypotensive (target systolic BP of 110–120 mm Hg). Intubation and control ventilation (16–20 breaths per minute or at rate to maintain $ETCO_2$ of 30–35 mm Hg). (Unequal pupils or dilated and fixed pupils and GSC 8 or less are suggestive of cerebral herniation.)
Pinpoint (with respiratory rate < 8)	Consider naloxone.
Dilated/reactive (with GCS < 8)	Give 100% oxygen. Consider intubation. Ventilate at 6–8 breaths per minute or to maintain $ETCO_2$ of 35–45.
GLASGOW COMA SCALE SCORE (for decreased LOC)	Give 100% oxygen. Do not let patient get hypotensive (target systolic BP of 110–120 mm Hg).
< 8	Maintain $ETCO_2$ of 30–35 mm Hg. Consider hyperventilation only if patient shows signs of cerebral herniation:
	– GCS < 8 with extensor posturing
	– GCS < 8 with pupillary asymmetry or nonreactivity
	– GCS < 8 with a subsequent drop of more than two points
ALL PATIENTS WITH DECREASED LOC	Check for medical identification devices. Obtain blood glucose level.

ITLS Primary Survey—Critical Information

If you ask the right questions, you will get the information you need to make the critical decisions necessary in the management of your patient. The following questions are presented in the order in which you should ask yourself as you perform the ITLS Primary Survey. This is the minimum information that you will need as you perform each step of the ITLS Primary Survey (Figure 3-1):

ITLS Patient Assessment

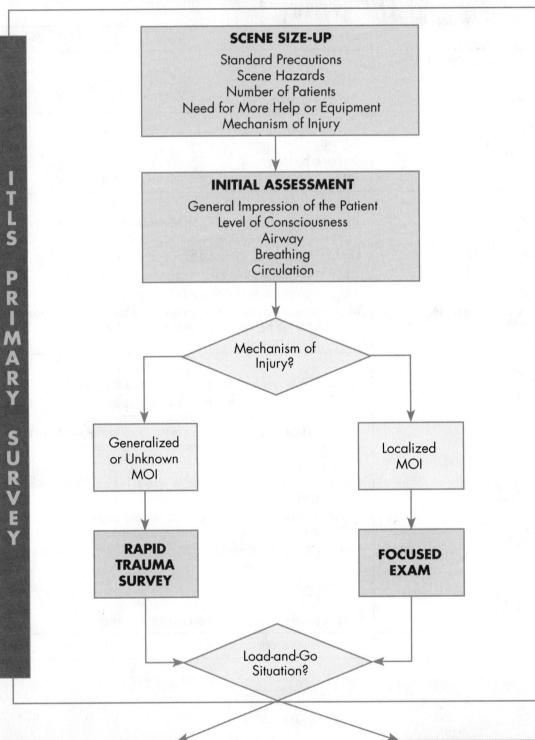

Figure 3-1 Steps in the assessment of the trauma patient.

Scene Size-up

- Have I taken standard precautions?
- Do I see, hear, smell, or sense anything dangerous?
- Are there any other patients?
- Are additional personnel or resources needed?
- Do we need special equipment?
- What is the mechanism of injury here?
- Is it generalized or focused?
- Is it potentially life threatening?

Initial Assessment

General Impression

- What is my general impression of the patient as I approach?
- Is there obvious life-threatening *external* bleeding that must be addressed now?

Level of Consciousness (AVPU)

- Introduce yourself, and say: "We are here to help you. Can you tell us what happened?"
- From the patient's response, what is the AVPU (alert, voice, pain, unresponsive) rating?

Airway

- Is the airway open and clear?
- Do I *hear* abnormal sounds such as snoring, gurgling, or stridor?

Breathing

- Is the patient breathing?
- What is the rate and depth of respiration?
- Is breathing labored?

Circulation

- Is there life-threatening external bleeding?
- What is the rate and quality of the pulse at the neck and wrist?
- What are the skin color, condition, and temperature?

Decision

- Is this a critical situation?
- Is spinal motion restriction indicated?
- Does the mechanism of injury or any initial assessment findings indicate the need for a rapid trauma survey?

Rapid Trauma Survey

(See Figure 3-2.)

Head and Neck

- Are there obvious wounds of the head or neck?
- Is there deformity or tenderness of the neck?
- Are the neck veins distended?
- Does the trachea look and feel midline or deviated?

PEARLS

ITLS Primary Survey

- Do not approach the patient until you have performed a scene size-up.
- Do not interrupt the ITLS Primary Survey except for immediate threats to life such as airway obstruction, cardiac arrest, severe hemorrhage, or if the scene becomes too dangerous. Team members may perform the necessary critical interventions while you complete the ITLS Primary Survey.
- Give any ventilation instructions as soon as you assess airway and breathing.
- Prophylactic hyperventilation is not recommended for patients with decreased level of consciousness. Use it only for head-injury patients who show signs of the cerebral herniation syndrome.
- Assist ventilations in anyone who is hypoventilating (less than eight breaths per minute, *moving little or no air,* or ETCO$_2$ of greater than 45). Confirm adequate tidal volume based on chest rise and fall.
- Give oxygen to all multiple-trauma patients. If in doubt or a pulse oximeter reading of less than 95 is present, give oxygen.
- Endotracheal tubes are the best method to protect the airway and provide ventilatory assistance to the adult patient. Other methods may be effective but are not as secure.
- *If spinal motion restriction (SMR) is indicated,* transfer the patient to the backboard as soon as the ITLS Primary Survey is completed.
- When the ITLS Primary Survey is completed, decide if the patient is critical or stable.
- Communicate with medical direction and the receiving facility early if you have a critical patient.

(continued on page 57)

Figure 3-2 The ITLS Primary Survey including the rapid trauma survey.

ITLS PRIMARY SURVEY

SCENE SIZE-UP
Standard Precautions
Hazards, Number of Patients, Need for additional resources,
Mechanism of Injury

- -

INITIAL ASSESSMENT
GENERAL IMPRESSION
Age, Sex, Weight, General Appearance, Position,
Purposeful Movement, Obvious Injuries, Skin Color
Life-threatening Bleeding (CABC)

LOC
(A-V-P-U)
Chief Complaint/Symptoms

AIRWAY
(CONSIDER C-SPINE CONTROL)
(Snoring, Gurgling, Stridor; Silence)

BREATHING
(**Present?** Rate, Depth, Effort)

CIRCULATION
(**Radial/Carotid Present?** Rate, Rhythm, Quality)
Skin Color, Temperature, Moisture; Capillary Refill
Has bleeding been controlled?

- -

RAPID TRAUMA SURVEY
HEAD AND NECK
Neck Vein Distention?
Tracheal Deviation?

CHEST
Asymmetry; (w/Paradoxical Motion?), Contusions, Penetrations,
Tenderness, Instability, Crepitation
Breath Sounds
(Present? Equal? If unequal: percussion)
Heart Tones

ABDOMEN
(Contusions, Penetration/evisceration; **Tenderness, Rigidity, Distention**)

PELVIS
Tenderness, Instability, Crepitation

LOWER/UPPER EXTREMITIES
Obvious Swelling, Deformity
Motor and Sensory

POSTERIOR
Penetrations, Obvious Deformity

If critical patient - transfer to ambulance to complete exam

If radial pulse present:
VITAL SIGNS
Measured Pulse, Breathing, Blood Pressure

If altered mental status:
PUPILS
Size? Reactive? **Equal?**

GLASGOW COMA SCALE
Eyes, Voice, Motor

Chest

- Is the chest symmetrical?
- If not, is there paradoxical movement?
- Is there any obvious blunt or penetrating trauma?
- Are there any sucking (open) wounds?
- Is there tenderness, instability or crepitation (TIC) of the *chest wall*?
- Are the breath sounds present and equal?
- If breath sounds are not equal, is the chest hyperresonant (pneumothorax) or dull (hemothorax) to percussion?
- Are heart sounds normal or abnormal (distant, muffled)?

Abdomen

- Are there obvious injuries or discoloration?
- Is the abdomen tender, rigid, or distended?

Pelvis

- Are there obvious wounds or deformity?
- Is there TIC?

Upper Legs

- Are there obvious wounds, swelling, or deformity?
- Is there TIC?

Lower Legs and Arms

- Are there obvious wounds, swelling, or deformity?
- Is there TIC?
- Can the patient feel/move fingers and toes?

Posterior

- This exam is performed during transfer to the backboard for *SMR or removal from backboard after movement of patient.*
- Are there any wounds, tenderness, or deformity of the patient's posterior side?

Decision

- Is there a critical situation?
- Should I move the patient to the ambulance now?
- Are there interventions that I must delegate or perform now?

History

- What is the SAMPLE history (if not already obtained)?
- Ascertain PQRST, if not done: provocation/palliation, quality, radiation, severity, and time.

Baseline Vital Signs

- Are the vital signs abnormal?
- What are the mental status, respirations, pulse, blood pressure, pulse oximetry, core temperature, and level of discomfort?

PEARLS
ITLS Primary Survey (*Continued*)

- If the patient has a critical trauma situation, load him or her into the ambulance and begin transport. (Transport the pregnant patient tilted slightly to the left.)
- If absolutely necessary, certain critical interventions may have to be done before transport. Remember that you are trading minutes of the patient's Golden Period for those procedures. Use good judgment. *They may include establishing an airway, ventilation, oxygen administration, control of serious external bleeding, sealing an open pneumothorax, decompression of a tension pneumothorax, stabilization of impaled objects, and packaging (with SMR when indicated) the patient for transport.*
- *For patients in traumatic cardiac arrest, address treatable causes and then determine whether to continue the resuscitation.*
- The indications to decompress a tension pneumothorax include signs of a tension pneumothorax and more than one of the following: respiratory distress and cyanosis, loss of radial pulse (obvious shock), loss of consciousness, or an obviously decreasing level of consciousness.
- Unless the patient is entrapped or the ambulance has not arrived on scene, start intravenous therapy while transporting the patient to the receiving facility.

Disability

Perform this exam now if there is altered mental status. Otherwise, postpone this exam until you perform the ITLS Secondary Survey. If the patient has an altered mental status, your questions are the following:

- Are the pupils equal and reactive?
- What is the Glasgow Coma Scale score?
- Are there signs of cerebral herniation (unresponsive, dilated pupil(s), hypertension, bradycardia, posturing)?
- Does the patient have a medical identification device?
- What is the finger-stick glucose test result?

Procedure

ITLS Ongoing Exam

During the ITLS class, short written scenarios will be used along with a model to simulate the patient. You will divide into teams to practice performing the ITLS Ongoing (reassessment) Exam, making critical decisions and interventions. Each member of the team must practice being team leader at least once. The critical information represents the answers you should be seeking at each step of the exam.

ITLS Ongoing Exam—Critical Information

The following questions are presented in the order in which should be asked as you perform the Ongoing Exam. *In an unstable multiple-trauma patient*, this is the minimum information that you will need as you perform each step of the exam (Figure 3-3).

Subjective Changes

- Ask the patient if they are feeling better or worse now.

Mental Status

- What is the level of consciousness (LOC)?
- What is pupillary size? Are they equal? Do they react to light?
- If altered mental status, what is the finger-stick glucose (if not already done), and what is the Glasgow Coma Scale score now?

Reassess ABCs

- Record vital signs (mental status, respirations, pulse, blood pressure, pulse oximetry, core temperature, and level of discomfort).

Airway

- Is the airway open and clear?
- Is the sound of breathing abnormal (snoring, gurgling, stridor)?
- If there are burns of the face, are there signs of inhalation injury?

Breathing and Circulation

- What is the rate and depth of respiration?
- What is the rate and quality of the pulse?

ITLS ONGOING EXAM

|

PATIENT HISTORY

Complete S.A.M.P.L.E. History if not already done

|

LOC

A-V/P-U

Pupils

|

If altered mental status:

Finger-stick Glucose

GLASCOW COMA SCALE

Eyes, Voice, Movement

VITAL SIGNS

Measured Pulse, Respiratory Rate, Blood Pressure

Pulse Oximeter, Cardiac Monitor, CO_2 Monitor, Temperature

|

AIRWAY

Patency? If burn patient assess for signs of inhalation injury

|

BREATHING

Present? Rate, Depth, Effort

|

CIRCULATION

Skin Color, Temperature, Moisture; Capillary Refill

|

BLEEDING STILL CONTROLLED?

|

Examine Neck

Obvious Wounds, Tenderness, Swelling

Neck Vein Distention? Tracheal Deviation?

|

Examine CHEST

Asymmetry (Paradoxical Motion?), Contusions, Penetrations,

Tenderness, Instability, Crepitation

|

BREATH SOUNDS

(Present? Equal? (If unequal: **Percussion**)

Heart Tones

|

Examine ABDOMEN

Contusions, Penetration/evisceration; Tenderness, Rigidity, Distension

|

Recheck Identified INJURIES

|

Check INTERVENTIONS

ET tube, Oxygen, IVs, seals on chest wounds, decompression needle,

splints & dressings, impaled objects, position of pregnant patients

|

Recheck MONITORS

Cardiac, Capnograph, Pulse Oximeter

Figure 3-3 The ITLS Ongoing Exam.

- What is the blood pressure?
- What are the skin color, condition, and temperature (capillary refill in children)?
- Is any external bleeding controlled?

Neck

- Are the neck veins normal, flat, or distended?
- If distended, is the trachea midline or deviated?
- Is there increased swelling of the neck?

Chest

- Are the breath sounds present and equal?
- If breath sounds are unequal, is the chest hyperresonant or dull?
- Are heart sounds still normal, or have they become muffled?

Abdomen

If mechanism suggests possible abdominal injury:

- Is there any tenderness?
- Is there abdominal guarding, distention or rigidity?

Assessment of Identified Injuries

- Have there been any changes in the condition of any of the injuries that have been found?

Checking All Completed Interventions

- Is the endotracheal tube still in the correct position?
- Is the oxygen rate correct?
- Is the oxygen tubing connected?
- Are the IVs running at the correct rate?
- Does the IV bag contain the correct fluid?
- Is the open chest wound still sealed?
- Is the decompression needle still working?
- Are any of the wound dressings blood soaked?
- Are the splints in the correct position?
- Is the impaled object still stabilized?
- Is the pregnant patient tilted 20 to 30 degrees to the patient's left?
- Is the cardiac monitor attached and working?
- Is the pulse oximeter attached and working?
- Is the capnograph attached and working?

PEARLS
ITLS Secondary Survey

- Critical patients get an ITLS Secondary Survey en route to the hospital if time permits.
- Stable patients may get an ITLS Secondary Survey at the scene.
- Transport immediately if your detailed exam reveals *any* of the critical trauma situations.
- Critical patients should not have traction splints applied at the scene. They take too long.

Procedure

ITLS Secondary Survey

During the ITLS class, short written scenarios will be used along with a model to simulate the patient. You will divide into teams to practice performing the ITLS Secondary Survey. Each member of the team must practice being team leader at least once. The critical information represents the answers you should be seeking at each step of the exam.

ITLS Secondary Survey—Critical Information

As a general rule, you should quickly repeat the initial assessment before you begin the ITLS Secondary Survey. You can do this as your teammate checks the vital signs. If you ask the right questions, you will get the information you need to make the critical decisions necessary in the management of your patient. The following questions are presented in the order in which you should ask yourself as you perform the ITLS Secondary Survey. This is the minimum information that you will need as you perform each step of the exam (Figure 3-4).

ITLS SECONDARY SURVEY

INITIAL ASSESSMENT

GENERAL IMPRESSION
Does the patient appear better, worse, or unchanged?

LOC
A-V/P-U

AIRWAY
(CONSIDER C-SPINE CONTROL)
Snoring, Gurgling, Stridor, etc.; Silence

BREATHING
Present? Rate, Depth, Effort

RADIAL PULSE – CAROTID if no radial
Present? Rate, Rhythm, Quality
Skin Color, Temperature, Moisture; Capillary Refill

BLEEDING STILL CONTROLLED?

DETAILED EXAM
PATIENT HISTORY
Complete S.A.M.P.L.E. History if not already done

VITAL SIGNS
Measured Pulse, Respiratory Rate, Blood Pressure
Consider Pulse Oximeter, Cardiac Monitor, CO_2 Monitor, Blood Sugar, Temperature, prn

GLASCOW COMA SCALE
(Eyes, Voice, Movement); Emotional State

Examine Head
DCAP-BLS, TIC
(Pupils, Battles Sign, Raccoon Eyes, Drainage from ears or nose

Examine Neck
DCAP-BLS, TIC Neck Vein Distention? Tracheal Deviation?

Examine CHEST
Asymmetry, Paradoxical motion, DCAP-BLS, TIC

BREATH SOUNDS
Present? Equal? (If unequal: Percussion) Abnormal Breath Sounds?
Heart Tones

Examine ABDOMEN
Contusions, Penetration/evisceration; Tenderness, Rigidity, Distension

Examine PELVIS
DCAP-BLS, TIC

Examine LOWER/UPPER EXTREMITIES
DCAP-BLS, TIC, Distal PMS

POSTERIOR
Examine only if not done in Primary Survey
DCAP-BLS, TIC

Figure 3-4 The ITLS Secondary Survey.

SAMPLE History

Complete the SAMPLE history now if you have not already done so.

- What is the patient's history?

Vital Signs and Repeat Initial Assessment

General Impression

- Does the patient appear better, worse, or unchanged?

Airway

- Is the airway open and clear?
- Is the sound of breathing abnormal (snoring, gurgling, stridor)?

Breathing

- What is the rate and depth of respiration?
- Is the breathing labored?

Circulation

- What is the pulse rate and blood pressure?
- What are the skin color, condition, and temperature (capillary refill in children)?
- Is all external bleeding still controlled?

Neurologic Exam

- What is the level of consciousness (LOC)?
- If altered mental status, what is the blood glucose (if not already done)?
- Are the pupils equal? Do they respond to light?
- Can the patient move the fingers and toes?
- Can the patient feel me touch the fingers and toes?
- What is the Glasgow Coma Scale score (if altered mental status)?

Detailed Exam

Head

- Are there deformities, contusions, abrasions, penetrations, burns, lacerations, and swelling (DCAP-BLS) or TIC of the face or head?
- Are Battle's sign or raccoon eyes present?
- Is there blood or fluid draining from the ears or nose?
- Is there pallor, cyanosis, or diaphoresis?

Neck

- Is there DCAP-BLS or TIC of the neck?
- Are the neck veins normal, flat, or distended?
- Is the trachea midline or deviated?

Chest

- Is there DCAP-BLS of the chest?
- Is there any TIC of the ribs?
- Are there any open wounds or paradoxical movement?
- Are the breath sounds present and equal?
- Are there abnormal breath sounds?
- If breath sounds are not equal, is the chest hyperresonant or dull?

- Are heart sounds normal or decreased?
- If patient is intubated, is the endotracheal tube still in good position?

Abdomen
- Is there DCAP-BLS of the abdomen?
- Is the abdomen tender, rigid, or distended?

Pelvis
If the pelvis has already been examined during the ITLS Primary Survey, no further exam should be done.

Lower Extremities
- Is there DCAP-BLS or TIC of the legs?
- Are there normal distal pulses, motor function, and sensation (PMS)?
- Is range of motion normal? (optional as appropriate)

Upper Extremities
- Is there DCAP-BLS of the arms?
- Is there normal PMS?
- Is range of motion normal? (optional as appropriate)

Procedure

Patient Assessment and Management

Short written trauma scenarios will be used along with a model to simulate the patient. You will be divided into teams to practice the management of simulated trauma situations using the principles and techniques taught in the course. You will be evaluated in the same manner on the second day of the course. You will be expected to use all the principles and techniques taught in this course while managing these simulated patients. To familiarize yourself with the evaluation procedure, you will be given a copy of a scenario and a grade sheet. Review Chapter 2 and the previous surveys in this chapter.

Ground Rules for Teaching and Evaluation

1. You will be allowed to stay together in several provider groups (different-size groups are permitted up to four) throughout the practice and evaluation stations.
2. You will have *multiple* practice scenarios. This allows each member of the team to be team leader once.
3. You will be evaluated as team leader at minimum one time.
4. You will assist as a member of the rescue team during the other scenarios in which another member of your team is being evaluated as team leader. You may assist, but the team leader must do all assessments. This gives you a total of six scenarios from which to learn: three practices, one evaluation, and two assists while others are evaluated.
5. Wait outside the door until the instructor comes out and gives you your scenario.
6. You will be allowed to look over your equipment before you start your exam.

7. Be sure to ask about scene safety if not provided in the scenario *and* to apply your personal protective equipment.

8. *Ask your instructor what you see as you approach. (What is my general impression?)*

9. If you have a live model to simulate the patient, you must talk to that person just as you would a real patient. It is best to explain what you are doing as you examine the patient. Be confident and reassuring.

10. You must ask your instructor for things you cannot find out from your patient. Examples are blood pressure, pulse, and breath sounds.

11. Wounds and fractures must be dressed or splinted just as if they were real. Procedures must be done correctly (such as blood pressure, log rolling, strapping, and splinting).

12. If you need a piece of equipment that is not available, ask your instructors. They may allow you to simulate the equipment.

13. During practice and evaluation, you may be allowed to go (or may be directed) to any station, but you cannot go to the same station twice.

14. You will be graded on the following:
    a. Assessment of the scene
    b. Assessment of the patient
    c. Management of the patient
    d. Efficient use of time
    e. Leadership
    f. Judgment
    g. Problem-solving ability
    h. Patient interaction

15. When you finish your testing scenario, there is to be no discussion of the case. If you have any questions, they will be answered after the faculty meeting at the end of the course.

Airway Management

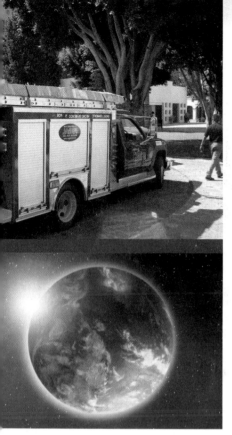

Kate Blackwelder

Kirk Magee, MD, MSc, FRCPC
Ronald D. Stewart, OC, BA, BSc, MD, FRCPC

Vie Aeree	Vía Aérea	Voie Respiratoire	Drogi oddechowe
Atemweg	Dišni put	مجرى الهواء	
disajni put	Dihalna pot	Légút	

Key Terms

Objectives

Upon successful completion of this chapter, you should be able to:

1. Describe the anatomy and physiology of the respiratory system.
2. Explain the importance of observation as it relates to airway control.
3. Describe methods to deliver supplemental oxygen to the trauma patient.
4. Briefly describe the indications, contraindications, advantages, and disadvantages of the following airway adjuncts: bag-valve masks, blind insertion airway devices, endotracheal intubation, flow-restricted oxygen-powered ventilation devices, nasopharyngeal airways, and oro-pharyngeal airways.
5. Describe the predictors of difficult mask ventilation and endotracheal intubation.
6. Describe apneic oxygenation and external laryngeal manipulation.
7. Describe the essential components of an airway kit.

Chapter Overview

ventilation: the movement of air or gases into and out of the lungs.

Of all the tasks expected of field teams who care for the trauma patient, none is more important than that of airway control. Maintaining an open airway and adequate **ventilation** in the trauma patient can be a challenge in any setting. It can be almost impossible in the adverse environment of the field with its poor lighting, the chaos that often surrounds the event, the position of the patient, and perhaps hostile onlookers.

Airway control is a task that you must master because it frequently cannot wait until you get to the hospital. Patients who are cyanotic, underventilated, or both are in need of immediate help—help that only you can give them in the initial stages of care. It falls to you, then, to be familiar with the basic structure and function of the airway and respiratory system, to be versed on how to achieve and maintain an open airway, and to know how to oxygenate and ventilate a patient.

Because of the unpredictable nature of the field environment, you will be called on to manage patient airways in almost every conceivable situation: in wrecked cars, dangling above rivers, in the middle of a shopping center, or at the side of a busy highway. You therefore need options and alternatives from which to choose. What will help one patient may not work for another. One patient may require a simple jaw-thrust maneuver to open an airway, whereas another may require a surgical procedure to prevent impending death.

Airway management is not simply "passing the tube." It is about maintaining and achieving effective oxygenation and ventilation. Whatever the methods required, you must always start with the basics. It is of little value—and in some cases it may be downright dangerous—to apply advanced techniques of airway control before beginning basic maneuvers. The discussion of airway control in the trauma patient will be rooted in several fundamental truths: Air should go in and out, oxygen is good, and blue is bad. Everything else follows from that.

This chapter begins with the basics (anatomy and physiology) and progresses through the concepts of the patent airway and basic techniques for artificial ventilation and on to advanced airway techniques and monitoring devices. It then reinforces what you have learned by allowing you to practice those techniques in the Airway Management Skill Station (Chapter 5).

Case Presentation

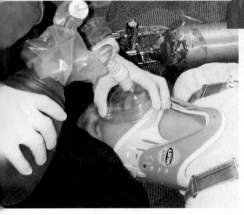

(Photo courtesy of Buddy Denson, EMT-P)

You are the lead emergency care provider in an ALS ambulance transporting a seriously injured motorcyclist to the trauma center. The ITLS Primary Survey and a rapid trauma survey identified the life-threatening external hemorrhage in the area of the left knee, now controlled by a tourniquet. Findings on exam also indicate possible head, chest, and abdominal injuries and concern for possible spine injury occasioned by a lack of movement in the lower extremities. The treatment performed and to be performed include SMR, supplemental oxygen, fluid administration, and reporting your ETA. Your partner is initiating two large-bore peripheral IVs, and you prepare to perform your ITLS Ongoing Exam, beginning with a repeat of the initial assessment.

You begin by noting the bleeding is still controlled by the tourniquet, but the patient is now unresponsive to pain. As you reassess the patient's airway and breathing, you note stridor upon inspiration.

Before proceeding, consider these questions: What is your first priority? What do you believe is the cause of this developing problem? What would you do next? Keep these questions in mind as you read through the chapter. Then, at the end of the chapter, find out how the emergency care providers managed this patient.

Anatomy and Physiology

The airway begins at the tip of the nose and the lips and ends at the alveolocapillary membrane, through which gas exchange takes place between the air sacs of the lungs (the alveoli) and the lungs' capillary network. The airway consists of chambers and pipes, which conduct air with its 21% oxygen content to the alveoli and carry away the waste, carbon dioxide, which diffuses from the blood into the alveoli.

Nasopharynx

The beginning of the respiratory tract (the nasal cavity and oropharynx) is lined with moist mucous membranes (Figure 4-1). This lining is delicate and highly vascular. It deserves all the respect that you can give it, which means you should prevent undue trauma by using liberally lubricated endotracheal tubes (ETTs) and avoiding unnecessary poking about. The nasal cavity is divided by a very vascular midline septum. On the lateral walls of the nose are "shelves" called the *turbinates*. Those projections can get in the way when ETTs or other devices need to be inserted into the nostrils. Carefully sliding a well-lubricated ETT's bevel along the floor or the septum of the nasal cavity will usually prevent traumatizing the turbinates.

Oropharynx

The teeth are the first obstruction we meet in the oral part of the airway. They may be more obstructive in some patients than in others. In any case, the same general principle always applies: Patients should have the same number and condition of teeth at the end of an airway procedure as they had at the beginning.

The tongue is mostly muscle and represents the next potential obstruction. It is attached to the jaw anteriorly and through a series of muscles and ligaments to the hyoid bone, a wishbone-like structure just under the chin from which the cartilage skeleton (the larynx) of the upper airway is suspended. The epiglottis also is connected to the hyoid, so elevating the hyoid will lift the epiglottis upward and open the airway further. When the patient is unconscious, the tongue loses muscle tone and can fall back against the posterior pharynx and obstruct the airway.

Hypopharynx

The epiglottis is one of the main anatomic landmarks in the airway. You must be familiar with it and be able to identify it by sight and by touch. It appears as a floppy piece of cartilage covered by mucosa—which is exactly what it is—and it feels like the tragus, the cartilage at the opening of the ear canal. It is thought to block the glottic opening when swallowing and is an important landmark when you must assume control of the airway.

The epiglottis is attached to the hyoid bone and thence to the mandible by a series of ligaments and muscles. In the unconscious patient, the tongue can produce some airway obstruction by falling back against the soft palate and even the posterior pharyngeal wall. However, it is the epiglottis that will produce complete airway obstruction in the supine unconscious patient whose jaw is relaxed and whose head and neck are in the neutral position. In such patients, the epiglottis will fall down against the glottic opening and prevent ventilation.

It is essential to understand this crucial anatomy when managing the airway. To ensure an open (patent) airway in an unconscious supine patient, displace the hyoid

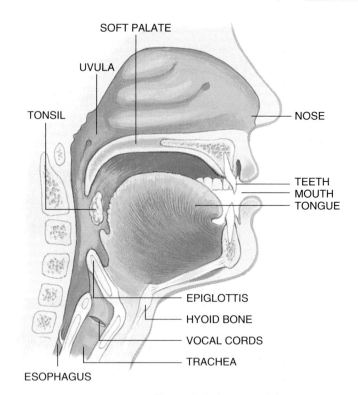

Figure 4-1 Anatomy of the upper airway. Note that the tongue, hyoid bone, and epiglottis are attached to the mandible by a series of ligaments. Lifting forward on the jaw will therefore displace all these structures anteriorly, opening the airway.

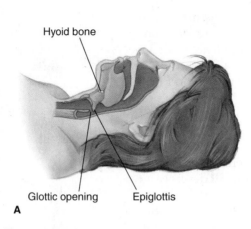

Figure 4-2a The epiglottis is attached to the hyoid and then to the mandible. When the mandible is relaxed and falls back, the tongue falls upward and against the soft palate and the posterior pharyngeal wall, whereas the epiglottis falls over the glottic opening.

Figure 4-2b Extension of the head and lifting the chin will pull the tongue and the epiglottis upward and forward, exposing the glottic opening and ensuring the patent airway. In the trauma patient, only the jaw, or chin and jaw, should be displaced forward, and the head and neck should be kept in alignment.

anteriorly by lifting forward on the jaw (chin lift, jaw thrust) or by pulling on the tongue. This will lift the tongue out of the way. It also will keep the epiglottis elevated and away from the posterior pharyngeal wall and glottic opening (Figure 4-2). Both nasotracheal and orotracheal intubation require elevation of the epiglottis, either by lifting the jaw forward (nasotracheal) or by a laryngoscope or the fingers when performing direct laryngoscopy or digital intubation.

Larynx

On either side of the epiglottis is a recess called the *pyriform fossa*. An endotracheal tube tip can end up in either one. Pyriform fossa placement of an endotracheal tube can be identified easily by "tenting" of the skin on either side of the superior aspect of the laryngeal prominence (Adam's apple) or by transillumination if a lighted stylet (or "lightwand") is being used to intubate.

The vocal cords are protected anteriorly by the thyroid cartilage, a box-like structure shaped like a C, with the open part of the C representing its posterior wall. That wall is covered with muscle. In some patients, the cords can close entirely in laryngospasm, producing complete airway obstruction. The thyroid cartilage can easily be seen in most people on the anterior surface of the neck as the laryngeal prominence. Manipulating the thyroid cartilage can help bring the vocal cords into view during endotracheal intubation. This is called **external laryngeal manipulation (ELM)**. The movement is usually pressing the thyroid cartilage backward against the esophagus and then upward and slightly to the patient's right side. This is also known as the BURP (back-up-right-pressure) maneuver and is different from the Sellick maneuver described next.

Inferior to the thyroid cartilage is another part of the larynx, the cricoid. The cricoid is a cartilage shaped like a signet ring with the ring in front and the signet behind. It can be palpated as a small bump on the anterior surface of the neck inferior to the laryngeal prominence. The esophagus is just behind the posterior wall of the cricoid cartilage. Pressure on the cricoid at the front of the neck will close off the

external laryngeal manipulation (ELM): a maneuver to improve visualization of the vocal cords during endotracheal intubation. Also called *BURP* (back-up-right-pressure).

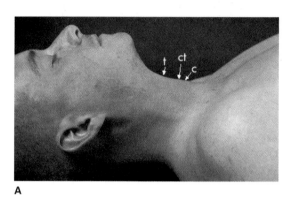

A

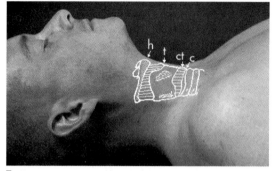

B

Figure 4-3a External view of the anterior neck, showing the surface landmarks for the thyroid cartilage (laryngeal) prominence, the cricothyroid membrane, and the cricoid cartilage.

Figure 4-3b Cutaway view showing the important landmarks of the larynx and upper airway: hyoid, thyroid cartilage, cricothyroid membrane, and cricoid cartilage.

esophagus to pressures as high as 100 cm H_2O. This is the Sellick maneuver. It was believed it would reduce the risk of gastric regurgitation during the process of intubation and to prevent insufflation of air into the stomach during positive pressure ventilation by mouth-to-mouth, bag-valve mask, or flow-restricted oxygen-powered ventilation device. Recent studies question the efficacy of the Sellick maneuver in preventing aspiration of stomach contents, and routine use is no longer recommended.

Connecting the inferior border of the thyroid cartilage with the superior aspect of the cricoid is the cricothyroid membrane. This membrane is a very important landmark through which you can gain direct access to the airway below the cords. You can palpate the cricothyroid membrane on most patients by finding the most prominent part of the thyroid cartilage. Then slide your index finger down until you feel a second "bump," just before your finger palpates the last depression before the sternal notch. That second bump is the cricoid cartilage. At its upper edge is the cricothyroid membrane (Figure 4-3). In some patients, especially those who have a thick neck, you may find the cricoid cartilage more easily by going from the sternal notch upward until you feel the first prominent cartilage "bump." Just over the "top" of this bump is the cricothyroid membrane. The sternal notch is an important landmark as well. It is the point at which the cuff of a properly placed endotracheal tube should lie (Figure 4-4). The sternal notch is readily palpated at the junction of the clavicles with the upper edge of the sternum.

Trachea and Bronchi

The tracheal rings (C-shaped cartilaginous supports for the trachea) continue beyond the cricoid cartilage. The trachea soon divides into the left and right mainstem bronchi. The point at which the trachea divides is called the *carina*. It is important to note that the right mainstem bronchus takes off at an angle slightly more in line with the trachea. As a result, ETTs or other foreign bodies usually end up in the right mainstem bronchus. One of the goals of a properly performed endotracheal intubation is to avoid a right (or left) mainstem bronchus intubation.

You should know how far some of the major anatomic landmarks are from the teeth. This knowledge will help you place an endotracheal tube at the correct level, and by remembering only three numbers you will be able to detect an ETT that is too far into the airway or not in far enough. The three numbers to remember are 15, 20, and 25. The first number, 15, is the distance (in centimeters) from the teeth to the vocal cords of the average adult. The number 20 (5 cm farther down the airway) is the sternal

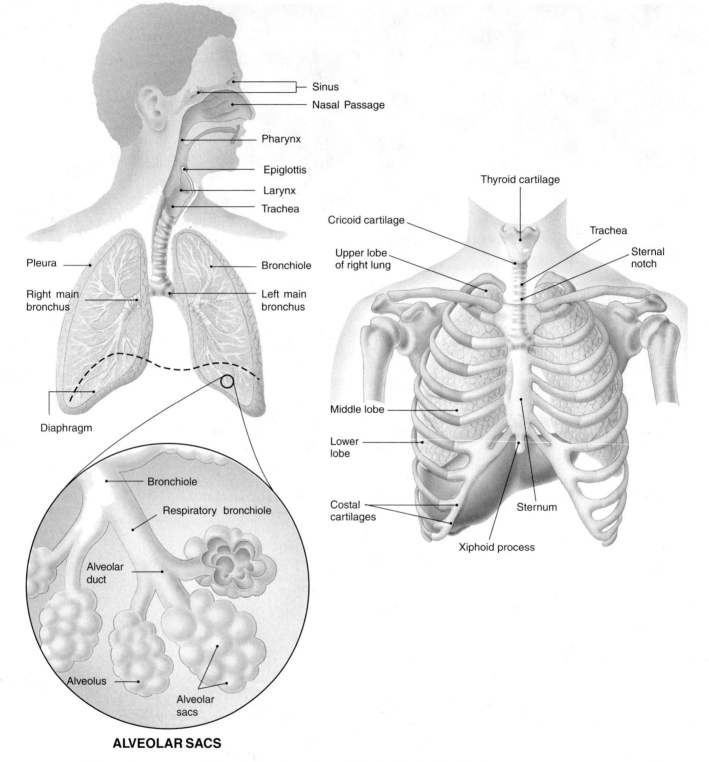

ALVEOLAR SACS

Figure 4-4 The respiratory system. Notice the sternal notch, at which point the clavicles join the sternum. It marks the position of the tip of a well-placed endotracheal tube.

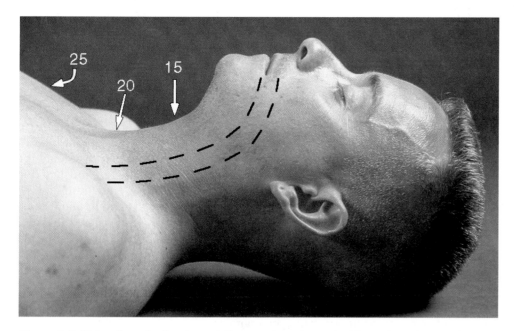

Figure 4-5 Major airway landmarks and distances from the teeth: 15 = 15 cm from teeth to cords, 20 = 20 cm from teeth to sternal notch, 25 = 25 cm from teeth to carina.

notch. About 5 cm farther again at 25 is the carina (Figure 4-5). Those are average distances and can vary by several centimeters. Another way to estimate correct depth is for the ETT mark at the teeth to be three times the diameter of the ETT (8.0 mm ETT should be no more than 24 cm at the teeth).

Extension or flexion of the head of an intubated patient will move the endotracheal tube up or down as much as 2 to 2.5 cm. As a result, ET tubes can easily become dislodged during patient movement. Detection of misplacement can be difficult unless you are monitoring oxygen saturation and expired CO_2. Taping the head down or guarding against movement will lessen the risk of ETT displacement. (This is even more important in children.) It also will reduce trauma to the tracheal mucosa. Less movement of the ETT will result in less stimulation to the patient's airway reflexes. It also may result in a more stable cardiovascular system and intracranial pressure in the patient.

To help protect the airway from becoming blocked and to reduce the risk of aspiration, the body has developed brisk reflexes that will attempt to expel any offending foreign material from the oropharynx, the glottic opening, or the trachea. Those areas are well supplied by sensitive nerves that can activate the swallowing, gag, and cough reflexes. Activation of swallowing, gagging, or coughing by stimulation of the upper airway can cause significant cardiovascular stimulation as well as elevation in intracranial pressure. You can protect patients from such unwanted effects by suppressing the reflexes through the use of topical lidocaine. (See Chapter 5.)

The Lungs

The lungs are the organs through which gas exchange takes place. They are contained within a "cage" formed by the ribs, and usually fill up the thoracic cavity. They are surrounded by a membrane, the pleura, which has both a visceral component covering the lungs and a parietal component, which lines the interior portion of the thoracic cage. Between these two pleural membranes is the pleural space, which is the potential space. The lungs have only one opening to the outside, the glottic opening, which is the space between the vocal cords. Expansion of the chest wall (the cage) and movement of the diaphragm downward cause the lungs to expand

patent airway: an open airway.

capnography: a noninvasive device that detects or measures the amount of carbon dioxide in the expired breath of a patient.

tidal volume: the amount of air that is inspired and expired during one respiratory cycle.

(because the pleural space is airtight), and as the pressure inside the chest is now lower than that outside the body, air rushes in through the glottis. The air travels down the smaller and smaller ETTs to the alveoli, where gas exchange (respiration) takes place. The volume of air that is in the trachea and bronchi where no gas exchange takes place is called "dead space."

The Patent Airway

One of the first maneuvers essential to caring for a patient is ensuring a patent or open airway. Without a patent airway, all other care is of little use. This must be done quickly because patients cannot tolerate hypoxia for more than a few minutes. The effect of hypoxia and inadequate ventilation in an unconscious injured patient can be devastating. If this is compounded by the absence of adequate perfusion, the patient is in even more difficult straits. Patients suffering from head trauma not only may have hypoxic brain damage from airway compromise but may also build up high levels of carbon dioxide that can cause dilation of the cerebral vessels, which leads to swelling and increased intracranial pressure.

Ensuring a patent airway in a patient can be a major challenge in the prehospital setting. Not only can trauma disrupt the anatomy of the face and airway, but it also can result in bleeding, which can lead to airflow obstruction and can obscure airway landmarks. Add to this the risk of cervical-spine injury, and the challenge is readily apparent. You also must remember that some airway maneuvers, including suction and insertion of nasopharyngeal and oropharyngeal airways, can stimulate a patient's protective reflexes and increase the likelihood of vomiting and aspiration, cardiovascular stimulation, and increased intracranial pressure.

The first step in providing a **patent airway** in the unconscious patient is to ensure that the tongue and epiglottis are lifted forward and maintained in that position. This is done by using the modified jaw-thrust or the jaw-lift maneuver (Figure 4-6). Either will prevent the tongue from falling backward against the soft palate or posterior pharyngeal wall. Either will pull forward on the hyoid, lifting the epiglottis up out of the way. Essential maneuvers for both basic and advanced airway procedures, when done properly, they will open the airway without tilting the head backward or moving the neck. You cannot clinically clear the cervical spine in an unresponsive patient (see Chapter 11), so do not hyperextend the neck to open the airway in unresponsive patients.

Constant vigilance and care are required to maintain a patent airway in your patient. Following are essentials for this task:

- *Observation.* Continual observation of the patient to anticipate problems, frequently requiring monitoring devices such as pulse oximetry and **capnography**
- *Suction.* An adequate suction device with large-bore tubing and attachment
- *Airway adjuncts*

Observation

The patient who is injured is at risk of airway compromise even if completely conscious and awake. This is partially due to the fact that many patients have full stomachs, are anxious, and are prone to vomiting. Some patients also will be bleeding into their oropharynx and thus swallowing blood. In view of these facts, you should constantly observe your patient for airway problems following injury. One team member must be responsible for both airway control and adequate ventilation for any patient who might be at risk of airway compromise.

The general appearance of a patient, the respiratory rate, and any complaints must be noted and addressed. In a patient who is breathing spontaneously, you must check frequently for adequate **tidal volume** by feeling over the mouth and nose and by observing chest wall movements. Bare the chest—at least below the breasts—is a

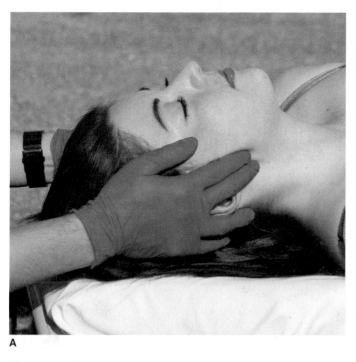

A

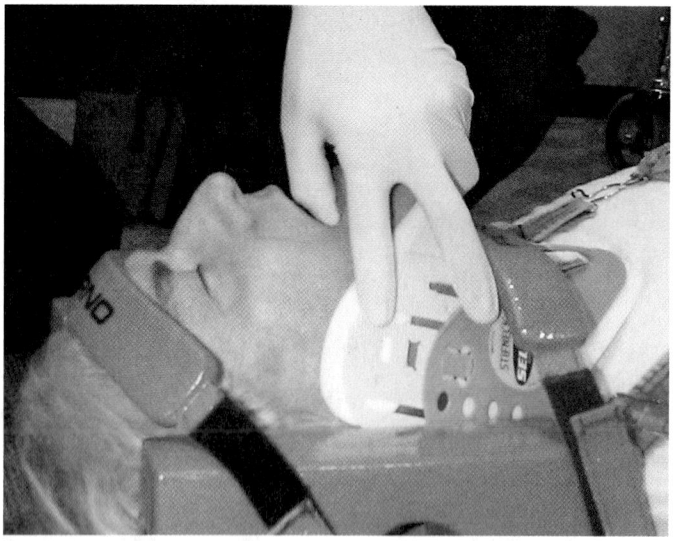

Figure 4-6a Opening the airway using a modified jaw-thrust maneuver. Maintain in-line stabilization while pushing up on the angle of the jaw.

B

Figure 4-6b Jaw lift. *(Photo courtesy of Buddy Denson, EMT-P)*

good rule to follow. Check the supplemental oxygen line periodically to ensure that oxygen is being delivered to the patient at a given flow rate or percentage.

Always immediately clear blood and secretions. You also must be alert for sounds that indicate trouble. Remember: Noisy breathing is obstructed breathing.

If the patient has an endotracheal tube in place, monitor **lung compliance** and search for the cause of any change in compliance. If possible, monitor endotracheal tube position by pulse oximetry and continuous expiratory CO_2 monitoring. (For more on capnography, see Chapter 5.) Use of waveform capnography is rapidly becoming the gold standard for monitoring ET tube placement during transport of critically ill patients and is strongly recommended in all intubated patients. By use of nasal sensors, capnography also can be used to monitor the ventilation status of the nonintubated patient. A trend toward elevation of the expired CO_2 is evidence that the patient is hypoventilating and will need ventilatory assistance. The use of capnography and pulse oximetry is recommended in all trauma patients. (See Chapter 5.)

lung compliance: the "give" or elasticity of the lungs

The development of confusion or combativeness can be a sign that the patient is hypoxic and needs an airway procedure such as ET intubation, or if intubated, the ETT may no longer be in the trachea and needs to be reinserted. Consider combative patients to be hypoxic until a systematic and rapid evaluation rules it out.

Suction

All patients who are injured and who have cervical motion-restriction devices in place should be considered at high risk for airway compromise. In addition, one of the greatest threats to the patent airway is that of vomiting and aspiration, particularly in patients who have recently eaten a large meal. As a result, portable suction devices are considered essential airway equipment for field trauma care. A portable suction device should have the following characteristics (Figure 4-7):

- It can be carried in an airway kit with an oxygen cylinder and other airway equipment. It should not be separated or stored remotely from oxygen. If it is, it would represent an "extra" piece of equipment requiring extra hands.

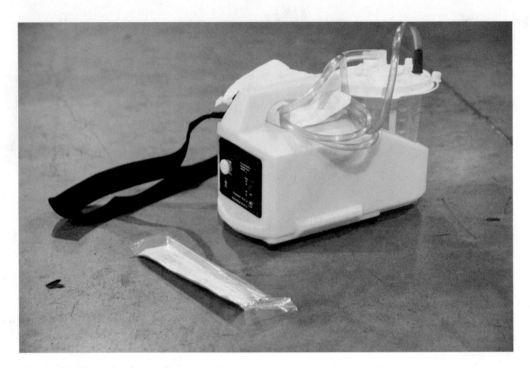

Figure 4-7 Example of a suction apparatus.

- It can be hand powered or battery powered rather than oxygen driven. You should always have a hand-powered suction as a backup if you use a battery-powered suction.
- It can generate sufficient suction and volume displacement to remove pieces of food, blood clots, and thick secretions from the oropharynx.
- It has tubing of sufficient diameter (0.8–1 cm) to handle whatever is suctioned from the patient.

Suction tips should be of large bore, such as the rigid tonsil-tip suckers that can handle most clots and bleeding. In some cases the suction tubing itself can be used to withdraw large amounts of blood or gastric contents. A 6 mm endotracheal tube can be used with a connector as a suction tip. The ETT's side hole removes the necessity for a proximal control valve to interrupt suction. Usually, the second emergency care provider (see Chapter 2) assumes responsibility for the airway. As the "VO" (vomit officer), the second emergency care provider must be constantly alert to prevent the patient from aspirating.

Airway Adjuncts

Equipment to help ensure a patent airway will include various nasopharyngeal airways (NPAs), oropharyngeal airways (OPAs), blind insertion airway devices **(BIADs)**, and endotracheal (ET) tubes. Insertion of these devices must be reserved for patients whose protective reflexes are sufficiently depressed to tolerate them. Care must be taken to avoid provoking vomiting or gagging because both occurrences are bad for these patients. (See Chapter 5.)

Nasopharyngeal Airways

Nasopharyngeal airways (NPAs) should be soft and of appropriate length. They are designed to prevent the tongue and epiglottis from falling against the posterior pharyngeal wall. (See Chapter 5 for insertion technique.) In a pinch, a 6 mm or 6.6 mm endotracheal tube can be cut and serve as an NPA. With light lubrication and gentle insertion, there should be few problems with this airway (Figure 4-8). However,

BIAD: a blind insertion airway device, such as the King Airway™, the i-Gel™ or LMA™ (laryngeal mask airway), which can be inserted without having to visualize the larynx. BIADs are also called *supraglottic airways*.

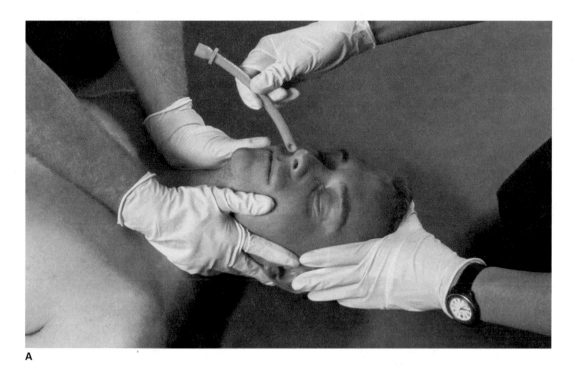

A

Figure 4-8a The nasopharyngeal airway is inserted with the bevel slid along the septum or floor of the nasal cavity.

bleeding and trauma to the nasal mucosa are common. Mild hemorrhage from the nose after insertion of the airway is not an indication to remove it. In fact, it is probably better to keep an NPA in place so as not to disturb the clot or reactivate the bleeding. The NPA will be better tolerated than the oropharyngeal airway adjunct and thus can usually be used in patients who still have a gag reflex. Note that patients on anticoagulants are at increased risk for nasal bleeding with insertion.

Oropharyngeal Airways

Oropharyngeal airways (OPAs) are designed to keep the tongue off the posterior pharyngeal wall and thereby help maintain a patent airway (Figure 4-9). Successful placement of an OPA should not give you a false sense of security. Patients who are easily able to tolerate an OPA should be considered candidates for endotracheal intubation because their protective reflexes are so depressed that they cannot protect their lower airways from aspiration. One OPA, the S.A.L.T.™ (supraglottic airway laryngopharyngeal tube) airway system is not only an OPA, but also, when inserted into the pharynx, serves as a guide to insert an endotracheal tube and then serves as the ET tube holder and protector (Figure 4-10).

Blind Insertion Airway Devices

Esophageal tracheal Combitube®, King LT-D™ airway, intubating laryngeal airway (ILA; air-Q™), i-Gel™, and the laryngeal mask airway (LMA™) are some of the blind insertion airway devices (BIADs) currently available. This means the EMS provider can properly insert the device without having to visualize the larynx.

BIADs are not as effective as endotracheal intubation in preventing aspiration but do provide effective ventilation and oxygenation. They are easier and faster to insert than an endotracheal tube. Previously, BIADs were regarded as "rescue airways" to be used when unable to intubate. These devices are now the initial invasive airway recommended in medical cardiac arrests by AHA/ILCOR. In many jurisdictions,

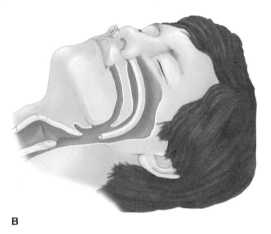

B

Figure 4-8b The nasopharyngeal airway rests between the tongue and the posterior pharyngeal wall.

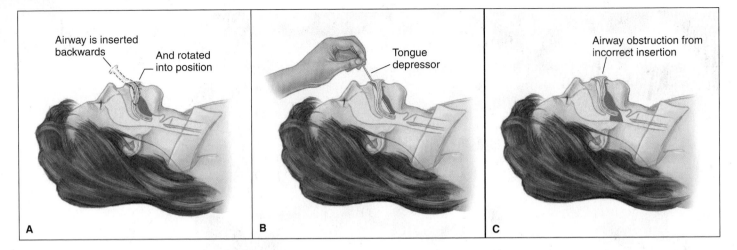

Figure 4-9 Insertion of an oropharyngeal airway.

supraglottic airway use is now a basic level skill. Evidence and experience suggest that single-tube devices such as the King LT-D™ and the LMA™ may be better suited for the prehospital environment than the more complicated esophageal tracheal Combitube®.

Endotracheal Tubes

Endotracheal intubation is the gold standard of airway care in patients who cannot protect their airways or in those needing assistance with breathing. However, it is not always the most appropriate choice for airway management in the prehospital setting. Several problems will face you when you decide to intubate a trauma patient. Intubation frequently must be done under the most difficult circumstances—on

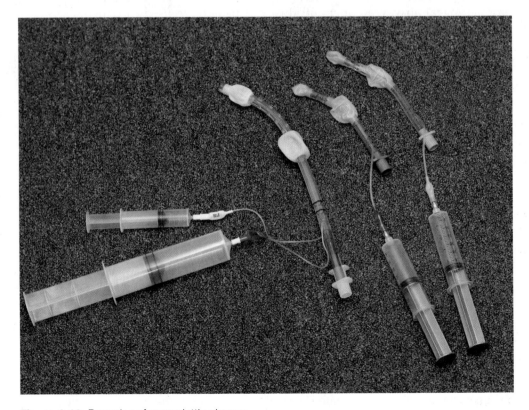

Figure 4-10 Examples of supraglottic airways.

the side of the road, in a crashed vehicle, or under a train. In addition, the patient may still have a gag reflex or the patient's spine may need to be motion restricted with a cervical collar or other equipment. This may so restrict movement and visualization of the airway that you have to consider alternative methods of intubation.

The original method of intubation was tactile or digital. That was changed by the invention of the laryngoscope, which allowed visualization of the upper airway and placement of the ETT under direct vision. The ability to see the actual passage of the ETT through the glottic opening rendered tactile orotracheal intubation obsolete, and its practice largely died out until interest in it was revived in the last two decades.

There are several choices to facilitate intubation in the trauma patient, ranging from awake intubation using topical anesthetics to deep sedation and **rapid sequence intubation (RSI)**. RSI (also referred to as **drug-assisted intubation (DAI)** refers to the use of sedatives and paralytic agents to quickly facilitate ETT placement and to minimize the risk of aspiration. These same medications can be used to allow placement of a BIAD (**rapid sequence airway [RSA]**), which is discussed in Chapter 5.

However, both deep sedation and RSI inhibit the normal muscle tone of the airway and thus may make it impossible to effectively mask-ventilate the patient. In this situation, it is necessary to immediately place an endotracheal tube to achieve successful ventilation, or failing this, alternative airways or a surgical airway may be required. For that reason, you must be very familiar with the predictors of difficult laryngoscopy and intubation before deciding to intubate a patient who is already breathing on his own. Remember, patients who have spontaneous yet inadequate respiratory effort are better off than the patient who has been given a paralytic and can be neither mask-ventilated nor intubated.

Although it is not possible to guess correctly every time, certain physical features allow you to predict which patients might potentially have difficult laryngoscopy and intubation. The mnemonic **MMAP** has been proposed to identify these features. The letters stand for:

M – *Mallampati.* The Mallampati score ranges from I to IV and is dependent on what structures can be viewed when the mouth is opened (Table 4-1). Generally, the higher the grade, the more difficult it will be to perform laryngoscopy.

M – *Measurement 3-3-1.* This measurement can aid in predicting the difficult airway. Ideally, you should be able to fit three fingers under the patient's chin between the hyoid bone and the mentum of the chin. The patient should be able to open his or her mouth so that three fingers fit between the upper and lower incisors. Last, the patient should be able to protrude the lower jaw such that the lower teeth are 1 cm beyond the upper teeth.

rapid sequence intubation (RSI) or drug-assisted intubation (DAI): a technique to improve the likelihood of intubating a difficult patient by administering a sedative and paralytic agent. Also called *rapid sequence induction.*

rapid sequence airway (RSA): the technique of administering a sedative and paralytic agent to allow insertion of a BIAD. Also called *pharmacologic assisted laryngeal airway (PALM).*

MMAP: a technique for predicting when a patient will be difficult to intubate; MMAP stands for Mallampati, measurement 3-3-1, atlanto-occipital extension, and pathology.

Table 4-1: Estimating Difficulty of Intubation

Mallampati Score

View pharynx with mouth open and tongue not protruding.

Scoring:

I. Entire tonsil or tonsillar bed is visible.

II. Upper half of tonsil or tonsillar bed is visible.

III. Soft and hard palate are clearly visible.

IV. Only hard palate is visible.

The higher the score, the higher the degree of difficulty.

A – *Atlanto-occipital extension.* In patients in whom cervical-spine injury is not suspected, the ability to extend the head at the atlanto-occipital junction to achieve the "sniffing position" will aid in visualizing the vocal cords.

P – *Pathology.* Finally, pathology refers to any clinical evidence of anatomic airway obstruction. Airway obstruction can result from medical or traumatic conditions, such as edema, infection, burns, and penetrating or blunt injuries. This is particularly important because upper airway obstructive pathology, often evidenced by stridor, is a relative contraindication to RSI.

As for all clinicians responsible for emergency airway management, the appropriate decision regarding whom and how to intubate will ultimately be related to several factors. These include the assessment of the patient and the particular clinical presentation, the skill set of the individual health-care professionals present, and the system in which they work. An additional factor unique to the prehospital setting is time. Ventilation with a bag-valve-mask device or BIAD and immediate transport of the patient may be a better option in certain instances than taking the additional time required to perform RSI. Remember, airway management can occur without RSI, but RSI cannot occur without airway management!

Although direct-vision orotracheal intubation should be considered the primary method of placing an ETT in the trachea, the procedure is not always easy, nor is it indicated in all patients. In the management of trauma patients particularly, options must be available to permit successful intubation in even the most challenging of situations and patients. There is evidence that the technique of direct-vision orotracheal intubation results in movement of the head and neck. The question therefore arises of whether the use of this method presents an added risk in possible cervical-spine injuries. Controversy exists about whether such movement is either substantial or of real clinical significance. In short, the method of intubation should be suited to each patient. Those with a low risk of cervical-spine injury can be intubated in the conventional way, using a laryngoscope. Intubation by video laryngoscopy, the nasotracheal route, the tactile or transillumination methods, or a combination should be reserved for patients with specific indication for alternative techniques. (See Chapter 5.)

Translaryngeal jet ventilation (TLJV) can provide a quick, reliable, and relatively safe temporary method of adequate oxygenation when the airway cannot be maintained because of obstruction or partial obstruction above the cords, and access below the level of the cords is needed. A special cannula is inserted through the cricothyroid membrane, and the patient is ventilated using a special manual jet ventilator device.

Supplemental Oxygen

Patients who are injured need supplemental oxygen, especially when they are unconscious. It is well recognized that patients suffering from head injury are frequently hypoxic. Furthermore, supplemental oxygen significantly reduces nausea and vomiting during ambulance transport. Supplemental oxygen can be supplied by a nasal cannula at 2 to 3 liters per minute (LPM) or a simple face mask run at 10 to 12 LPM. A simple face mask can provide the patient with about 40% to 50% oxygen. Nonrebreathing masks with a reservoir bag and oxygen flow rates into the bag of 12 to 15 LPM can provide 60% to 90% oxygen to the patient. They are recommended for all trauma patients requiring supplemental oxygen, especially if hypoxic. Nasal oxygen cannula are well tolerated by most patients, but provide only about 25% to 30% oxygen to the patient. They are recommended for patients who have a stable airway or who cannot tolerate an oxygen mask. They are also useful for passive oxygenation prior to intubation by setting flow rates over 10 LPM.

Supplemental oxygen must be used to ensure adequate oxygenation when you perform positive pressure ventilation. Oxygenation should be supplemented during mouth-to-mask ventilation by running oxygen at 10 to 12 LPM through the oxygen nipple attached to most masks or by placing the oxygen tubing under the mask and running it at the same rate. Alternatively, you can increase the oxygen percentage delivered during mouth-to-mask breathing by placing a nasal cannula on yourself. This increases the delivered oxygen percentage from 17% to about 30%.

Bag-valve-mask devices or resuscitator bags with a large (2.5 liters) reservoir bag and an oxygen flow rate of 12 to 15 LPM will increase the delivered oxygen from 21% (air) to 90% or 100%. Adding a reservoir bag to a bag-valve mask will increase the delivered oxygen from 40% or 50% to 90% or 100% and thus always should be used.

A **flow-restricted oxygen-powered ventilation device (FROPVD)** will provide 100% oxygen at a flow rate of 40 LPM at a maximum pressure of 50 cm ± 5 cm water.

As this book goes to press, emerging research, primarily in nontrauma patients, raises concerns that too much oxygen may be detrimental. It is well established that hypoxia, especially in head-injured patients, can increase mortality. The new research should make us focus on ensuring adequate oxygenation and ventilation by using pulse oximetry and end-tidal CO_2 monitoring and monitor carefully the oxygen delivered to the patient.

flow-restricted oxygen-powered ventilation device (FROPVD): an artificial ventilation device that provides 100% oxygen at a flow rate of 40 L/min at a maximum pressure of 50 ± 5 cm water.

Ventilation

Normal Ventilation

The movement of air or gases into and out of the lungs is called *ventilation*. This should not be confused with respiration, which is the exchange of oxygen at the alveoli. At rest, adults normally take in about 400 to 600 cc air with each breath. This is called the *tidal volume*. Multiplying that value by the number of breaths per minute (the respiratory rate) gives the **minute volume**, the amount of air breathed in (and, of course, out) each minute. This is an important value and is normally 5–12 liters per minute. **Normal ventilation** by healthy lungs will produce an oxygen level of about 100 mm Hg in the blood and a carbon dioxide level of 35 to 45 mm Hg. A carbon dioxide level below 35 mm Hg indicates hyperventilation, and values greater than 45 mm Hg indicate **hypoventilation**.

The clinical terms *hypoventilation* and *hyperventilation* do not refer to oxygenation but to the level of carbon dioxide maintained. It is easier for carbon dioxide to diffuse across the alveolocapillary membrane of the lungs than it is for oxygen to do so. This makes it easier to excrete carbon dioxide than to oxygenate the blood. Thus, if the chest or lungs are injured, the body may be able to maintain normal levels of carbon dioxide in the blood and yet the cells can be hypoxic. A patient with a contused lung might have a respiratory rate of 36, a carbon dioxide level of 30 mm Hg, and an oxygen level of only 80 mm Hg. Although hyperventilating, this person is still hypoxic. He or she does not need to breathe faster, but needs instead supplemental oxygen. When in doubt, give your patient oxygen.

Devices to measure oxygen saturation (**pulse oximeters**) have been available for several years, and expired CO_2 monitors (capnographs) are now available for prehospital use. Pulse oximeters measure oxygen saturation and should be used on almost all trauma patients, whereas CO_2 monitors are most useful for continuously monitoring endotracheal tube placement (though they have many other uses. (See Chapters 8 and 10.) These devices will be discussed in Chapter 5.

minute volume: the volume of air breathed in and out in one minute. This varies from 5 to 12 liters per minute.

normal ventilation: the movement of air into and out of the lungs is able to maintain the carbon dioxide level between 35 and 45 mm Hg.

hypoventilation: the movement of air into and out of the lungs is unable to maintain the carbon dioxide level below 45 mm Hg.

pulse oximeter: a noninvasive device for measuring the oxygen saturation of the blood.

Positive Pressure (Artificial) Ventilation

Normal breathing takes place because the negative pressure inside the (potential) pleural space "draws" air in through the upper airway from the outside. In any patient who is unable to do this, or whose airway needs protecting, you may need to actively force air or oxygen in through the glottic opening. This is called *intermittent positive pressure ventilation (IPPV)*. IPPV in trauma patients can take various forms, from mouth-to-mouth to bag-valve-mask-endotracheal tube ventilation. NOTE: Simply "pumping" air into the oropharynx is no guarantee that it will go through the glottic opening and into the lungs.

The oropharynx leads to the esophagus. Pressure in the oropharynx of greater than 25 cm H_2O will open the esophagus and lead to air entering the stomach (gastric insufflation). Bag-valve masks and FROPVDs can produce pressures greater than 25 cm H_2O, especially if the bag is squeezed rapidly and forcefully.

When you need to ventilate a patient using IPPV, you should know approximately what the delivered volume is. Delivered volume is how much air volume you are delivering with each breath you give. You can estimate the minute volume by multiplying delivered volume by the ventilatory rate. A FROPVD that delivers oxygen at the rate of 40 LPM will have a delivered volume of about 700 cc each second that the valve is activated. Because the FROPVD delivers this volume at a pressure of 50 cm H_2O, it almost guarantees gastric insufflation and all the complications resulting from it. Bag-valve-mask ventilation has similar challenges because pressures generated by squeezing the bag may equal or exceed 60 cm H_2O. Steady compression of the bag compared to very forceful, rapid compression results in lower peak airway pressures and reduces insufflation of air into the stomach.

Delivered volumes are usually less with bag resuscitators than with FROPVDs. There are two reasons for this. The average resuscitator bag holds only 1,800 cc of gas, which is the absolute limit to the volume that could be delivered if you were able to squeeze the bag completely. Using one hand, the best an average adult can squeeze is approximately 1,200 cc. Most people will squeeze only 800 to 1,000 cc with one hand. The other reason for greater delivered volumes with FROPVDs is that they have a trigger that allows the rescuer to hold a mask on the face with both hands, thus decreasing mask leak. These volumes do exceed normal tidal volumes, which in an adult is about 500 cc (pediatric patients: 10 cc/kg). Keep in mind that these volumes, delivered from the ventilating port of these devices, equal the volumes delivered to the patient only if an endotracheal tube is in place. In other words, they do not take into account mask leak. When performing IPPV with a mask, keep the following essentials in mind:

- Supplemental oxygen must be provided for the patient during IPPV.
- Suction must be immediately available.
- Ventilation must be done carefully to avoid gastric distention and to reduce the risk of regurgitation and possible aspiration. You can help prevent these complications by timing ventilation with the patient's native respiration.
- Pulse oximetry and end-tidal CO_2 monitoring (capnography) are the most reliable methods of monitoring effectiveness of ventilation. The pulse oximeter measures the oxygen saturation of the blood, and the capnograph measures the CO_2 level in the expired air. Use the end-tidal CO_2 level to judge whether to increase or decrease the rate of ventilation. If you adjust your respiratory rate to keep the expired CO_2 level between 35 and 45, you can be sure you are neither hypo- nor hyperventilating the patient.

In the case of bag-valve-mask breathing, up to 40% mask leak can be expected. Balloon-mask designs can reduce this, and a two-person technique, in which one rescuer holds the mask in place with both hands while a second squeezes the bag, may better ensure adequate delivered volumes. You must deliver the appropriate tidal volume as well as account for any air lost to mask leak.

During the stress of an emergency situation, you will tend to ventilate patients at an increased rate. Your pulse oximeter and end-tidal CO_2 monitor are most important in getting the correct rate and volume for each patient. Your objective is to avoid hypoventilation and hyperventilation. The two key numbers for airway management are keeping oxygen saturation at about 95% and an end-tidal CO_2 of 35 to 40 mm Hg.

Compliance

When air, or air containing oxygen, is delivered by positive pressure into the lungs of a patient, the "give," or elasticity, of the lungs and chest wall will influence how easy it will be for the patient to breathe. If you are performing mask ventilation, a normal elasticity of the lungs and chest wall will allow air to enter the glottic opening, and little gastric distention should result. However, if the elasticity is poor, ventilation will be harder to achieve and gastric distention more likely. The ability of the lungs and chest wall to expand and therefore ventilate a patient is known as *compliance*. It is simpler to speak of "good compliance" or "bad compliance" rather than "high" or "low" compliance because the latter terms can be somewhat confusing.

Compliance is an important concept because it governs whether or not you can adequately ventilate a patient. Compliance can become bad (that is, low) in some disease states of the lung or in patients who have an injury to the chest wall. In cardiac arrest, compliance will become bad due to poor circulation to the muscles. This makes ventilating the patient all the more difficult. With an endotracheal tube in place, the patient's compliance becomes an important clinical sign and may reveal airway problems. Keep in mind that with an endotracheal tube in place and with bag-valve-mask ventilation, you have a kind of "pressure-detection" device much like a tire-pressure gauge. That is, you can feel compliance worsening or improving with your fingers and hand. A worsening of compliance may be the first sign of a tension pneumothorax. Poor compliance also will be felt in right (or left) mainstem bronchus intubation; pulling back on the ETT will result in an immediate improvement in the ability to ventilate (that is, better compliance).

Ventilation Techniques

Mouth-to-Mouth

Mouth-to-mouth ventilation is an old and effective method, with the advantage of requiring no equipment and a minimum of experience and training. Delivered volumes are consistently adequate because mouth seal is effectively and easily maintained. In addition, compliance can be felt more accurately, and high oropharyngeal pressures are therefore less likely. This method is rarely used because of the concern of disease transmission. However, it is appropriate for some patients, especially those with whom you are familiar (such as family members). Because of its effectiveness and universal availability, you should be familiar with the technique.

Mouth-to-Mask

Though not quite as effective as mouth-to-mouth ventilation, mouth-to-mask ventilation can overcome the slight risk of disease transmission by interposing a face mask between your mouth and that of the patient. Commercially designed pocket face masks, which fold into a small case that can be carried in your pocket, are particularly suited for the initial ventilation of many types of patients. Some have a side port for supplemental oxygen. Pocket ventilating masks have consistently been shown to deliver larger volumes than bag-valve-mask devices and do so with a greater percentage of oxygen than mouth-to-mouth ventilation. Mouth-to-mask ventilation has significant advantages over bag-valve-mask devices and should be more widely used. (See Chapter 5.)

Flow-Restricted Oxygen-Powered Ventilating Device

In the past, the high-pressure, oxygen-powered ventilators (demand valves) were considered too dangerous to use in multiple-trauma patients. Experience with the newer FROPVDs that meet American Heart Association guidelines (oxygen flow rate of 40 liters per minute at a maximum pressure of 50 ± 5 cm H_2O) suggests that

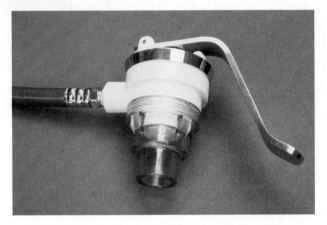

Figure 4-11 The flow-restricted oxygen-powered ventilation device. This valve delivers a set flow of 40 liters per minute at a maximum pressure of 50 ± 5 cm H_2O. Do not use it unless it meets these standards and the system medical director approves.

these may now be the equal of bag-valve-mask devices for ventilation (Figure 4-11). They have the advantage of delivering 100% oxygen and allowing use of two hands while using face mask ventilation. FROPVDs are no worse than bag-valve masks at producing gastric distention. However, because it is more difficult to feel lung compliance when ventilating with the FROPVD, there is still some controversy about its use. FROPVD ventilation, like bag-valve-mask ventilation, can cause or worsen a pneumothorax. Follow your medical director's advice on the use of an FROPVD.

Bag-Valve-Mask Device

The bag-valve mask (BVM), a descendant of the anesthetic bag, is a fixed-volume ventilator with an average delivered volume of about 800 cc of air or oxygen. With a two-handed squeeze, over 1 liter can be delivered to the patient. It should be used with a reservoir bag or tubing. Plain bag-valve masks without reservoir bag or tubing can only deliver 40% to 50% oxygen and thus should be replaced with reservoir bags.

The most important problem associated with the bag-valve-mask device is the volume delivered. Mask leak is a serious problem, decreasing the volume delivered to the oropharynx by sometimes 40% or more. In addition, old masks of conventional design have significant dead space beneath them, thus increasing the challenge to provide an adequate volume to the patient. The balloon mask has a design that eliminates dead space beneath the mask and provides an improved seal over the nose and mouth. It has been shown in mannequin studies to decrease mask leak and to improve ventilation. It is recommended particularly for trauma patients (Figure 4-12).

A better seal can sometimes be obtained, and sufficient volumes delivered, in either the balloon or conventional mask, with the use of extension tubing attached to the ventilating port of the bag-valve-mask device. This permits the mask to be better seated on the face without a levering effect from the rigid ventilating port connector that tends to unseat the mask. With the extension in place, the bag can be more easily compressed, even against the knee or thigh, thus increasing the delivered volume and overcoming any mask leak (Figure 4-13). The two-person technique where one person holds the mask seal and another ventilates is another way to improve ventilations where mask seal is an issue or hand size is small. Capnography should be used to ensure adequate ventilation and prevent inadvertent hyperventilation.

Effective ventilation with a bag-valve mask requires a high degree of skill and is not without problems. Prehospital personnel must be prepared for situations where mask ventilation is difficult and be able to respond to these challenges. Predictors of difficult mask ventilation can be remembered using the "BOOTS" mnemonic:

B – Beards

O – Obesity

O – Older patients

T – Toothlessness

S – Snores or stridor

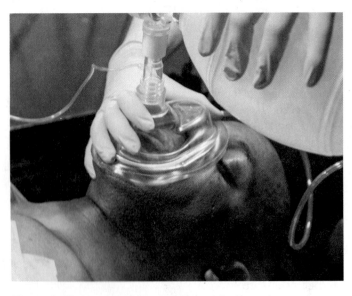

Figure 4-12 Appropriate hand placement for bag-valve-mask ventilation.

All these signs suggest that the patient will not be easy to mask ventilate. Facial hair and the lack of teeth make mask seal more difficult. Obesity increases both lung and chest compliance. In older patients and in those in whom cervical-spine control is essential, it is more difficult to get proper head and neck positioning. Finally, the presence of snoring or stridor or wheezes should alert the rescuer to the presence of airway obstruction and the need to extend expiratory time for patients with obstructed airway disease.

If unable to ventilate a patient using a bag-valve mask, the first step should be to reposition the airway by performing an exaggerated head-tilt/chin-lift (if not contraindicated by possible neck injury) and an aggressive jaw-thrust. Insert an OPA or NPA. If you are still unsuccessful, the next step is to initiate two-person bag-valve-mask ventilation with extra emphasis on the jaw-thrust maneuver to maximize airway opening. If cricoid pressure is being applied, ease up or release entirely. Consider changing the mask size or type. Continued problems with mask ventilation should prompt the consideration of airway obstruction as a potential cause. Ultimately, the placement of a "rescue" ventilation device (BIAD, such as laryngeal mask airway) or endotracheal tube may be required to definitively ventilate the patient in the worst-case scenario (Figure 4-14).

Airway Equipment

The most important rule to follow in regard to airway equipment is that it should be in good working order and immediately available. It will do the patient no good if you have to run back to the ambulance to get the suction apparatus. In other words, be prepared. This is not difficult. Five basic pieces of equipment are necessary for the initial response to all prehospital trauma calls. They are

- Personal protection equipment (See Chapter 1.)
- Patient transfer device (backboard or scoop)
- Appropriate-size rigid cervical extrication collar
- Airway kit (See the following information.)
- Trauma box (See Chapter 1.)

The airway kit should be completely self-contained and should contain everything needed to secure an airway in any patient. Equipment now available is lightweight and portable. Oxygen cylinders are aluminum, and newer suction devices are less bulky and lighter. It is no longer acceptable to have suction units that are bulky and stored separately from a source of oxygen. Suction units should be contained in a kit with oxygen and other essential airway tools. A lightweight airway kit should consist of the following (Figure 4-15):

- Oxygen D cylinder, preferably aluminum
- Portable battery-powered and hand-powered suction units
- Oxygen cannulae and masks
- Oropharyngeal and nasopharyngeal airways
- Endotracheal intubation kit, with both adult and pediatric laryngoscope blades and ET tubes
- Gum elastic bougie

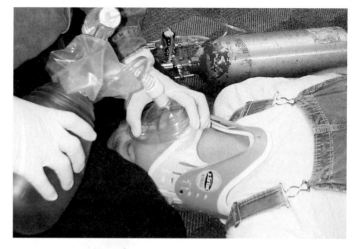

Figure 4-13 A ventilating port extension attached to a ventilating bag permits a better mask seal and therefore greater delivered volumes. There is more dead space when using extension tubing, so a higher volume of air must be given. Compressing the bag against the thigh, as shown here, will also increase the delivered volume. *(Photo courtesy of Buddy Denson, EMT-P)*

Increasing Difficulty

- Reposition
- OPA/NPA
- Two-person bag
- Consider obstruction
- BIAD
- Laryngoscopy and intubation

Figure 4-14 Response to difficult bag-valve-mask ventilation.

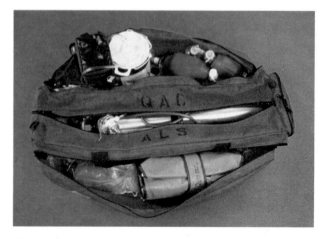

Figure 4-15 An airway kit containing the essentials for airway management. Note that portable suction is included in this design. The total weight (with aluminum "D" oxygen cylinder) is approximately 10 kg (22 lb), about the same as a steel "E" cylinder.

- Rescue airway device such as the esophageal tracheal Combitube®, King LT-D™ airway, intubating laryngeal airway (ILA/air-Q™), or laryngeal mask airway (LMA™)
- Bag-valve-mask ventilating device (with reservoir bag)
- Pocket mask with supplemental oxygen intake
- Pulse oximeter
- CO_2 monitor (preferably a waveform capnograph, which allows you to analyze airway problems)
- Translaryngeal oxygen cannula and manual ventilator or a cricothyrotomy kit

The contents of the airway kit are critical. Check all equipment each shift, and have a card attached to be initialed by the person checking it.

Case Presentation (continued)

You are the lead emergency care provider in an ALS ambulance transporting a seriously injured motorcyclist to the trauma center. A tourniquet is controlling bleeding in the area of the left knee, and exam findings indicate possible, head, chest, and abdominal injuries, with concern for spine injury. The patient is unresponsive. Noting the development of stridor, along with a decrease in tidal volume in your patient, you immediately have your partner set up suction and begin to assist respirations with a bag-valve mask, while preparing to perform orotracheal intubation. (If you were not trained in this procedure, you would immediately contact medical direction for advice on the nearest facility capable of handling this problem.) You also have equipment ready should he need to perform a needle cricothyrotomy.

After testing your equipment, you insert the laryngoscope, confirm the absence of a gag reflex, and insert the endotracheal tube through the patient's vocal cords into the mainstem bronchus. Then, instructing your partner to ventilate the patient, you listen with your stethoscope first over the epigastrium, where you hear no sounds, and then over the lungs, where you hear good breath sounds on the left side. (The patient most likely has a pneumothorax on the right.) You then inflate the cuff.

With the airway now established, you instruct your partner to assist ventilations with 100% oxygen at one 500 cc breath every eight seconds. You check a pulse oximeter reading, attach an end-tidal CO_2 detector, and instruct your partner to maintain ventilation to achieve an end-tidal CO_2 of 35 to 40.

You then reassess the patient, after which you will recontact the trauma center to update them on his status and your ETA.

Summary

Trauma patients provide the greatest challenge in airway management. To be successful you must have a clear understanding of the anatomy of the airway and be proficient in techniques to open and maintain your patient's airway. You must have the correct equipment organized in a kit that is immediately available when you begin assessment of the trauma patient. To provide adequate ventilation for your patient, you must understand the concepts of tidal volume, minute volume, and lung compliance. Finally, you must become familiar with the various options for monitoring and control of the airway and develop and maintain expertise in performing using them.

Bibliography

American College of Emergency Physicians Policy Statement. Verification of endotracheal tube placement. Revised and approved by the ACEP Board of Directors, April 2009. American College of Emergency Physicians website, Policy Statements page, 2014. Accessed January 4, 2015, at http://www.acep.org/Clinical---Practice-Management/Verification-of-Endotracheal-Tube-Placement/

Biebuyck, J. F., and J. L. Benumouf. "Management of the Difficult Adult Airway with Special Emphasis on Awake Intubation." *Anesthesiology* 75 (1991): 1087–1110.

Bledsoe B. E., E. Anderson, R. Hodnick, L. Johnson, and E. Dievendorf. "Low-Fractional Oxygen Concentration Continuous Positive Airway Pressure Is Effective in the Prehospital Setting." *Prehospital Emergency Care* 16, no. 2 (April–June 2012): 217–21.

Donald M.J., and B. Paterson. "End Tidal Carbon Dioxide Monitoring in Prehospital and Retrieval Medicine: A Review." *Emergency Medicine Journal* 23, no. 9 (September 2006): 728–30.

Driscoll, R. "Emergency Oxygen Use." *BMJ* website, October, 2012; 345. doi:10.1136/bmj.e6856

Hüter L., K. Schwarzkopf, J. Rödiger, N. P. Preussler, and T. Schreiber. "Students Insert the Laryngeal Tube Quicker and More Often Successful Than the Esophageal-Tracheal Combitube in a Manikin." *Resuscitation* 80, no. 8 (August 2009): 930–34.

Kilgannon, J. H., A. E. Jones, J. E. Parillo, R. P. Dellinger, B. Milcarek, K. Hunter, N. I. Shapiro, S. Trzeciak, and Emergency Medicine Shock Research Network (EMShockNet) Investigators. "Relationship Between Supranormal Oxygen Tension and Outcome After Resuscitation from Cardiac Arrest." *Circulation* 123, no. 23 (June 14, 2011): 2717–22.

Kober, A., R. Fleischackl, T. Scheck, F. Lieba, H. Strasser, A. Friedmann, and D. I. Sessler. "A Randomized Controlled Trial of Oxygen for Reducing Nausea and Vomiting During Emergency Transport of Patients Older Than 60 Years with Minor Trauma." *Mayo Clinical Proceedings* 77, no. 1 (January 2002): 35–38.

Kovacs, G., and A. Law. *Airway Management in Emergencies.* 2nd ed. New York: McGraw-Hill. 2011.

Langeron, O., E. Masso, C. Huraux, M. Guggiari, A. Bianchi, B. Coriat, and B. Riou. "Prediction of Difficult Mask Ventilation." *Anesthesiology* 92, no. 5 (May 2000): 1229–36.

Lecky F., D. Bryden, R. Little, N. Tong, and C. Moulton. "Emergency Intubation for Acutely Ill and Injured Patients." *Cochrane Database of Systematic Reviews* 2 (April 16, 2008): CD001429.

McNulty, P. H., N. King, S. Scott, G. Hartman, J. McCann, M. Kozak, C. E. Chambers, L. M. Demers, and L. I. Sinoway. "Effects of Supplemental Oxygen Administration on Coronary Blood Flow in Patients Undergoing Cardiac Catheterization." *American Journal of Physiology: Heart and Circulatory Physiology* 288, no. 3 (March 2005): H1057–H1062.

Morrison, L., C. D. Deakin, et al. "Advanced Life Support: 2010 International Consensus on Cardiopulmonary Resuscitation and Emergency Cardiovascular Care Science with Treatment Recommendations." *Circulation* 122: S345–S421.

Moss, R., K. Porter, and I. Greaves. "Pharmacologically Assisted Laryngeal Mask Insertion: A Consensus Statement." *Emergency Medicine Journal* 30, no. 12 (December 2013): 1073–75.

Mosesso, V. N., K. Kukitsch, J. Menegazzi, and J. Mosesso. "Comparison of Delivered Volumes and Airway Pressures When Ventilating Through an Endotracheal Tube with Bag-Valve versus Demand-Valve." *Prehospital and Disaster Medicine* 9, no. 1 (January–March 1994): 24–28.

O'Connor, R. E., and R. A. Swor. "Verification of Endotracheal Tube Placement Following Intubation: National Association of EMS Physicians Standards and Clinical Practice Committee." *Prehospital Emergency Care* 3, no. 3 (July–September 1999): 248–50.

Peters, J., and N. Hoogerwerf. "Prehospital Endotracheal Intubation; Need for Routine Cuff Pressure Measurement?" *Emergency Medicine Journal* 30, no. 10 (October 2013): 851–53.

Ravussin, P., and J. Freeman. "A New Transtracheal Catheter for Ventilation and Resuscitation." *Canadian Anaesthetists' Society Journal* 32, no. 1 (January 1985): 60–64.

Robinson, N., and M. Clancy. "In Patients with Head Injury Undergoing Rapid Sequence Intubation, Does Pretreatment with Intravenous Lignocaine/Lidocaine Lead to an Improved

Neurological Outcome? A Review of the Literature." *Emergency Medicine Journal* 18, no. 6 (November 2001): 453–57.

Salem, M. R., A. Y. Wong, M. Mani, and B. A. Sellick. "Efficacy of Cricoid Pressure in Preventing Gastric Inflation During Bag-Valve-Mask Ventilation in Pediatric Patients." *Anesthesiology* 40, no. 1 (January 1974): 96–98.

Sivestri, S., G. A. Ralls, B. Krauss, J. Thundiyil, S. G. Rothrock, A. Senn, E. Carter, and J. Falk. "The Effectiveness of Out-of-Hospital Use of Continuous End-Tidal Carbon Dioxide Monitoring on the Rate of Unrecognized Misplaced Intubation Within a Regional Emergency Medical Services System." *Annals of Emergency Medicine* 45, no. 5 (May 2005): 497–503.

Stewart, R. D., R. M. Kaplan, B. Pennock, et al. "Influence of Mask Design on Bag-Mask Ventilation." *Annals of Emergency Medicine* 14 (1985): 403–6.

Stockinger, Z. T., and N. E. McSwain Jr. "Prehospital Endotracheal Intubation for Trauma Does Not Improve Survival over Bag-Valve-Mask Ventilation." *Journal of Trauma* 56, no. 3 (March 2004): 531–36.

Tumpach E. A., M. Lutes, D. Ford, and E. B. Lerner. "The King LT versus the Combitube: Flight Crew Performance and Preference." *Prehospital Emergency Care* 13, no. 3 (July–September 2009): 324–28.

Ufbert J. W., J. S. Bushra, D. J. Karras, W. A. Satz, and F. Kueppers. "Aspiration of Gastric Contents: Association with Prehospital Intubation." *American Journal of Emergency Medicine* 23, no. 3 (May 2005): 379–82.

Wang, H. E., T. A. Sweeney, R. E. O'Conner, and H. Rubinstein. "Failed Prehospital Intubations: An Analysis of Emergency Department Courses and Outcomes." *Prehospital Emergency Care* 5, no. 2 (April–June 2001): 131–41.

Weingart, S. D., and R. M. Levitan. "Preoxygenation and Prevention of Desaturation during Emergency Airway Management." *Annals of Emergency Medicine* 59, no. 3 (March 2012): 165–75.

White, S. J., R. M. Kaplan, and R. D. Stewart. "Manual Detection of Decreased Lung Compliance as a Sign of Tension Pneumothorax." (abstr.) *Annals of Emergency Medicine* 16 (1987): 518.

Get more information about this course by calling
ITLS International at 888-495-4875
(outside the United States call +1-630-495-6442) or visit

www.itrauma.org

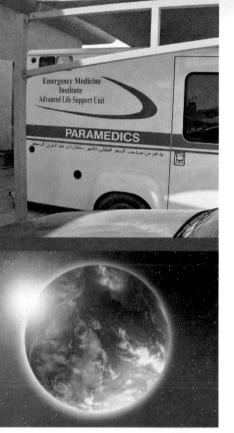

Kate Blackwelder

Airway Skills

S. Robert Seitz, M.Ed, RN, NRP
Bob Page, MEd, NRP, CCP, NCEE
Roy L. Alson, PhD, MD

Vie Aeree	Vía Aérea	Voie Respiratoire	Drogi oddechowe
Atemweg	Dišni put	مجرى الهواء	disajni put
Dihalna pot	Légút		

Objectives

Upon successful completion of this chapter, you should be able to:

1. Suction the airway.
2. Insert a nasopharyngeal and oropharyngeal airway.
3. Use the pocket mask.
4. Use the bag-valve mask.
5. Use the pulse oximeter.
6. Perform airway management utilizing supraglottic airway devices.
7. Prepare for endotracheal intubation.
8. Perform laryngoscopic orotracheal intubation.
9. Perform nasotracheal intubation.
10. Confirm placement of the endotracheal tube (ETT).
11. Use capnography to confirm placement of the ETT.
12. Anchor the ETT.
13. Understand the use of medications to assist with intubation.

Chapter Overview

Loss of airway is one of the leading causes of preventable trauma death. It is imperative that emergency care providers know how to assess and manage the airway in the trauma patient. This chapter reviews the necessary skills to open and stabilize the airway of the trauma patient. It is essential that during airway management all team members communicate clearly with each other to ensure a smooth process and successful outcome. One should never be in a rush to secure an airway; finesse is often more important than force during airway procedures.

Basic Airway Management

Procedures

Suctioning the Airway

1. Attach the suction connecting tubing to the suction machine.
2. Turn the device on and test it.
3. Insert the suction tip through the nose (soft or whistle tip catheter) or mouth (soft or rigid) without activating the suction.
4. Open the patient's mouth, if needed, using a tongue blade. If using the scissors method, be aware that patients can still bite down as a reflex.
5. Activate the suction, and withdraw the suction tube.
6. Repeat the procedure as necessary.

Note that although the intent is to suction foreign matter (Figure 5-1), air and oxygen also are being suctioned out of the patient. Never suction for greater than 15 seconds. After suctioning, reoxygenate the patient as soon as possible.

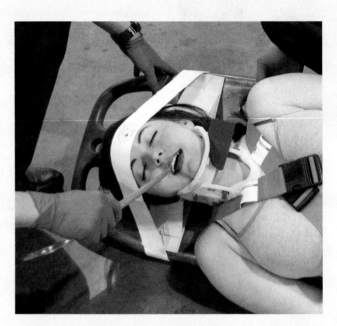

Figure 5-1 Suctioning material from the oropharynx using a Yankauer suction tip.

Inserting the Nasopharyngeal Airway (NPA)

The nasopharyngeal airway (NPA) is made to go into the right nostril. Consider using an alternative to the NPA if the patient has facial fractures or raccoon eyes. To insert the NPA into the patient's right nostril follow these steps:

1. Choose the appropriate size. It should be as large as possible but still fit easily through the patient's external nares. The size of the patient's little finger can be used as a rough guide (Figure 5-2).

2. Measure the NPA from the nare to the tip of the ear lobe to ensure it is the correct length.
3. Lubricate the tube with a water-based lubricant.
4. Insert the tube straight back through the right nostril along the floor of the nose with the beveled edge of the airway toward the septum.
5. Gently pass it into the posterior pharynx with a slight rotating motion until the flange rests against the nares.

Note that if resistance to passage of the NPA is felt, DO NOT FORCE the NPA in, as injury may occur.

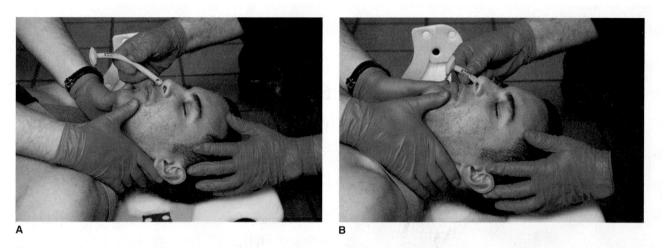

A   **B**

Figure 5-2 The nasopharyngeal airway should be the largest size that will easily fit through the external nares. *(Photos courtesy of Lewis B. Mallory, MBA, REMT-P)*

Remove NPA and attempt insertion in the other nostril. To insert the NPA into the left nostril:

1. Turn the airway upside down so that the bevel is toward the septum.
2. Insert straight back through the nostril until you reach the posterior pharynx.
3. Turn the airway over 180 degrees and insert it down the pharynx.

Note that if the tongue is occluding the airway, a jaw thrust or chin lift must be performed to allow the nasopharyngeal airway to go under the tongue (Figure 5-3).

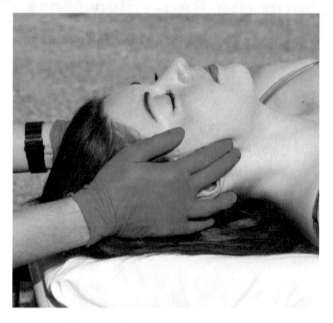

Figure 5-3 Opening the airway using a modified jaw-thrust maneuver. Maintain in-line stabilization while pushing up on the angle of the jaw.

Inserting the Oropharyngeal Airway (OPA)

1. Choose the size oropharyngeal airway (OPA) that is appropriate for the patient. The distance from the corner of the mouth to the lower part of the external ear or to the angle of the jaw is a good estimate (Figure 5-4).
2. In the unresponsive patient, open the patient's mouth with a scissor maneuver (Figure 5-5), a jaw lift (Figure 5-6), or a tongue blade. If you are placing your fingers in the patient's mouth, use caution because broken teeth and biting can cause injury.

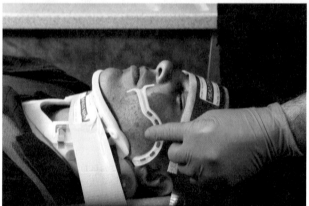

Figure 5-4 The distance from the corner of the mouth to the lower part of the external ear or to angle of the jaw is a good estimate for the correct size oropharyngeal airway. *(Photo courtesy of Lewis B. Mallory, MBA, REMT-P)*

(continued)

Procedure (*continued*)

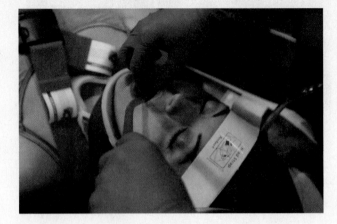

Figure 5-5 Scissors maneuver being used to open mouth for suctioning. Use same maneuver to open mouth to insert an oropharyngeal airway.

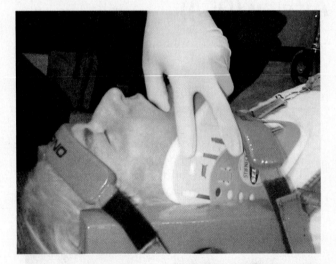

Figure 5-6 Jaw lift. *(Photo courtesy of Buddy Denson, EMT-P)*

3. Insert the airway gently without pushing the tongue back into the pharynx. (See Chapter 4, Figure 4-9.)
   a. Insert the airway under direct vision, using a tongue blade. This is the preferred method and is safe for adults and children.
   b. Insert the airway upside down or sideways and rotate into place after tip of airway passes the tongue. This method should *not* be used for children.
4. If the OPA causes gagging, remove it and replace it with an NPA. The presence of a gag reflex is a contraindication to use of an OPA.

Using a Pocket Mask with Supplemental Oxygen

1. Stabilize the patient's head in a neutral position.
2. Connect the oxygen tubing to the oxygen cylinder and the mask.
3. Open the oxygen cylinder, and set the flow rate to a minimum of 15 liters per minute
4. Open the patient's mouth.
5. Insert an OPA or NPA, if available. Otherwise use the chin-lift or jaw-thrust maneuver to open the airway.
6. Place the mask on the face, and establish a good seal. Make sure the mask is the proper size for your patient. The mask should cover the nose and mouth and make a good seal. Facial hair, lack of teeth, obesity, or advanced age may make it difficult to get a good mask seal.
7. Ventilate mouth-to-mask with enough volume (8–10 mL per kg body weight) *to cause adequate chest rise.* Ventilate at a rate of 8 to 10 breaths per minute. The inspiratory phase should last 1.5 to 2 seconds. Let the patient exhale before giving the next breath.

Using the Bag-Valve Mask

1. Stabilize the patient's head in a neutral position.
2. Connect the oxygen, connecting tubing to the bag-valve-mask system and oxygen cylinder.
3. Attach the oxygen reservoir to the bag-valve mask.
4. Open the oxygen cylinder, and set the flow rate to minimum of 15 liters per minute.
5. Select the proper size mask, and attach it to the bag-valve-mask device. The mask should go from the bridge of the nose to the chin.
6. Open the patient's mouth.
7. Insert an OPA (or an NPA, if the patient has a gag reflex).
8. If available, apply a capnography cannula or attach an airway adapter between the bag and the mask (Figure 5-7).
9. Place the mask on the patient's face, and have your partner establish and maintain a good seal. Facial hair, lack of teeth, obesity, or advanced

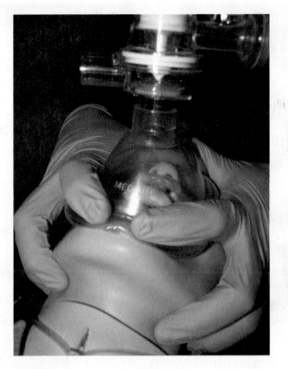

Figure 5-7 A capnography nasal cannula can be placed under the mask of the DVM. *(Photo courtesy of Roy L. Alson, PhD, MD, FACEP, FAAEM)*

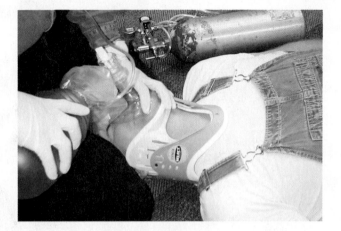

Figure 5-8 To make a proper seal, place the thumb over the nose and index finger over chin while the rest of the fingers are in contact with the mandible. *(Photo courtesy of Buddy Denson, EMT-P)*

age might make it difficult to get a good mask seal.

10. Using both hands, ventilate at a rate of 8 to 10 breaths per minute. If you are getting good bilateral chest rise, you are giving adequate tidal volume. Calculated tidal volume is 8-10 mL per kg body weight. Use capnography to ensure adequate ventilation and prevent inad-

vertent hyperventilation. As a general rule, keep the end-tidal CO_2 (ETCO$_2$) between 35 and 45 mm Hg.

11. If you are forced to ventilate without the assis tance of another emergency care provider, use one hand to maintain a face seal and the other hand to squeeze the bag. This may decrease the volume of ventilation because less volume is produced by only one hand squeezing the bag. Watch for chest rise to ensure adequate ventilation volume. To make a proper seal, place the thumb on the mask over the nose and index finger on the mask over the chin while the rest of the fingers are in contact with the mandible (Figure 5-8).

The Pulse Oximeter

A pulse oximeter is a noninvasive photoelectric device that measures the oxygen saturation of hemoglobin and pulse rate in the peripheral circulation. It consists of a portable monitor and a sensing probe that clips onto the patient's finger, toe, or earlobe (Figure 5-9). The probe sends two beams of light, red and infrared, and the percentage of hemoglobin saturation is then calculated based on the nonabsorbed light that reaches the photodetector. The device displays the pulse rate and the arterial oxygen saturation in a percentage value (% SaO$_2$). Certain toxins (such as carboxyhemoglobin, the result of carbon monoxide inhalation) can falsely elevate the percentage of saturation. This useful device should be used on all patients who have any type of respiratory compromise. The pulse oximeter is useful to assess the patient's respiratory status, the effectiveness of oxygen therapy, and the effectiveness of bag-valve-mask or flow-restricted oxygen-powered ventilation device (FROPVD) ventilation.

Remember that the device measures percentage of hemoglobin carrying oxygen (SaO$_2$), not the arterial partial pressure of oxygen (PaO$_2$). The hemoglobin molecule

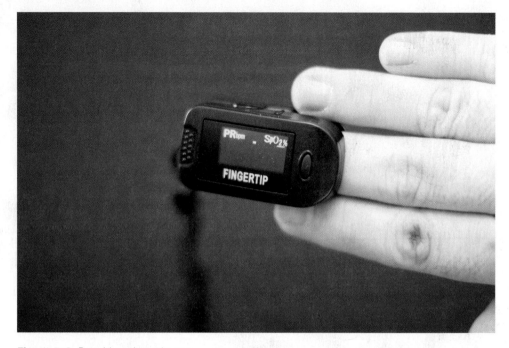

Figure 5-9 Portable pulse oximeter.

is so efficient at carrying oxygen that it is 90% saturated (90% SaO_2) when the partial pressure of oxygen in the blood is only 60 mm Hg (100 mm Hg is normal). If you are accustomed to thinking about PaO_2 (where 90–100 mm Hg is normal), then you may be fooled into thinking that an SaO_2 pulse oximeter reading of 90% is normal when it is actually critically low. As a general rule, any pulse oximeter reading below 92% is cause for concern and requires some sort of intervention (such as opening the airway, suction, oxygen, assisted ventilation, intubation, decompression of tension pneumothorax). A pulse oximeter reading below 90% is critical and requires immediate intervention to maintain adequate tissue oxygenation. Try to maintain a pulse oximeter reading of 95% or higher. However, do not withhold oxygen from a patient with a pulse oximeter reading above 95% who also shows signs and symptoms of hypoxia or difficulty breathing.

The following are conditions that make the pulse oximeter reading unreliable:

- *Poor peripheral perfusion* (shock, vasoconstriction, hypotension). Do not attach the sensing probe onto an injured extremity. Try not to use the sensing probe on the arm you are using to monitor blood pressure. Be aware that the pulse oximeter reading will go down while the blood pressure cuff is inflated.

- *Hyperventilation.* An $ETCO_2$ less than 25 mm Hg can lead to alkalosis, causing oxygen to bind tightly to hemoglobin and not releasing it for use. This leads to tissue hypoxia with a falsely high (even 100%) pulse oximetry reading.

- *Hypoventilation.* High $ETCO_2$ (above 50 mm Hg) can lead to acidosis. Acidosis causes oxygen to bind loosely and reduces the amount carried to the cells. This gives a low pulse oximeter reading that does not respond to O_2 therapy.

- *Severe anemia or exsanguinating hemorrhage.*

- *Hypothermia.* Vasoconstriction causes decreased blood flow to the probe site on the extremities.

- *Excessive patient movement.*

- *High ambient light* (bright sunlight, high-intensity light on area of the sensing probe).

- *Nail polish or a dirty fingernail,* if you are using a finger probe. Use acetone to clean the nail before attaching the probe.

- *Carbon monoxide poisoning*. This will give falsely high readings because the sensing probe cannot distinguish between oxyhemoglobin and carboxyhemoglobin. If carbon monoxide poisoning is suspected, you must use a specific monitor and sensor to measure levels (see Chapter 16).
- *Cyanide poisoning*. Cyanide poisons at the cellular level prevent the cells from using oxygen to make energy. Because the body is not using oxygen, the circulating blood will usually be 95% to 100% saturated. However, the patient will still be dying from lack of oxygen (at the cellular level).

To use the pulse oximeter, turn on the device, clean the area that you are to monitor (earlobe, fingernail, or toenail), and attach the sensing clip to the area. Remember that although very useful, the pulse oximeter is just another tool to help you assess the patient. Like all tools, it has limitations, as noted earlier, and should not replace careful physical assessment.

Blind Insertion Airway Devices

Introduced in the early 1970s, blind insertion airway devices (BIADs), also known as supraglottic airways (SGA), were designed for use by EMS personnel who were not trained to intubate the trachea. Emergency care providers now routinely use these devices in managing airways. Reasons for use include ease of placement as an initial advanced airway intervention or as a backup device for failed endotracheal intubation attempts. Devices such as Combitube®, Rusch Easy Tube®, LMA®, I-Gel®, and King LT-D® airway are classified as single- or double-lumen devices. They are all designed to be inserted into the pharynx without the need for a laryngoscope to visualize where the tube is going. Many of them have a tube with an inflatable cuff that is designed to seal the esophagus, thus helping to prevent vomiting and aspiration of stomach contents, as well as preventing gastric distention during bag-valve-mask or FROPVD ventilation. Others use the distal end of the device to occlude the esophagus. It also was thought that by sealing the esophagus, more air would enter the lungs, and ventilation would be improved.

The devices have their own dangers and require careful evaluation to be sure they are in the correct position. This class of airway is now referred to as *supraglottic airways*. None of the BIADs are equal to the ETT, which has become the invasive airway of choice for advanced EMS providers. In many systems, basic life support level providers are permitted to use BIADs.

King LT-D™ Airway

The King LT-D™ airway is a single lumen device inserted into the esophagus. It is designed with an esophageal and pharyngeal cuff, which inflate simultaneously. Once inflated, the patient is ventilated through the single tube (Figure 5-10). With the airway in place, you may be able to insert a bougie or a fiberoptic bronchoscope through the ventilating tube and swap the airway for an ETT, though it is not always successful. There is also an LTS-D™ airway that has a port through which you can insert a gastric tube to decompress the stomach. It is inserted in exactly the same way as the King LT-D™ airway. When using the King LT-D™, just as you would any BIAD, you must be sure that you are ventilating the lungs and not the stomach. The King LT-D™ is available in five sizes for patients greater than 35 inches (90 cm) to six feet (183 cm) or more in height.

Essential Points You must remember six essential points about the King LT-D™ airway. They are as follows:

- Use the King LT-D™ airway only in patients who are unresponsive and without protective (gag) reflexes.
- Do not use it in any patient with injury to the esophagus (such as caustic ingestions)
- Do not use it in patients who are less than 35 inches (90 cm) tall.

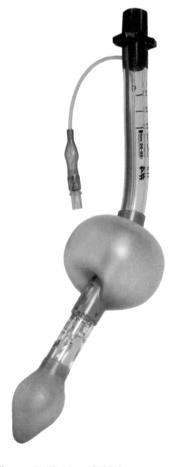

Figure 5-10 King LT-D™ airway.

- Pay careful attention to proper placement. Unrecognized intratracheal placement of the tube is a rare but lethal complication that produces complete airway obstruction. Such an occurrence is not always easy to detect, and the results are catastrophic. Capnography is recommended for confirmation of all supraglottic airway placement.
- You must insert it gently and without force.
- If the patient regains consciousness, you must remove the airway because it will cause retching and vomiting.

Procedure

Inserting the King LT-D™ Airway

1. Select the correct size King LT-D airway™.
   - Size 2 (green connector color) is for children 35 to 45 inches (90 to 115 cm) in height or who weigh 12 to 25 kg.
   - Size 2.5 (orange connector color) is for children 41 to 51 inches (105 to 130 cm) in height or who weigh 25 to 35 kg.
   - Size 3 (yellow connector color) is for adults 4 to 5 feet (122 to 155 cm) in height.
   - Size 4 (red connector color) is for adults 5 to 6 feet (155 to 180 cm) in height.
   - Size 5 (purple connector color) is for adults greater than 6 feet (>180 cm) in height.

2. Test the cuff inflation system for air leaks.

3. Apply a water-soluble lubricant to the distal tip.

4. Hold the airway at the connector with your dominant hand. With the neck stabilized in a neutral position, hold the mouth open, and apply a chin lift with your nondominant hand. Using a lateral approach, introduce the tip into the mouth (Figure 5-11).

5. Advance the tip behind the base of the tongue while rotating the tube back to the midline so that the blue orientation line faces the chin of the patient (Figure 5-12).

6. Without exerting excessive force, advance the tube until the base of the connector is aligned with the patient's teeth or gums (Figure 5-13).

7. Hold the KLT 900™ cuff pressure gauge in the nondominant hand, and inflate the cuffs of the King LT-D™ with air to a pressure of 60 cm H_2O (Figure 5-14). If a cuff pressure gauge is not available and a syringe is being used to inflate the King LT-D™, inflate cuffs with the minimum volume necessary to seal the airway at the peak

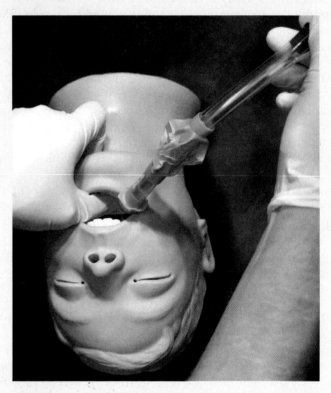

Figure 5-11 Hold the KLT-D™ with dominant hand. With nondominant hand, open mouth and apply chin lift. Using a lateral approach, introduce tip into mouth.

ventilatory pressure employed (just seal volume). Typical sizing and inflation volumes are as follows:

- Size 2 (green), 35 to 45 inches (90 to 115 cm), 25 to 35 mL
- Size 3 (orange), 41 to 51 inches (105 to 130 cm), 30 to 40 mL
- Size 3 (yellow), 4 to 5 feet (122 to 155 cm), 45 to 60 mL

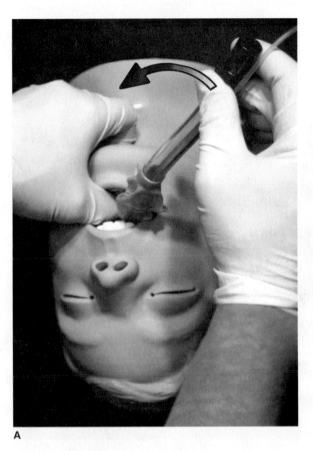

A

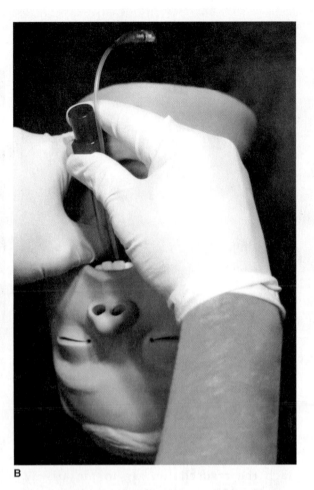

B

Figure 5-12 Advance the tip behind the base of the tongue while rotating the tube back to the midline so that the blue orientation line faces the chin of the patient.

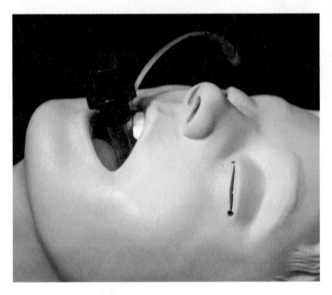

Figure 5-13 Gently advance the tube until the base of connector is aligned with teeth or gums.

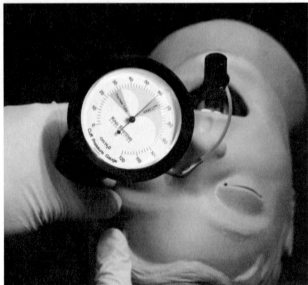

Figure 5-14 Holding the KLT 900 Cuff Pressure Gauge in nondominant hand, inflate the cuffs of the King LT-D™ with air to a pressure of 60 cm H_2O.

(continued)

Procedure (*continued*)

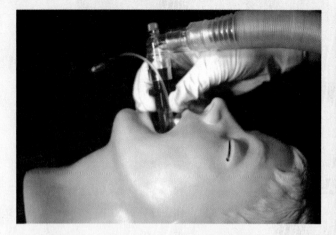

Figure 5-15 Attach the bag-valve mask to the airway. While bagging the patient, gently withdraw the tube until ventilation becomes easy. Adjust cuff inflation if necessary to obtain a seal of the airway.

- Size 4 (red), 5 to 6 feet (155 to 180 cm), 60 to 80 mL
- Size 5 (purple), greater than 6 feet (> 180 cm), 70 to 90 mL

8. Attach the resuscitator bag to the airway. While bagging the patient, gently withdraw the tube until ventilation becomes easy and free flowing (Figure 5-15). Adjust cuff inflation if necessary to obtain a seal of the airway at the peak ventilatory pressure employed. You must see the chest rise, hear breath sounds, feel good compliance, and hear no breath sounds over the epigastrium to be sure that the King LT-D™ airway is correctly placed. However, capnography remains the most reliable way to

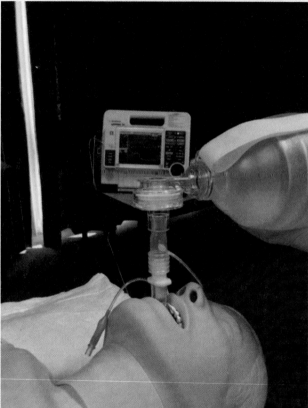

Figure 5-16 Capnography used on a King Airway®. *(Courtesy of Bob Page, MEd, NRP, CCP, NCEE)*

confirm and monitor the position of the tube (Figure 5-16).

Like the other BIADs, if the patient becomes conscious, you must remove the airway. Extubation is likely to cause vomiting, so be prepared to suction the pharynx and turn the backboard.

Esophageal Tracheal Combitube™

This class of airway is now referred to as supraglottic airways. None of the BIADs are equal to the ETT, which has become the invasive airway of choice for advanced EMS providers.

The Combitube™ has a double lumen. The two lumens are separated by a partition. (See Figure 5-17.) The port notated as #1 is slightly longer in length at the proximal end and sealed at the distal end of the tube with openings in the area of the posterior pharynx. Port #2 is slightly shorter at the proximal end and opens at the distal end of the tube. Approximately 85% of the time insertion of the Combitube™ results in the distal end being placed in the esophagus. With inflation of the distal and pharyngeal balloons, ventilation through port #1 results in air exiting the side of the tube into the pharynx. As the esophagus and oral and nasopharyngeal openings are

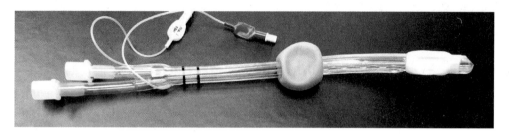

Figure 5-17 The Combitube™ is a dual-lumen supraglottic airway. The two black rings should be positioned at the teeth. *(Photo courtesy of Roy Alson, PhD, MD, FACEP, FAAEM)*

occluded by the balloons, air will enter through the glottic opening into the lungs. Secretions and blood found in the pharynx may still enter the airway.

When insertion of the tube results in a tracheal position, port #2 is ventilated with air being directly delivered through the trachea to the lungs.

Please note that there are two sizes to the Combitube™, small adult (SA), designated for individuals between 4 and 5 ½ feet (122 to 168 cm), and the Combitube™ for use with individuals 5 feet and taller. As with the other BIADs, confirmation of air reaching the lungs and not the stomach is paramount. Selection of the incorrect port for ventilating the patient will result in inadequate ventilation and oxygenation.

Essential Points You must remember five essential points about the Combitube™. They are as follows:

- Use the Combitube™ only in patients who are unresponsive and who have no protective airway reflexes.
- Do not use it in any patient who has an injury to the esophagus (such as caustic ingestions) or in children who are younger than 15. Pay attention to tube sizing because use in individuals shorter than 4 feet (122 cm) is not recommended.
- Pay careful attention to proper placement. Unrecognized intratracheal placement is a lethal complication that results in complete airway obstruction, which is not always easily detected. Use of capnography to confirm airway placement and monitor position of the device is recommended because auscultation and chest wall movement may be unreliable in the prehospital setting.
- You must insert the tube gently and without force, utilizing lubrication to facilitate the procedure.
- If the patient regains consciousness, you must remove the Combitube™ because it will cause retching and vomiting. Be prepared to suction the oral cavity and pharynx as needed.

Procedure

Inserting the Esophageal Tracheal Combitube™

1. With the neck stabilized in a neutral position, insert the tube blindly, watching for the two black rings on the Combitube™ that are used for measuring the depth of insertion. The rings should be positioned between the teeth and the lips (Figure 5-18).

2. Use the larger syringe to inflate the pharyngeal cuff with the appropriate amount of air for the size being utilized. *Do not* hold the Combitube™ while inflating the pharyngeal balloon. As inflation occurs, the Combitube™ will seat itself in the posterior pharynx behind the hard palate.

(continued)

Procedure (*continued*)

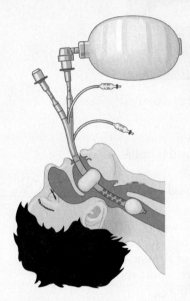

Figure 5-18 Esophageal placement of the Combitube™—ventilate through tube 1.

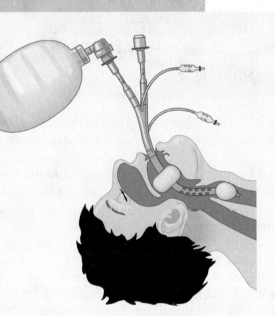

Figure 5-19 Tracheal placement of the Combitube™—ventilate through tube 2.

3. Use the smaller syringe to fill the distal cuff with the appropriate amount of air for the size being utilized.

4. Initial ventilation is attempted through port #1. You must see the chest rise, hear breath sounds, feel good compliance, and hear no breath sounds over the epigastrium to be sure that you are ventilating the lungs.

5. If you do not see the chest rise, hear breath sounds, and feel good compliance, and if you hear breath sounds over the epigastrium, the tube has been placed in the trachea (Figure 5-19). In this case, change ventilation to the second port marked as #2. Again, you must check to see the chest rise, hear breath sounds, feel good compliance, and hear no breath sounds over the epigastrium to be sure that you are ventilating the lungs. Use capnography to confirm and monitor correct placement.

Like the other BIADs, if the patient becomes conscious, you must remove the Combitube™. Extubation is likely to cause vomiting, so be prepared to suction the pharynx upon removal.

Laryngeal Mask Airway (LMA™)

This section describes the insertion of the laryngeal mask airway (LMA™). There are various other devices available that utilize a similar approach by placing a mask over the glottic opening. The user should follow the recommendations from the manufacturer for insertion of the device they are using.

The LMA™ was developed for use as an alternative to the face mask for achieving and maintaining control of the airway during routine anesthetic procedures in the operating room. Because it does not protect the airway against vomiting and aspiration, the LMA™ was meant to be used in patients who had been fasting and thus had an empty stomach. It was later found to be useful in the emergency situation when intubation is not possible and the patient cannot be ventilated with a bag-valve mask. It may prevent a surgical procedure to open the airway.

The LMA™ is another supraglottic airway (BIAD) but differs from the Combitube™ and King LT-D™ in that it was never designed to seal the esophagus and was not originally meant for emergency use.

Essential Points

- Use the LMA™ only in patients who are unresponsive and without protective reflexes. If the patient still has a gag reflex, the LMA™ may cause laryngospasm or vomiting.

- Do not use it in any patient who has injury to the esophagus (such as caustic ingestions)

- Lubricate only the posterior surface of the LMA™ to avoid blockage of the aperture or aspiration of the lubricant.

- Patients should be adequately monitored (constant visual monitoring, cardiac monitor, and if possible, pulse oximeter) at all times during LMA™ use.

- To avoid trauma to the airway, force should never be used during LMA™ insertion.

- Never overinflate the cuff after insertion. Overinflation may cause malposition, loss of seal, or trauma. Cuff pressure should be checked periodically, especially if nitrous oxide is used.

- If airway problems persist or ventilation is inadequate, the LMA™ should be removed and reinserted or an airway established by other means.

- The LMA™ does not prevent aspiration if the patient vomits. The presence of a nasogastric tube does not rule out the possibility of regurgitation and may even make regurgitation more likely because the tube makes the esophageal sphincter incompetent.

- If the patient regains consciousness, you must remove the LMA™ because it will cause retching and vomiting.

Procedure

Inserting the Laryngeal Mask Airway (LMA™)

Scan 5-1 illustrates this procedure.

1. With the neck stabilized in a neutral position, ventilate with a mouth-to-mask or bag-valve-mask technique. Suction the pharynx before insertion of the airway.

2. Remove the valve tab and check the integrity of the LMA™ cuff by inflating with the maximum volume of air (Table 5-1).

3. Using the syringe included with the LMA™, the cuff of the LMA™ should be tightly deflated, so

LMA Size	Patient Size	Maximum Cuff Volumes (Air Only)
1	Newborn and infants up to 5 kg or 11 lb	4 mL
1.5	Infants 5–0 kg or 11–22 lb	7 mL
2	Children 10–20 kg or 22–44 lb	10 mL
2.5	Children 20–30 kg or 22–65 lb	14 mL
3	Children > 30 kg (65 pounds) and small adults	20 mL
4	Normal and large adults	30 mL
5	Large adults	40 mL

Table 5-1: Cuff Volumes for LMA Pro Seal™

Adapted from *LMA™ Quick Reference Guide.* San Diego, CA: LMA North America, 2010.

(*continued*)

Procedure (*continued*)

that it forms a flat oval disk with the rim facing away from the aperture. This can be accomplished by pressing the mask with its hollow side down on a sterile flat surface (Scan 5-1-1). Use the fingers to guide the cuff into an oval shape and attempt to eliminate any wrinkles on the distal edge of the cuff. A completely flat and smooth leading edge facilitates insertion, avoids contact with the epiglottis, and is important to ensure success when positioning the device (Scan 5-1-2).

4. Lubricate the posterior surface of the LMA™ with a water-soluble lubricant just before insertion.

5. Preoxygenate (do not hyperventilate) the patient.

6. If there is no danger of spine injury, position the patient with the neck flexed and the head extended. If the mechanism of injury suggests the potential for spine injury, the patient's head and neck must be maintained in a neutral position.

7. Hold the LMA™ like a pen, with the index finger placed at the junction of the cuff and the tube (Scan 5-1-3). Under direct vision, press the tip of the cuff upward against the hard palate and flatten the cuff against it (Scan 5-1-4). The black line on the airway tube should be oriented anteriorly toward the upper lip.

8. Use the index finger to guide the LMA™, pressing upward and backward toward the ears in one smooth movement (Scan 5-1-5). Advance the LMA™ into the hypopharynx until definite resistance is felt (Scan 5-1-6).

9. Before removing the index finger, gently press down on the tube with the other hand to prevent the LMA™ from being pulled out of place (Scan 5-1-7).

10. Without holding the tube, inflate the cuff with just enough air to obtain a seal. The maximum volumes are shown in Table 5-1. When inflating, the LMA™ may move slightly as it seats. Holding the tube will prevent this movement and not allow a seal over the glottic opening.

11. Connect the LMA™ to the bag-valve mask and employ manual ventilation of less than 20 cm H_2O. (This precludes use of an FROPVD, unless you use one that allows you to set the pressure.) As with the supraglottic airways (BIADs), you must see the chest rise, hear breath sounds, feel good compliance, and hear no breath sounds over the epigastrium to be sure that the LMA™ is correctly placed. However, this confirmation method can be unreliable, so use of capnography to confirm and monitor tube position is recommended.

12. Insert a bite block (not an oropharyngeal airway), and secure the LMA™ with tape or a commercial tube holder (Scan 5-1-8). Remember that the LMA™ does not protect the airway from aspiration. If the patient becomes conscious, the LMA™ must be removed. Extubation is likely to cause vomiting, so be prepared to suction the pharynx and turn the backboard.

Pharmacologically Assisted Laryngeal Mask (PALM) Insertion

Airway management is a key intervention to ensure good patient outcome. Accumulating information from studies suggests that intubation in the field can in some populations worsen outcomes. This is felt to be due to hypoxia occurring during prolonged intubation attempts. As previously mentioned, BIADs can provide effective airways in trauma patients. A major contraindication for their use is an intact gag reflex. In the PALM technique, sedation and paralytics are administered, as in drug-assisted intubation (DAI), to achieve conditions that allow the insertion of an LMA™ (or other BIAD).

The assessment for a difficult airway is the same as with intubation as is the preparation of the device, medications, rescue airway plan, and preoxygenation. (See section on drug assisted intubation that follows.) The emergency care provider must be

SCAN 5-1 Insertion of the Laryngeal Mask Airway

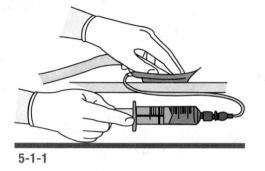

5-1-1

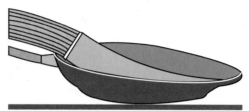

5-1-2

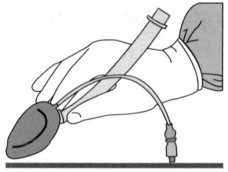

5-1-3

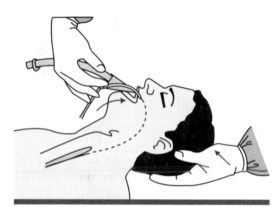

5-1-4

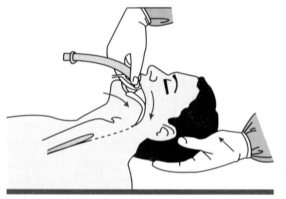

5-1-5

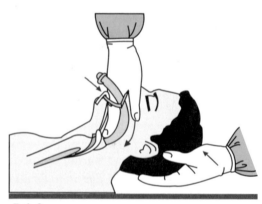

5-1-6

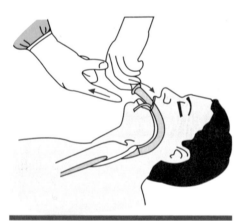

5-1-7

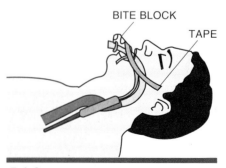

BITE BLOCK

TAPE

5-1-8

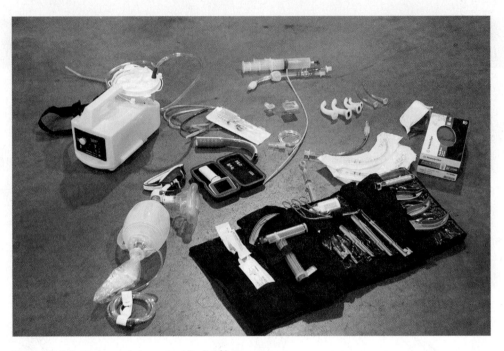

Figure 5-20 Equipment necessary for intubation.

absolutely sure that the airway can be maintained with a bag-valve mask in case insertion of the BIAD is unsuccessful.

Confirmation of the airway is best achieved by use of capnography as described elsewhere in the text. A major advantage to this technique is that it is more rapid than endotracheal intubation, decreasing the risk of hypoxia.

Advanced Airway Management

Preparation for Intubation

Whatever the method of intubation used, both patients and emergency care providers should be prepared for the procedure. The following equipment is considered basic to all intubation procedures (Figure 5-20):

- *Gloves.* Protective gloves such as latex or nitrile examining gloves (not necessarily sterile) should be worn for all intubation procedures.
- *Eye protection.* Providers must wear goggles or face shield.
- *Oxygenation devices.* All patients should be ventilated by way of a bag-valve mask or should breathe high-flow oxygen (at least 12 liters per minute) for several minutes prior to the attempt, using either a face mask or via nasal cannula. This will "wash out" residual nitrogen in the lungs and decrease the risk of hypoxia during the intubation process. Apneic oxygenation is discussed in the section on drug-assisted intubation.

Check all oxygenation devices, and keep them at hand in an organized kit (Figure 5-21). For laryngoscopic intubation, the ETT should be held in a "field hockey stick" or open "J" shape by a malleable stylet that is first lubricated and inserted until the distal end is just proximal to the side hole of the ETT. Check the cuff of the ETT by inflating it with 10 cc of air. Completely remove the air, and leave the syringe filled with air attached to the pilot tube. Lubricate the cuff and distal end of the tube.

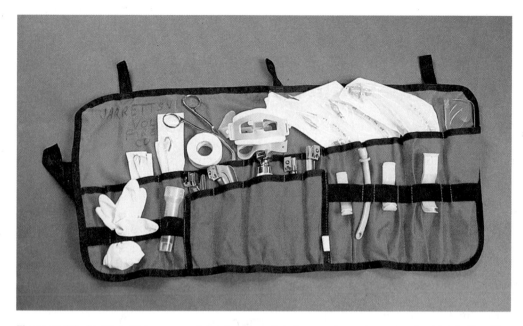

Figure 5-21 An intubation wrap contains the essentials for carrying out endotracheal intubation. The kit folds on itself and is compact and portable. When opened, it provides a clean working surface.

Have the capnography unit turned on and the waveform visible on the monitor. Record the baseline waveform and CO_2 levels while oxygenating the lungs prior to intubation.

The suction unit must be immediately at hand.

An assistant should be available to help in the procedure. The assistant can help hold the head and neck in a neutral position or perform external laryngeal manipulation to help make the cords visible to the emergency care provider.

Laryngoscopic Orotracheal Intubation

For laryngoscopic orotracheal intubation, the upper airway and the glottic opening are visualized, and the tube is slipped gently through the cords. The advantages of this method include the ability to see obstructions and to visualize the accurate placement of the tube. It has the disadvantage of requiring a relatively relaxed patient without anatomic distortion and with minimal bleeding or secretions.

The equipment needed for a laryngoscopic orotracheal intubation includes the following:

- Straight (Miller) or curved (Macintosh) blade and laryngoscope handle, all in good working order (checked daily), in multiple sizes including pediatric sizes.
- Transparent ETT, 28 to 33 cm in length and 7, 7.5, or 8 mm in internal diameter for the adult patient. Pediatric size tubes should also be available.
- Stylet to help mold the tube into a configuration to make insertion easier.
- Water-soluble lubricant. There is no need for it to contain a local anesthetic.
- 10 or 12 cc syringe for inflating the balloon
- Magill forceps
- Tape and tincture of benzoin or ETT holder
- Suction equipment in good working order with catheters and Yankauer tonsil sucker.
- Pulse oximeter and capnography unit
- A bougie (tracheal tube introducer) for difficult intubations

Procedure

Laryngoscopic Orotracheal Intubation

Intubation in the trauma patient differs from the usual endotracheal intubation in that the patient's neck must be stabilized in the neutral position during the procedure. This does make it more difficult to visualize the vocal cords during laryngoscopy. After ventilation and initial preparations, the following steps should be carried out (Figure 5-22; Scan 5-2):

1. An assistant stabilizes the head and neck, and counts slowly aloud to 30 (at your request).

2. In the supine patient, lift the chin, and slide the blade into the right side of the patient's mouth. Push the tongue to the left, and "inch" the blade down along the tongue in an attempt to see the epi-

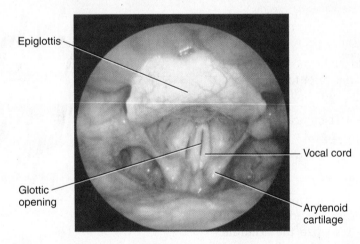

Figure 5-22 Landmarks during intubation.

Epiglottis

Glottic opening

Vocal cord

Arytenoid cartilage

glottis. A key maneuver must be performed here: The blade must pull forward (up) on the tongue to lift up the epiglottis and bring it into view.

3. Use the laryngoscope blade to lift the tongue and epiglottis up and forward in a straight line. "Levering" the blade is an error and can result in broken teeth and other trauma. The laryngoscope is essentially a "hook" to lift the tongue and epiglottis up and out of the way so that the glottic opening can be identified. Remember that the Miller (straight) blade is used to lift the epiglottis directly, whereas the Macintosh (curved) blade is inserted into the vallecula and lifts the epiglottis indirectly.

4. Advance the tube along the right side of the oropharynx once the epiglottis is seen. When the glottic opening (or even just the arytenoid cartilages) is identified, pass the tube through to a depth of about 5 cm beyond the cords. The mark on the tube that is even with the teeth should be three times the diameter of the ET tube. Thus, an 8.0 mm tube in an adult should be at 24 cm.

5. While the tube is still held firmly, remove the stylet, inflate the cuff, attach a bag-valve mask, and check the tube for placement using the immediate confirmation protocol given in the paragraphs that follow.

6. Begin ventilation using adequate oxygen concentration and tidal volume. Maintain an ETCO$_2$ level between 35 and 45 mm Hg.

For difficult intubations where you cannot see the cords or where the angle is such that it is difficult to advance the tube through the cords, a tracheal tube introducer (also called a bougie or gum elastic bougie) can be very helpful (Scan 5-3). Insert the bougie through the cords, and then slip the tube over the bougie and slide it down through the cords. This technique works best when the intubating emergency care provider keeps the blade inserted and the assistant threads the ET tube onto the bougie and holds the end of the bougie. The intubating emergency care provider then threads the ET tube down the bougie through the cords. By maintaining direct visualization, the chance of the ET tube becoming caught on the tongue or epiglottis is reduced. Then remove the bougie and perform the procedural steps 5 and 6 listed earlier.

If still having difficulty visualizing the vocal cords, the emergency care provider can take his right hand and, using gentle pressure, manipulate the thyroid (laryngeal) cartilage to bring the vocal cords into view. This process is known as *external laryngeal manipulation (ELM)*. The assistant is then instructed to maintain the positioning

SCAN 5-2 Laryngoscopic Orotracheal Intubation

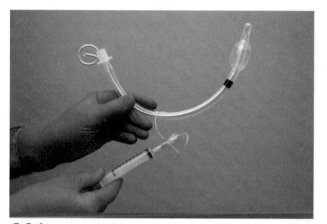

5-2-1 Assemble, prepare, and test all equipment.
(Photo courtesy of Louis B. Mallory, MBA, REMT-P)

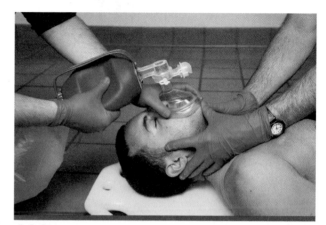

5-2-2 Position the patient's head and ventilate him with 100% oxygen. Do not hyperventilate. *(Photo courtesy of Louis B. Mallory, MBA, REMT-P)*

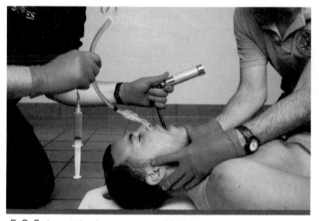

5-2-3 Insert the laryngoscope blade. *(Photo courtesy of Louis B. Mallory, MBA, REMT-P)*

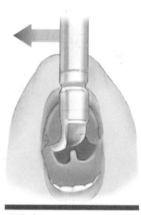

5-2-4 Lift the tongue and epiglottis to bring the glottic opening into view.

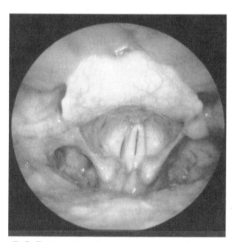

5-2-5 Visualize the cords and glottic opening, and insert the ET tube with stylet through the cords.

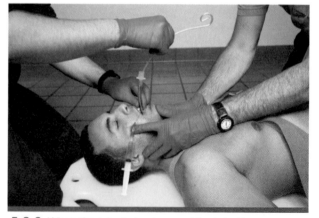

5-2-6 When the tube is in place and firmly held, remove the stylet. *(Photo courtesy of Louis B. Mallory, MBA, REMT-P)*

(continued)

SCAN 5-2 Laryngoscopic Orotracheal Intubation (*continued*)

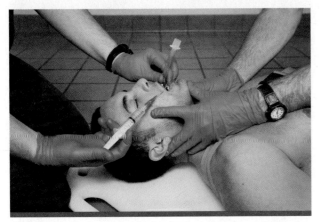

5-2-7 Continuing to hold tube firmly, inflate the cuff with 5 to 10 cc of air. *(Photo courtesy of Louis B. Mallory, MBA, REMT-P)*

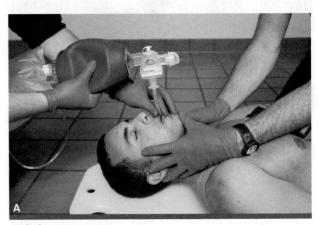

5-2-8a If capnography is not available, begin ventilation with colorimetric CO_2 detector. *(Photo courtesy of Louis B. Mallory, MBA, REMT-P)*

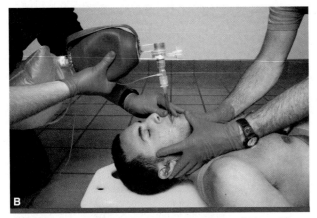

5-2-8b If capnography is available, begin ventilation with capnography monitor. *(Photo courtesy of Louis B. Mallory, MBA, REMT-P)*

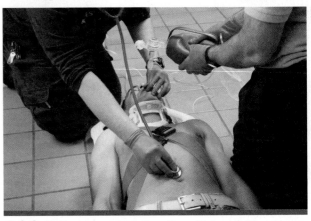

5-2-9 Perform manual confirmation of tube position using a stethoscope. *(Photo courtesy of Louis B. Mallory, MBA, REMT-P)*

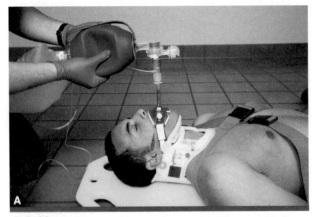

5-2-10a Secure the tube in place and continue ventilating.
(Photo courtesy of Louis B. Mallory, MBA, REMT-P)

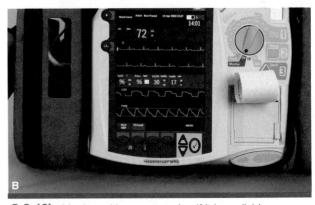

5-2-10b Monitor with capnography, if it is available.
(Photo courtesy of Louis B. Mallory, MBA, REMT-P)

SCAN 5-3 Orotracheal Intubation Using Bougie

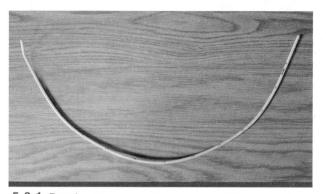

5-3-1 Bougie. *(Photo courtesy of Stanley Cooper, EMT-P)*

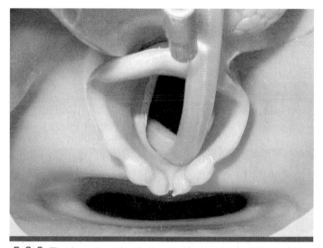

5-3-3 The bougie going between the cords and through the glottic opening. *(Photo courtesy of Roy Alson, PhD, MD, FACEP, FAAEM)*

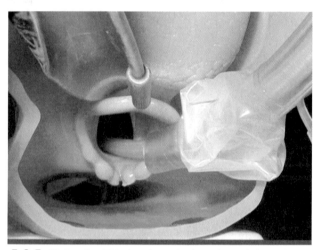

5-3-5 Sliding the ET tube down the bougie and through the cords. *(Photo courtesy of Roy Alson, PhD, MD, FACEP, FAAEM)*

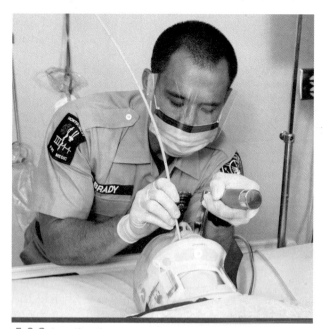

5-3-2 Inserting the bougie into the trachea. *(Photo courtesy of Stanley Cooper, EMT-P)*

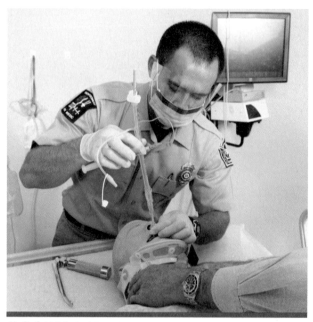

5-3-4 While holding the bougie firmly, slide the ET tube over the bougie and into the trachea. *(Photo courtesy of Stanley Cooper, EMT-P)*

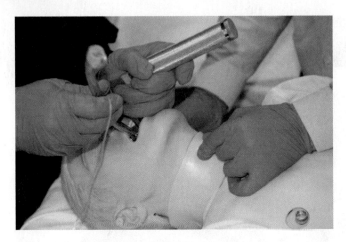

Figure 5-23 External laryngeal manipulation (ELM). Grasp the thyroid cartilage, and move the larynx around to better visualize the vocal cords. *(Photo courtesy of Bob Page, MEd, NRP, CCP, NCEE)*

of the cartilage, and the emergency care provider passes the tube. (See Figure 5-23.)

Nasotracheal Intubation

The nasotracheal route of endotracheal intubation in a prehospital setting may be justified when you cannot open the adult patient's mouth because of clenched jaws and when you cannot ventilate the patient by other means. The disadvantages of this method are its relative difficulty, depending as it does on the appreciation of the intensity of the breath sounds of spontaneously breathing patients, the longer duration to achieve intubation, and the need for the patient to be breathing on his own. It is a blind procedure and as such requires extra skill and care to successfully perform proper intratracheal placement. With the advent of pharmacologically assisted intubation, this technique is being used less frequently. Facial fractures, head injury, and a patient who is taking anticoagulants are all relative contraindications to using nasotracheal intubation.

Guidance of the tube through the glottic opening is a question of you perceiving the intensity of the sound of the patient breathing out. You can, with some difficulty, guide the tube toward the point of maximum intensity and slip it through the cords. You can hear and feel the breath sounds better with your ear placed against the proximal opening of the tube.

Emergency care providers must always be cautious and wear personal protective equipment when performing this procedure. Commercial adaptors are now available to do this without contaminating yourself or your equipment (Figure 5-24).

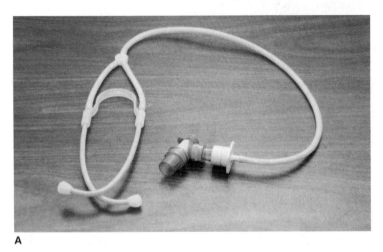

A

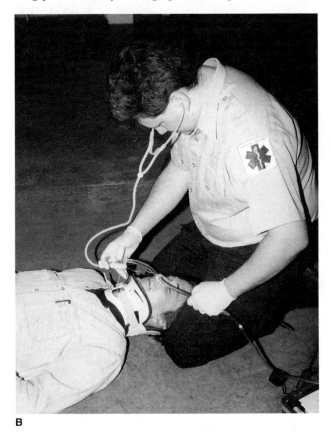

B

Figure 5-24 (A) Example of a commercial nasotracheal tube auscultation device (Burden nasoscope) used to (B) better hear breath sounds while inserting the nasotracheal tube. *(Photos courtesy of Brant Burden, EMT-P)*

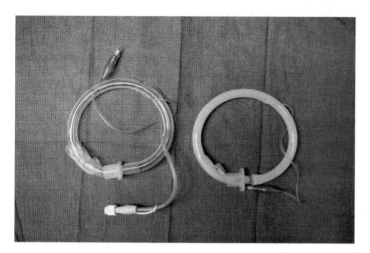

Figure 5-25 Prepare a tube for nasotracheal intubation by inserting the distal end of a 7 mm tube into its proximal opening, thus molding it into a formed circle. *(Photo courtesy of Stanley Cooper, EMT-P)*

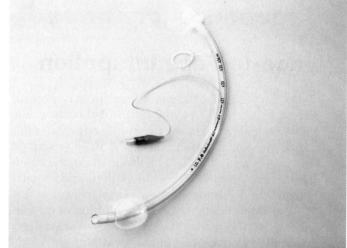

Figure 5-26 Commercial ET tube made for performing nasotracheal intubation. *(Image used with permission from Nellcor Puritan Bennett LLC, Boulder, Colorado, doing business as Covidien)*

The success of this method also will depend on an anterior curve to the tube that will prevent it from passing into the esophagus. Prepare two tubes prior to carrying out the intubation attempt. Insert the distal end of the 7 mm tube into its proximal opening, thus molding it into a formed circle (Figure 5-25). Preparing two tubes allows the immediate use of the second, more rigid tube should the first plastic tube become warm with body temperature, thus losing its anterior curve. Some commercial ETTs can be made to assume this curved shape by pulling on an embedded nylon cord (Figure 5-26). Displacing the tongue and jaw forward also can help in achieving placement because this maneuver lifts the epiglottis anteriorly out of the way of the advancing tube. Please use caution when pulling on this cord because an overzealous tug can cause the tip of the tube to miss the mark or come out of the patient's mouth.

Procedure

Nasotracheal Intubation

1. Perform routine preparation procedures.
2. Lubricate the cuff and distal end of a 7 mm or 7.5 mm ETT. With the bevel against the floor or septum of the nasal cavity, slip the tube distally through the largest naris. Insert along the floor of the nasal cavity at a 90-degree angle to the face.
3. When the tube tip reaches the posterior pharyngeal wall, take great care on "rounding the bend," and then direct the tube toward the glottic opening.
4. By watching the neck at the laryngeal prominence, you can judge the approximate placement of the tube. Tenting of the skin on either side of the prominence indicates that the tube is caught up in the pyriform fossa, a problem solved by slight withdrawal and rotation of the tube to the midline.

Bulging and anterior displacement of the laryngeal prominence usually indicate that the tube has entered the glottic opening and has been correctly placed. At this point the patient, especially if not deeply comatose, will cough, strain, or both. This may be alarming to the novice emergency care provider, who might interpret this as laryngospasm or misplacement of the tube. The temptation may be to pull the tube and ventilate because the patient may not breathe immediately. Holding your hand or ear over the opening of the tube to detect airflow may reassure you that the tube is correctly placed, and you may inflate the cuff and begin ventilation.

5. Confirm tube placement using the immediate confirmation protocol listed in the following section.

(continued)

Procedure (*continued*)

Face-to-Face Intubation

On occasion the location of the victim may prevent access to his head to allow for intubation from the conventional position. A face-to-face approach (also called the tomahawk method) has been described and used successfully. Using this method, the emergency care provider faces the patient and usually utilizes the Macintosh (curved) laryngoscope blade. An assistant maintains a neutral position of the cervical spine, if possible. The emergency care provider holds the laryngoscope in his hand with the blade end of the handle emerging from the thumb side of the fist, so that the blade can "hook" the tongue.

Preparation of equipment is as previously mentioned, including having mechanical suction immediately available. Entering from the right side of the mouth, the tongue is swept to the left of the mouth, and the jaw and tongue are pulled toward the emergency care provider, allowing for visualization of the larynx and insertion of the ET tube. This technique is very effective with patients in a seated position, such as one trapped in a motor vehicle. It also can be used with morbidly obese patients on whom the emergency care provider is not able to generate sufficient leverage to move the jaw forward.

Confirmation of Tube Placement

One of the greatest challenges of intubation is ensuring the correct intratracheal placement of ETTs. An unrecognized esophageal intubation is a lethal complication of this life-saving procedure. Every effort must be made to avoid this catastrophe, and a strict protocol must be followed to reduce the risk. The emergency care provider should remain vigilant in noting the depth marking at the mouth or nose and to continually reassess the tube to ensure that it has not moved or become dislodged. The emergency care provider should perform ongoing confirmation of the tube placement and also document this on the appropriate form.

Although the most reliable method of ensuring proper placement is actually visualizing the tube passing through the glottic opening, even this is not 100% sure. In fact, it is only reliable for the moment you see it. The gold standard for confirming and monitoring ETT placement is waveform capnography. (See later discussion.) If you do not have capnography available, the following protocol may be used but is not 100% reliable. When you use this protocol, you should recognize the unreliable nature of auscultation as the sole method of confirming intratracheal placement.

Correct intratracheal placement is indicated by the following initial signs:

- An anterior displacement of the laryngeal prominence is visible or felt as the tube is passed distally.
- Adequate chest rise occurs with each ventilation.
- Auscultation of breath sounds as described later.
- There is coughing, bucking, or straining on the part of the patient who is not sedated and paralyzed. Note: Phonation—any noise made with the vocal cords—is absolute evidence that the tube is in the esophagus, and the tube should be removed immediately.
- There is normal compliance with bag ventilation. (The bag does not suddenly "collapse," but rather there is some resilience to it and resistance to lung inflation.)
- No cuff leak is seen after inflation. (Persistent leak indicates esophageal intubation until proven otherwise.)
- There is breath condensation on the tube with each ventilation—not a very reliable method.

The following procedure should then be carried out immediately to prove correct placement.

Procedure

Confirmation of Tube Placement

1. Auscultate three sites as shown in Figure 5-27.
   a. Epigastrium—the most important—should be silent, with no sounds heard.
   b. Right and left midaxillary lines to confirm equal breath sounds and to ensure tube is not in right mainstem bronchi.

2. Inspect for full movement of the chest with ventilation.

3. Check position using one of the CO_2 detecting devices or a suction bulb or syringe AKA esophageal detector device (EDD).

4. Watch for any change in the pulse oximeter reading or in the patient's skin color. Also observe the ECG monitor for changes.

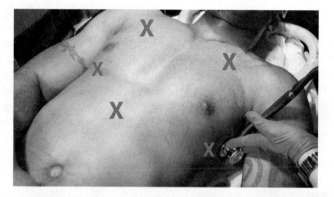

Figure 5-27 Sites to auscultate when performing immediate confirmation of ET tube placement are marked by a red X. They include the lateral chest, anterior chest, and epigastrium.

Commercial suction bulbs or EDDs have been used for confirmation of tube placement (Figure 5-28). Recent research suggests that they are less reliable than capnography, which has become the gold standard for confirming initial tube placement. (Capnography is the best method for confirming ET placement and allows for constant monitoring of tube position.)

To use a bulb detector, squeeze the bulb and insert the end onto the 15 mm adapter on the ETT. *Do this before you inflate the cuff on the ETT.* Release the bulb. If the tube is in the trachea, the bulb will expand immediately. If the tube is in the esophagus, the bulb will remain collapsed. If you are using a syringe with an adapter to the ETT, you will be able to withdraw the EDD syringe plunger easily when the tube is in the trachea, but you will not be able to withdraw the plunger if the tube is in the esophagus.

Note that the literature about the bulb detector and the EDD warn that patients with obstructed airway diseases, congestive heart failure, obesity, pregnancy, or right mainstem intubation may have a false-positive reading due to decreased air available

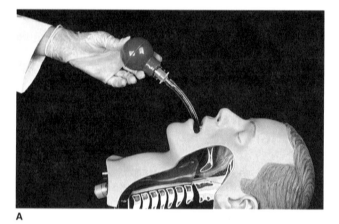
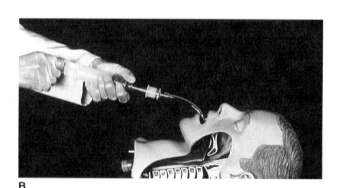

A   B

Figure 5-28 (A) Esophageal intubation detector device bulb style. (B) Esophageal intubation detector device, syringe style.

for aspiration. Some studies have shown poor sensitivity with children under one year of age and with patients in cardiac arrest.

Commercial CO_2 detectors also are available to attach in-line between the ETT and the bag-valve mask. Three different kinds are available: qualitative (colorimetric) CO_2 detectors, quantitative CO_2 monitors, and quantitative waveform CO_2 monitors. (See the detailed discussion of the monitors in the following section, "Using Capnometry and Capnography to Confirm and Monitor ET Tube Position.")

Apply the protocol for confirmation of tube placement immediately following intubation. If you are using a quantitative CO_2 monitor or quantitative waveform CO_2 monitor, then you may continue monitoring ET tube position with those devices. If you are not using one of those devices, then repeat the ET tube position reconfirmation protocol after several minutes of ventilation. Thereafter, repeat the reconfirmation protocol after movement of the patient from the ground to the stretcher, after loading onto the ambulance, when you perform the ITLS Secondary Survey and ITLS Ongoing Exam, and immediately prior to arrival at the hospital.

Procedure

Reconfirming ET Tube Position

1. Auscultate the sites shown in Figure 5-29.
   a. Epigastrium—should be silent with no sounds heard.
   b. Right and left midaxillary lines
   c. Right and left apex
   d. Sternal notch—"tracheal" sounds should be readily heard here.

2. Inspect the chest for full movement of the chest with ventilation.

3. Use adjuncts such as CO_2 detectors (or a suction bulb, if part of local protocol) to help confirm placement.

Any time placement is still in doubt despite the preceding protocol, visualize directly or remove the tube. Never assume that the tube is in the right place. Always be sure, and record that the protocol has been carefully followed.

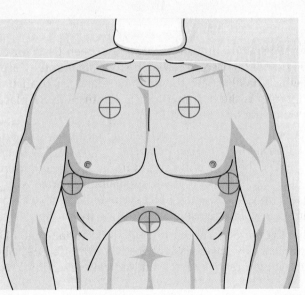

Figure 5-29 Sites to auscultate when performing reconfirmation of ET tube placement.

Using Capnometry and Capnography to Confirm and Monitor ET Tube Position

Capnometry represents a major clinical upgrade in the assessment and monitoring of the ventilatory status of the patients. It is important for you to understand the differences between simple detection of ETCO2 called colorimetric or qualitative capnometry, quantitative capnometry (a value without a waveform), and the most useful and diagnostic form known as quantitative waveform capnography.

Colorimetric CO_2 detectors (qualitative capnometry) are simple devices designed to detect $ETCO_2$ (Figure 5-30). They do not accurately measure the amount of CO_2. Typically, the devices use a special piece of "litmus paper" that changes color from purple to yellow as it detects CO_2. If a device of this type is used as a confirming device, you must be aware of the following:

- It may not be accurate in poor perfusion states, such as shock or cardiac arrest, due to very small amounts of CO_2 returning to the lungs. In those cases, another confirming device is necessary. In cases of cardiac arrest, best results will be obtained if good compressions are being done at the time the device is used.
- Although the device will change color upon exposure to CO_2, to ensure that any trapped CO_2 in the stomach is purged, it is necessary to give six ventilations prior to confirming that the ETT is in the trachea.
- If the device gets wet with gastric contents, blood, or secretions, it will no longer function correctly.
- Once intubated, the device may be used intermittently as part of the confirmation process only because it will stay yellow after a few minutes of continuous exposure to CO_2.
- Because the device only detects $ETCO_2$ and does not provide a quantifiable measure, it cannot be used to monitor ventilation.

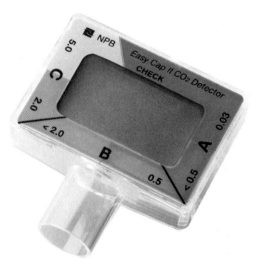

Figure 5-30 Colorimetric CO_2 detector.

(Image used by permission from Nellcor Puritan Bennett LLC, Boulder, Colorado, doing business as Covidien)

Quantitative capnometry actually measures the amount of CO_2 in expired air ($ETCO_2$). More than just detection, the device can be used to monitor the adequacy of ventilations and help the provider to accurately "titrate" the $ETCO_2$ levels in patients where CO_2 levels are critical, such as those with closed head injuries. They are often combined with a pulse oximeter. Quantitative capnometry refers to $ETCO_2$ measurement without a waveform. If the devices are used to confirm tube placement, you must be aware of the following limitations:

- Cardiac arrest patients have a low $ETCO_2$ that is commonly < 20 mm Hg, depending on how long they have been in arrest and how effective resuscitation efforts are.
- Colorimetric devices can detect esophageal CO_2, so six breaths are necessary to actually confirm tracheal position with CO_2 from the lung.
- In cases of cardiac arrest, best results are obtained if good compressions are being performed while the device is being used.

Quantitative waveform capnography is the ultimate confirmation device and is a standard of care in surgical suites and many EMS systems. The devices not only detect and measure the $ETCO_2$ but also provide you with a diagnostic waveform that can confirm (by the shape of the waveform) endotracheal placement even in low perfusion states. The waveforms will appear within two seconds of the actual breath. Furthermore, the devices can be built into existing cardiac monitors, which will allow you to continuously monitor the waveform and value (Figure 5-31). They also will allow you to print out a real-time waveform that is time and date stamped for absolute documentation of correct tube placement.

Capnography has many other uses in nonintubated patients, including perfusion monitor, airway monitor, and ventilation monitor. In using capnography to confirm ETT placement, you must be aware of the following limitations:

- Like all CO_2 detection devices, low perfusion states will result in low CO_2 readings and subsequently small waveforms (Figure 5-32). In arrest situations, good compressions should be done as the waveforms are being evaluated. This will increase the size of the waveform.

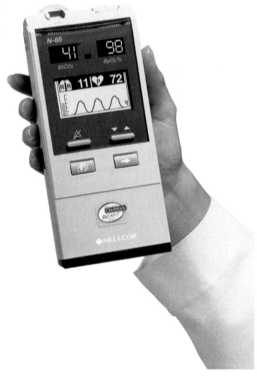

Figure 5-31 Quantitative waveform CO_2 monitor incorporated into cardiac monitor. *(Image used by permission from Nellcor Puritan Bennett LLC, Boulder, Colorado, doing business as Covidien)*

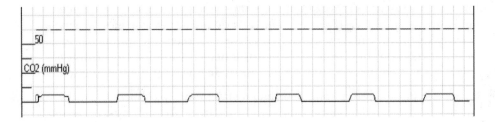

Figure 5-32 Small capnography means poor perfusion.

- To use the devices in conjunction with your cardiac monitors, you must enable the waveform display on the monitor screen before intubation. A delay of 10 to 30 seconds for warm-up (depending on the monitor) will ensue if you wait to activate it after placing the tube. For best results, have the capnography waveform default when the monitor is turned on.

Procedure

Confirming and Monitoring ET Tube Placement with Capnography

1. Prepare all equipment for intubation. Turn on the monitor, and attach the capnography filter line or wires to it. (This will vary depending on the brand of capnograph.) It is advisable to apply and record baseline capnography during preoxygenation prior to an intubation attempt to prevent inadvertent hyperventilation.

2. Place the ETT, and inflate the cuff. In cases of arrest, compressions should *not* be interrupted to perform this procedure.

3. Attach the capnography airway adapter on the ETT, and then attach the bag-valve mask to the airway adapter (Figure 5-33).

4. Ventilate the patient, and observe the waveform. The presence of a "square" pattern confirms tracheal placement (Figure 5-34). Print out the waveform, if possible (for documentation). If the waveform is nonexistent or appears in gross and irregular waveform patterns, the tube is possibly in the esophagus or hypopharynx. In pediatrics, small tube size may limit CO_2 readings because some air may go around the tube and, thus, is not detectable by the capnogram. Use a cuffed tube in those cases, and the waveform and CO_2 readings should improve.

5. Listen for breath sounds midaxillary on each side to rule out right mainstem intubation.

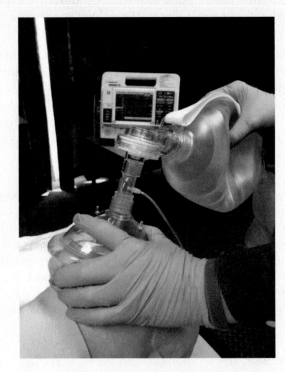

Figure 5-33 A capnography airway adapter is placed between the mask and the bag. This allows continuous measurement and reduces risk of hypoventilation or hyperventilation. *(Photo courtesy of Bob Page, MEd, NRP, CCP, NCEE)*

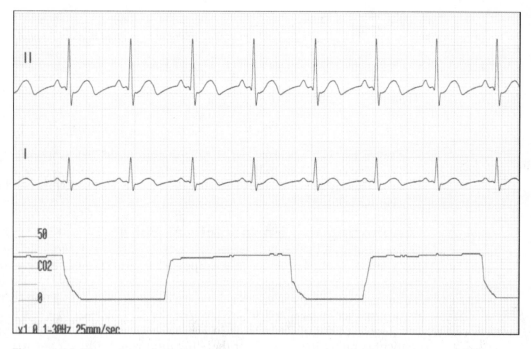

Figure 5-34 "Square" waveform is normal.

6. Secure the tube, and continually monitor the waveforms during transport. Carefully watch the $ETCO_2$ value to avoid inadvertent hypo- or hyperventilation (Figure 5-35).

7. On arrival at the receiving facility, print out another waveform (if available) to prove correct placement at the time of patient transfer.

8. On your run report, document the visualization of the vocal cords, attach the waveform printout(s) or document the presence, or upload the data to your electronic patient care record, if your EMS service uses such devices, and document equal breath sounds.

Capnography can also be used on a BIAD such as King Airway®, LMA®, Combitubes®, or others to confirm those and to monitor ventilations through these devices.

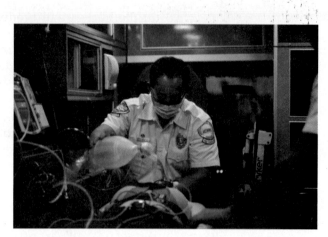

Figure 5-35 Monitoring the intubated patient.

Troubleshooting While Monitoring

- *Complete loss of waveform.* Apnea, or tube is dislodged or obstructed, or air may be leaking around the cuff.
- *Waveforms and values getting smaller.* Hyperventilation (check the depth and rate of ventilation) or hypoperfusion (shock, or loss of pulses). Remember, it is very easy to hyperventilate an intubated patient because the ventilating bag is not squeezed as fast or deep as it is with bag-valve-mask-only techniques. Also, airway pressure increases in the lungs following intubation. It is expected that hypoperfusion will have hypocapnia. However, rarely will you have hypoperfusion with normal or high $ETCO_2$.

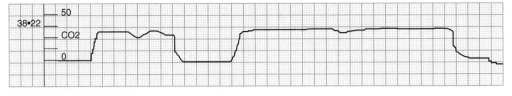

Figure 5-36 Capnogram showing a curare cleft. This may not be visible on the monitor, so it is important to print out the waveform. *(Photo courtesy of Bob Page, MEd, NRP, CCP, NCEE)*

- Waveform with a "curare cleft." Note the undulation in the waveform. This represents the diaphragm starting to recover from the effects of a neuromuscular blockade. This sign should alert you that the patient will probably need to be sedated (Figure 5-36).

Anchoring the Endotracheal Tube

Anchoring an ETT can be a frustrating exercise. Not only does it require some fine movements of the hands when you appear to be all thumbs, but it is also difficult to perform when ventilation, movement, or extrication is being carried out. Keep one thing in mind: There is no substitute for the human anchor. That is, an emergency care provider is assigned to ensure that the ETT is held fast and that it does not migrate in or out of the airway. To lose a tube can be a catastrophe, especially if the patient is rather inaccessible or the intubation was a difficult one to perform.

Fixing the ETT in place is important for several reasons. First, movement of the tube in the trachea will produce more mucosal damage and may increase the risk of postintubation complications. In addition, movement of the tube will stimulate the patient to cough, strain, or both, leading to cardiovascular and intracranial pressure changes that could be detrimental. Most important, there is a greater risk in the prehospital setting of dislodging a tube and losing control of the airway if it is not anchored solidly in place.

The ETT can be secured in place by either tape, umbilical tape made of woven cotton, or a commercially available tube holder. Although taping a tube in place is convenient and relatively easily done, it is not always effective. There is often a problem with the tape sticking to skin wet with rain, blood, airway secretions, or vomitus. If you are using tape, several principles should be followed:

- Insert an oropharyngeal airway to prevent the patient from biting down on the tube.
- Dry the patient's face and apply tincture of benzoin to better ensure proper adhesion of the tape.
- Carry the tape right around the patient's neck when anchoring the tube. Do not move the neck. Do not tie it so tight that it occludes the external jugular veins. Alternatively, you can secure the tube to the maxilla with the tape.
- Anchor the tube at the corner of the mouth, not in the midline.

Because of the difficulty of fixing the tube in place with tape, it may be better to use a commercial ETT holder that uses a strap to fix the tube in a plastic holder, which also acts as a bite block (Figure 5-37). Because flexion or extension of the patient's head can move the tube in or out of the airway by 2 or 3 cm, it is good practice to restrict head and neck movement of any patient who has an ETT in place. (This is even more important in children.) If the patient is spinal motion restricted because of the risk of cervical-spine injury, flexion and extension of the neck should be less of a concern.

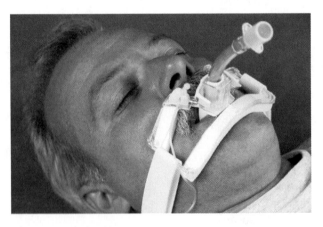

Figure 5-37 A commercial endotracheal tube holder.

Drug-Assisted Intubation (DAI)

Also known as medically assisted airway management (MAAM) or rapid sequence intubation [RSI]), this technique uses medications to sedate and relax the patient allowing for better visualization of the airway and increased success in intubating the patient. However, because the patient is rendered apneic, the emergency care provider must be able to provide airway and ventilation for the patient. Not all EMS systems allow use of paralytic drugs and may instead utilize sedation only to assist with intubation.

The importance in appropriately managing the airway of the trauma patient cannot be overemphasized. Loss of airway remains the leading cause of early preventable trauma deaths, and hypoxia has been shown to worsen outcomes for trauma patients, especially those with closed head injury. The indications for active airway management and the options managing the airway are well covered in Chapter 4. All emergency care providers should be familiar with the materials in Chapter 4 and this chapter and be able to apply the care described.

When EMS first obtained the ability to perform endotracheal intubation, it was essentially performed on "dead" patients, patients who were unresponsive and apneic. Not all patients fit this situation, and airway management of patients who were agitated, were combative, or had airway trauma had to wait until they deteriorated and became unresponsive.

It is important to remember that all airways managed in the field meet the American Society of Anesthesiology's definition of a difficult airway. Thus the emergency care provider must have many tools in the toolbox available to manage the airway of the trauma patient.

For many years EMS has made use of DAI to address such issues as the agitated and combative patient needing active airway management. The old term *rapid sequence intubation* is a misnomer because the procedure is certainly not rapid (Figure 5-38). Because of this, it can adversely affect patient outcome by prolonging scene time. Unless there is a critical need, the procedure should be performed during transport. In the urban setting where there are short transport times the need for a definitive airway should be balanced against use of other airway methods and the impact on transport times.

A variant of the practice of rapid sequence induction (RSI) used by anesthesiologists when confronted with a nonfasting patient, the DAI technique allows the emergency care provider to achieve conditions that improve the likelihood of intubating the patient, while minimizing the risks of aspiration by rapidly administering a sedative and paralytic to improve intubating conditions. In some jurisdictions, a paralytic is not used, and benzodiazepines and opiates in combination are administered to achieve intubating conditions.

Multiple studies have shown that EMS personnel can be effectively taught to use DAI and apply it in the field setting. Other studies have shown a potential for prolonged hypoxia during this procedure, so constant recording of pulse oximetry reading should be done, and there should be a strict quality improvement program that monitors intubation time, oxygenation of the patient, and scene time.

The actual technique of DAI is quite simple. The difficult part for EMS personnel is to recognize the patient who should not undergo DAI. The worst thing you can do in airway management is take a spontaneously breathing patient and place him into a "can't intubate and can't ventilate" situation. All personnel who utilize DAI should be familiar with and able to use one of the many supraglottic (blind insertion) airway devices (BIADs) and also should be able to perform a cricothyroidotomy if unable to ventilate or intubate the patient.

Last (but most important of all), all EMS personnel should be able to manage an airway using a bag-valve mask. Remember BLS comes before ALS. Some EMS

Drug-Assisted Intubation

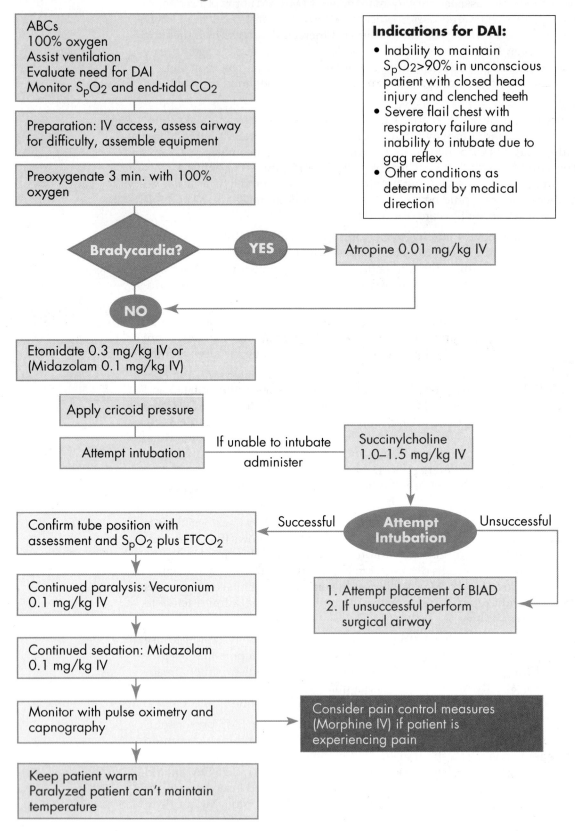

Figure 5-38 Steps in drug-assisted intubation.

providers erroneously see the use of DAI and even intubation as a measure of prestige. It is simply one of many tools available to manage an airway. The real trick is to choose the right one for your patient and correctly apply it. The other key to airway management is to have a backup plan ready to go just in the first approach does not work.

Performance of DAI in the field remains controversial. Some studies have shown worse outcomes in patients (especially serious head injuries) who undergo DAI in the field, and this is attributed to longer scene times as well as hypoxia during intubation. Other studies question whether this delay is significant. Also there is the related issue of transport times. Short times to definitive trauma care may allow for less-invasive airway management, as long as the airway can be kept open and adequate ventilation and oxygenation ensured.

Other concerns raised with this technique include skill retention on the part of field providers, something that is an issue for many of the advanced procedures performed by EMS.

The decision to implement the use of DAI by an EMS system should be carefully reviewed, especially with respect to issues of skill retention, transport times, and the availability of alternative airway methods. Any system using DAI must have in place a strong educational and quality improvement program.

The ideal approach uses the six Ps: preparation, preoxygenation, premedicate, paralyze, pass the tube, and confirm position. They are as follows:

- *Preparation.* First, evaluate the difficulty you may experience when you try to intubate. Do this by using the Mallampati score. (See Chapter 4, Table 4-1.) If the patient appears to be particularly difficult to intubate, you (and the patient) would be better served using a supraglottic BIAD or bag-valve mask than struggling with a paralyzed, apneic, hypoxic patient. If you decide to perform DAI, you should have a plan for an escape airway should intubation be unsuccessful. All necessary equipment, including suction, should be readily available and checked.

  Proper positioning is an important part of preparation. Although the EMS environment often precludes placing the patient at a good height on a stretcher in the sniffing position, any steps you can take to better position yourself so that you have the best view are helpful. Given that many of your patients are in spinal motion restriction, one positioning step you can take, just prior to intubation, is to remove or loosen the cervical collar and apply in-line stabilization. This will allow you to move the jaw forward and improve visualization of the cords.

  For obese patients, elevating the head of the bed while maintaining in-line spinal alignment may improve visualization of the airway and a successful intubation. Attempt to position the patient with the head of the bed elevated so that the suprasternal notch of the sternum is level with the opening of the ear canal.

- *Preoxygenation.* Because the patient will be rendered apneic, hypoxia will rapidly follow. To extend the time for intubation, nitrogen in the lungs is "washed out" by having the patient breathe 100% oxygen for two to three minutes. Washout of the nitrogen allows the patient to tolerate up to five minutes of apnea (only two to three minutes in children) during intubation without becoming hypoxic. In patients with airway compromise or other problems, ventilations can be assisted, though care should be made not to ventilate with too much force, thus reducing the risk of insufflating air into the stomach and thus regurgitation of stomach contents leading to aspiration. Previously, application of cricoid pressure (Sellick's maneuver) was thought to help reduce this, as well as reduce risk of aspiration as the lower esophageal sphincter relaxes after administration of paralytics. Recent studies have questioned the utility of cricoid pressure, and it should not be used. All patients should be placed on a cardiac monitor, a pulse oximeter, and a capnometer at this time, if not previously done.

Another useful technique to increase the time until the patient becomes critically hypoxic is apneic oxygenation. Instilling oxygen via a nasal cannula (> 8 liters per minute) maintains a high oxygen concentration gradient from the nasopharynx down to the alveoli. As oxygen is absorbed in the alveoli, more oxygen moves down this gradient into the alveoli, even if there is no ventilation. However, because there is no ventilation, carbon dioxide levels in the blood do rise, and with the hypercarbia, the patient does become acidotic.

- *Premedicate.* Both the act of intubation and some paralytics can raise intracranial pressure. Though advocated in the past, use of IV lidocaine prior to intubation has been found to be of no benefit in the field setting. Pediatric patients given succinylcholine may develop bradycardia. Most experts feel that pediatric patients and those adults receiving a repeat dose of succinylcholine should receive 0.1 mg/kg of atropine. Remember also in the pediatric patient that the use of a length-based system, such as the Broselow™ tape, can decrease dosing errors. Depolarizing paralytic agents like succinylcholine can cause fasciculations, which can cause a rise in both intracranial pressure and intraocular pressure as well as be uncomfortable for the patient. To prevent fasciculations, a nondepolarizing paralytic agent such as vecuronium at 0.01 mg per kg body weight can be given at three minutes prior to administering the depolarizing paralytic agent. Because it adds time to the process in what is often a time-critical situation, many field providers omit this step.

  The last premedication is the sedative. This ensures that the patient is not awake while paralyzed. Benzodiazepines such as versed at 0.1 mg per kg body weight can be used, although etomidate (0.3 mg per kg body weight) is a more common sedative agent and has the advantage of having minimal effects on hemodynamics. Some trauma surgeons do not support use of etomidate due to reported adrenal suppression, with even a single dose.

  Ketamine, a dissociative anesthetic agent, is another useful sedation agent for intubation. It is given at 1-2 mg per kg body weight. It is very effective with agitated patients, has some analgesic effects, and is less likely to depress the patient's respirations compared to other sedatives. Increased intracranial pressure is considered a relative contraindication to the use of ketamine, but as stated in Chapter 10, hypoxia markedly worsens the outcome of traumatic brain injuries.

- *Paralyze.* Two types of paralytics are available. A depolarizing agent, such as succinylcholine is the preferred agent due to rapid onset of action and rapid degradation. At a dose of 1 to 1.5 mg per kg body weight (2 mg per kg body weight in children), intubating conditions are achieved within 90 seconds of administration and is cleared within five minutes. Contraindications to use of depolarizing agents are listed in Table 5-2.

  Nondepolarizing agents have a longer onset and paralysis lasts longer. The fastest acting agent is rocuronium (0.5 mg per kg body weight adult; 0.75 mg per kg body weight in children). Vecuronium 0.1 mg per kg body weight can be used to maintain paralysis after intubation is successful. To reduce fasciculation a

---

Table 5-2: Contraindications for Use of Succinylcholine

- History of Malignant Hyperthermia
- Burns > 24 hours old
- Crush injury > 24 hours old
- Stroke, cord injury > 7 days, < 6 months
- Sepsis > 7 days
- Myopathies, denervating diseases

Table 5-3: Suggested Drug-Assisted Intubation Timeline

Time	Action
	Identify need for intubation
	Brief history if possible to rule out contraindications
−7 minutes	Prepare equipment and patient
−5 minutes	Preoxygenate
−3 minutes	Pretreat and sedate (note that pretreatment with defasciculating agent can be omitted)
0	Paralyze
0.75 to 1.5 minutes	Pass the tube
1.5 to 2 minutes	Confirm position
2 minutes	Postintubation care

pre-administration dose of 0.01 mg/kg may be delivered prior to the administration of a depolarizing agent.

- *Pass the tube.* Once intubating conditions are achieved, pass the tube. Aids in the process include the use of a stylet, the gum elastic bougie, and external laryngeal manipulation.
- *Confirm position.* Use techniques previously described. Use of capnography is mandatory so that inadvertent tube dislodgement can be detected. See the suggested timeline for DAI in Table 5-3.

Fiberoptic and Video Intubation

In the last decade there has been an exponential growth in the number and type of devices designed to improve visualization of the larynx and cords during intubation. For example, fiberoptic endoscopic intubation has been used for many years in the operating room. However, the size and complexity of the equipment limited its applicability in the field setting. Some of today's new systems use a variant of the optical scopes, which allows direct visualization of the cords and passage of the ET tube off the scope into the cords (Figure 5-39). Other systems make use of newly developed miniature video cameras that have the image projected on the screen that is either attached to the scope or adjacent to it (Figure 5-40).

Studies have shown an excellent success rate with many of the devices, and they have been proven to be very helpful in intubation of patients with difficult airways. The major drawback with many of the systems has been the cost of the equipment. However, as more manufacturers enter the market, the cost per unit continues to decrease, and with that, more of those types of devices will be in field use.

At this time, the use of the devices should not be considered a standard of care in the field setting nor do the authors of this text favor any particular system. For emergency response organizations that have adopted intubating devices, their use should be incorporated into airway management protocols. If available during training courses, personnel should be trained in the use of the devices, so long as such training does not detract from the instruction in the conventional devices used for airway management and stabilization.

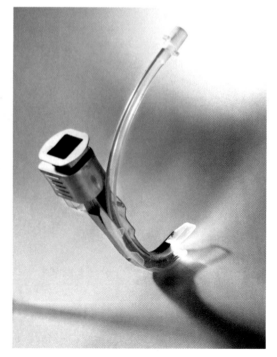

Figure 5-39 Example of fiberoptic intubation device (Airtraq Optical Laryngoscope). (Airtraq® is a registered trademark of Prodol Meditec S.A. Las Arenas Vizcaya Spain)

Figure 5-40 (A) Example of video intubation device (Glidescope Ranger). *(Photo courtesy of Verathon©)* (B) Example of a provider utilizing a King Vision Video Laryngoscope™.

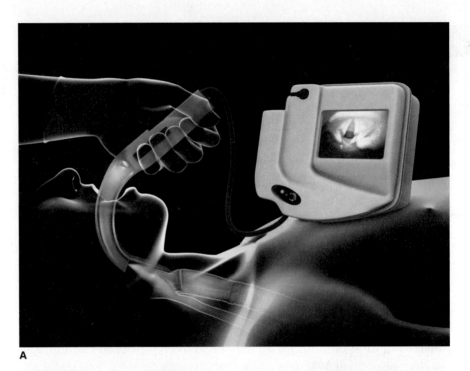

A

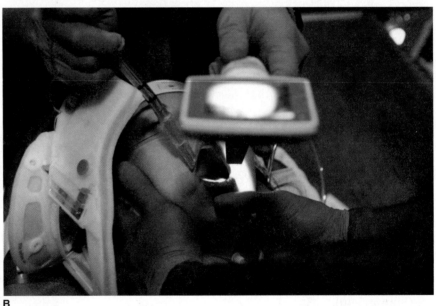

B

Bibliography

Davis, D. P., D. B. Hoyt, M. Ochs, D. Fortlage, T. Holbrook, L. K. Marshall, and P. Rosen. "The Effect of Paramedic Rapid Sequence Intubation on Outcome in Patients with Severe Traumatic Brain Injury." *Journal of Trauma* 54, No. 3 (March 2003): 444–53.

McGill, J. "Airway Management in Trauma: An Update." *Emergency Medicine Clinics of North America* 25, No. 3 (August 2007): 603–22.

Moss, R., K. Porter, I. Greaves, and Consensus Group Faculty of Pre-Hospital Care. "Pharmacologically Assisted Laryngeal Mask Insertion: A Consensus Statement." *Emergency Medicine Journal* 30, No. 12 (December 2013): 1073–75.

Orebaugh, S. L., and P. E. Bigeleisen. "Part II: Difficult Airway Management: Recognition, Training and Management," Chapters 9–15. In *Atlas of Airway Management: Tools and Techniques*. Philadelphia: Lippincott Williams and Wilkins, 2012.

Robinson, N., and M. Clancy. "In Patients with Head Injury Undergoing Rapid Sequence Intubation, Does Pretreatment with Intravenous Lignocaine/Lidocaine Lead to an Improved Neurological Outcome? A Review of the Literature." *Emergency Medicine Journal* 18, No. 6 (November 2001): 453–57.

Sivestri, S., G. A. Ralls, B. Krauss, J. Thundiyil, S. G. Rothrock, A. Senn, E. Carter, and J. Falk. "The Effectiveness of Out-of-Hospital Use of Continuous End-Tidal Carbon Dioxide Monitoring on the Rate of Unrecognized Misplaced Intubation Within a Regional Emergency Medical Services System." *Annals of Emergency Medicine* 45, No. 5 (May 2005): 497–503.

Takeda, T., K. Tanigawa, H. Tanaka, Y. Hayashi, E. Goto, and K. Tanaka. "The Assessment of Three Methods to Verify Tracheal Tube Placement in the Emergency Setting." *Resuscitation,* 56, no. 2 (February 2003): 153–57.

Walls, R. M, and M. F. Murphy. *Manual of Emergency Airway Management*, 4th ed. Philadelphia: Lippincott Williams and Wilkins, 2012.

Wang, H. E., D. F. Kupas, D. Hostler, R. Cooney, D. M. Yealy, and J. R. Lave. "Procedural Experience with Out-of-Hospital Endotracheal Intubation." *Critical Care Medicine* 33, no. 8 (August 2005): 1718–21.

Wang, H. E., D. P. Davis, R. E. O'Connor, and R. M. Domeier. "Drug Assisted Intubation in the Prehospital Setting (Joint Position Statement by NAEMSP and ACEP)." *Prehospital Emergency Care* 10, no. 2 (April–June 2006): 261–71.

Weingart, S. D., and R. M. Levitan. "Preoxygenation and Prevention of Desaturation During Emergency Airway Management." *Annals of Emergency Medicine* 59, No. 3 (March 2012): 165–75.

6

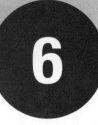

Thoracic Trauma

Graciela M. Bauzá, MD
Andrew B. Peitzman, MD, FACS

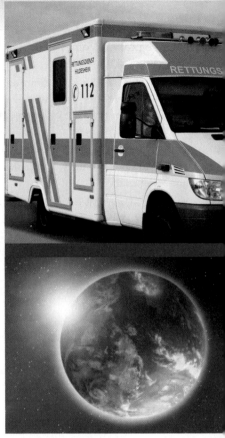

Trauma Toracico   Traumatismo Torácico   Traumatisme Thoracique

Urazy klatki piersiowej   Thorax Trauma   Ozljeda prsnog koša

إصابات القفص الصدري   torakalna trauma

Poškodbe prsnega koša   Mellkasi sérülés

(Ambulance photo © Maria P., Fotolia, LLC)

Key Terms

Beck's triad, *p. 137*
flail chest, *p. 129*
massive hemothorax, *p. 133*
mediastinum, *p. 126*
open pneumothorax, *p. 131*
paradoxical pulse, *p. 137*
pericardial tamponade, *p. 137*
pleural space, *p. 125*
simple pneumothorax, *p. 142*
tension pneumothorax, *p. 135*

Objectives

Upon successful completion of this chapter, you should be able to:

1. Identify the major symptoms of thoracic trauma.
2. Describe the signs of thoracic trauma.
3. List the immediate life-threatening thoracic injuries.
4. Define flail chest in relation to associated physical findings and management.
5. Explain the pathophysiology and management of an open pneumothorax.
6. Explain the hypovolemic and respiratory compromise pathophysiology and management in massive hemothorax.
7. Describe the clinical signs of a tension pneumothorax in conjunction with appropriate management. Contrast those with the clinical signs of massive hemothorax.
8. List three indications to perform emergency chest decompression.
9. Identify the physical findings (including Beck's triad) of cardiac tamponade.
10. Explain the cardiac involvement and management associated with blunt injury to the chest.

Chapter Overview

The thoracic cage protects multiple vital organs, including the lungs, heart, great vessels, and spinal cord, as well as the liver, stomach, spleen, pancreas, kidneys, and transverse colon. Injury to those organs can result in early death. However, when thoracic injuries are recognized and treated appropriately, many patients will survive.

Injuries to the chest may be caused by motor-vehicle collisions (MVCs), motorcycle collisions (MCCs), falls, firearms, knives, crush, and other blunt and penetrating mechanisms. It is common in the multiple-trauma patient and responsible for 20% to 25% of all trauma-related deaths. When the mechanism suggests thoracic trauma, you must quickly assess for life-threatening injuries (causing hypoxia or hemorrhage), perform life-saving maneuvers, and transport the patient to the appropriate trauma center without delaying care. This chapter will discuss critical injuries to the chest and associated organs and the interventions that may give the patient the best chance for survival.

Case Presentation

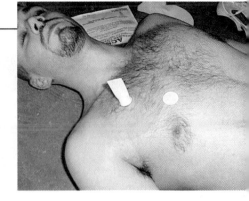

You are the lead emergency care provider transporting a motorcyclist involved in a multiple-vehicle, multiple-patient collision to the closest trauma center. The motorcyclist is critically injured with a major hemorrhage to the left leg controlled with a tourniquet, possible right pneumothorax, blunt traumatic brain injury, and intra-abdominal injury. During transport he developed airway problems and required intubation, which was successfully performed. Having re-established an airway, the lead emergency care provider performs the ITLS Ongoing Exam. The patient remains unresponsive. While the second emergency care provider assists ventilation to maintain a rate of one breath every eight seconds and an ETCO$_2$ of 35 to 40 mm Hg, the lead emergency care provider notes that the patient exhibits some cyanosis around the mouth. Upon questioning, the second emergency care provider, who is ventilating the patient, observes that the patient is becoming increasingly difficult to ventilate.

Before proceeding, consider these questions: How would you approach this situation? Because the patient's condition seems to have changed, what is the next thing you would do? Keep these questions in mind as you read through the chapter. Then, at the end of the chapter, find out how the emergency care providers managed this patient.

The Thorax

Anatomy

The ribs, 12 pairs of them, encircle the thoracic organs from spine to sternum (Figure 6-1). The chest wall is comprised of skin, subcutaneous tissue, muscle, ribs, and the neurovascular bundle (Figure 6-2). Note that the neurovascular bundle runs around the lower border of the ribs. This is an important anatomical feature if you have to perform needle decompression of the chest.

The structures within the chest but above the diaphragm include the lungs, the lower trachea and mainstem bronchi, the heart and great vessels, and the esophagus. The adult thoracic cavity can hold up to three liters of blood on each side. This means that half of the circulating blood volume (6 liters or 12 units) can end up in either the right or left hemithorax without any sign of external bleeding.

The lungs are a pair of spongy and elastic organs lined by the pleura, a thin slippery membrane. The visceral pleura lines the lungs directly, whereas the parietal pleura makes up the inner lining of the chest wall. Together they form the **pleural space**,

pleural space: the potential space between the visceral and parietal pleura within the thorax. In disease or injury states, this space can fill with air, fluid, or blood.

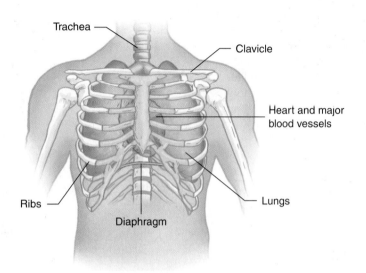

Trachea

Clavicle

Heart and major
blood vessels

Lungs

Ribs

Diaphragm

Figure 6-1 Thorax.

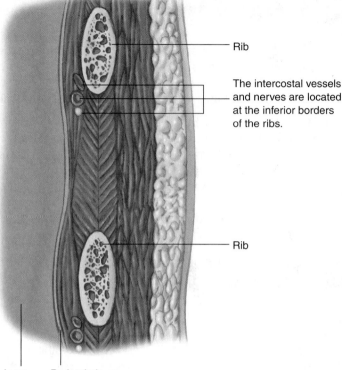

Rib

The intercostal vessels
and nerves are located
at the inferior borders
of the ribs.

Rib

Lung   Parietal pleura

Figure 6-2 Rib with intercostal vessels and nerves.

mediastinum: the anatomic region within the thorax, located between the lungs, that contains the heart and great vessels, trachea, major bronchi, and the esophagus.

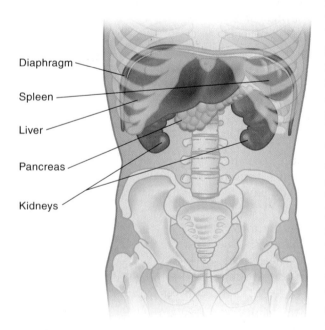

Diaphragm

Spleen

Liver

Pancreas

Kidneys

Figure 6-3 Intrathoracic abdomen.

a potential space in which air (pneumothorax), fluid, or blood (hemothorax) can accumulate.

Within the midline of the thoracic cavity is the **mediastinum**, which includes the heart, the aorta and pulmonary artery, superior and inferior vena cava, trachea, major bronchi, and the esophagus. Having a higher likelihood of being fatal, penetrating injuries that traverse the mediastinum are particularly dangerous because in this area the heart, great vessels, and tracheobronchial structures are close together. Penetrating injuries to the anterior chest, between the nipples, below the clavicles, and above the costal margins, have a high chance of injuring the important mediastinal organs. (This area is called the "Box of Death.") Deceleration injuries such as in head-on collisions or falls from a height are also of concern because they can result in fatal thoracic aortic injuries. Prompt management and transport of these patients can be life saving.

The lower aspect of the chest protects the upper abdominal organs (stomach, spleen, liver, kidneys, and pancreas), which are divided from the thoracic cavity by the diaphragm (Figure 6-3). The diaphragm (a thin sheet of muscle) has its origin on the lower six ribs and the xiphoid process of the sternum. Its main function is ventilation and is innervated by the phrenic nerve, which begins at cervical levels C3 to C5. This is very important because a cervical spinal-cord injury below the fifth cervical vertebrae will cause paralysis from the neck down, yet allow the victim to continue to breathe using the diaphragm. In contrast, a spinal-cord injury above the third cervical vertebrae will render the patient unable to breathe at all due to loss of innervation of the phrenic nerve. Because of the movement of the diaphragm with respiration, any blunt or penetrating injury between the nipples (T4, or fourth intercostal space) and the 12th rib may cause both intrathoracic and intra-abdominal injuries, depending on where the diaphragm is in the respiratory cycle when the injury occurs.

Pathophysiology

In the trimodal distribution of trauma deaths (immediate, hours, and weeks after injury), injuries to the chest are responsible for most deaths at the scene (immediate deaths) and many of those within a few hours (early deaths). Deaths at the scene (immediate deaths) usually involve disruption of the heart or great vessels. The second peak of deaths (early deaths) is usually due to airway obstruction, tension pneumothorax, hemorrhage, or cardiac tamponade. Only 10% to 15% of patients with chest trauma will require operative intervention. This means that timely prehospital care can save lives.

Chest injury may be the result of different mechanisms. Blunt trauma is the result of rapid deceleration, shearing forces, and crush injuries. Typically, the aorta, lungs, ribs, and less commonly the heart and esophagus can be injured in predictable fashion from blunt trauma. Conversely, penetrating trauma injuries are unpredictable. A bullet can be erratic and cause damage beyond its path, depending on the energy transferred, bullet path, and deformation. (See Chapter 1.) The depth and direction of knife wounds are difficult to assess on external examination alone. However, obvious trajectory of a penetrating injury can at least suggest the organs most likely to be at risk of injury.

When evaluating the trauma patient, always follow the ITLS Primary Survey as discussed in Chapter 2. The ITLS Primary Survey is designed to identify life-threatening injuries, and thoracic injuries make up the majority of those. Injuries to the organs within the thoracic cavity may result in decreased oxygenation and massive hemorrhage, both of which can lead to tissue hypoxia (shock) and death. Tissue hypoxia can result from the following:

- Inadequate oxygen delivery to the tissues secondary to airway obstruction
- Hypovolemia from blood loss
- Ventilation/perfusion mismatch from lung parenchymal injury
- Compromise of ventilation and/or circulation from a tension pneumothorax
- Pump failure from severe myocardial injury or pericardial tamponade

Emergency Care of Chest Injuries

The major symptoms of chest injury are shortness of breath and chest pain. The signs indicative of chest injury found upon inspection include chest wall contusion, open wounds, subcutaneous emphysema, hemoptysis, distended neck veins, tracheal deviation, asymmetrical chest movement including paradoxical motion, cyanosis, and shock. In addition, palpation may reveal tenderness, instability, and crepitus (TIC). Listen to the lung fields for the presence and equality of breath sounds. Using the ITLS Primary Survey, including the rapid trauma survey, will guide you in an organized fashion to discovery of those injuries (Figure 6-4).

Life-threatening thoracic injuries should be identified immediately during the ITLS Primary Survey. Major thoracic injuries to identify are listed next and may be remembered as the "deadly dozen":

ITLS Primary Survey
- Airway obstruction
- Flail chest
- Open pneumothorax

PEARLS
Penetrating Chest Wounds
Patients who have penetrating chest trauma and shock are at the top of the list of load-and-go patients. Nothing should delay transport.

ITLS PRIMARY SURVEY

SCENE SIZE-UP
Standard Precautions Hazards, Number of Patients, Need for additional
resources, **Mechanism of Injury**

INITIAL ASSESSMENT
GENERAL IMPRESSION
Age, Sex, Weight, General Appearance, Position,
Purposeful Movement, Obvious Injuries, Skin Color
Life-threatening Bleeding

LOC
A-V-P-U
Chief Complaint/Symptoms

AIRWAY
(CONSIDER C-SPINE CONTROL)
Snoring, Gurgling, Stridor; Silence

BREATHING
Present? Rate, Depth, Effort

CIRCULATION
Radial/Carotid Present? Rate, Rhythm, Quality
Skin Color, Temperature, Moisture; Capillary Refill
Has bleeding been controlled?

RAPID TRAUMA SURVEY
HEAD and NECK
Wounds?
Neck Vein distention? Tracheal Deviation?

CHEST
Asymmetry (Paradoxical Motion?), Contusions, Penetrations, Tenderness, Instability, Crepitation
Breath Sounds
Present? Equal? (If unequal: percussion)
Heart Tones

ABDOMEN
Contusions, Penetration/Evisceration; Tenderness, Rigidity, Distension

PELVIS
Tenderness, Instability, Crepitation

LOWER/UPPER EXTREMITIES
Obvious Swelling, Deformity
Motor and Sensory

POSTERIOR
Obvious wounds, Tenderness, Deformity

If radial pulse present:
VITAL SIGNS
Measured Pulse, Breathing, Blood Pressure

If altered mental status: Brief Neurological exam
PUPILS
Size? Reactive? **Equal?**

GLASGOW COMA SCALE
Eyes, Voice, Motor

Figure 6-4 ITLS Primary Survey.

- Massive hemothorax
- Tension pneumothorax
- Cardiac tamponade

ITLS Secondary Survey or during hospital evaluation
- Myocardial contusion
- Traumatic aortic rupture
- Tracheal or bronchial tree injury
- Diaphragmatic tears
- Pulmonary contusion
- Blast injuries

Airway Obstruction

Airway management remains a major challenge in the care of any multiple-trauma patient. Hypoxia secondary to airway obstruction (foreign body, tongue, aspiration of vomitus, or blood) is a common cause of preventable trauma death. Management of the airway has been discussed in Chapter 4, so nothing further is added here other than to stress its importance.

Flail Chest

Flail chest occurs with the fracture of two or more adjacent ribs in two or more places (Figure 6-5), causing instability of the chest wall and paradoxical movement of the "flail segment" in a spontaneously breathing patient. The unstable section of ribs will suck in when the patient breathes in and will push out when the patient breathes out (Figure 6-6). Positive pressure ventilation reverses the movement of the flail segment. Flail segments are not usually seen in the posterior chest because the heavy back muscles usually prevent movement of a flail segment. Patients with a flail chest are at risk for development of a hemothorax or pneumothorax. Because of the forces involved to cause a flail chest, these patients usually develop a pulmonary contusion (Figures 6-7 and 6-8).

Large flails decrease the ability of the patient to create a negative intrathoracic pressure, and thus the patient may not be able to

PEARLS
Rib Fractures
Multiple rib fractures with or without flail chest can cause hypoxia from mechanical ventilatory problems as well as pulmonary contusion. The patient, especially the older patient, must be closely monitored for hypoxia and respiratory failure. Monitoring with pulse oximetry and capnography is very helpful.

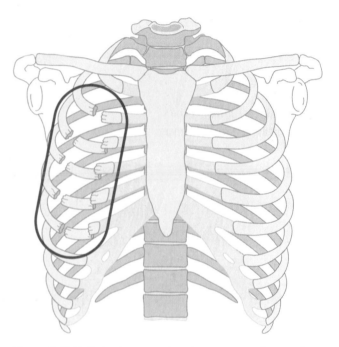

Figure 6-5 Flail chest occurs when two or more adjacent ribs fracture in two or more places.

flail chest: the fracture of two or more adjacent ribs in two or more places, causing instability of the chest wall and paradoxical movement of the "flail segment" in a spontaneously breathing patient.

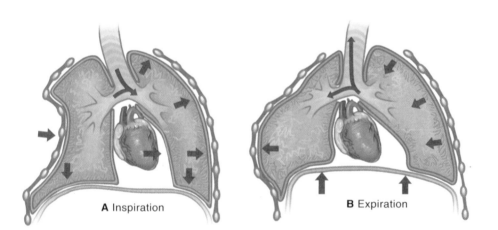

Figure 6-6 Pathophysiology of flail chest showing paradoxical motion.

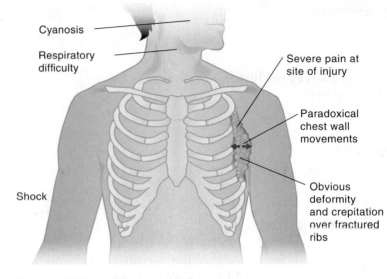

Figure 6-7 Physical findings of flail chest.

Figure 6-8 Flail chest may be identified during the ITLS Primary Survey.

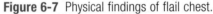

FLAIL CHEST

SCENE SIZE-UP
T-bone collision? Intrusion of door?

INITIAL ASSESSMENT
LOC
Often unconscious
Airway
Possibly snoring or gurgling
Breathing
Apneic, or shallow and guarded; often NO tidal volume
Pulses
Rapid/thready
Skin cool/clammy; cyanotic

RAPID TRAUMA SURVEY
Neck Veins
Flat
Trachea
Midline
Chest
Asymmetrical with paradoxical motion on affected side
Breath Sounds
Usually decreased on affected side (may be heard on both sides)
Abdomen
Pain of broken ribs may mask abdominal tenderness
Check carefully

PEARLS
C-spine and Penetrating Chest Trauma

Spinal motion restriction (SMR) is not indicated in patients with isolated penetrating chest and abdominal trauma, unless it involves the bony spine. Performing cervical-spine motion restriction increases scene time and can worsen outcome.

ventilate and may be in marked respiratory distress. Movement of broken ribs is very painful and will contribute to the difficulty with ventilation.

Large flails are best treated with endotracheal intubation and assisted ventilation with positive end-expiratory pressure (PEEP). For smaller flails, oxygen and continuous positive airway pressure (CPAP) ventilation may be sufficient.

Procedure

Management of Flail Chest

1. Ensure an open airway.
2. Assist ventilation, if it is inadequate.
3. Administer high-flow oxygen.
4. A large flail segment can be stabilized with a bulky dressing to decrease pain associated with rib motion during respirations (Figure 6-9). When the patient needs to be log rolled, roll him or her onto the uninjured side.
5. Patients with a flail chest should be "load and go."
6. Transport rapidly to the appropriate hospital.
7. Notify medical direction early.
8. Consider intubation early to provide PEEP. CPAP could be used here if available.
9. Administer adequate pain relief, avoiding respiratory depression.
10. If shock is present, use care to prevent fluid overload, which could worsen hypoxemia.

Remember that intubation and positive pressure ventilation are the best way to stabilize a flail chest,

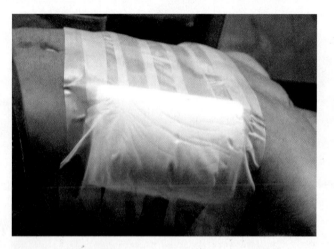

Figure 6-9 Stabilization of a flail chest.

but they may be very difficult in the field if the patient still has a gag reflex. Drug-assisted intubation (DAI) is useful here if available. Also keep in mind that a pneumothorax and pulmonary contusions are associated with a flail chest. Be alert for development of tension pneumothorax and/or hypoxia.

Open Pneumothorax

An **open pneumothorax** is the result of accumulation of air in the potential space between the visceral and parietal pleura secondary to injury. This results in at least a partial collapse of the lung. As the lung tightly adheres to the pleura, it is rare for the lung itself not to have some damage from a penetrating chest wound.

An open or sucking chest wound (>3 cm in diameter) remains open to the atmosphere. The persistent open wound equalizes intrathoracic pressure and atmospheric pressures, resulting in partial or complete lung collapse. The size of the pneumothorax and resultant symptoms are usually proportional to the size of the chest wall defect (Figures 6-10 and 6-11). Normal ventilation involves the creation of negative intrathoracic pressure by diaphragmatic contraction to draw air into the airways and lungs. If the open wound is greater than two-thirds the diameter of the trachea, air will follow the path of least resistance through the chest wall defect into the intrathoracic space, resulting in severe hypoxia and hypoventilation as the chest bellows is compromised.

open pneumothorax: accumulation of air in the pleural space secondary to penetrating injury presenting as an open or sucking chest wound (>3 cm in diameter).

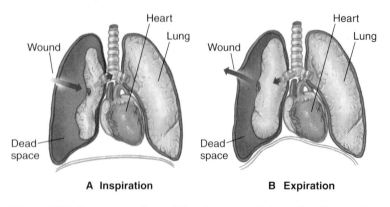

Figure 6-10 Open pneumothorax. If the chest wound is larger than the opening to the trachea, air will preferentially go into the pleura space rather than the lung.

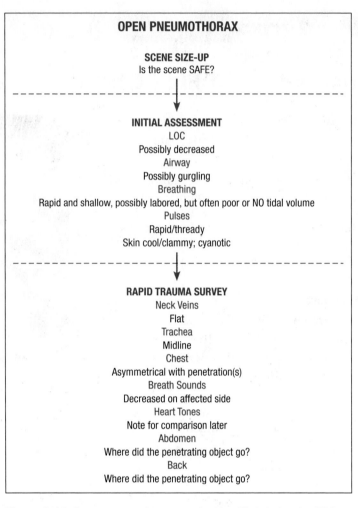

Figure 6-11 Open pneumothorax may be identified during the ITLS Primary Survey.

Procedure

Management of Open Pneumothorax

1. Ensure an open airway.

2. Administer high-flow oxygen. Assist ventilation as necessary.

3. Initially, seal the wound with your gloved hand. Then place a commercial chest seal over the defect (Figure 6-12). (A chest seal with an exit valve is needed, such as Asherman Chest Seal, Bolin Chest Seal, or Halo vent.) Alternatively, you may make a seal from a sterile occlusive dressing taped on three sides to act as flutter-type valve (Figure 6-13). Do not tape on all four sides because that could convert an open pneumothorax into a tension pneumothorax.

4. Load and go.

5. Insert a large-bore IV.

6. Monitor the heart, and note heart tones for comparison later.

7. Monitor oxygen saturation with a pulse oximeter and end-tidal CO_2 with capnography (if available).

8. Transport rapidly to the appropriate hospital.

9. Notify medical direction early.

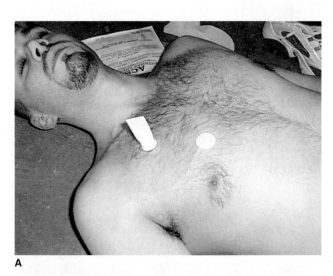

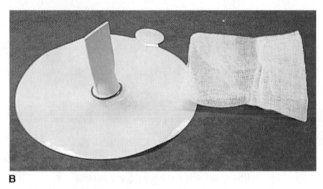

Figure 6-12 (A) Sealing a sucking chest wound with (B) the Asherman Chest Seal. *(Photo B courtesy of Teleflex Incorporated, all rights reserved. No other use shall made of the image without the prior written consent of Teleflex Incorporated.)*

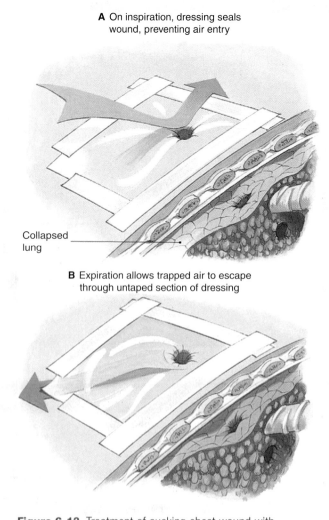

A On inspiration, dressing seals wound, preventing air entry

Collapsed lung

B Expiration allows trapped air to escape through untaped section of dressing

Figure 6-13 Treatment of sucking chest wound with impervious dressing taped on three sides to allow air to escape but not enter.

Massive Hemothorax

Blood in the pleural space is a hemothorax (Figure 6-14). A **massive hemothorax** occurs as a result of at least a 1,500 mL blood loss into the pleural space within the thoracic cavity. Each thoracic cavity may contain up to 3,000 mL of blood. Massive hemothorax is more often due to penetrating trauma than to blunt trauma, but either injury may disrupt a major pulmonary or systemic vessel. As blood accumulates within the pleural space, the lung on the affected side is compressed.

Signs and symptoms of massive hemothorax are produced by both hypovolemia and respiratory compromise. The patient may be hypotensive from blood loss and compression of the heart or great veins. Anxiety and confusion are produced by hypovolemia and hypoxemia. Clinical signs of shock may be apparent. The neck veins are usually flat secondary to profound hypovolemia, but may very rarely be distended due to mediastinal compression. Other signs of hemothorax include decreased breath sounds and dullness to percussion on the affected side. The massive hemothorax may be identified during the ITLS Primary Survey. (See Table 6-1 for comparison of tension pneumothorax and massive hemothorax.)

massive hemothorax: the presence of at least 1,500 mL of blood loss into the pleural space of the thoracic cavity.

Figure 6-14 Physical findings of massive hemothorax.

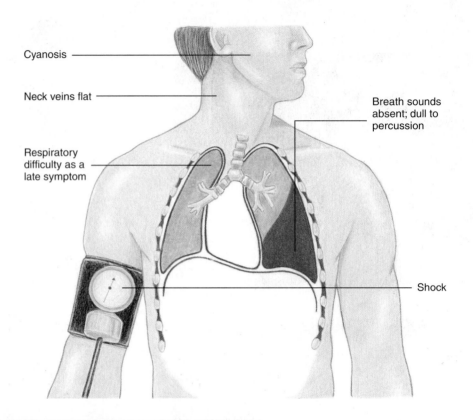

Cyanosis

Neck veins flat

Respiratory difficulty as a late symptom

Breath sounds absent; dull to percussion

Shock

Table 6-1: Primary Survey of Tension Pneumothorax Contrasted to Massive Hemothorax		
	Tension Pneumothorax	**Massive Hemothorax**
Scene size-up	Seat belt? Steering wheel?	Scene safe? Penetrating vs. blunt trauma
Level of consciousness	Decreased	Decreased
Breathing	Rapid/shallow; labored	Rapid/shallow; labored
Pulses	Weak/thready; absent radials	Weak/thready; absent radials
Skin	Cool/clammy/diaphoretic; cyanotic	Cool/clammy/diaphoretic; pale/ashen
Neck	Neck vein distension; possible tracheal deviation (rare)	Neck veins flat; trachea midline
Breath sounds	Decreased or absent breath sounds on affected side	Decreased or absent breath sounds on affected side
Percussion note	Hyperresonant on affected side	Dull on affected side

Procedure

Management of Massive Hemothorax

1. Secure an open airway.
2. Apply high-flow oxygen.
3. Load and go.
4. Notify medical direction early.
5. Treat for shock. Replace volume carefully after IV insertion en route. Try to keep the blood pressure just high enough to maintain perfusion. Target blood pressure is 80 to 90 mm Hg systolic. Although the major problem in massive hemothorax is usually hemorrhagic shock, elevating the blood pressure will increase the bleeding into the chest.
6. Observe closely for the possible development of a tension hemopneumothorax, which would require acute chest decompression.

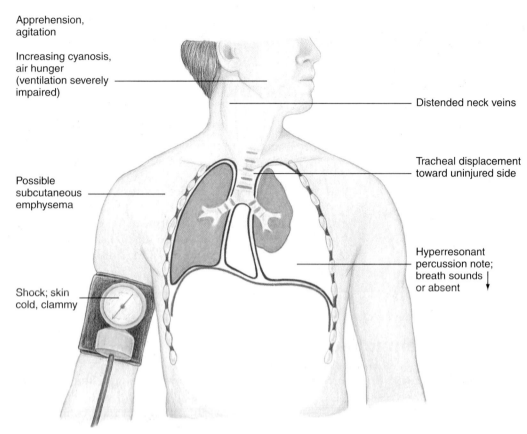

Apprehension, agitation

Increasing cyanosis, air hunger (ventilation severely impaired)

Distended neck veins

Tracheal displacement toward uninjured side

Possible subcutaneous emphysema

Hyperresonant percussion note; breath sounds ↓ or absent

Shock; skin cold, clammy

Figure 6-15 Physical findings of tension pneumothorax.

tension pneumothorax: a condition in which air continuously leaks out of the lung into the pleural space. The air continues to accumulate without means of exit, resulting in increasing intrathoracic pressure on the affected side and eventual collapse of the superior and inferior vena cava as well as the lung.

Tension Pneumothorax

A pneumothorax is accumulation of air in the potential space between the visceral and parietal pleura, resulting in complete lung collapse. In a **tension pneumothorax**, air continues to accumulate without means of exit, resulting in increasing intrathoracic pressure on the affected side, displacing the heart and trachea to the opposite side, and collapsing the superior and inferior vena cava, thus occluding venous return to the heart (Figure 6-15).

Clinical signs of a tension pneumothorax include dyspnea, anxiety, tachypnea, distended neck veins, and possibly tracheal deviation away from the affected side. Auscultation will reveal diminished breath sounds on the affected side and will be accompanied by hyperresonance when percussed (Figure 6-16). Shock with hypotension will follow. In a retrospective review of 108 EMS patients diagnosed with tension pneumothorax and requiring needle decompression, none were recorded as having a deviated trachea, so one must rely on the other physical findings of tension pneumothorax as well as mechanism of injury.

The development of decreased lung compliance (difficulty in squeezing the bag-mask device) in the intubated patient should always alert you to the possibility of a tension pneumothorax. Intubated patients with a history of chronic obstructive pulmonary disease (COPD) or asthma are at increased risk for development of tension pneumothorax from positive pressure ventilation. Any patient receiving positive pressure ventilation who develops a pneumothorax is presumed to have a tension pneumothorax, and immediate intervention is necessary to decompress.

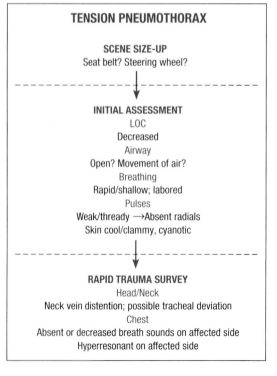

TENSION PNEUMOTHORAX

SCENE SIZE-UP
Seat belt? Steering wheel?

INITIAL ASSESSMENT
LOC
Decreased
Airway
Open? Movement of air?
Breathing
Rapid/shallow; labored
Pulses
Weak/thready →Absent radials
Skin cool/clammy, cyanotic

RAPID TRAUMA SURVEY
Head/Neck
Neck vein distention; possible tracheal deviation
Chest
Absent or decreased breath sounds on affected side
Hyperresonant on affected side

Figure 6-16 The tension pneumothorax may be identified during the ITLS Primary Survey.

Procedure

Management of Tension Pneumothorax

1. Establish an open airway.
2. Administer high-flow oxygen.
3. Decompress the affected side of the chest, if indicated. The indication for performing emergency chest decompression is the presence of a tension pneumothorax with decompensation as evidenced by more than one of the following:
   a. Respiratory distress and cyanosis
   b. Loss of the radial pulse (late shock)
   c. Decreasing level of consciousness

4. Load and go.
5. Rapidly transport to the appropriate hospital.
6. Notify medical direction early.

If you are not authorized to decompress the chest, the patient must be transported rapidly to the hospital so decompression can be performed. A chest tube will be necessary on arrival to the hospital. Needle decompression is a temporary, but life-saving, measure. (See Chapter 7.)

Cardiac Tamponade

The pericardial sac is an inelastic membrane that surrounds the heart. If blood collects rapidly between the heart and pericardium from a cardiac injury, the ventricles of the heart will be compressed, making the heart less able to refill, and cardiac output falls. A small amount of pericardial blood (as little as 50 cc) may compromise cardiac filling and cause signs of **pericardial tamponade** (Figure 6-17).

Figure 6-17 Pathophysiology and physical findings of cardiac tamponade.

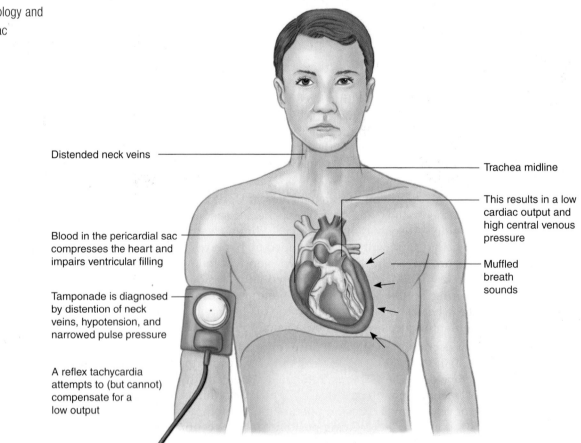

Distended neck veins

Trachea midline

This results in a low cardiac output and high central venous pressure

Blood in the pericardial sac compresses the heart and impairs ventricular filling

Muffled breath sounds

Tamponade is diagnosed by distention of neck veins, hypotension, and narrowed pulse pressure

A reflex tachycardia attempts to (but cannot) compensate for a low output

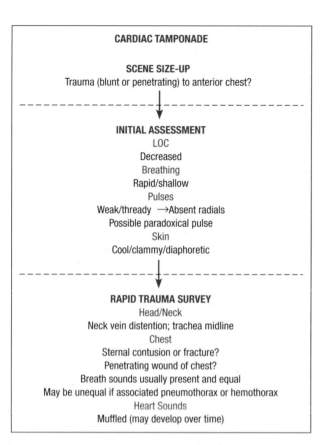

Figure 6-18 Cardiac tamponade may be identified during the ITLS Primary Survey.

pericardial tamponade: the rapid collection of blood between the heart and pericardium from a cardiac injury. The accumulating blood compresses the ventricles of the heart preventing the ventricles from filling between contractions and causing cardiac output to fall.

Beck's triad: the three clinical signs of cardiac tamponade (distended neck veins, muffled heart sounds, and *hypotension*).

paradoxical pulse: a clinical sign of cardiac tamponade. It is an exaggeration of the normal variation of the strength of the pulse during the inspiratory phase of respiration, in which the blood pressure decreases as one inhales and increases as one exhales. The paradox is that, in the case of a pericardial tamponade with decreased cardiac output, the palpated radial pulse disappears during inspiration. Also called *pulsus paradoxus.*

Identification of cardiac tamponade classically relies on the presence of hypotension with narrow pulse pressure and **Beck's triad**, a combination of distended neck veins, muffled heart sounds, and hypotension. Muffled heart sounds may be very difficult to appreciate in the prehospital setting, but if you briefly listen to the heart when performing the ITLS Primary Survey, you may notice a change later. Beck's triad is seen in fewer than half of patients with cardiac tamponade, so maintain a high index of suspicion in patients with the appropriate mechanism. With cardiac tamponade, you may note a decrease in the pulse pressure, which is the difference between the systolic and diastolic blood pressures, as the tamponade progresses. Pulsus paradoxus, or **paradoxical pulse**, may be noted. This is where the radial pulse is not felt with inspiration.

The major differential diagnosis in the field is tension pneumothorax. With cardiac tamponade, the patient will be in shock with equal breath sounds and a midline trachea (Figure 6-18), unless there is an associated pneumothorax or hemothorax.

Other life-threatening thoracic injuries may not be apparent during the ITLS Primary Survey, or at all in the prehospital environment. However, you should remain alert for clues, which may point to the following conditions.

Procedure

Management of Cardiac Tamponade

1. Ensure an open airway.
2. Administer high-flow oxygen.
3. Load and go.
4. Transport rapidly to the appropriate hospital.
5. Notify medical direction early.

(continued)

Procedure (*continued*)

6. Monitor the heart early, especially with chest pain or an irregular pulse.

7. If available, perform a 12-lead ECG (including V4R).

8. Treat for shock. An intravenous infusion of electrolyte solution (en route) may increase the filling of the heart and increase cardiac output. However, because there may be associated intrathoracic bleeding, give only enough fluid to maintain perfusion. Target blood pressure is 80 to 90 mm Hg systolic.

9. Treat dysrhythmias as they present.

10. Watch for other complications, including hemothorax and pneumothorax.

11. If permitted under your scope of practice, pericardiocentesis can be life saving in tamponade.

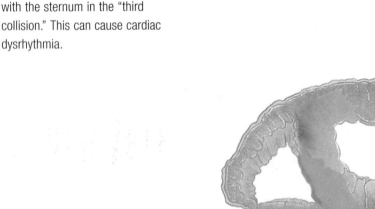

BODY COLLISION

Figure 6-19 Pathophysiology of blunt cardiac injury, a collision of the heart against the sternum.

Figure 6-20 Myocardial contusion most frequently affects the right atrium and ventricle as they collide with the sternum in the "third collision." This can cause cardiac dysrhythmia.

Myocardial Contusion

Blunt cardiac injury (BCI) includes a number of diagnoses, including myocardial contusion, dysrhythmias, acute heart failure, valvular injury, or cardiac rupture. The mechanism is blunt trauma to the anterior chest as in a deceleration motor-vehicle collision or a fall from a height. Among them, myocardial contusion is something that you may suspect and possibly identify as a result of your ITLS Secondary Survey.

Myocardial contusion is a potentially lethal lesion that is the result of a blunt chest injury. Blunt injury to the anterior chest is transmitted via the sternum to the heart, which lies immediately posterior to it (Figure 6-19). Cardiac injuries from this mechanism may include valvular rupture, pericardial tamponade, or cardiac rupture, but contusion of the right atrium and right ventricle occurs most commonly (Figure 6-20). This bruising of the heart is basically the same

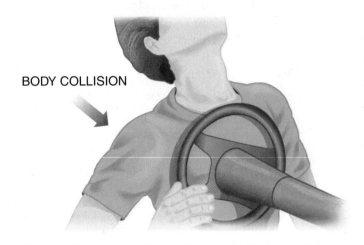

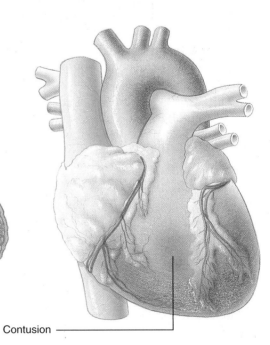

Contusion

injury as an acute myocardial infarction and likewise presents with chest pain, dys-rhythmias, or cardiogenic shock (rare). It may not develop immediately after injury but can develop over time.

Cardiac contusion should be suspected if the patient complains of chest pain, has an otherwise unexplained irregular pulse, and exhibits neck vein elevation, especially in the presence of blunt force trauma to the anterior chest (bruised or flail sternum). Those signs are similar to pericardial tamponade and cannot be differentiated in the field, so they are treated the same. If available, a 12-lead ECG should be performed, which may indicate an injury pattern to the right ventricle (STEMI in leads II, III, aVr, V1, and V4R). Premature ventricular contractions are the most common cardiac dysrhythmia seen on the monitor of patients who have a myocardial contusion.

Procedure

Management of Cardiac Contusion

1. Ensure an open airway.
2. Administer high-flow oxygen.
3. Load and go.
4. Transport rapidly to the appropriate hospital.
5. Notify medical direction early.
6. Apply cardiac monitor, especially with chest pain or an irregular pulse.
7. If available, perform a 12-lead ECG (including V4R).
8. Treat for shock. An intravenous infusion of electrolyte solution (en route) may increase the filling of the heart and increase cardiac output. However, because there may be associated intrathoracic bleeding, give only enough fluid to maintain a pulse (80 to 90 mm Hg systolic).
9. Treat dysrhythmias as they present based on AHA/ILCOR guidelines.
10. Watch for other complications, including hemothorax and pneumothorax.

Traumatic Aortic Rupture

Traumatic aortic rupture is a tear in the wall of the aorta. Eighty-five percent of tears occur at the ligamentum arteriosum or the take-off of the left subclavian artery. Most patients with traumatic aortic rupture (80%) die at the scene. These are usually free ruptures. For the 10% to 20% who do not exsanguinate immediately, the aortic tear will be contained temporarily by surrounding tissue and adventitia. However, usually this will rupture within hours unless recognized and surgically repaired. Identifying a contained thoracic aortic laceration is impossible in the field, so you should have a high index of suspicion for it if the patient has a mechanism of rapid deceleration.

This injury should be suspected in patients with a blunt mechanism associated with rapid deceleration, such as falls from a height and high-speed motor-vehicle collisions (front and lateral impacts, ejected occupants). There may be no symptoms, or the patient may complain of chest pain or scapular pain. Be suspicious if the patient has asymmetric blood pressure measurements in upper extremities, or upper extremity hypertension, widened pulse pressure, and diminished lower extremity pulses.

Procedure

Management of Potential Aortic Tears

1. Ensure an open airway.
2. Administer high-flow oxygen.
3. Rapidly transport to the appropriate hospital.
4. Establish vascular access, but limit fluid administration.
5. Monitor the heart. The mechanism of injury is the same as for myocardial contusion.
6. If available, perform a 12-lead ECG (including V4R)
7. Notify medical direction early.

Tracheal or Bronchial Tree Injury

Tracheobronchial injuries may result in partial or complete disruption of the airway. Injury is localized within 2 cm of the carina in up to 80% of cases. These injuries usually cannot be diagnosed in the field but will present with dyspnea and pneumothorax. Victims may suffer a penetrating or blunt mechanism such as motor-vehicle collision or crush injury to the chest and exhibit dyspnea, subcutaneous emphysema associated hemo/pneumothorax, and deformed chest.

Diaphragmatic Tears

Tears in the diaphragm may result from a severe blow to the abdomen. A sudden increase in intra-abdominal pressure, such as a seat-belt injury or a kick to the abdomen, may tear the diaphragm and allow herniation of the abdominal organs into the thoracic cavity. This occurs more commonly on the left than the right because the liver protects the right hemidiaphragm. Blunt trauma produces large radial tears in the diaphragm. Penetrating trauma also may produce holes in the diaphragm, but these tend to be small.

Traumatic diaphragmatic hernia is difficult to diagnose even in the hospital. The herniation of abdominal contents into the thoracic cavity may cause marked respiratory distress. Upon examination, the breath sounds may be diminished, and infrequently, bowel sounds may be heard when the chest is auscultated. The abdomen may appear scaphoid (sunken) if a large quantity of abdominal contents is in the chest. If traumatic diaphragmatic hernia is suspected and the patient requires a needle decompression for a tension pneumothorax, perform the decompression at the second intercostal space, midclavicular line, not at the lateral site.

Procedure

Management of Diaphragmatic Rupture

1. Ensure an open airway.
2. Assist ventilation as necessary
3. Administer high-flow oxygen.
4. Transport the patient to the appropriate hospital.
5. Treat for shock. Insert an IV en route. Associated injuries are common and hypovolemia may occur.
6. Notify medical direction early.

Pulmonary Contusion

Pulmonary contusion is a very common chest injury. It is caused by hemorrhage into lung parenchyma secondary to blunt force trauma or penetrating injury such as a missile. It occurs commonly with flail segment or multiple rib fractures. A pulmonary contusion takes hours to develop and rarely develops during prehospital care, unless there is a very long transport, secondary transport during a transfer to a trauma center, or delayed discovery of the victim. Children may have severe pulmonary contusions without rib fractures due to the flexibility of the chest wall. Contusion of the lung may produce marked hypoxemia.

Management consists of intubation and/or assisted ventilation if indicated, oxygen administration, transport, and IV insertion.

Blast Injuries

With the increase in terrorism, understanding blast injury is important. The magnitude of the blast wave depends on the size of the explosion and the environment in which it occurs. Closed spaces, such as buses, produce highly lethal blast injuries. (See Chapter 1.)

The mechanism of injury by explosion is due to three to five factors:

- *Primary.* This is the initial air blast. A primary blast injury is caused solely by the direct effect of blast overpressure on tissue. Air is easily compressible, unlike water. As a result, a primary blast injury almost always affects air-filled structures such as the lungs, ears, and gastrointestinal tract. Depending on the pressure wave, there may be pulmonary contusions, pneumothorax, tension pneumothorax, or arterial gas embolus.
- *Secondary.* The patient is struck by material (shrapnel) propelled by the blast force.
- *Tertiary.* The patient's body is thrown by the pressure wave and impacts the ground or another object. These injuries, including crush injury, also are seen from structural collapse.
- *Quaternary.* This is thermal burns from the explosion, radiation from radiological material that was dispersed by the explosion (dirty bomb), or respiratory injuries from inhalation of toxic dust or fumes.
- *Quinary.* This is reported as a hyperinflammatory state caused by chemicals used in making a bomb or added to the bomb (another form of dirty bomb).

Procedure

Management of the Blast Injury Patient

1. Place yourself, other responders, and equipment in a safe location. Be aware of secondary devices.
2. Triage patients per multiple-casualty injury (MCI) protocol. Patients who have primary blast injury have a high mortality.
3. Ensure an open airway.
4. Administer high-flow oxygen. Be aware that positive pressure ventilation may lead to or worsen pneumothorax or tension pneumothorax.
5. Load and go critical patients to appropriate level of care.
6. Manage the other injuries found.
7. Obtain venous access.
8. Notify medical direction.

Other Chest Injuries

Impaled Objects

Penetrating objects, such as a knife, may cause impalement injuries of the chest. With the exception of the face (cheek), where the object causes airway compromise, impaled objects should not be removed in the field. Stabilize the object, ensure an airway, insert an IV, and transport the patient.

Traumatic Asphyxia

Traumatic asphyxia is an important set of physical findings (Figure 6-21). However, the term *traumatic asphyxia* is a misnomer because the condition is not caused by asphyxia. The syndrome results from a severe compression injury to the chest, such as from a steering wheel, conveyor belt, or heavy object. The sudden compression of the heart and mediastinum transmits this force to the capillaries of the neck and head. These patients appear similar to those who have been strangulated, with cyanosis and swelling of the head and neck. The tongue and lips are swollen, and conjunctival hemorrhage is evident. The skin below the level of the crush injury to the chest will be normal in appearance unless there are other problems.

Traumatic asphyxia indicates the patient has suffered a severe blunt thoracic injury, and major thoracic injuries are likely to be present. Management includes airway maintenance, IV access, treating other injuries, and rapid transport.

Simple Pneumothorax

Simple pneumothorax may result from blunt or penetrating trauma. Fractured ribs are the usual cause in blunt trauma. Pneumothorax is caused by accumulation of air within the potential space between the visceral and parietal pleura. The lung may be totally or partially collapsed as the air continues to accrue in the thoracic cavity. In a healthy patient this should not acutely compromise ventilation, if a tension pneumothorax does not evolve. Patients with less respiratory reserve may not tolerate even a simple pneumothorax.

Clinical findings that suggest a pneumothorax include pleuritic chest pain, dyspnea, decreased breath sounds on the affected side, and tympany to percussion. Close observation is required in anticipation of the patient developing a tension pneumothorax.

PEARLS

Simple Pneumothorax

Reassess patients with chest injuries frequently to prevent progression of a simple pneumothorax or open pneumothorax to a tension pneumothorax. The pulse oximeter and waveform capnography can be helpful.

simple pneumothorax: the presence of air in the pleural space that causes the lung to separate from the chest wall and can compromise the mechanics of breathing.

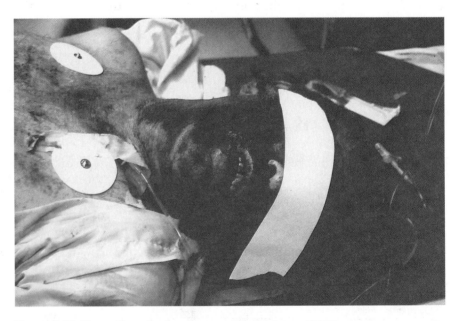

Figure 6-21 Traumatic asphyxia. *(Courtesy of Stanley Cooper, EMT-P)*

Any patient with a simple pneumothorax who undergoes intubation and positive pressure ventilation must then be treated as a tension pneumothorax.

Sternal Fractures

Sternal fractures indicate the patient has suffered marked blunt trauma to the anterior chest. These patients should be presumed to have a myocardial contusion. Diagnosis of sternal fracture may be made by palpation.

Simple Rib Fracture

Simple rib fracture is the most frequent injury to the chest. If the patient does not have an associated pneumothorax or hemothorax, the major problem is pain. This pain will prohibit the patient from breathing adequately. Upon palpation, the area of rib fracture will be tender and may be unstable. Give oxygen and monitor for pneumothorax or hemothorax while encouraging the patient to breathe deeply. It is reasonable to give medication for pain management. Elderly patients with multiple rib fractures have an increased risk for hypoxemia.

Case Presentation (continued)

The lead emergency care provider now notes that the carotid pulse is weaker and that radial pulses are no longer palpable. Removing the C-collar, he observes that the patient has engorged neck veins, and his trachea is deviated to the left. Reassessment of the chest reveals that the right side still does not move and seems enlarged, even exhibiting intercostal bulging. Breath sounds are still absent on the right though heard on the left. Percussion on the right side of the chest reveals a drum-like note (hyperresonance).

The lead emergency care provider concludes that the patient has progressed to a tension pneumothorax, and with the decreased level of consciousness, the cyanosis, and the loss of radial pulses, he decides to decompress the chest. The lead emergency care provider inserts a specifically designed needle decompression device into the second intercostal space just over the third rib on the right side, at the midclavicular line. A loud hiss of air is heard, indicating successful decompression. The emergency care provider then re-evaluates the patient, finding the patient easier to ventilate, the disappearance of cyanosis, flat neck veins, and the return of radial pulses. Although the chest no longer appears hyperinflated, he auscultates and confirms breath sounds on the left only (indicating a *simple* pneumothorax on the right). After repeating vital signs, the emergency care provider updates the receiving facility of the change in the patient's condition and their ETA to the facility.

Summary

Chest injuries are common in multiple-trauma patients. Many of the injuries are life threatening. If you follow the ITLS Primary Survey, you will be able to identify most of them. These are often load-and-go patients. Primary goals in treating the patient with chest trauma are the following:

- Ensure an open airway while protecting the cervical spine.
- Administer high-flow oxygen and ventilate if necessary.
- Stabilize flail segments.

- Seal sucking chest wounds.
- Decompress the chest if needed.
- Load and go to appropriate level of care.
- Obtain venous access.
- Transport to appropriate level of care.
- Notify medical direction.

The thoracic injuries discussed are life threatening, but treatable by prompt intervention and transport to the appropriate level of care. Early recognition along with appropriate interventions and rapid transport may be life saving.

Bibliography

American College of Surgeons Committee on Trauma. "Thoracic Trauma." In *Advanced Trauma Life Support*, 9th ed., 94–110. Chicago: American College of Surgeons, 2012.

Asensio, J. A., F. N. Mazzini, and T. Vu. "Thoracic Injuries." In *The Trauma Manual: Trauma and Acute Care Surgery*, 4th ed., edited by A. B. Pietzman, M. Rhodes, C. W. Schwab, D. M. Yealy, and T. C. Fabian, 327–366. Philadelphia: Lippincott Williams & Williams, 2013.

Ball, C. G., A. D. Wyrzykowski, A. W. Kirkpatrick, C. J. Dente, J. M. Nicholas, J. P. Salomone, G. S. Rozycki, J. B. Kortbeek, and D. V. Feliciano. "Thoracic Needle Decompression for Tension Pneumothorax: Clinical Correlation with Catheter Length." *Canadian Journal of Surgery* 53, no. 3 (June 2010): 184–188.

"CDC Blast Injury Mobile Application." CDC Emergency Preparedness and Response Web page. Last reviewed June 30, 2104. Accessed January, 2015, at http://emergency.cdc.gov/masscasualties/blastinjury-mobile-app.asp

DePalma R. G., D. G. Burris, H. R. Champion, and M. J. Hodgson. "Blast Injuries." *New England Journal of Medicine* 352 (March 31, 2005): 1335–1342.

Harcke, H. T., L. A. Pearse, A. D. Levy, J. M Getz, and S. R. Robinson. "Chest Wall Thickness in Military Personnel: Implications of Needle Thoracentesis in Tension Pneumothorax." *Military Medicine* 172, no. 12 (December 2007): 1260–1263.

Lee, C., M. Revell, K. Porter, and R. Steyn. "The Prehospital Management of Chest Injuries: A Consensus Statement; Faculty of Pre-hospital Care, Royal College of Surgeons of Edinburgh." *Emergency Medicine Journal* 24, no. 3 (March 2007): 220–224

Livingston, D. H., and C. J. Hauser. "Chest Wall and Lung." In *Trauma*, 6th ed., edited by D. V. Feliciano, K. L. Mattox, and E. E. Moore, 525–552. New York: McGraw-Hill, 2008.

Netto, F. A., H. Shulman, S. B. Rizoli, L. N. Tremblay, F. Brenneman, and H. Tien. "Are Needle Decompressions for Tension Pneumothoraces Being Performed Appropriately for Appropriate Indications?" *American Journal of Emergency Medicine* 26, no. 5 (June 2008): 597–602.

Get more information about this course by calling
ITLS International at 888-495-4875
(outside the United States call +1-630-495-6442) or visit

www.itrauma.org

Thoracic Trauma Skills

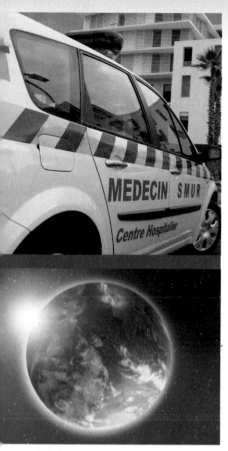

S. Robert Seitz, MEd, RN, NRP
Arthur Proust, MD, FACEP

Trauma Toracico	Traumatismo Torácico	Traumatisme Thoracique
Urazy klatki piersiowej	Thorax Trauma	Ozljeda prsnog koša
إصابات القفص الصدري	torakalna trauma	Poškodbe prsnega koša
Mellkasi sérülés		

(Ambulance photo © yannik LABBE, Fotolia, LLC)

Objectives

Upon successful completion of this chapter, you should be able to:

1. Explain the advantages, disadvantages, and complications of needle decompression of a tension pneumothorax by the anterior approach and the lateral approach.
2. Describe the indications for emergency decompression of a tension pneumothorax.
3. Perform needle decompression of a tension pneumothorax by either the anterior or lateral approach.

Chest Decompression

For many years needle decompression of a tension pneumothorax has been advocated as a life-saving procedure, and the anterior approach (second or third intercostal space, midclavicular line) has been most commonly used by emergency care providers. Multiple studies also have been published showing that the catheters being used with the anterior approach were too short to decompress the chest. It is recommended that the anterior approach utilize a large-bore catheter needle (8 French or about 14 gauge) and 6 to 9 cm long (2.5 to 3.5 inches).

Tactical medicine courses that emphasize management of penetrating injuries associated with tension pneumothorax have encouraged performing needle chest decompression laterally. This is for two reasons: First is the belief that a lateral approach is more likely to ensure successful entry of the catheter into the pleural space. Second is the ability to perform the procedure quickly without removal of body armor. The indications for needle chest decompression are the same, regardless of a tactical or civilian environment.

Some courses recommend the fourth intercostal space (between fourth and fifth ribs) in the anterior axillary line (AAL), whereas other courses advocate use of the third intercostal space laterally. Either lateral location will be effective, assuming that the needle enters the pleural space. There is theoretically less risk of damaging solid organs (liver, spleen) in the third intercostal space compared to the fourth intercostal, and it may also be more rapidly accessible in a tactical or combat environment.

Prehospital systems utilizing ultrasound have the advantage of performing an extended focused assessment with sonography in trauma (E-FAST) when the exam for pneumothorax is performed. The presence of a sliding lung sign (SLS), where the two pleural layers are seen to move across each other, rules out a pneumothorax, thereby reducing unnecessary needle chest decompression procedures.

Because there are advantages and disadvantages to each decompression site, this chapter covers lateral and anterior anatomical positions. However, the anterior approach is preferred for civilian (nontactical) EMS performing needle decompression because the number of complications and disadvantages with the lateral approach outweigh its benefits. Follow your EMS system protocol and consult your service medical director for guidance about which site to use routinely.

Indications to Perform Chest Decompression

As with all advanced procedures, this technique must be permitted by local protocol, or you must obtain medical direction before performing the procedure. The conservative management of tension pneumothorax is oxygen, ventilatory assistance, and rapid transport. The indication for performing emergency decompression is the presence of a tension pneumothorax (listed later) with decompensation as evidenced by any of the following:

- Respiratory distress and cyanosis
- Signs of shock
- Decreasing level of consciousness

Performing a Chest Decompression by the Anterior Approach

Advantages
- The anterior site is preferred by many because, in the supine patient, air in the pleural space tends to accumulate anteriorly. Thus, there is a better chance of having the air in the pleural space removed when the anterior approach to decompressing is used. It is also easier to access when the patient is on the ambulance stretcher.

- Monitoring of the site is easier when the anterior approach is used because the catheter is not as likely to be unintentionally dislodged when the patient is moved or if the patient moves an arm.

Disadvantages and Complications

- Unless a needle of proper length is used, it is likely that the needle will not reach the pleural space, and the tension pneumothorax will not be decompressed. The recommended catheter length is 6 to 9 cm (2.5 to 3.5 inches; Figure 7-1).

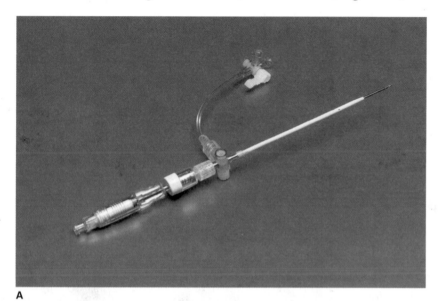

A

Figure 7-1a Examples of catheters long enough to decompress a tension pneumothorax: In this photo, a Turkel safety needle. *(Courtesy of Covidien. Covidien and ™ marked brands are trademarks of Covidien AG.)*

B

Figure 7-1b An ARS needle for decompression. *(© 2020 North American Rescue, LLC)*

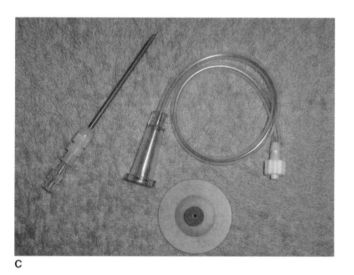

C

Figure 7-1c A Cook pneumothorax needle (has wire coil inside to prevent kinking). *(Courtesy of Stanley Cooper, EMT-P)*

- If the insertion of the needle is medial to the midclavicular line (nipple line), there is danger of cardiac puncture or blood vessel laceration.
- Laceration of the intercostal vessels may cause hemorrhage. The intercostal artery and vein run around the inferior margin of each rib. Poor needle placement can lacerate one of these vessels.
- Creation of a pneumothorax can occur if one is not already present. If your assessment was incorrect, you could give the patient a pneumothorax when you insert the needle into the chest.
- Laceration of the lung is possible. Poor technique or inappropriate insertion (no pneumothorax present) can cause laceration of the lung, with subsequent bleeding and an air leak.
- Risk of infection is a consideration. Adequate skin preparation with an antiseptic will usually prevent this.

Procedure

Performing Decompression by the Anterior Approach

1. Assess the patient to make sure that his or her condition is due to a tension pneumothorax. Signs of tension pneumothorax are the following:
   a. Absent or decreased breath sounds on the affected side
   b. Decreased level of consciousness (LOC)
   c. Respiratory distress; tachypnea
   d. Weak/thready pulses; possible absent radial pulse
   e. Skin cool, clammy, diaphoretic; pale or cyanotic
   f. Neck vein distention (may not be present if there is associated severe hemorrhage)
   g. Possible tracheal deviation away from the side of the injury (late sign and often not present)
   h. Decreased level of consciousness (LOC)
   i. Tympanic sound (hyperresonance) to percussion on the affected side
2. Give the patient high-flow oxygen and ventilatory assistance.
3. Determine that indications for emergency decompression are present. Then, if required, obtain medical direction to perform the procedure.
4. *Anterior site for decompression:* Expose the side of the tension pneumothorax, and identify the second intercostal space on the anterior chest at the midclavicular line. This may be done by feeling for "angle of Louis," the bump located on the sternum about a quarter of the way from the

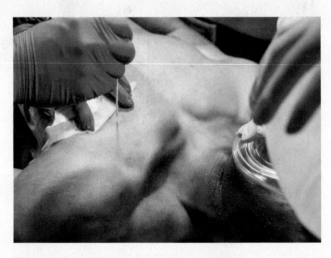

Figure 7-2 Anterior approach for needle decompression. Note the distended neck veins.

suprasternal notch (Figure 7-2). The insertion site should be slightly lateral to the midclavicular line (nipple line) to avoid cardiac or major vascular complications in the mediastinum.

5. Quickly prepare the area with an antiseptic.
6. Remove the plastic cover from a 14 gauge or larger catheter that is 6 to 9 cm long (8 French, 9 cm Turkel Safety Needle, 14-gauge, 8.25 cm ARS decompression needle, 8.5 French, 6 cm Cook pneumothorax needle, or 14 gauge, 8 cm angiocath). Insert the needle into the second intercostal space at a 90-degree angle to the

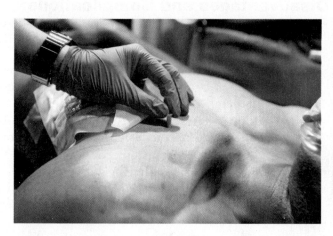

Figure 7-3 Insert the catheter at a 90-degree angle over the superior border of the third rib into the second intercostal space.

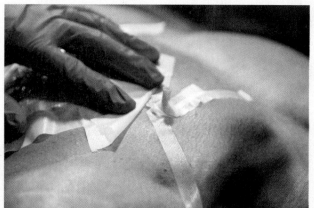

Figure 7-4 Advance the catheter into the chest. There may be a rush of air as the pressure is relieved. Secure the catheter with tape.

superior border of the third rib to avoid the neurovascular bundle (Figure 7-3). Direction of the bevel of the needle is irrelevant to successful results. Be very careful not to angle the needle toward the mediastinum (medially). As the needle enters the pleural space, you may be able to feel a "pop." If a tension pneumothorax is present, a hiss of air may be audible as the thoracic pressure is relieved. You will not hear this sound if you use a syringe as a handle for the needle or leave the end plug in place. When using an over-the-needle catheter, advance the catheter into the chest (Figure 7-4). Remove the needle, and leave the catheter in place. To avoid dislodgement the catheter hub may be stabilized to the chest with tape.

7. Place a one-way valve on or over the decompressing needle. The Asherman chest seal will go over the needle to provide a one-way valve and to protect the needle from accidently being dislodged. Other one-way valves are available or can be made, but should be tested before using. (A needle through the finger of a rubber glove will not work as a one-way valve.) Younger, healthy patients will tolerate having no valve at all on the decompressing needle.

8. Leave the plastic catheter, and secure it in position until it is replaced by a chest tube at the hospital.

9. Some emergency care providers find it helpful to take a small syringe to which is added a few milliliters of saline and attach it to the needle hub before insertion. The syringe can be used as a handle during insertion. Drawing back on the syringe plunger as you advance, you will aspirate air when you reach the pleural cavity, which will be seen as air bubbles in the saline.

10. Intubate the patient if indicated. Monitor closely for recurrence of the tension pneumothorax, and repeat decompression procedure if signs redevelop.

Performing a Chest Decompression by the Lateral Approach

Advantages

- The lateral chest wall is thinner than the anterior chest wall (averages 2.6 cm, or about 1 in.), so you are more likely to decompress the pneumothorax with a shorter needle and less likely to inadvertently cause hemorrhage from vascular structures.

- The military and tactical medical personnel prefer the lateral approach because in a tactical situation it has the advantage of allowing decompression while keeping body armor in place.

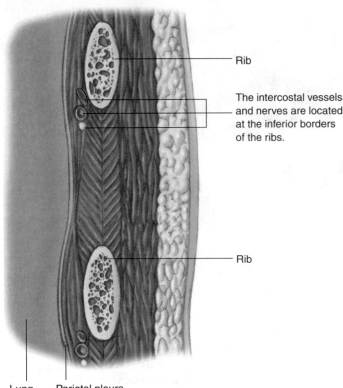

The intercostal vessels and nerves are located at the inferior borders of the ribs.

Rib

Rib

Lung   Parietal pleura

Figure 7-5 Rib with intercostal vessels and nerves.

Disadvantages and Complications

- The decompression catheter is more likely to be dislodged when moving the patient or if the patient moves an arm. Using the Asherman chest seal (or similar device) for a one-way valve also will provide some protection against dislodgement of the decompression catheter.

- It can be difficult to reach this area when the patient is in the ambulance (especially if the tension pneumothorax is on the right).

- Laceration of the intercostal vessels may cause hemorrhage. The intercostal artery and vein run around the inferior margin of each rib (Figure 7-5). Poor needle placement can lacerate one of these vessels.

- If performing the lateral approach, inserting the needle too low can lacerate the liver or spleen, and inserting the needle too high can lacerate the axillary artery, vein, or network of nerves known as the *brachial plexus.*

- Creation of a pneumothorax can occur if one is not already present. If your assessment was incorrect, you could give the patient a pneumothorax when you insert the needle into the chest.

- Laceration of the lung is possible. Poor technique or inappropriate insertion (no pneumothorax present) can cause laceration of the lung, with subsequent bleeding and an air leak.

- Increased risk of the catheter kinking has been reported with this approach, partially and/or temporarily occluding the catheter during transport. This may contribute to the redevelopment of the tension pneumothorax.

- Risk of infection is a consideration. Adequate skin preparation with an antiseptic will usually prevent this.

Procedure

Performing a Chest Decompression by the Lateral Approach

1. Assess the patient to make sure that his or her condition is due to a tension pneumothorax. Signs of tension pneumothorax are the following:

   a. Absent or decreased breath sounds on the affected side
   b. Decreased level of consciousness (LOC)
   c. Respiratory distress; tachypnea
   d. Weak/thready pulses; possible absent radial pulse
   e. Skin cool, clammy, diaphoretic; pale or cyanotic
   f. Neck vein distention (may not be present if there is associated severe hemorrhage)
   g. Possible tracheal deviation away from the side of the injury (late sign and often not present)
   h. Decreased level of consciousness (LOC)
   i. Tympanic sound (hyperresonance) to percussion on the affected side

2. Give the patient high-flow oxygen and ventilatory assistance.

3. Determine that indications for emergency decompression are present. Then, if required, obtain medical direction to perform the procedure.

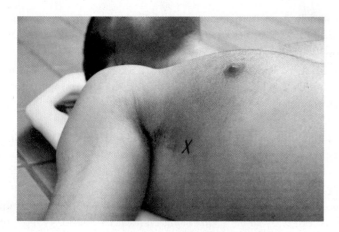

Figure 7-6 Determine that the patient has a tension pneumothorax, and mark the site for needle decompression using the lateral approach. *(Photo courtesy of Louis B. Mallory, MBA, REMT-P)*

4. *Lateral site for decompression*: Expose the side of the tension pneumothorax, and identify the intersection of the nipple (fourth rib) and anterior axillary line on the same side as the pneumothorax (Figure 7-6).

5. Quickly prepare the area with an antiseptic.

6. Remove the plastic cap from a 14 gauge catheter needle that is at least 2 inches or 5 cm long, and insert the needle into the intercostal space at a 90-degree angle to the superior border of the fourth rib to avoid the neurovascular bundle (Figure 7-7).

   If the patient is muscular or obese, you may need to use a 6 to 9 cm catheter needle. Direction of the bevel is irrelevant to successful results. As the needle enters the pleural space, there will be a "pop." If a tension pneumothorax is present, there will be a hiss of air as the pneumothorax is decompressed. When using an over-the-needle catheter, advance the catheter into the chest. Remove the needle, and leave the catheter in place. The catheter hub must be stabilized to the chest with tape.

7. Place a one-way valve on or over the decompressing needle. The Asherman chest seal will go over the needle to provide a one-way valve and to protect the needle from accidently being dislodged. Other one-way valves are

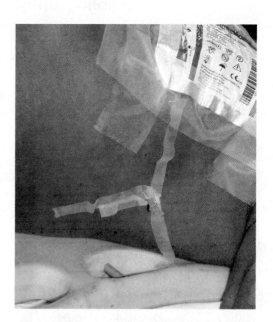

Figure 7-7 Needle decompression by the lateral approach. Advance the catheter into the chest, and secure with tape.

available or can be made, but should be tested before using. (A needle through the finger of a rubber glove will not work as a one-way valve.) Young, healthy patients will tolerate having no valve at all on the decompressing needle.

8. Leave the plastic catheter and secure it in position until it is replaced by a chest tube at the hospital.

9. Some emergency care providers find it helpful to take a small syringe to which is added a few milliliters of saline and attach it to the needle hub before insertion. The syringe can be used as a handle during insertion. Drawing back on the syringe plunger as you advance, you will aspirate air when you reach the pleural cavity, which will be seen as air bubbles in the saline.

10. Intubate the patient if indicated. Monitor with capnography when available. Monitor closely for recurrence of the tension pneumothorax, as an increase in the CO_2 is an early sign the catheter is kinked or a tension pneumothorax is reoccurring.

Bibliography

Asensio, J. A., F. N. Massini, and T. Vu. "Thoracic Injuries." In *The Trauma Manual: Trauma and Acute Care Surgery*, 4th ed., Edited by A. B. Peitzman, M. Rhodes, G. W. Schwab, D. M. Yealy, and T. C. Fabian, 327–56. Philadelphia: Lippincott Williams & Wilkins, 2013.

Ball, C. G., A. D. Wyrzykowski, A. W. Kirkpatrick, C. J. Dente, J. M. Nicholas, J. P. Salomone, G. S. Rozycki, J. B. Kortbeek, and D. V. Feliciano. "Thoracic Needle Decompression for Tension Pneumothorax: Clinical Correlation with Catheter Length." *Canadian Journal of Surgery* 53, no. 3 (June 2010): 184–88.

Beckett, A., E. Savage, D. Pannell, S. Acharya, A. Kirkpatrick, and H. C. Tien. "Needle Decompression for Tension Pneumothorax in Tactical Combat Casualty Care: Do Catheters Placed in the Midaxillary Line Kink More Often Than Those in the Midclavicular Line?" *Journal of Trauma* 71, no. 5, Suppl. 1 (November 2011): S408–S412.

Blaivas, M. "Inadequate Needle Thoracostomy Rate in the Prehospital Setting for Presumed Pneumothorax: An Ultrasound Study." *Journal of Ultrasound in Medicine* 29, no. 9 (September 2010): 1285–89.

Butler, F. K. "Tactical Combat Casualty Care: Update 2009." *Journal of Trauma* 69, Suppl. 1 (July 2010): S10–S13.

Committee on Trauma, American College of Surgeons. "Chest Trauma Management." In *Advanced Trauma Life Support*, 9th ed., 118-21. Chicago: American College of Surgeons, 2012.

Harcke, H. T., L. A. Pearse, J. M. Getz, and S. R. Robinson. "Chest Wall Thickness in Military Personnel: Implications of Needle Thoracentesis in Tension Pneumothorax." *Military Medicine* 172, no. 12 (December 2007): 1260–63.

Lee, C., M. Revell, K. Porter, and R. Steyn. "The Prehospital Management of Chest Injuries: A Consensus Statement. Faculty of Pre-hospital Care, Royal College of Surgeons of Edinburgh." *Emergency Medicine Journal* 24, no. 3 (March 2007): 220–24.

Netto, F. A., H. Shulman, S. B. Rizoli, L. N. Tremblay, F. Brenneman, and H. Tien. "Are Needle Decompressions for Tension Pneumothoraces Being Performed Appropriately for Appropriate Indications?" *American Journal of Emergency Medicine* 26, no. 5 (June 2008): 597–602.

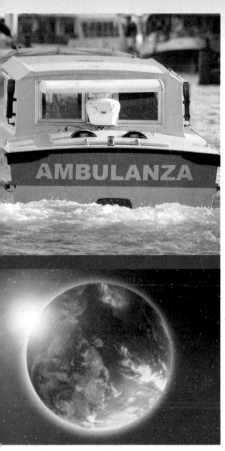

8

Shock

Raymond L. Fowler, MD, FACEP
Paul E. Pepe, MD, MPH, FACEP, FCCM
John T. Stevens, EMT-P
Mario Luis Ramirez, MD, MPP
Howard Mell, MD, MPH

Shock	Shock	Choc	Wstrząs	Schock
Šok	الصدمه	šok	Šok	Sokk

Key Terms

capillary refill time (CRT), *p. 158*
cardiogenic shock, *p. 157*
distributive shock, *p. 161*
hemorrhagic shock, *p. 160*
hemostatic agents, *p. 168*
hypovolemic shock, *p. 156*
mechanical shock, *p. 157*
neurogenic shock, *p. 154*
pulse pressure, *p. 157*
tranexamic acid, *p. 172*
vasoconstriction, *p. 156*

Objectives

Upon successful completion of this chapter, you should be able to:

1. List the four components of the vascular system necessary for normal tissue perfusion.
2. Describe the symptoms and signs of shock in the order that they develop, from the very least to the very worst.
3. Describe the four common clinical shock syndromes.
4. Explain the pathophysiology of hemorrhagic shock, and compare it to the pathophysiology of mechanical and neurogenic shock.
5. Describe the management of the following:
   a. Hemorrhage that can be controlled
   b. Hemorrhage that cannot be controlled
   c. Nonhemorrhagic shock syndromes
6. Discuss the use of hemostatic agents for uncontrolled extremity hemorrhage.
7. Discuss the current indications for the use of IV fluids in the treatment of hemorrhagic shock.
8. Describe when it is appropriate to use tranexamic acid (TXA) in the management of hemorrhage.

Chapter Overview

The management of shock has been the subject of intensive research for decades. As a result, changes continue to be made in the recommendations for prehospital treatment of the patient with hemorrhagic shock. The experience of the U.S. military and its coalition partners in the Iraq and Afghanistan wars has led to new thinking in the management of life-threatening hemorrhage. This chapter reviews present knowledge. It also offers the results of recent research about the pathophysiology and treatment of shock in the trauma patient and in patients with various other shock states.

Case Presentation

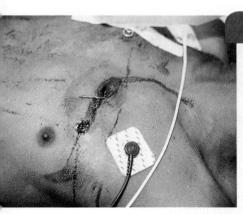

(© Edward T. Dickinson, MD)

An ALS ambulance has been dispatched to a construction site, where a worker tripped and fell onto a piece of concrete reinforcement bar sticking out of the ground. His coworkers pulled him off the bar and called for EMS. The scene size-up reveals that the fire department is on scene, there are no other hazards, and they are giving the worker oxygen by mask. There is a single male patient who is sitting on the tailgate of a pickup truck, holding his chest. Because the scene is safe and the mechanism of injury (puncture/stab wound) is readily apparent, the team dons personal protective equipment. As they approach the patient, each carries essential trauma care equipment.

Before proceeding, consider these questions: How would you approach this patient? What type of assessment would you perform? What would you do first? Is this a load-and-go situation? What potential injuries could this patient have? Keep these questions in mind as you read through the chapter. Then, at the end of the chapter, find out how the emergency care providers managed this patient's care.

Basic Pathophysiology

The normal perfusion of body tissues requires four intact components. They are as follows:

- Intact vascular system to deliver oxygenated blood throughout the body: the blood vessels
- Adequate air exchange in the lungs to allow oxygen to enter the blood: oxygenation
- Adequate volume of fluid in the vascular system: red blood cells and plasma
- Functioning pump: the heart

neurogenic shock: shock caused by spinal injury in which the spinal connections to the adrenal glands and to the blood vessels are interrupted and the vasoconstrictors, epinephrine and norepinephrine, are not produced. Without the vasoconstrictors the blood vessels dilate and redistribute blood flow to a larger vascular volume causing a relative hypovolemia and the heart muscle cannot be stimulated to contract harder and faster.

It is important to remember that blood pressure requires a "steady state" activity of all the preceding factors. The heart must be pumping, the blood volume must be adequate, the blood vessels must be intact, and the lungs must be oxygenating the blood. An important formula regarding the maintenance of blood pressure should be fresh in the mind of every emergency care provider:

$$\text{Blood Pressure} = \text{Cardiac Output} \times \text{Peripheral Vascular Resistance}$$

In addition, the formula for cardiac output is written as follows:

$$\text{Cardiac Output} = \text{Heart Rate} \times \text{Stroke Volume}$$

Stroke volume is the amount of blood the heart pushes out with each contraction. Thus, if cardiac output falls (either due to dropping or a very fast heart rate or lowered stroke volume) or if peripheral vascular resistance falls (such as in the dilated arteries that occur in **neurogenic shock**), then blood pressure will fall.

The preservation of these components can be related to the basic rules of shock management, which are the following:

- Control bleeding where possible.
- Maintain the airway.
- Maintain oxygenation and ventilation.
- Maintain circulation through an adequate heart rate and intravascular volume.

You should be aware that when you give positive pressure ventilation with a bag-valve mask, you raise the pressure inside the chest and can decrease the amount of blood returning to the heart, which will result in a decreased cardiac output.

The term *shock* describes a condition that occurs when the perfusion of the body's tissues with oxygen, electrolytes, glucose, and fluid becomes inadequate to meet the body's needs. Several processes cause this drop in perfusion. For example, the loss of red blood cells in hemorrhaging patients results in less oxygen transport to the body tissues. Decreased circulating blood volume leads to decreased delivery of glucose, fluid volume, and electrolytes to the cells. Those circulatory disturbances result in the cells of the body becoming "shocked," and grave changes in body tissue begin to occur. Eventually, severe cell damage or cell death follows.

When deprived of oxygen, cells begin to stop using aerobic respiration and switch to anaerobic respiration, which makes energy for the body less efficiently and produces toxic by-products such as lactic acid. The anaerobic processes may postpone cellular death for a time. However, the lack of oxygen is compounded by those toxic by-products because they can poison certain cellular functions, such as the production of energy by mitochondria. Eventually, accumulating lactic acid in the blood and organs creates a systemic acidosis that further disrupts cellular activity. Respiratory muscle function also weakens, respiratory failure develops, and hypoxia worsens.

Inadequate oxygen delivery causes the body to respond with increased activity of the sympathetic nervous system (increased sympathetic tone), resulting in the increased release of circulating catecholamines (epinephrine and norepinephrine). Those hormones increase both the rate and strength of the heart's contractions and constrict peripheral arterial blood vessels. The midbrain responds to the progressive hypoxia and acidosis with an increase in the respiratory rate.

Shock begins with an injury. It then spreads through the body as a multisystem insult to major organs. Specific symptoms result, symptoms that you can detect at the bedside as the patient becomes progressively sicker. Thus, shock is a cellular process with systemic clinical manifestations. Whereas your examination of the patient with shock may show paleness, diaphoresis, and tachycardia, at the cellular level, the patient's cells are starving for oxygen and nutrients. Shock, therefore, is a condition in which poor tissue perfusion can severely and permanently damage the organs of the body, causing disability or death. The clinical signs and symptoms of shock imply that critical processes are threatening every vulnerable cell in the patient's body, particularly those in vital organs.

Finally, the part of shock that field personnel do not usually see occurs after the patient is admitted to the hospital. Days after suffering severe hemorrhagic shock in the field, the patient may develop multisystem organ failure in the intensive care unit. So, discovering a patient in shock, treating according to current guidelines, and rapid transport of the patient to the appropriate hospital facility are essential aspects of saving the patient's life.

Assessment of Shock

Shock produces signs and symptoms you can observe during patient assessment. The initial diagnosis of the shock state often can be made from the physical exam findings. Although blood pressure should be monitored frequently to help determine whether

PEARLS
Basic Rules

Shock kills. Look for early signs of shock, and manage it appropriately. The basic rules of shock management are:

- Maintain the airway.
- Maintain oxygenation and ventilation.
- Control bleeding where possible.
- Maintain circulation through an adequate heart rate and intravascular volume.

or not organ perfusion is adequate, remember that hypotension is a late sign, indeed a sign that the body's vascular system has decompensated and the patient is near death. Assessment tools other than measuring the blood pressure must be used to recognize early shock in the trauma patient.

The blood pressure required to maintain adequate perfusion varies among people. The question, "How low can you go?" while maintaining adequate perfusion has not yet been answered. It is known that the healthy young patient often can maintain adequate perfusion of critically important tissue despite severe hypotension. In contrast, older patients, hypertensive patients, and those with head injury often cannot tolerate hypotension for even short periods. It is vital that you work with your medical director to stay up to date on recommendations for shock management as new research is published.

Although this chapter is about trauma, shock is a clinical condition associated with medical problems as well. Following is a discussion of shock syndromes, many of which are caused by traumatic conditions. The take-home point, though, is that *the shock state is one of low tissue perfusion*. There are some differences in the body's response to different kinds of shock, and there also are some similarities. For example, the stabbed and bleeding patient in hemorrhagic shock often shows many of the same signs as the burned or dehydrated patient with low blood volume not due to hemorrhage.

Compensated and Decompensated Shock

Generally, the onset of the signs and symptoms of **hypovolemic shock** (including hemorrhagic shock) occur in the following order: compensated shock and then decompensated shock.

Compensated Shock

During compensated shock, the body is still able to maintain perfusion by compensatory mechanisms and will present with the following signs and symptoms, often in this order of progression:

- *Weakness and lightheadedness*—caused by decreased blood volume
- *Pallor* (pale, lack of color in the skin)—caused by catecholamine-induced **vasoconstriction** and/or loss of circulating red blood cells. In persons of color this may be better seen in the palms and nailbeds.
- *Tachycardia* (elevated heart rate)—caused by the effect of catecholamines on the heart as the brain increases the activity of the sympathetic nervous system
- *Diaphoresis* (sweating)—caused by the effects of catecholamines on sweat glands
- *Tachypnea* (elevated respiratory rate)—caused by the brain elevating the respiratory rate under the influence of stress, catecholamines, acidosis, and hypoxia
- *Decreased urinary output*—caused by hypovolemia, hypoxia, and circulating catecholamines. This is a consideration in interfacility transfers in patients with a urinary catheter in place. Normal urinary output is 0.5 to 1 mL/kg/minute. So, for a 60-minute interfacility transport of a trauma patient, who has a Foley catheter in place and weighs 132 lb (60 kg), you would expect to see between 30 and 60 mL of urine produced during that period. Output less than that could indicate the patient is getting worse, even if blood pressure is still relatively normal. Empty the catheter bag at the start of the transport. The urine collected when catheter was first placed should not count in the hourly total.
- *Weakened peripheral pulses*—the "thready" pulse (meaning "threadlike") is caused by the arteries shrinking in width as intravascular volume is lost
- *Thirst*—caused by hypovolemia (especially with relatively low fluid amounts in the blood vessels)

Note: The signs and symptoms listed here are in the order of progressive "compensation," as the body attempts to deal with the cause of shock. Beginning with the next sign, hypotension, the body is no longer able to maintain perfusion, and the shock condition becomes "decompensated."

Decompensated Shock

When the body is no longer able to maintain perfusion and the compensatory mechanisms begin to fail, decompensated shock develops, and the following signs and symptoms appear:

- *Hypotension*—caused by hypovolemia, either absolute or relative (see later paragraphs for a discussion of relative hypovolemia), or by the diminished cardiac output seen in "obstructive," "**mechanical shock**," or **cardiogenic shock**
- *Altered mental status* (confusion, restlessness, combativeness, unconsciousness)—caused by decreased cerebral perfusion, acidosis, hypoxia, and catecholamine stimulation
- *Cardiac arrest*—caused by critical organ failure secondary to blood or fluid loss, hypoxia, and occasionally arrhythmia caused by catecholamine stimulation and/or low perfusion

To summarize, many of the symptoms of shock of any etiology—including the classic hemorrhagic shock picture—are caused by the release of catecholamines. When the brain senses that perfusion to the tissues is insufficient, messages are sent down the spinal cord to the sympathetic nervous system and the adrenal glands, causing a release of catecholamines (epinephrine and norepinephrine) into the circulation as part of the body's efforts to improve perfusion. The circulating catecholamines cause tachycardia, anxiety, diaphoresis, and vasoconstriction. This narrowing of the small arteries (the arterioles in the periphery of the arterial vascular system) shunts blood away from the skin and intestines to the heart, lungs, and brain.

Close monitoring early in the shock syndrome may allow you to detect an initial rise in blood pressure due to shunting, though this does not always happen. The **pulse pressure** is the pressure driving blood through the vascular system. It is calculated by subtracting the diastolic blood pressure from the systolic. It is usually about 40 mm Hg (blood pressure of 120/80 equals pulse pressure of 40). There will almost always be an initial narrowing of the pulse pressure because vasoconstriction raises the diastolic pressure more than the systolic. The shunting of blood from the skin and the loss of circulating red blood cells cause the pallor commonly seen in shock.

Decreased perfusion causes weakness initially and then, later, an alteration in the level of consciousness (confusion, restlessness, or combativeness) and worsening skin pallor. Development of confusion, restlessness, or combativeness always should alert you to possible hypoxia or shock. As shock continues, the prolonged tissue hypoxia leads to worsening acidosis, which can ultimately cause a loss of response to catecholamines, worsening the drop in blood pressure. This is often the point at which the patient in "compensated" shock suddenly "crashes" (decompensates). Eventually, the hypoxia and acidosis cause cardiac dysfunction, including cardiac arrest and, ultimately, death.

Although the individual response to post-traumatic hemorrhage may vary, many patients have the following classic patterns of "early" and "late" shock:

- *Early shock.* This is the loss of approximately 15% to 25% of blood volume. That is enough to stimulate slight to moderate tachycardia, pallor, narrowed pulse pressure, thirst, weakness, and possibly delayed capillary refill. In "early shock," the body is "compensating" for the physical insult that is causing the problem (hemorrhage, dehydration, tension pneumothorax, and so on).

mechanical shock: shock produced by conditions that affect the ability of the heart to pump blood; caused by a damaged heart (myocardial contusion) or by conditions preventing the filling of the heart (pericardial tamponade, tension pneumothorax).

cardiogenic shock: shock produced by conditions that impair the ability of the heart to pump blood, such as a myocardial contusion (bruise) or heart attack.

pulse pressure: the pressure driving blood through the vascular system. It is calculated by subtracting the diastolic from the systolic blood pressures (SBP − DBP = PP).

- *Late shock.* Late shock is the loss of approximately 30% to 45% of the blood volume. It is enough to cause hypotension as well as the other symptoms of hypovolemic shock listed earlier. When "late shock" occurs, it means the body's ability to compensate for the physical insult has failed. As mentioned earlier, hypotension is the first sign of "late shock." The hypotensive patient, then, is near death. Aggressive assessment and management must be provided to prevent the death of the patient.

Note that during the initial assessment, early shock presents as a fast pulse with pallor and diaphoresis. In contrast, late shock may present as weak pulse or loss of the peripheral pulse. A useful tip to remember is that the lowest pressure at which the radial pulse can usually be felt by the examiner begins at a systolic pressure of about 80 mm Hg, the femoral pulse can initially be felt at a systolic pressure of about 70 mm Hg, and the carotid pulse can initially be felt at a systolic pressure of about 60 mm Hg. Thus, if you had a trauma victim with a carotid pulse but no radial pulse, you could estimate that the patient's systolic pressure was between 60 and 80 mm Hg. One scientific study suggests that those numbers may even be slightly high. Nevertheless, weakened pulses, taken together with other signs of shock, should lead you quickly to suspect decompensated shock. The aggressiveness with which you treat it will depend on a number of factors. You will be guided by the patient's systolic blood pressure as well as respiratory rate, pulse rate, level of consciousness, and any obvious bleeding.

capillary refill time (CRT): a test for perfusion performed by pressing on the palm of the hand or sides of the fingertips and noting how quickly color returns to the blanched area. The test is suspicious for shock if the blanched area remains pale for longer than 2 seconds. It has been found to be unreliable for early shock and neurogenic shock.

Prolonged **capillary refill time (CRT)** was previously thought to be very useful for detecting early shock. CRT is tested by pressing on the palm of the hand or the sides of the fingertips. For a small child, CRT may be checked by squeezing the whole foot and looking to see how quickly color returns to the ball of the foot. The test is suspicious for shock if the blanched area remains pale for longer than 2 seconds. Scientific evaluation of this test has shown it to have a high correlation with late shock but to be of little value for detecting early shock. The test was associated with both frequent false-positive and false-negative results. Low blood volume, cold temperatures, and catecholamine-induced vasoconstriction can all cause decreased perfusion of the capillary bed in the skin and thus cause results that cannot be reliably trusted. Measurement of capillary refill may be useful for small children in whom it is difficult to get an accurate blood pressure, but it is of little use for detecting early shock in adults.

Evaluation of Tachycardia

One of the first signs of illness, and arguably one of the most common, is that of tachycardia. You will frequently be confronted with the patient who has an elevated pulse rate, and you must make some sort of determination about the cause.

First, you should always identify why a patient has tachycardia. An elevated pulse rate (generally considered to be above 100 in an adult and higher at younger ages) is never normal. Humans can transiently raise their pulses in the setting of anxiety, but such elevation quickly returns to normal or fluctuates in rate, depending on the waxing and waning of the anxiety state.

Second, remember that an elevated pulse rate is one of the first signs of shock. Any adult trauma patient with a sustained pulse rate above 100 must be suspected of having occult hemorrhage until proven otherwise. During the ITLS Primary Survey, a pulse rate greater than 120 should be a red flag for possible shock.

Finally, some patients who are in shock may not develop tachycardia. Patients with traumatic hypotension may develop a "relative bradycardia." Up to 20% of patients with bleeding into the abdomen may not show tachycardia. The patient in neurogenic shock may have a relatively normal or even slow pulse rate while being hypotensive. Always take into consideration the injured patient's medications because they can affect the intrinsic heart rate. Beta-blockers or calcium channel blocking medications, commonly used for hypertension or heart disease, might prevent the patient from developing a tachycardia even with severe blood loss. The presence of such medications in the patient's possession or medical history should always alert the emergency

PEARLS
Tachycardia

A persistently elevated pulse rate while at rest is always an indication of something medically wrong with the patient, including the possibility of occult hemorrhage. Absence of tachycardia does not rule out shock, however. Patients on medications such as beta-blockers may not become tachycardic.

care provider to evaluate all hemodynamic parameters, not just heart rate alone. So, the absence of tachycardia in an injured patient does not always rule out shock.

Children are unable to increase their stroke volume, so their cardiac output is very dependent on their heart rate (cardiac output = stroke volume × heart rate). Children in decompensated shock may develop bradycardia, which can have a devastating effect on their ability to maintain blood flow to their vital organs.

Capnography

The heart delivers oxygen and nutrients to the cells of the body by way of blood vessels. The cells "burn" the nutrients in the presence of oxygen to produce energy, water, and carbon dioxide (CO_2). The water and CO_2 move into the bloodstream, the CO_2 being carried to the lungs, mostly as dissolved bicarbonate ions, for excretion during exhalation. CO_2, then, is the exhaled by-product of metabolism. To put it another way, the level of exhaled CO_2 indicates how brightly the fire of metabolism is burning in the cells.

When measured moment to moment at the airway, the level of CO_2 being excreted may be graphed as a waveform and can give some measure of the patient's underlying metabolic rate. Devices are now commonly available, either separately or on ECG monitors, that measure exhaled CO_2 levels and display them as a waveform. The typical exhaled CO_2 is approximately 35 to 45 mm Hg. Falling measured CO_2 indicates that either the patient is hyperventilating (from anxiety or acidosis) or the amount of oxygen being supplied to the cells is falling. You might say it this way: A falling exhaled CO_2 level suggests that the fire of metabolism in the patient's cells may be burning low.

Patients in shock have decreased oxygen being supplied to their cells. This is either because they have lost blood through hemorrhage and the heart is not circulating it effectively, or a lung injury may be present (such as severe pulmonary contusion or from aspiration of stomach contents). Thus, if you are monitoring a patient either in shock or at risk of going into shock, monitor the level of exhaled CO_2 as part of your overall care. A level of exhaled CO_2 that falls much below 35 mm Hg—especially if it falls into the 20s or below—may be an indication of circulatory collapse and thus can be an additional warning sign of worsening shock. (See Chapter 5, Figures 5-30 and 5-31.)

The Shock Syndromes

Although the most common shock state seen in trauma patients is associated with hemorrhage and the accompanying hypovolemia, there are actually four major classifications of shock. Those "types" of shock relate directly to the blood pressure equation discussed earlier in this chapter (Blood Pressure = Cardiac Output × Peripheral Vascular Resistance). The four shock states can be categorized according to their causes as follows:

- *Low-volume shock* (absolute hypovolemia) is caused by hemorrhage or other major body fluid loss (diarrhea, vomiting, and "third spacing" due to burns, peritonitis, and other causes). Think of this as the tank is no longer full.

- *Distributive shock* (relative hypovolemia) is caused by spine injury, vasovagal syncope, sepsis, and certain drug overdoses that dilate the blood vessels (the arterioles) and redistribute blood flow to a larger vascular volume, thus causing reduced pressure in the vascular system (low blood pressure). Think of this as the tank has increased in size without having more fluid placed into it. This type of shock is also called *high-space shock*.

- *Mechanical shock*, also known as obstructive shock, is a form of shock that is caused by an actual physical blocking of the large blood vessels in the chest. Examples include conditions preventing the filling of the heart (pericardial tamponade and/or tension pneumothorax) or something obstructing blood flow through the lungs (massive pulmonary embolism). Think of this as blood flow into the heart or lungs being blocked.

PEARLS
Capnography

Falling height of the capnography waveform may be one of the first indicators that a patient is going into a shock state.

• *Cardiogenic shock* is produced by a problem with the heart itself (a "pump" problem, if you remember the equation). This type of shock is caused by a damaged heart, such as in the setting of a severe myocardial contusion or an acute myocardial infarction, both of which can reduce the heart's ability to pump, thus dropping blood pressure. The signs and symptoms of cardiogenic shock may be similar to those of obstructive shock. Think of this as the pump is not working as well as it should.

There are some notable differences in the appearance of patients with these conditions, and it is critical that you be aware of the signs and symptoms that accompany each one.

Low-Volume Shock (Absolute Hypovolemia)

hemorrhagic shock: shock caused by blood loss resulting in insufficient blood within the vascular system.

Loss of blood from injury is called *post-traumatic hemorrhage*. In addition to head injury, **hemorrhagic shock** is a leading cause of preventable death from injury. The volume that the vascular system can hold is many liters more than what actually flows through the vasculature. The sympathetic nervous system keeps the vessels constricted, which reduces the potential vascular volume and maintains blood pressure high enough to perfuse vital organs. If blood volume is lost, "sensors" in the major vessels signal the adrenal gland and the nerves of the sympathetic nervous system to secrete catecholamines. They cause vasoconstriction and thus further shrink the vascular space and maintain perfusion pressure to the brain and heart. If blood loss is minor, the sympathetic system can shrink the vascular space enough to maintain blood pressure and provide for vital organ perfusion. If blood loss is severe, though, the vascular space cannot be shrunk down enough to maintain blood pressure, and hypotension and reduced organ perfusion result.

Normally, the blood vessels are elastic and are distended by the volume within them. This produces a radial artery pulse that is full and wide. Blood loss allows the artery to shrink in width, becoming more threadlike in size. The term *thready pulse* means that the actual width of the artery shrinks, becoming barely wider than a thread, and often more difficult to feel.

Hypovolemic shock victims usually have tachycardia, are pale, and have flat neck veins. So, if you find a trauma victim with a fast heart rate, who is pale, with weak radial pulses and flat neck veins, this patient is probably bleeding from some injury, either internally or externally (or possibly both).

Remember always that absolute hypovolemic shock can be the result of conditions other than hemorrhage caused by trauma. The patient with severe diarrhea (such as from common viral conditions or from some disease as deadly as cholera) can experience hypovolemic shock. A bowel obstruction from a surgical condition, as another example, can cause profuse vomiting, dehydration, and ultimately shock. It is common to see patients who have some sort of severe internal gastrointestinal bleeding (such as ruptured esophageal varices) who may present in hypovolemic hemorrhagic shock of a nontraumatic cause. So, the emergency care provider finding a weak, pale, and tachycardic patient with flat neck veins and no evident source of trauma must broaden clinical suspicion while searching for other causes of this shock syndrome and while also avoiding delays in transport.

Absolute hypovolemic shock may be identified in your patient during the ITLS Primary Survey (Figure 8-1).

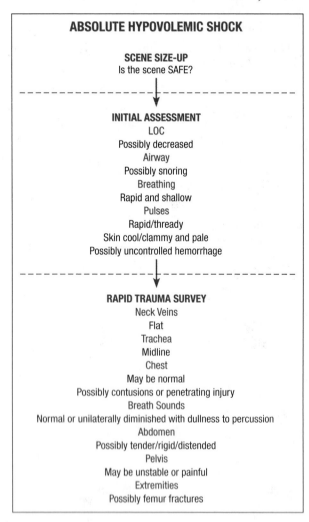

ABSOLUTE HYPOVOLEMIC SHOCK

SCENE SIZE-UP
Is the scene SAFE?

INITIAL ASSESSMENT
LOC
Possibly decreased
Airway
Possibly snoring
Breathing
Rapid and shallow
Pulses
Rapid/thready
Skin cool/clammy and pale
Possibly uncontrolled hemorrhage

RAPID TRAUMA SURVEY
Neck Veins
Flat
Trachea
Midline
Chest
May be normal
Possibly contusions or penetrating injury
Breath Sounds
Normal or unilaterally diminished with dullness to percussion
Abdomen
Possibly tender/rigid/distended
Pelvis
May be unstable or painful
Extremities
Possibly femur fractures

Figure 8-1 Absolute hypovolemic shock may be identified during the ITLS Primary Survey.

High-Space Shock (Relative Hypovolemia)

As mentioned earlier, the volume that the blood vessels can hold is many liters more than the blood volume in the blood vessels. The average-size adult has around 5 liters (10 units) of blood in the vascular system. However, the vascular system could hold as many as 25 liters (50 units) of blood, if the arterioles were to fully dilate and allow the high pressure arterial blood to flow out into the low pressure capillary network. Again, it is the steady-state action of the sympathetic nervous system that keeps the arterioles of the vascular bed constricted in the normal state, keeping most of the blood in the arteries, distending the usually elastic arterial system, and maintaining perfusion to the heart and brain. Anything that interrupts the outflow from the sympathetic nervous system and causes the loss of normal vasoconstriction allows the vascular space to dilate, becoming much "too large" for the amount of blood in the vascular system. If blood vessels dilate, the 5 liters (10 units) or so of blood flowing through the normal adult's vascular space may not be sufficient to maintain blood pressure and vital tissue perfusion. The condition causing the vascular space to be too large for a normal amount of blood has been called "high-space shock," or relative hypovolemia (also known as vasodilatory shock or **distributive shock**). Although several causes of high-space shock exist (such as sepsis syndrome and drug overdose), neurogenic shock, commonly called spinal shock, is addressed here because it may be caused by trauma.

The nerves of the sympathetic nervous system come off the spinal cord in the thoracic (chest) and lumbar area. This is why the sympathetic nervous system is often called the "thoracolumbar autonomic nervous system." Neurogenic shock occurs most typically after an injury to the spinal cord. An injury to the neck can damage the spinal cord in that area, preventing the brain from being able to send out sympathetic nervous system signals. Thus, a cervical spinal-cord injury can prevent the brain from raising the pulse rate, from raising the strength of the heart's contraction, or from constricting the peripheral arterioles (the vessels that maintain blood pressure). Although circulating catecholamines already present in the bloodstream may preserve the blood pressure for a short time, the disruption of the sympathetic nervous system outflow from the spinal cord results in loss of the normal vascular tone and in the inability of the body to compensate for any accompanying hemorrhage.

The clinical presentation of neurogenic shock differs from hemorrhagic shock in that there is no catecholamine release and thus no pallor (vasoconstriction), tachycardia, or sweating. The patient will have a decreased blood pressure, but the heart rate will be normal or slow, and the skin is usually warm, dry, and pink. The patient also may have accompanying paralysis or sensory deficit corresponding to the spinal-cord injury. You also may see a lack of chest wall movement and only simple diaphragmatic movement when the patient is asked to take a deep breath. This diaphragmatic breathing is seen as a protrusion of the abdomen during inspiration. In males, priapism (prolonged erection of the shaft of the penis) may be present.

A key point is that neurogenic shock does not have the typical picture of hemorrhagic shock, even when associated with severe bleeding. A careful neurologic assessment is essential. Do not rely on the classic signs and symptoms of shock to identify internal bleeding or accompanying hemorrhage-associated shock in patients with neurogenic shock. Neurogenic shock patients may "look better" than their actual condition really is and can be some of the most difficult patients to accurately assess.

Finally, trauma patients with altered mental status, including coma, can make assessment difficult in terms of determining the cause of the hypotension. Just remember: If you see shock in a trauma patient with a normal or slow pulse and no other obvious cause, think about neurogenic shock as a potential cause, especially if there is evident injury to the head and/or neck.

distributive shock: state that results from the loss of ability of the small arterial vessels to regulate distribution of blood, leading to inadequate tissue perfusion. Because of the loss of vascular resistance and vasodilatation, it is often referred to as "warm" shock.

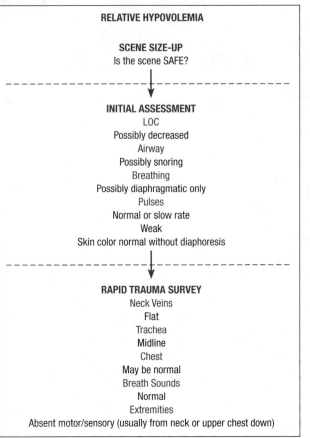

RELATIVE HYPOVOLEMIA

SCENE SIZE-UP
Is the scene SAFE?

- -

INITIAL ASSESSMENT
LOC
Possibly decreased
Airway
Possibly snoring
Breathing
Possibly diaphragmatic only
Pulses
Normal or slow rate
Weak
Skin color normal without diaphoresis

- -

RAPID TRAUMA SURVEY
Neck Veins
Flat
Trachea
Midline
Chest
May be normal
Breath Sounds
Normal
Extremities
Absent motor/sensory (usually from neck or upper chest down)

Figure 8-2 Relative hypovolemia due to neurogenic (spinal) shock may be identified during the ITLS Primary Survey.

PEARLS
Mechanical or Distributive Shock

Look for signs of mechanical or distributive shock, especially if there is no bleeding.

Certain drug overdoses and chemical exposures also can result in shock from arterial vasodilatation causing a relative hypovolemia. Very often injuries result after such overdoses, and their effect on typical clinical signs and symptoms (like neurogenic shock) should be considered. Examples of drug overdoses and chemical exposures that may produce the relative hypovolemia syndrome include nitroglycerin, beta-blockers and calcium channel blockers, other antihypertensive medications, cyanide, and even the ethyl alcohol found in legal alcoholic beverages.

Whereas the patient with neurogenic shock (due to spinal-cord injury) has a slow heart rate, has pink, warm skin, and has flat neck veins, patients with medical causes of high-space shock (such as certain drug overdoses, cyanide, sepsis) will show similar signs, but they usually have a fast heart rate. The physical evaluation of these patients may give signs difficult to interpret. Calcium channel blocker or beta-blocker poisonings often produce bradycardia, whereas nitroglycerin overdose might produce tachycardia. In these patients, taking a good history is essential. Be sure to get information from others who may know the patient, including what medications the patient may be taking. This information may be life saving.

Relative hypovolemia due to neurogenic (spinal) shock may be identified in your patient during the ITLS Primary Survey (Figure 8-2).

Mechanical (or Obstructive) Shock

The heart is a pump. Like any pump, it has a "power" stroke and a "filling" stroke, just like a piston moving up and down in the cylinder of a motor. In the normal adult's resting state, the heart pumps out about 5 liters of blood per minute. This means, of course, that the heart also must take in about 5 liters of blood per minute. Therefore, any traumatic or medical condition that slows or prevents the venous return of blood can cause shock by lowering cardiac output and thus oxygen delivery to the tissues. Likewise, anything that obstructs the flow of blood to or through the heart can cause shock.

Traumatic conditions that can cause mechanical shock are tension pneumothorax and cardiac tamponade:

- *Tension pneumothorax* is so named because of the high air tension (pressure) that can develop in the pleural space (between the lung and chest wall) due to a lung or chest-wall injury. This very high positive pressure collapses the low-pressure superior and inferior vena cava, preventing the return of venous blood to the heart. The resulting "backup" of blood presents is seen as distended neck veins. Shifting of mediastinal structures also may lower venous return by impinging on the superior and inferior vena cava, also causing a deviation of the trachea away from the affected side (rarely seen clinically). Decreased venous return results in lower cardiac output and the development of shock. Also, decreased blood flow through the lungs can result in hypoxia, ultimately causing cyanosis of the patient's skin. (See Figure 8-3 and Chapters 6 and 7 for a complete description of the signs, symptoms, and treatment of tension pneumothorax.)

- *Cardiac tamponade*, or "pericardial tamponade," of a traumatic nature occurs when blood fills the "potential" space between the heart and the pericardium, squeezing the heart and preventing the heart from filling (Figure 8-4). Just as the "squeezing" of the superior and inferior vena cava present as distended neck veins in the patient who has tension pneumothorax, the "squeezing" of the heart during tamponade produces the same sign. This decreased filling of the heart causes cardiac

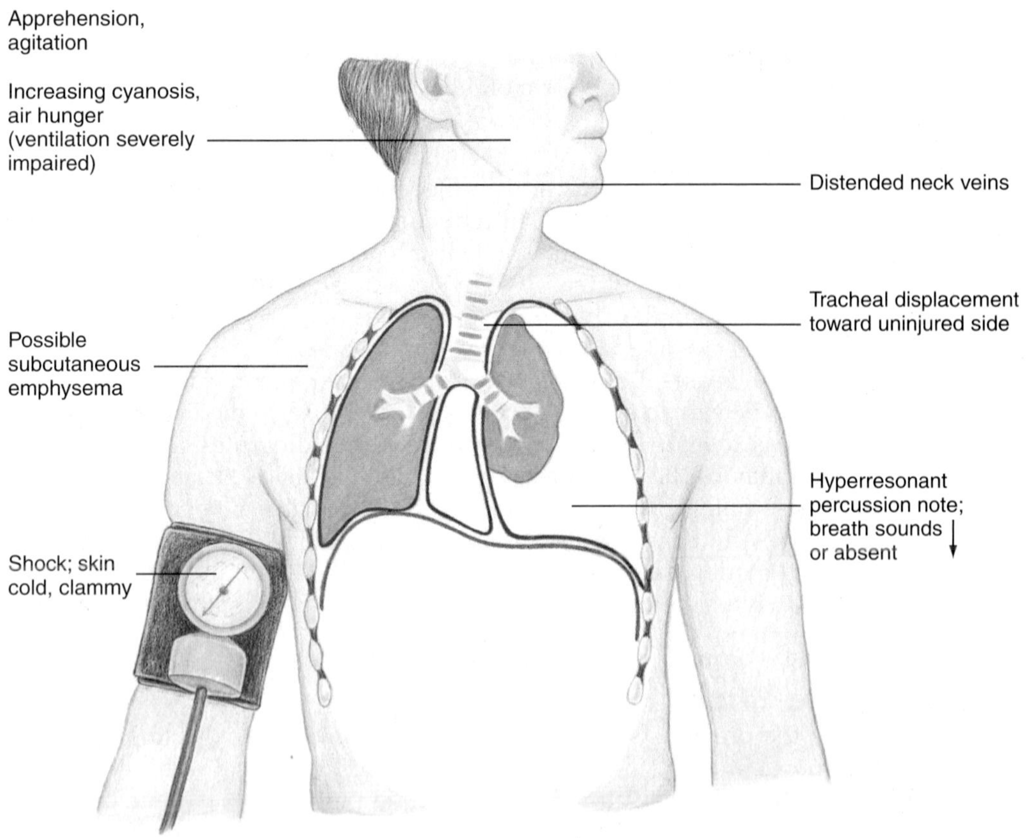

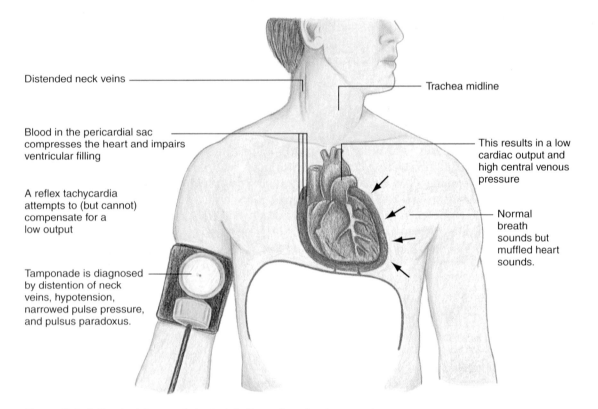

Apprehension, agitation

Increasing cyanosis, air hunger (ventilation severely impaired)

Possible subcutaneous emphysema

Shock; skin cold, clammy

Distended neck veins

Tracheal displacement toward uninjured side

Hyperresonant percussion note; breath sounds ↓ or absent

Figure 8-3 Physical findings of tension pneumothorax.

Distended neck veins

Blood in the pericardial sac compresses the heart and impairs ventricular filling

A reflex tachycardia attempts to (but cannot) compensate for a low output

Tamponade is diagnosed by distention of neck veins, hypotension, narrowed pulse pressure, and pulsus paradoxus.

Trachea midline

This results in a low cardiac output and high central venous pressure

Normal breath sounds but muffled heart sounds.

Figure 8-4 Pathophysiology and physical findings of cardiac tamponade.

output to fall, resulting in the development of shock. As with tension pneumothorax, cyanosis may occur during cardiac tamponade also due to decreased blood flow through the lungs from this form of mechanical shock.

Pericardial tamponade may occur in more than 75% of cases of penetrating cardiac injury. The signs of tamponade have been labeled "Beck's triad," consisting of hypotension, distended neck veins, and muffled heart tones. A "pulsus paradoxus" may be present, which is an abnormal reduction in the patient's pulse pressure during inspiration. (When a normal patient inhales, the pulse weakens slightly during inspiration, usually less than 10 mm Hg; a pulsus paradoxus is the marked dropping off of the strength of the pulse during inspiration.) Scene interventions should be avoided if the diagnosis of cardiac tamponade is suspected because time wasted on scene increases the chances of death for the patient. If it is within your scope of practice, perform a pericardiocentesis. Otherwise, immediate transport to a facility that has the capability to perform a pericardiocentesis or pericardial decompression may be the only life-saving measure available. Using intravenous fluids to increase filling pressure of the heart may possibly be of some value in tamponade, but IV fluids might also worsen the condition if there is an additional internal exsanguinating injury. Use of IV fluids in this situation should be during transport and only at the order of medical direction. (See Chapter 6 for a more complete discussion.)

Cardiogenic Shock

As discussed in the previous section, the heart is a pump, and its pumping action produces the output of blood into the vascular system. The typical cardiac output of blood in the normal resting adult is 5 liters of blood per minute. If some condition causes the heart to lose pumping strength, then the amount of blood being circulated would be reduced. This is precisely what happens when the heart muscle itself is damaged. Pumping strength is reduced, cardiac output falls, and blood pressure goes down. Such a condition is called *cardiogenic shock*. Be aware that cardiogenic and mechanical shock may present with similar findings during the physical assessment. Because of how the heart is situated in the chest, with the right ventricle more anterior than the left, the right ventricle is a common location for myocardial contusions. The right ventricle may not pump as well, and this results in a decrease in preload for the left ventricle. Because of the decreased preload, there is decreased output from the left ventricle and cardiac output and peripheral perfusion drops.

In the trauma patient, the significant causes of cardiogenic shock are the following:

- *Myocardial contusion.* Direct trauma to the heart can injure it, damaging the muscle and reducing pumping strength, a condition called myocardial contusion. Myocardial contusion can result in diminished cardiac output because of this heart muscle damage, as well as possibly causing cardiac dysrhythmia (Figures 8-5 and 8-6). Myocardial contusion often cannot be differentiated from cardiac tamponade in the field. Therefore, rapid transport, supportive care, and cardiac monitoring are the mainstays of therapy.

- *Myocardial infarction (MI).* Though this is a medical cause of loss of heart muscle strength, the emergency care provider must remember that cardiogenic shock must be considered in the hypotensive and usually tachycardic patient who presents with chest pain. Especially in older patients, an MI may be the precipitating cause of the traumatic event.

A word of caution is needed here. Patients with shock from both mechanical and cardiogenic causes can be very near death. Delay on scene can prevent salvage of the patient because the time from development of a traumatic cardiac tamponade to circulatory arrest may be as little as 5 to 10 minutes. Survival following traumatic circulatory arrest due to tamponade, even in the best of trauma systems, is rarely achieved if pericardiocentesis is not performed within 5 to 10 minutes. Anything that

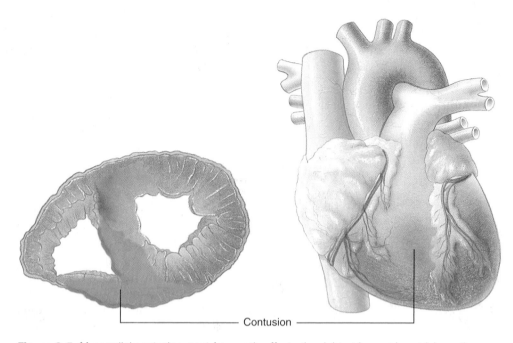

Figure 8-5 Myocardial contusion most frequently affects the right atrium and ventricle as they collide with the sternum.

delays transport to definitive care, such as taking the time to package the patient on a backboard, increases mortality.

Mechanical and cardiogenic shock states are caused by a diminished cardiac output rather than blood loss. Thus, these patients usually have a different appearance upon assessment than hemorrhagic shock patients. Because the cardiac output is diminished, the blood backs up into the venous system, resulting in distended neck veins. The lungs are not being perfused well, causing the patient to become dyspneic and cyanotic. Because the patient is in shock with an intact spinal cord, catecholamines are released, and the patient develops tachycardia and diaphoresis. Thus, mechanical shock patients are cyanotic with distended neck veins and tachycardia, as are patients with cardiogenic shock. A post-trauma patient with these signs is near death, requiring rapid transport to a trauma center. In the setting of a tension pneumothorax, needle decompression of the affected side of the thorax can be life saving.

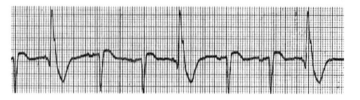

Figure 8-6 Myocardial contusion may cause ventricular ectopy.

Mechanical (obstructive) shock may be identified in your patient during the ITLS Primary Survey (Figure 8-7).

Management and Treatment
General Management of Post-Traumatic Shock States

Management of post-traumatic shock states includes the following:

- *Control bleeding.* Red blood cells are necessary to carry oxygen. Control of bleeding must be obtained either by direct pressure, tourniquet, hemostatic agent, or rapid transport to surgery.
- *Administer high-flow oxygen.* Patients in shock need oxygen supplementation. Evaluation of skin color in shock patients may not tell you what the patient's oxygen requirement is. Generally, patients in hemorrhagic shock are pale. Cyanosis (from mechanical or cardiogenic shock states) is an extremely late sign of hypoxemia and

PEARLS
Hemorrhage

Control hemorrhage. If it cannot be done in the field, the patient needs to be in the operating room as soon as possible.

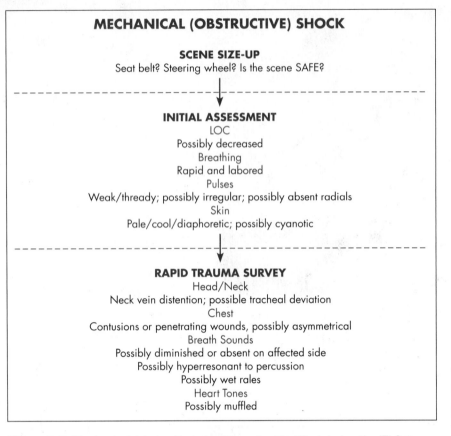

MECHANICAL (OBSTRUCTIVE) SHOCK

SCENE SIZE-UP
Seat belt? Steering wheel? Is the scene SAFE?

INITIAL ASSESSMENT
LOC
Possibly decreased
Breathing
Rapid and labored
Pulses
Weak/thready; possibly irregular; possibly absent radials
Skin
Pale/cool/diaphoretic; possibly cyanotic

RAPID TRAUMA SURVEY
Head/Neck
Neck vein distention; possible tracheal deviation
Chest
Contusions or penetrating wounds, possibly asymmetrical
Breath Sounds
Possibly diminished or absent on affected side
Possibly hyperresonant to percussion
Possibly wet rales
Heart Tones
Possibly muffled

Figure 8-7 Mechanical (obstructive) shock may be identified during the ITLS Primary Survey.

may not occur at all if there has been extensive blood loss. Indeed, a patient has to have at least 5 grams of deoxygenated hemoglobin (Hgb) per 100 mL of blood (normal Hgb is 14 grams per 100 mL) for cyanosis to occur. Someone bleeding to death, literally, may not have enough hemoglobin around to manifest cyanosis. So, it is safe to say regardless of the patient's skin color, you should give high-flow oxygen to all patients at risk for shock. Try to maintain a pulse oximeter reading of about 95%.

- *Load and go.* Trauma patients in shock from any cause are considered to be in the load-and-go category. Transport as soon as you finish the ITLS Primary Survey (initial assessment and rapid trauma survey). Almost all critical interventions should be done in the ambulance. (See Chapter 2.)

Treatment of Post-Traumatic Hemorrhage

Specific prehospital management of the patient in shock remains both controversial and the subject of ongoing research. There is no question of the need for control of hemorrhage, supplemental oxygen, and early transport, but the indications for most other therapies are still being debated. Hypertonic saline has been proposed as an alternative resuscitation fluid. It is believed that lower volumes of fluid can be given to achieve restoration of circulatory volume. However, studies have shown that low-volume resuscitation with hypertonic saline in patients in severe hemorrhagic shock generally show no significant benefit over conventional IV fluids. Further studies designed to identify the "best" resuscitation fluid, including how much fluid should be administered, are ongoing at this time

Since the early days of modern shock treatment (about the middle of the 20th century), intravenous crystalloid solutions (and sometimes colloid) have been tested and/or utilized to reverse the effects of hypovolemia. In addition, it has been previously proposed that intra-abdominal and pelvic bleeding may possibly be diminished by use of the pneumatic antishock garment (PASG) or military antishock trousers (MAST). Research showed that the PASG seemed to cause a higher death rate when the garment was applied to patients with uncontrolled internal bleeding.

Patients in hypovolemic shock due to hemorrhage may be generally thought of as falling into one of the following two categories: those with bleeding you can control (such as many extremity injuries) and those with bleeding you cannot control (such as hemorrhage from internal injuries).

Hemorrhage That Can Be Controlled

A patient with controllable bleeding is fairly easy to manage. Most bleeding can be stopped with direct pressure. In some situations (usually blast or tactical injuries), there may be life-threatening hemorrhage you cannot control with direct pressure. In these most extreme circumstances, you should not hesitate to apply a tourniquet. A tourniquet is rarely needed, but when it is needed, it should be applied quickly. Commercially manufactured tourniquets are preferable to devices that might be used as a tourniquet but are not manufactured for that purpose. Tourniquets must be used as part of a predeveloped hemorrhage control protocol from your medical director or your EMS agency.

If the patient has clinical evidence of shock that persists after direct control of the bleeding, you should take the steps outlined in the "Procedure" that follows.

Procedure

Managing Shock When Bleeding Has Been Controlled

1. Put the patient's body in a horizontal position.
2. Administer high-flow oxygen, preferably using a nonrebreather mask with a reservoir.
3. Transport to definitive care immediately in a safe, rapid manner.
4. Obtain IV access with large-bore catheters (16 gauge or greater if possible). Consider intraosseous (IO) vascular access if the patient is critical and you are unable to quickly establish an intravenous line. IO flow rate is substantially faster using the large adult needle and a pressure bag. (See Chapter 9.)
5. Give normal saline as a bolus (500 to 1,000 mL in adults, 20 mL/kg in pediatric patients) rapidly and then repeat the ITLS Ongoing Exam. When bleeding is controlled, it is permissible to attempt to normalize blood pressure, unlike the situation of uncontrolled bleeding. If shock symptoms persist, continue to administer fluid in boluses and reassess. In some cases of very severe hemorrhage—because of the substantial loss of red blood cells and markedly impaired oxygen delivery to the tissues—shock signs and symptoms may persist despite hemorrhage control and IV volume infusion. These patients need the rapid transfusion of blood and blood products.
6. Place the patient on an ECG monitor early during evaluation and treatment.
7. Apply pulse oximetry and, if available, waveform capnography.
8. Perform ITLS Ongoing Exams, and observe closely, especially for any return of bleeding.

Hemorrhage That Cannot Be Controlled

External Hemorrhage A patient with external hemorrhage that cannot be controlled by direct pressure must be rapidly transported to an appropriate facility where necessary procedures to gain surgical hemostasis can be performed. Although most physicians advocate fluid resuscitation to treat hemorrhagic shock, you must remember that elevating blood pressure can increase uncontrolled hemorrhage. To manage this patient, you should take the following steps.

PEARLS
IV Access

Do not waste scene time to establish IV access. Consider the use of IO vascular access if the patient is critical and you cannot obtain peripheral IV access.

Procedure

Managing Shock Due to Exsanguinating External Hemorrhage That You Cannot Control

1. Apply direct pressure on the bleeding site (femoral artery or facial hemorrhage, for example). Substantial pressure may be required. Release of direct pressure may result in the continuation of bleeding.
2. Place the patient in a horizontal position.

Procedure (*continued*)

3. Do not hesitate to apply a tourniquet to a bleeding extremity to stop severe bleeding that cannot be otherwise controlled. Commercially manufactured tourniquets are preferable to devices that might be used as a tourniquet but are not manufactured for that purpose. Tourniquets must be used as part of a predeveloped hemorrhage control protocol from your medical director or your EMS agency.

4. If you cannot stop severe bleeding with pressure and cannot use a tourniquet (groin, axilla, neck, face, scalp), you may use one of the **hemostatic agents** such as QuikClot® Combat Gauze, Hemcon Dressing, or Celox™, if available. (See Chapter 14.) Pack the hemostatic agent in the wound, and hold firm pressure. Always remember that the hemostatic agent is an "adjunct" to assist in controlling hemorrhage, not a hemorrhage control by itself. The agents must be part of an overall hemorrhage control protocol authorized by the medical director or by system protocol.

5. Administer high-flow oxygen through a nonrebreather mask with a reservoir.

6. Transport immediately in a prompt but safe manner.

7. Gain IV access when en route. Consider IO vascular access if patient is critical and you are unable to establish an intravenous line. IO flow rate is substantially faster using the large adult needle placed in the humeral head.

   a. Give only enough normal saline to maintain a blood pressure high enough for adequate peripheral perfusion. Maintaining peripheral perfusion may be defined as producing a peripheral pulse (such as a radial pulse), maintaining consciousness (assuming a traumatic brain injury is not also present), and maintaining an adequate blood pressure. The definition of an adequate blood pressure ("How low can you go?") remains controversial and will continue to be subject to change based on ongoing research, as previously mentioned. Certainly most young patients can maintain adequate perfusion with a blood pressure of 80 to 90 mm Hg systolic, but some experts now advocate even lower pressures. Keep in mind that a higher systolic pressure may be required in the setting of head injury with increased intracranial pressure and in patients who have a history of hypertension. (See Chapter 10.) Rely on local medical direction or EMS agency policy for guidelines in this area.

   b. Early blood transfusion is the most important fluid replacement in severe cases.

   c. Finally, as discussed earlier, research continues trying to find the "best" resuscitation fluid. Rely on local medical direction or EMS agency for guidelines about using any resuscitation fluid.

8. Monitor the heart, and apply pulse oximetry and waveform capnography (if available).

9. Perform ITLS Ongoing Exams, and observe closely.

Note: Hemorrhage control should remain the priority, when help is not available and when other procedures interrupt. In the case of wounds with exsanguinating hemorrhage, the military has changed the initial assessment from ABC (airway, breathing, and circulation) to CABC, making control of the hemorrhage the first priority. ITLS also has refined its approach to hemorrhage. It specifies that upon approaching the patient, if the emergency care provider encounters life-threatening external hemorrhage, immediate efforts to control the bleeding must be undertaken. (See Chapter 2.)

---

hemostatic agents: chemical or physical agents that help stop hemorrhage by facilitating clotting of the blood at the bleeding site.

Internal Hemorrhage The patient with uncontrolled internal hemorrhage is the classic critical trauma victim who will almost certainly die unless you promptly transport to an appropriate facility for rapid operative hemostasis (control of bleeding). The results of the most current medical research on the management of patients with exsanguinating internal hemorrhage is that there exists no substitute for gaining surgical control of bleeding. Research into the administration of IV fluids to patients with uncontrolled hemorrhage has indicated the following:

- The use of large amounts of IV fluids in the setting of uncontrolled internal hemorrhage may increase internal bleeding and mortality through raising the blood pressure, which may increase bleeding as well as dilute clotting factors in the blood. Furthermore, IV fluids carry almost no oxygen and are not a replacement for red blood cells. Early blood transfusion is very important in severe cases of hemorrhagic shock.

- Do not delay in providing rapid transport of such patients unless absolutely unavoidable, as in the case of a patient requiring prolonged extrication or in a tactical setting where transport is delayed. Always document such circumstances carefully in the patient care report.

- Moribund trauma patients (ones in very deep shock with blood pressures under 50 mm Hg systolic and therefore no pulses can be felt) often die. Fluid administration is indicated to maintain some degree of circulation, according to current understanding. Treatment of this extreme amount of hemorrhage may override the concerns for increased hemorrhage secondary to the use of these interventions. However, this approach is still controversial. Local medical direction or EMS agency policy should guide such therapy pending further research.

The recommendations, therefore, for a patient with probable exsanguinating internal hemorrhage are as follows.

Procedure

Managing Shock Due to Internal Hemorrhage

1. Transport immediately and in a rapid, safe manner.
2. Place the patient in a horizontal position.
3. Administer high-flow oxygen.
4. Gain IV access with large-bore catheters. Consider IO vascular access if unable to quickly establish an intravenous line, remembering the improved flow rate of the IO placed into the humeral head.
5. Administer sufficient normal saline to maintain peripheral perfusion, following local or EMS agency medical direction policies. Maintaining peripheral perfusion is generally defined as giving enough fluid—usually in boluses—to return a peripheral pulse, such as a radial pulse. However, many research experts now recommend that fluid resuscitation be kept to a minimum until hemorrhage control is obtained (operative intervention). Regardless, it would seem prudent to give sufficient fluid to maintain level of consciousness in the patient who has no traumatic brain injury. Hemostatic agents are not indicated for internal hemorrhage.
6. Monitor the heart, and apply pulse oximetry and waveform capnography (where available).
7. Perform ITLS Ongoing Exams, and observe closely.

Patients who have blunt injuries can lose a significant amount of blood and fluid from the intravascular space, including into the sites of large-bone fractures (hematoma and edema). This loss can be enough to cause shock, though the blood loss from the fractures tends to be self-limited. Pelvic fractures, however, are a *very important exception*. Pelvic fractures can result in exsanguination and death, so any suspicion for a pelvic fracture (especially one that appears severe or even unstable) is a sign that this patient may become unstable very quickly. Many EMS agencies now carry pelvic binders for these patients, which can reduce the risk of exsanguination post application. (See Chapter 14.)

The blunt injury trauma patient may sustain a tear of a large internal blood vessel or a laceration or avulsion of an internal organ. In this setting raising the blood pressure through fluid administration prior to surgical intervention may result in accelerated bleeding or a secondary hemorrhage. Therefore, if an internal hemorrhage is not suspected (patient is alert and oriented and has no apparent chest, abdominal, or pelvic injuries), IV fluids may be used judiciously for hypotension associated with large-bone fractures and/or externally controlled hemorrhage.

In the case of a severe mechanism of injury or inability to assess the patient, use IV fluids with caution. As indicated earlier, administering enough fluids to maintain peripheral perfusion and mental status seems to be a reasonable course, remembering that early blood transfusion, when available, is the most appropriate fluid replacement of severe blood loss. Frequent patient assessments and local EMS medical direction should guide therapy.

Special Situations in Hypovolemic Shock

Head Injury

The patient with severe head injury (Glasgow Coma Scale score of 8 or less) and shock is a special situation. (See Chapter 10.) These patients do not tolerate hypotension. Therefore, if necessary, adults with suspected hemorrhagic shock in addition to head injury should be fluid resuscitated to a blood pressure of 100 mm Hg systolic to maintain a cerebral perfusion pressure of at least 60 mm Hg. (See Chapter 10.)

Nonhemorrhagic Hypovolemic Shock

The patient who has low-volume shock syndrome not due to hemorrhage can generally be managed in the same manner as a patient with shock due to bleeding that can be controlled. An example of this type of patient would be one with shock due to fluid loss from burns or severe diarrhea. Hypovolemic shock is a common cause of death in these patients. Because the loss of volume in this case is not from an injured vascular system, it is reasonable to treat such patients with aggressive volume replacement to restore vital signs toward normal. Just beware: Hemorrhagic shock due to a bleeding internal organ (such as a bleeding ulcer or a ruptured ectopic pregnancy) may be rapidly lethal. The bleeding may not be at all apparent from the physical exam. So, if you see signs of shock present, follow the basic rules of shock management until you have explained the cause. For example, an unconscious, pale young woman of childbearing age who has a rapid, weak pulse with no obvious cause for her abnormal vital signs is bleeding to death from a ruptured ectopic pregnancy until proved otherwise.

Treatment of Nonhemorrhagic Shock Syndromes

Treatments for the other shock syndromes, namely, mechanical, cardiogenic, and high-space (vasodilatory) shock are different from hemorrhagic shock. All patients require high-flow oxygen, rapid transport, supine positioning, and IV line placement (usually en route).

Mechanical (or Obstructive) Shock

The patient with mechanical shock must first be accurately assessed to attempt to determine the cause of the problem. The patient with tension pneumothorax needs prompt decompression of the elevated pleural pressure. (See Chapter 7 for indications and procedure for decompression.)

The patient with suspected pericardial tamponade must undergo immediate pericardiocentesis, if it is within your scope of practice. If not, then the patient must be rapidly transported to an appropriate facility because the time from onset of tamponade to the time of cardiac arrest can be a matter of minutes (one of the ultimate load-and-go situations). Although anecdotal support exists for use of an intravenous volume challenge as a temporizing measure, no clear evidence exists that such treatment will improve survival. Use of IV fluids in this situation should be during transport and only on the order of medical direction. Obtaining IV access certainly should not delay direct transport or airway/oxygen interventions. Consider IO vascular access if you are unable to quickly establish an intravenous line. Bear in mind that trauma is not the only cause of tamponade. Metastatic cancer and other diseases such as pericarditis resulting in pericardial effusion also may cause tamponade.

Cardiogenic Shock

Myocardial contusion rarely causes shock. Recent reports indicate that most myocardial contusions cause little or no clinical findings. However, severe contusion may cause acute heart failure, manifested by distended neck veins, tachycardia, cyanosis, and possibly arrhythmias. These are similar signs as are seen with pericardial tamponade. These patients require rapid transport for proper care. Give high-flow oxygen, and perform cardiac monitoring on the patient with suspected myocardial contusion. IV fluids may cause worsening of the patient's condition.

High-Space (or Vasodilatory) Shock

High-space shock, in theory, resembles controlled hemorrhage, in that there is relative hypovolemia with an "intact" vascular system (no "leaks"). Therefore, initial management includes IV fluid boluses. Consider IO vascular access if the patient is critical and you are otherwise unable to establish an intravenous line. The patient with vasodilatory shock may benefit from various therapies, including administration of glucagon and vasopressors for beta-blocker or calcium channel blocker overdoses as well as prompt early volume resuscitation. Septic patients need IV fluid, vasopressors, and appropriate antibiotics.

Finally, in the absence of a head injury, the patient's level of consciousness is a useful monitor of the success or failure of resuscitation. Be alert for possible occult internal injuries, and keep in mind that raising the blood pressure may increase internal bleeding in that situation.

Areas of Current Study

Much work continues into finding the "ideal resuscitation fluid." Even after decades of research, it is not at all clear at this time what the best initial resuscitation fluid is. It remains quite reasonable to begin with normal saline as a resuscitation fluid for trauma, with the understanding that patients in shock due to hemorrhagic causes need blood and blood products.

The Resuscitation Outcomes Consortium (ROC) recently completed a study called "PROPPR," examining what the ratio of "blood administration" to "blood product" administration should be. Although beyond the scope of this chapter, this is an important area that will continue to guide emergency medicine and surgery in the resuscitation of these patients.

It was mentioned earlier that hypertonic saline resuscitation was not found to be beneficial by the ROC in patients with severe hemorrhagic shock. This treatment seems to work by mobilizing internal, interstitial fluid (fluid found between the cells but outside the vascular space) into the vascular system. The ROC trial found that some hemorrhagic shock patients receiving hypertonic saline appeared to be clinically better on arrival to the emergency department. Overall, though, the mortality rate of the patients was not changed from those receiving conventional fluid therapy.

Methods of evaluating and monitoring patients in traumatic shock continue to be developed. One promising method that is undergoing clinical evaluation is the use of "lactate levels" in the prehospital arena to monitor patients in shock. Recent work by the ROC suggests that elevated lactate levels detected early in a trauma patient's course may be predictive of a patient who will require more aggressive resuscitative measures. Lactate, a by-product of anaerobic metabolism, is produced by cells during the "compensated" phase of shock, an early indication of decreased tissue perfusion found even before hypotension develops. This finding suggests that field measurement of lactate may help predict developing shock. Indeed, lactate measurement might take its place beside the usual vital signs (P, R, T, BP, pulse oximetry, capnography) and devices such as 12 ECG acquisition in the field as an early monitor for the critically ill patient.

It should be stressed that hemostatic agents should be used only in the setting of an overall hemorrhage control protocol and not as agents that control bleeding by themselves. This is an area in which the hemostatic agent of choice seems to change frequently, so consult your medical director or agency protocols for current recommendations.

Tourniquets are life-saving devices, and their introduction and training should be part of the education of all EMS personnel. The rapid control of massive external bleeding—by tourniquets if necessary—is a critical and now widely accepted part of patient care, though they must be part of an overall hemorrhage control protocol. Tourniquets should be used early, and they should be tight enough on the affected extremity so that the bleeding is controlled, which may eliminate the pulse in the extremity distal to the tourniquet. It is likely best to use the tourniquet higher up on the extremity, and a second one can be applied if the first one is insufficient to control bleeding. A second tourniquet should be applied just below the first one.

The role of hypothermia in the care of critically ill patients is being evaluated. In the setting of the return of spontaneous circulation after nontraumatic cardiac arrest, therapeutic hypothermia appears to be beneficial. The trauma patient, however, appears to suffer from being cold. Trauma resuscitation rooms are often kept at body temperature (to the discomfort of some members of the resuscitation team, who are in gowns). IV fluids may be warmed to try to help maintain the patient's body temperature. The benefit at this time of warming IV fluids in the first few minutes of resuscitation in the field are unknown as far as actually improving survival in the prehospital environment and remains an important area of study.

The use of waveform capnography is important in managing the critically ill patient. However, in patients with both hemorrhagic shock and traumatic brain injury, waveform capnography may not be reliable for managing ventilator rate settings. Presumably the reason for that is, in shock, the amount of carbon dioxide actually being produced by the cells of the body versus what is being returned to the lungs in a hypotensive state is unpredictable. So, on these particular patients, decisions about ventilator settings are apparently best made using conventional arterial blood gas analyses. This has very little application to prehospital care but might be important in interfacility transfers of critically ill trauma patients.

tranexamic acid (TXA): a synthetic analog of the amino acid lysine. An antithrombolytic agent, it works by blocking the activation of plasminogen to plasmin, which normally breaks down clots in the body. It has been used in surgery to reduce blood loss, particularly in obstetric, gynecologic, and orthopedic procedures. Recently, there has been interest in the use of this medication to reduce bleeding in trauma.

A substantial derangement of the body's clotting control mechanisms often occurs in the critically ill trauma patient. As many as 25% to 40% of severely traumatized patients develop abnormalities. Shock causes acidosis, exacerbated by hypothermia, ultimately resulting in "fibrinolysis," which can break down clots that may have formed in bleeding vessels and organs. If such "hyperfibrinolysis" develops in the severely traumatized patient, the mortality rate can exceed 70%. **Tranexamic acid (TXA)** is a drug that "blocks fibrinolysis," which blocks clot breakdown. Binding to a clot precursor called "plasminogen," the chemical "blocks plasminogen–fibrin interaction" and has been shown to reduce bleeding post trauma.

TXA is not a new drug. TXA has been in wide use to control operative bleeding in obstetrical/gynecological, orthopedic, and cardiovascular surgery for many years. Its safety profile is very favorable and is well described in the literature. At the molecular level, TXA binds to a lysine-binding site on plasminogen. When this TXA-bound plasminogen combines with endogenous tissue plasminogen activator (tPA), the plasmin that is created is inactive and cannot break down fibrin clots. Thus, TXA augments the body's natural response to bleeding. It is important to note that TXA is not thrombogenic; that is, it does not create clots. Thus, does not cause a deep venous thrombosis or pulmonary embolism.

Two separate randomized, placebo-controlled, double-blinded studies (CRASH-2 in 2010 and MATTERS in 2012) have demonstrated the safety and efficacy of TXA in this role. A Cochrane review published in 2011 found that TXA reduced mortality from hemorrhage without increasing risk of adverse events. The World Health Organization, the British National Health Service, the Tactical Combat Casualty Care program, and the Royal Flying Doctors Service endorse TXA use for trauma patients.

A study published in the *Lancet* in 2010 from a trial called CRASH 2 looked at over 20,000 trauma patients in Africa, Asia, and Europe. It demonstrated a modest survival benefit for TXA if given in the dose of a gram over the first 10 minutes and then a gram over the next eight hours. However, the CRASH 2 data from that trial have been restudied, finding that the risk of death from bleeding was reduced by about one-third if the TXA was given early (within three hours) but when given after three hours increased the risk of death from bleeding by as much as 40%. Morrison et al. studied injured U.S. military personnel in Afghanistan requiring transfusion and demonstrated that the use of TXA dramatically reduced mortality. Survival in soldiers requiring massive transfusions was increased by a factor of 7.2. Not all studies show such a major improvement, and not all show a reduction in blood transfusion. In fact, patients who received transfusions of two or more units of red blood cells showed no decrease in mortality from receiving TXA.

Studies that look at the impact of TXA on trauma survival are ongoing as this text goes to print. They may help further identify which patients would benefit the most from use of TXA.

Emergency care providers who are managing the severely injured trauma patient need to understand that TXA use has been extensively studied and is actively used in many trauma centers at this time. The position of ITLS on the use of TXA is: ITLS believes that there is sufficient evidence to support the use of TXA in the management of traumatic hemorrhage in the adult patient, pursuant to system medical control approval. Following initial resuscitation, including control of external bleeding and stabilization of airway, consideration should be given to administration of TXA during early stages of transport.

The following approach is suggested for TXA use.

- TXA should be given (1 g over 10 minutes loading dose, followed as soon as practical by 1 g over 8 hours) to all significantly injured trauma patients *who are not anticipated to require massive transfusion* (>2,000 mL or 8 units of pRBCs) or *operative management.*

- TXA should be given (1 g over 10 minutes loading dose, followed as soon as practical by 1 g over 8 hours) to all significantly injured trauma patients *who are anticipated to require massive transfusion* (>2,000 mL or 8 units of pRBCs) or *operative management when the patient cannot be transported to a trauma center within one hour of injury.*

- Whenever possible, the TXA should be initiated within one hour of injury because TXA demonstrates greatest benefit when administered in this time frame. TXA should be held if administration cannot be initiated within three hours of injury (because administration after this time has been associated with adverse outcomes).

- When a significantly injured trauma patient who is anticipated to require massive transfusion (>2,000 mL or 8 units or pRBCs) presents to, or can be transferred within one hour of injury to, a tertiary trauma center, that institution's massive transfusion protocol should be followed. Such protocols may or may not include TXA. Although there are data to suggest that TXA has a positive synergistic effect with cryoprecipitate, direct comparisons to the transfusion of blood, plasma, and platelets (the so-called 1:1:1 protocols) are not available.

- When a significantly injured trauma patient who is anticipated to require operative management presents to, or can be transferred within one hour of injury to, a tertiary trauma center, the preoperative initiation of TXA should be at the discretion of the attending trauma surgeon

Note: There are currently no data on the use of TXA in pediatric trauma patients.

Last, a 2012 review paper looked at the literature surrounding the routine use of the Trendelenburg position in the trauma patient. Long a staple of field care of the trauma patient, there has also been concern about the effect of abdominal contents interfering with respiratory efforts. After an exhaustive review of the subject, the authors state that there is no evidence to recommend the routine use of the Trendelenburg position for treating hypovolemia or hypotension.

Case Presentation (continued)

An ALS ambulance has been called to a construction site, where a single male victim has had an isolated penetrating wound to the chest. The scene size-up reveals the fire department on scene, ensuring no hazards. Because the scene is safe and the mechanism of injury (stab/puncture wound) is readily apparent, the team dons personal protective equipment and each carries their essential trauma care equipment as they approach the patient. The patient, a male in his 20s, is sitting on the tailgate of a pickup truck and holding his right anterior chest. He states that he tripped and fell onto the rebar, which went into his chest but did not come out the back. His coworkers pulled him up off the bar and brought him over to the office. The patient denies any other injuries and says it hurts to breathe.

The lead emergency care provider begins the initial assessment. The general impression is not good. The patient is awake and answering appropriately. He is pale and diaphoretic, but there is no obvious external bleeding. Respiration appears to be slightly fast, but depth appears normal. When his hand is removed from his right chest, there is a single small puncture wound at about the fourth intercostal space and anterior axillary line. The wound is bleeding. The radial pulse seems a little fast but strong. The team leader asks rescuer 2 to apply a nonrebreather oxygen mask and then apply an occlusive dressing over the chest wound. Because of the nature of the injury the lead emergency care provider decides to do a focused exam, which shows the airway is normal, with good movement of air and a normal speaking voice. The neck veins are flat, and the trachea is in the midline. The breath sounds are decreased on the right and dull to percussion. Heart sounds are normal but fast. The abdomen is soft and nontender. There are no other wounds. The patient is placed on a stretcher (no backboard or SMR) and immediately moved to the ambulance.

Vital signs are pulse 120–130, respiration 24/minute, and blood pressure 104/84. He is treated with 100% oxygen by nonrebreather mask. Two large-bore IVs are started during transport, but because the blood pressure is greater than 90 mm Hg, the flow rate is set just fast enough to keep the vein open. There is concern about causing worsening of the intrathoracic bleeding. Because of the penetrating wound to the chest, the EMS crew decides to transport the patient to the Level 2 trauma center across town, which is eight miles away (13 km) rather than the community hospital, which is three miles (3 km) away.

The history reveals the following:

S — Slight pain in the wound site

A — None

M — None

P — No history of serious illness

L — Ate breakfast three hours before and had a coffee about an hour ago

E — States he was carrying a tool box, tripped on a rock, and landed on the rebar. His coworkers pulled him off.

While the second emergency care provider applies a cardiac monitor and a pulse oximeter (95% on 100% oxygen), the team leader performs an ITLS Ongoing Exam. The patient is becoming restless but is still oriented and cooperative, airway is still normal with slight tachypnea, but the pulse is now thready and more rapid (around 140 beats/minute on monitor). The patient is still diaphoretic and is noticeably pale.

The neck veins are flat, and the trachea is midline. Breath sounds are normal on the left and still decreased on the right with dullness to percussion. Heart sounds are rapid and not muffled.

The second emergency care provider reports the blood pressure is now 80/60 mm Hg. The fluid rate is increased to maintain the blood pressure above 80 mm Hg systolic, and the team leader immediately notifies medical direction that they will be arriving in five minutes with a young male who has shock from a possible massive hemothorax. Medical command advises to watch the vital signs and hold fluids unless the systolic blood pressure is less than 80 mm Hg.

The ITLS Secondary Survey was not performed because they arrived at the emergency department before they had time to do one. Immediately on arrival in the emergency department, a chest tube was inserted and 1,600 cc of blood obtained. There was only slight bleeding after this, so the blood was autotransfused and the patient observed. Imaging of the chest and abdomen failed to show other injuries, and the patient's bleeding stopped without surgery. He had an uneventful recovery.

This is one of the few examples of a focused exam being adequate for a trauma patient. Note that even a focused exam required that both the chest and the abdomen be examined because the diaphragm rises so high in the chest that a midchest stab-type wound may go through the diaphragm and cause abdominal injuries. IV fluids should only be used to maintain systolic pressure of 80 to 90 mm Hg.

Summary

A patient with shock must be diagnosed early. The early signs and symptoms of shock may be subtle, and when the later signs such as hypotension develop, the patient may be near death. The importance of careful assessment and reassessment cannot be overemphasized. You must understand the risk of any of the shock states to your patient. Further, you need to study and memorize the shock syndromes, especially in regard to the rapid provision of the proper treatment for such conditions as internal hemorrhage, pericardial tamponade, and tension pneumothorax. Finally, you should be aware of the controversy on the use of IV fluid resuscitation for cases of uncontrolled hemorrhage. Rely on your EMS system's medical direction or EMS agency protocols to help keep you current on the standard of care in these areas.

Bibliography

Baraniuk, S., Tilley, B. C., et al. "Pragmatic Randomized Optimal Platelet and Plasma Ratios (PROPPR) Trial: Design, Rationale, and Implementation." *Injury*, 45, no. 9 (September 2014): 1287.

Bickell, W. H., M. J. Wall Jr., P. E. Pepe, R. R. Martin, V. F. Ginger, M. K. Allen, and K. L. Mattox. "Immediate Versus Delayed Fluid Resuscitation for Hypotensive Patients with Penetrating Torso Injury." *New England Journal of Medicine*, 331, no. 17 (October 1994): 1105–1109.

Bulger, E. M., S. May, J. D. Kerby, S. Emerson, I. G. Stiell, M. A. Schreiber, K. J. Brasel, S. A. Tisherman, R. Coimbra, S. Rizoli, et al. "Out-of-Hospital Hypertonic Resuscitation After Traumatic Hypovolemic Shock: A Randomized, Placebo Controlled Trial." *Annals of Surgery*, 253, no. 3 (March 2011): 431–441.

Champion, H. R. "Combat Fluid Resuscitation: Introduction and Overview of Conferences." *Journal of Trauma*, 54, Suppl. 5 (May 2003): S1–S12.

Chiara, O., P. Pelosi, L. Brazzi, N. Bottino, P. Taccone, S. Cimbanassi, M. Segala, L. Gattinoni, and T. Scalea. "Resuscitation from Hemorrhagic Shock: Experimental Model Comparing Normal Saline, Dextran, and Hypertonic Saline Solutions." *Critical Care Medicine*, 31, no. 7 (July 2003): 1915–1922.

CRASH-2 Trial Collaborators. "Effects of Tranexamic Acid on Death, Vascular Occlusive Events, and Blood Transfusion in Trauma Patients with Significant Hemorrhage (CRASH-2): A Randomized, Placebo-Controlled Trial." *Lancet*, 376, no. 9734 (July 3, 2010): 23–32.

CRASH-2 Trial Collaborators. "The Importance of Early Treatment with Tranexamic Acid in Bleeding Trauma Patients: An Exploratory Analysis of the CRASH-2 Randomised Controlled Trial." *Lancet*, 377, no. 9771 (March 26, 2011): 1096–1101.

Demetriades, D., L. S. Chan, P. Bhasin, T. V. Berne, E. Ramicone, F. Huicochea, G. Velmahos, E. E. Cornwell, H. Belzberg, J. Murray, and J. A. Asensio. "Relative Bradycardia in Patients with Traumatic Hypotension." *Journal of Trauma*, 45, no. 3 (September 1998): 534–539.

Dunn, C. J., and K. L. Goa. "Tranexamic Acid: A Review of Its Use in Surgery and Other Indications." *Drugs*, 57, no. 6 (June 1999): 1005–1032.

Haut, E. R., B. T. Kalish, D. T. Efron, A. H. Haider, K. A. Stevens, A. N. Kieninger, E. E. Cornwell 3rd, and D. C. Chang. "Spine Immobilization in Penetrating Trauma: More Harm Than Good?" *Journal of Trauma*, 68, no. 1 (January 2010): 115–121.

Kowalenko, T., S. Stern, S. Dronen, and X. Wang. "Improved Outcome with Hypotensive Resuscitation of Uncontrolled Hemorrhagic Shock in a Swine Model." *Journal of Trauma*, 33, no. 3 (September 1992): 349–353.

Kragh, J. F., M. L. Littrel, J. A. Jones, T. J. Walters, D. G. Baer, C. E. Wade, and J. B. Holcomb. "Battle Casualty Survival with Emergency Tourniquet Use to Stop Limb Bleeding." *Journal of Emergency Medicine*, 41, no. 6 (December 2011): 590–597.

Mapstone, J., I. Roberts, and P. Evans. "Fluid Resuscitation Strategies: A Systematic Review of Animal Trials." *Journal of Trauma*, 55, no. 3 (September 2003): 571–589.

Mattox, K. L., W. Bickell, P. E. Pepe, J. Burch, and D. Feliciano. "Prospective MAST Study in 911 Patients." *Journal of Trauma*, 29, no. 8 (August 1989): 1104–1112.

Moore, E. E. "Blood Substitutes: The Future Is Now." *Journal of the American College of Surgeons*, 196, no. 1 (January 2003): 1–16.

Morrison, J. J., J. J. Dubose, T. E. Rasmussen, and M. J. Midwinter. "The Military Application of Tranexamic Acid in Trauma Emergency Resuscitation (MATTERs) Study." *Archives of Surgery*, 147, no. (February 2012): 113–119.

Pena, S. B., and A. R. Larrad. "Does the Trendelenburg Position Affect Hemodynamics? A Systematic Review." *Emergencias*, 24, no. 2 (April 2012): 143–150.

Roberts, I., H. Shakur, K. Ker, and T. Coats, on behalf of the CRASH-2 Trial Collaborators. "Antifibrinolytic drugs for acute traumatic injury." Cochrane Database of Systematic Reviews, Issue 12. Art. No. CD004896 (2012).

Schriger, D. L., and L. J. Baraff. "Capillary Refill—Is It a Useful Predictor of Hypovolemic States?" *Annals of Emergency Medicine*, 20, no. 6 (June 1991): 601–605.

Warner, K. J., J. Cuschieri, B. Garland, D. Carlbom, D. Baker, M. K. Copass, G. J. Jurkovich, and E. M. Bulger. "The Utility of Early End-Tidal Capnography in Monitoring Ventilation Status After Severe Injury." *Journal of Trauma*, 66, no. 1 (January 2009): 26–31.

Valle, E. J., C. J. Allen, R. M. Van Haren, J. M. Jouria, H. Li, A. S. Livingstone, N. Namias, C. I. Schulman, and K. G. Proctor. "Do All Trauma Patients Benefit from Tranexamic Acid?" *Journal of Trauma and Acute Care Surgery*, 76, no. 6 (June 2014): 1373–1378.

Get more information about this course by calling
ITLS International at 888-495-4875
(outside the United States call +1-630-495-6442) or visit

www.itrauma.org

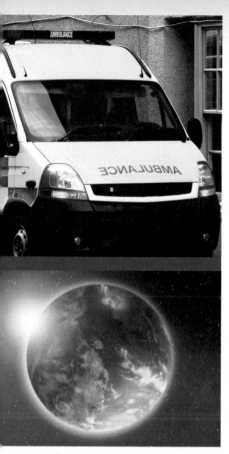

9

Vascular Access Skills

S. Robert Seitz, MEd, RN, NRP
Kyee Han, MD, FRCS, FCEM

Fluid Resuscitation	Infusione di Liquidi	Reanimación con Líquidos
Réanimation fluide	Płynoterapia (Resuscytacja płynowa)	Volumentherapie
Nadoknada tekućine	الإنعاش بالسوائل	nadoknada tečnosti
Tekočinska reanimacija	Folyadék reszuszcitáció	

(Ambulance photo © TA Craft Photography, Fotolia, LLC)

Objectives

Upon successful completion of this chapter, you should be able to:

1. Perform the technique of cannulation of the external jugular vein.
2. Recite indications for the use of intraosseous infusion.
3. Perform intraosseous infusion using the EZ-IO® Drill for tibial and humeral sites.
4. Perform intraosseous infusion using FAST Responder™ device at sternal site.
5. Use length-based resuscitation tape to estimate the weight of a child.

All advanced students of this course are expected to be familiar with the technique of inserting an IV cannula in the veins of the lower arm or antecubital space; thus, these sites will not be discussed here.

Cannulation of the External Jugular Vein

The external jugular vein runs in a line from the angle of the jaw to the junction of the medial and middle third of the clavicle (Figure 9-1). This vein is usually easily visible through the skin. Pressing on it just above the clavicle will make it more prominent. It runs into the subclavian vein.

Indication for cannulation of the external jugular vein is the pediatric or adult patient who needs IV access and in whom no suitable peripheral vein is found.

Procedure

Performing External Jugular Cannulation

1. The patient must be in the supine position, preferably head down, to distend the vein and to prevent air embolism.

2. If no suspicion of cervical-spine injury exists, turn the patient's head to the opposite side. If there is a danger of cervical-spine injury, one emergency care provider must stabilize the head (it must not be turned) while the IV is being started. The cervical collar should be opened or the front removed during the procedure.

3. Quickly prepare the skin with an antiseptic, and then align the cannula with the vein. The needle will be pointing toward the clavicle at the junction of the middle and medial thirds.

4. With one finger, press on the vein just above the clavicle. This should make the vein more prominent.

5. Insert the needle into the vein at about the midportion, and cannulate in the usual way.

6. If not already done, draw a 30 mL sample of blood and store it in the appropriate tubes (if the hospital will accept blood drawn in the field).

7. Connect the intravenous, and tape down the line securely. If there is danger of cervical-spine injury, a cervical collar can be applied over the IV site.

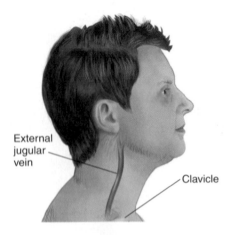

Figure 9-1 Anatomy of the external jugular vein.

External jugular vein

Clavicle

Intraosseous Infusion

The technique of bone marrow infusion of fluid and drugs is not new. It was first described in 1922 and in the 1930s and 1940s was used commonly as an alternative to IV infusion of crystalloids, drugs, and blood. The technique was "rediscovered" in 1985 by James Orlowski, MD, on a trip to India. Studies have confirmed it to be a fast, safe, and effective route to infuse medications, fluids, and blood. It is an established standard in pediatric advanced life support and now is a recommended primary vascular access site in the American Heart Association and European Resuscitation Council Guidelines.

Intraosseous (IO) infusion can be used for giving medications in both adults and children. It is now an early second-line choice for venous vascular access following two attempts at peripheral venous cannulation in adults as well. With pressures of 300 mm Hg applied to the infusion bag or pump, adequate flow rates of 150 mL/minute can be achieved for crystalloids. IO infusion has the advantage of being quick and simple to perform while providing a stable (anchored in bone) access that is not easily dislodged during transport.

Indications

Indications for the use of IO infusion include the pediatric or adult patient who is in cardiac arrest and in whom you cannot quickly obtain peripheral venous access, or the patient with hypovolemic shock and difficult intravenous placement. It is indicated for any patient who needs drugs or fluids within five minutes, when a peripheral intravenous cannula cannot be placed in two attempts or 90 seconds.

Contraindications

Contraindications for intraosseous infusion include local infection at the selected site for insertion, fractures in the selected limb, a prosthesis, recent (24 hours) IO access in the same extremity, osteogenesis imperfecta, and the absence of anatomical landmarks or excessive tissue at the site of insertion.

Recommended Sites

Sites recommended for an intraosseous infusion include the following:

* *Proximal tibia*, approximately 2 cm below the patella and approximately 2 cm (depending on the patient's anatomy) medial to the tibial tuberosity, or one finger breadth medial to the tibial tuberosity. This is often the easiest site to locate.
* *Proximal humerus*, laterally over most prominent aspect of the greater tubercle. Positioning of the patient is important. Ensure that the patient's hand is resting on the abdomen and that the elbow is adducted. Slide your thumb up the anterior shaft of the humerus until you feel the greater tubercle; this is the surgical neck. The insertion site is approximately 1 cm (depending on the patient's anatomy) above the surgical neck.
* *Distal tibia*, two finger breadths or 3 cm proximal to the most prominent aspect of the medial malleolus. Place one finger over the medial malleolus. Move approximately 2 cm (depending on the patient's anatomy) proximal, and palpate the anterior and posterior borders of the tibia to ensure that your insertion site is on the flat central aspect of the bone.

Potential Complications

Complications are rare. However, good aseptic technique is important, just as it is with IV therapy. Potential complications of IO infusion include extravasation, compartment syndrome, dislodgment, fracture, failure (device or user in origin), pain, and infection (adult infection rates < 0.6 %; retrospective analysis).

PEARLS
Low Infusion

* If infiltration occurs (rare), do not reuse the same bone. Another site must be selected because fluid will leak out of the original hole made in the bone. If this occurs, apply a pressure dressing and secure it with an elastic bandage.
* Never place an IO line in a fractured extremity. If the femur is fractured, use the other leg.

Procedure

Performing IO by Use of EZ-IO® Device (Adult or Child)

The equipment needed to perform IO by use of EZ-IO® device is as follows:

* EZ-IO® driver
* EZ-IO® AD, EZ-IO® LD, or EZ-IO® PD needle set
* Antiseptic swab, such as alcohol or Betadine®

* EZ-Connect® or standard extension set
* Two 10 mL syringes
* Normal saline (or suitable sterile fluid)
* Pressure bag or infusion pump
* 2% lidocaine for IV/IO use (preservative free, epinephrine free)

Procedure

Insertion of IO Needle by Use of the EZ-IO® System

Determine the need for this procedure. Obtain permission from medical direction if required. If the patient is conscious, advise him of emergent need for this procedure and obtain informed consent. To perform the insertion (Scan 9-1):

1. Wear approved personal protective equipment (PPE).

2. Determine EZ-IO® AD, EZ-IO® AD, or EZ-IO® PD indications.

3. Rule out contraindications.

4. Locate an appropriate insertion site.

5. Prepare the insertion site, using aseptic technique, and then allow it to dry.

6. Prepare the EZ-IO® driver (power or manual) and the appropriate needle set.

   a. EZ-IO® 15 mm for 3 to 39 kg (less than 16 pounds)

   b. EZ-IO® 25 mm for 40 kg (more than 16 pounds) and greater

   c. EZ-IO® 45 mm for 40 kg and greater with excessive tissue

7. Stabilize the site to prepare to insert the appropriate needle set.

8. Remove the needle cap. Insert the EZ-IO® needle into the selected site. (Keep your hand and fingers away from the needle.) Position the driver at the insertion site with the needle set at a 90-degree angle to the bone surface.

9. Gently pierce the skin with the needle until the needle touches the bone. The black line on the needle should be visible. Penetrate the bone cortex by squeezing the driver's trigger and applying gentle, consistent, steady downward pressure. (Allow the driver to do the work.) Do not use excessive force. In some patients insertion may take 10 seconds. If the driver sounds like it is slowing down during insertion, reduce the pressure on the driver to allow the RPMs of the needle tip to do the work. If the battery fails, you may manually finish inserting the needle just as you would a manual IO needle.

10. Release the driver's trigger and stop the insertion process when a sudden "give or pop" is felt on entry into the medullary space or when desired depth is obtained.

11. Remove the EZ-IO® driver from the needle set while stabilizing the catheter hub.

12. Remove the stylet from the catheter by turning counterclockwise. Place the stylet in the shuttle or an approved sharps container.

13. Confirm placement. Connect the primed EZ-Connect®. Syringe bolus (flush) the EZ-IO® catheter with the appropriate amount of normal saline (10 mL for adults and 5 mL for children). Remember: no flush = no flow!

14. If the patient is responsive to pain or complains of pain when you flush the marrow cavity, slowly (in 0.2 mL increments), administer the appropriate dose of preservative-free (for IV/IO use) lidocaine 2% (20 mg/mL) IO to anesthetize the IO space. (IO infusion causes severe pain in alert patients.) Follow local protocols when administering medicine.

    a. 2–4 mL (20–40 mg) for adults

    b. 0.5 mg/kg (0.025 mL per kg) for children

    Then wait 15 to 30 seconds for the lidocaine to take effect.

15. Begin the infusion. Utilize pressure—up to 300 mm Hg (pressure bag or infusion pump)—for continuous infusion.

16. Dress the site, secure the tubing, and apply the wristband (document time and date) as directed by local protocols.

17. Monitor the EZ-IO® site and the patient's condition.

To remove the catheter, start by supporting the patient's leg. Simultaneously, connect a sterile Luer-Lok™ syringe to the hub of the catheter. Once connected, rotate the syringe and catheter clockwise while gently pulling. When the catheter has been removed, immediately place it in an appropriate biohazard container. Do not leave the EZ-IO® catheter in place for more than 24 hours.

SCAN 9-1 Insertion of IO Needle by Use of Easy-IO System

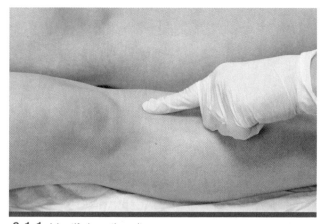

9-1-1 Identify insertion site. *(Photo courtesy of Vidacare Corp)*

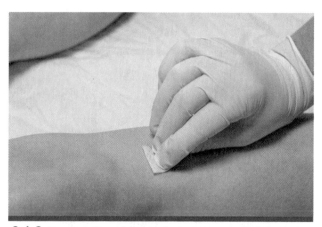

9-1-2 Prepare site using aseptic technique and allow to dry. *(Photo courtesy of Vidacare Corp)*

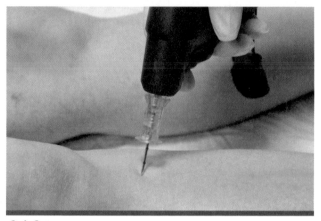

9-1-3 Insert the needle at a 90-degree angle to the bone surface. Keep your hand and fingers away from the needle. *(Photo courtesy of Vidacare Corp)*

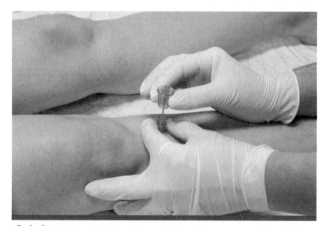

9-1-4 While stabilizing the catheter hub, remove the stylet from the catheter by turning counterclockwise. *(Photo courtesy of Vidacare Corp)*

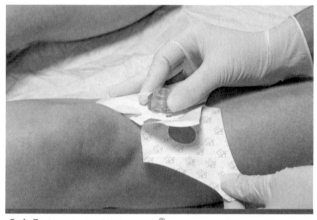

9-1-5 Attach the EZ-Connect® and secure the needle. *(Photo courtesy of Vidacare Corp)*

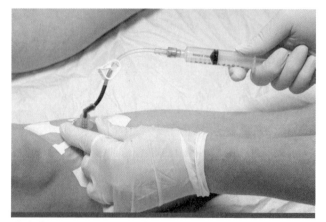

9-1-6 Confirm the placement of the needle by aspirating blood from the marrow cavity. You may not be able to aspirate marrow; however, if the catheter flushes easily and without infiltration, it is okay to use. *(Photo courtesy of Vidacare Corp)*

(continued)

SCAN 9-1 Insertion of IO Needle by Use of Easy-IO System (*continued*)

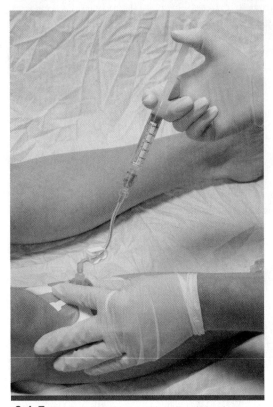

9-1-7 Flush the catheter with saline (10 mL adults, 5 mL children). *(Photo courtesy of Vidacare Corp)*

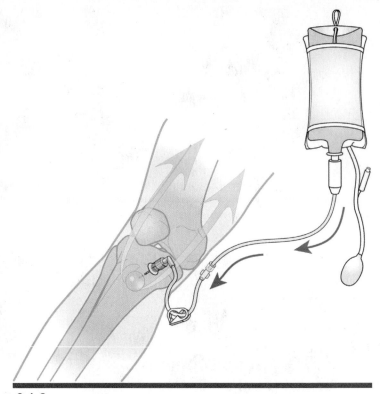

9-1-8 Connect IV infusion. *(Image courtesy of Vidacare Corp)*

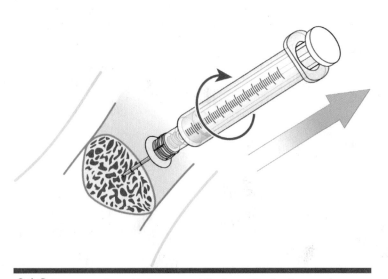

9-1-9 To remove the catheter, support the leg while simultaneously connecting a sterile Luer-Lok™ syringe to the hub of the catheter. Rotate the syringe and catheter clockwise while gently pulling. *(Image courtesy of Vidacare Corp)*

Procedure

Performing Manual IO Infusion in a Child

1. Determine the need for this procedure. Obtain permission from medical direction if required.

2. Have all the equipment needed ready prior to bone penetration.
   a. 16-18 gauge IO needles
   b. 5 mL and 10 mL syringes
   c. Antiseptic solution to prep the skin
   d. IV tubing and IV fluids
   e. Tape and dressing material to secure the IO needle
   f. Blood pressure cuff or commercial pressure device to infuse fluid under pressure

3. Identify the site, which is the proximal tibia, two finger breadths below the tibial tuberosity, either midline or slightly medial to the midline (Figure 9-2).

4. Prep the skin with an appropriate antiseptic (very important).

5. Obtain the proper needle. The needle must have a stylet so that it does not become plugged with bone. Although 13-, 18-, and 20-gauge spine needles will work, they are difficult and uncomfortable to grip during the insertion process. Long spine needles tend to bend easily, so if you use spine needles, try to obtain the short ones. The preferred needle is a 14–18 gauge IO needle, but bone marrow needles also can be used.

6. Using aseptic technique. Insert the needle into the bone marrow cavity perpendicular to the skin (Figure 9-2). Advance it to the periosteum.

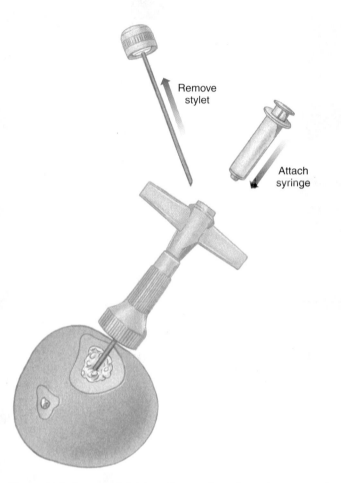

Figure 9-3 Remove stylet from the needle and attach syringe.

Penetrate the bone with a slow boring or twisting motion until you feel a sudden "give or pop" (decrease in resistance) as the needle enters the marrow cavity. This can be confirmed by removing the stylet and aspirating blood and bone marrow (Figures 9-3 and 9-4). You may not be able to aspirate marrow; however, if the catheter flushes easily and without infiltration, it is okay to use.

7. Syringe bolus (flush) the IO catheter with 5 mL of normal saline. Remember: no flush = no flow!

8. If the child is responsive to pain or complains of pain when you flush, slowly (0.2 mL increments) administer a 0.5 mg/kg (0.025 mL per kg) dose of preservative-free (for IV/IO use)

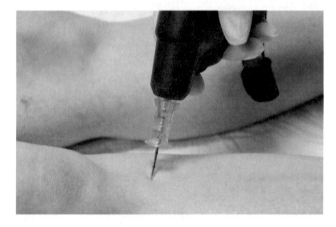

Figure 9-2 Insertion site for intraosseous infusion needle in the proximal tibia. *(Photo courtesy of Vidacare Corp)*

(continued)

Procedure (*continued*)

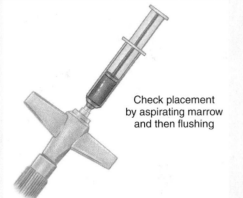

Check placement by aspirating marrow and then flushing

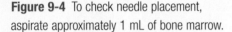

Figure 9-4 To check needle placement, aspirate approximately 1 mL of bone marrow.

lidocaine 2% (20 mg/mL) IO to anesthetize the IO space. A 10-kg child would get 0.25 mL (5 mg of 2% lidocaine). Wait 15 to 30 seconds for the lidocaine to take effect. Assess for potential IO complications. Follow local protocols for medication administration.

9. Attach standard IV tubing, and infuse the fluid and/or medications (Figure 9-5). To obtain an adequate flow rate you may have to infuse fluid under pressure. Use of a pressure infusion bag or securing an inflated blood pressure cuff around the IV bag will assist in maximizing the fluid infusion.

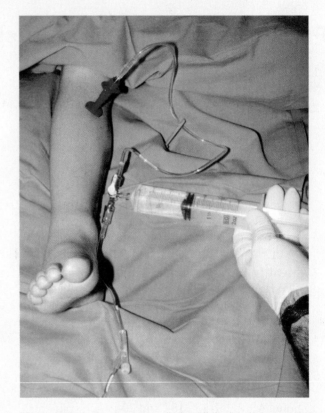

Figure 9-5 Intraosseous needle in child's tibia being used for fluid infusion. *(Photo courtesy of Bob Page, MEd, NRP, CCP, NCEE)*

10. Tape the tubing to the skin and secure the bone marrow needles as if to secure an impaled object. (Use gauze pads taped around the insertion site.)

FAST Responder™ Intraosseous Device

The FAST Responder™ intraosseous device is designed for rapid sternal intraosseous access for the purpose of infusing fluid and medication directly into the bone marrow of the manubrium. Bone marrow flows into the vascular system and the manubrium is especially effective due to close proximity to central circulation. It does feature a depth control that reduces risk of overpenetration.

Indications are similar to other intraosseous devices in patients 12 years of age and older (adolescent to adult).

The insertion site is the manubrium of sternum, 15 mm below the sternal notch in the midline. The bone thickness at the insertion site is 13.30 mm, and the risk of overpenetration is less than 1 in 1,000,000.

The device relies on operator force only. It is not spring-loaded, battery dependent, or pneumatic. Its downward force pushes the steel infusion tube tip through soft tissue into bone and when the steel tip is just inside marrow space, the infusion tube automatically separates from the introducer. The bone probe needles ensures proper depth control only; it does not enter the bone This mechanism prevents overpenetration.

Procedure

Inserting the FAST Responder™ Intraosseous Device

1. Expose the sternum, and locate the sternal notch.
2. Clean the insertion site with an antiseptic.
3. Remove the adhesive liner with the locking pin.
4. Position yourself. Stand/kneel at the head or the side of patient, or as you are comfortable.
5. Place the device. Align the target foot notch with the patient's sternal notch and the introducer (the device handle) perpendicular to the manubrium. Verify placement in the correct location.
6. Push the FAST Responder™ down perpendicular to the sternum completely to deploy the infusion tube.
7. Pause and pull back. Withdraw the FAST Responder™ device straight back while holding down the target foot. Support comes out with the infusion tube.
8. Discard the device following your contaminated sharps protocols.
9. Prepare. Connect the IV line directly to the Luer-Lok, and clip the strain relief hook to the target foot.
10. Optional: According to local protocol, flush with fluid to clear line, and confirm placement by aspiration.
11. Optional: Remove the liner from the protective dome and apply the dome over the target foot infusion site.

Remember the six Ps: position yourself relative to the patient, place the device, push to deploy, pause (hold target foot), pull back the device, and prepare (connect fluid source).

Fluid flow rates are as follows: gravity, 30 to 80 mL/minute; pressure infuser to 120 mL/minute; syringe, 150 to 250 mL/minute.

Procedure

Removing the FAST Responder™ Intraosseous Device

1. Remove the protective dome from the target foot.
2. Turn off the source of fluid, and disconnect the IV line.
3. Grasp the infusion tube with your fingers or clamp and pull perpendicular to manubrium until the entire infusion tube emerges from the patient's chest. Using the tube to pull, pull in one continuous motion until the device is removed.
4. Peel off the target foot following your contaminated sharps protocol.

Precautions/warnings include all of the following: Trauma, infection, or burns at the insertion site may preclude use of the FAST device. Safety with very severe osteoporosis has not been proven. Use in patients who have had a recent sternotomy may prove less effective. The function of the device may be affected by fracture of the sternum or vascular injury, which may compromise the integrity of the manubrium or its vascularization.

Length-Based Resuscitation Tapes

Calculation of the volume of fluid resuscitation or the dose of an IV medication for the pediatric patient depends on the patient's weight. In an emergency situation the age and weight of a child may not be known. The weight of a child is directly related to his length, and resuscitation tapes (Broselow® tape or SPARC system) have been developed to estimate a child's weight by measuring his length. The tapes list precalculated doses of IV fluids and emergency drugs for each weight range (Figure 9-6). They also include the correct sizes of emergency equipment and supplies for each weight range.

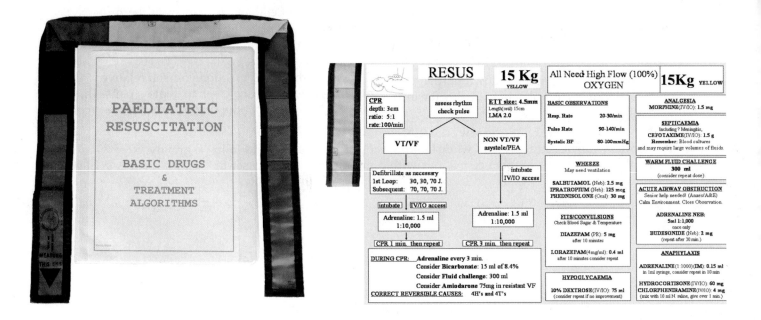

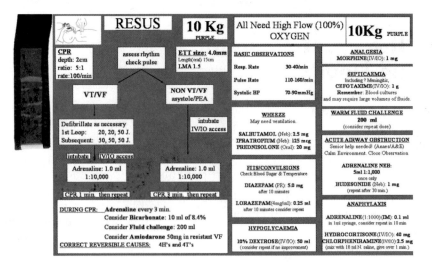

Figure 9-6 SPARC system has color-coded tape and booklet of precalculated doses of fluids and medications. *(Photos courtesy of Kyee Han, MD)*

Procedure

Estimating a Child's Weight with a Length-Based Resuscitation Tape

1. Place the patient in the supine position.
2. Using the tape, measure the patient from the crown to the heel. The red end with an arrow goes at the child's head. (See Figure 9-7.)
3. Note the box on the tape where the child's heel falls. With the SPARC system, match the color of the tape where the child's heel falls with the same colored area of the booklet.
4. If the measurement falls on a line, the box or colored panel proximal to the line is used to generate the fluid volume, drug doses, and sizes of equipment needed for resuscitation.
5. The tape may be disinfected if it becomes contaminated.

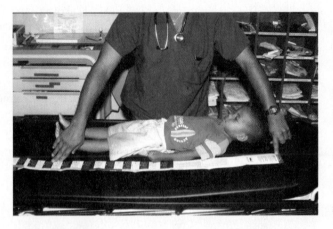

Figure 9-7 Measure the patient from crown to heel to read precalculated doses of fluids and medications. *(Photo courtesy of James Broselow, MD)*

Bibliography

American Heart Association. "2010 Guidelines for Cardiopulmonary Care Resuscitation (CPR) and Emergency Cardiovascular Care (ECC) Science," Part 8 and Part 14. *Circulation*, 122, no. 18, Suppl. 3 (November 2, 2010).

Cooper, B. R., P. F. Mahoney, T. J. Hodgetts, and A. Mellor. "Intra-osseous Access (EZ-IO®) for Resuscitation: UK Military Combat Experience." *Journal of the Royal Army Medical Corps*, 153, no. 4 (December 2007): 314–16.

Cotton, B. A., R. Jerome, B. R. Collier, S. Khetarpal, M. Holevar, B. Tucker, S. Kurek, N. T. Mowery, K. Shah, W. Bromberg, et al. "Guidelines for Prehospital Fluid Resuscitation in the Injured Patient." *Journal of Trauma*, 67, no. 2 (August 2009): 389–402.

Day, M. W. "Intraosseous Devices for Intravascular Access in Adult Trauma Patients." *Critical Care Nurse*, 31, no. 2 (April 2011): 76–89.

Fowler, R., J. V. Gallagher, S. M. Isaacs, E. Ossman, P. Pepe, and M. Wayne. "The Role of Intraosseous Vascular Access in the Out-of-Hospital Environment (Resource Document to NAEMSP Position Statement)." *Prehospital Emergency Care*, 11, no. 1 (January–March 2007): 63–66.

Kapoor, D., and M. Singh. "Novel Rapid Infusion Device for Patients in Emergency Situations." *Scandinavian Journal of Trauma, Resuscitation, and Emergency Medicine*, 19 (June 2011): 35.

Kovar, J., and L. Gillum. "Alternate Route: The Humerus Bone—A Viable Option for IO Access." *Journal of Emergency Medical Services (JEMS)*, 35, no. 8 (August 2010): 52–59.

Myers L. A., C. S. Russi, and G. M. Arteaga. "Semiautomatic Intraosseous Devices in Paediatric Prehospital Care Replacing a Manual Intraosseous (IO) Device Improves the Success Rate for Attempts at Vascular Access." *Prehospital Emergency Care*, 15, no. 4 (October–December 2011): 473–76.

Pasley, J., C. Miller, J. Dubose, S. Shackelford, R. Fang, K. Boswell, C. Halcome, J. Casey, M. Cotter, M. Matsuura, N. Relph, et al. "Intraosseous Infusion Rates Under High Pressure: A Cadaveric Comparison of Anatomic Sites." Presented at the Eastern Association for the Surgery of Trauma (EAST), Scientific Session III-A Clinical Science, 27th Scientific Assembly, January 16, 2014, Naples, FL.

Paxton, J. H., T. E. Knuth, and H. A. Klausner. "Proximal Humerus Intraosseous Infusion: A Preferred Emergency Venous Access." *Journal of Trauma*, 67, no. 3 (September 2009): 606–11.

Revell, M., K. Porter, and I. Greaves. "Fluid Resuscitation in Prehospital Trauma Care: A Consensus View." *Emergency Medicine Journal*, 19, no. 6 (November 2002): 494–98.

Soreide, E., and C. D. Deakin. "Pre-hospital Fluid Therapy in the Critically Injured Patient: A Clinical Update." *Injury*, 36, no. 9 (September 2005): 1001–10.

Sunde, G. A., B. E. Heradstvert, B. H. Vikenes, and J. K. Heltne. "Emergency Intraosseous Access in a Helicopter Emergency Medical Service: A Retrospective Study." *Scandinavian Journal of Trauma, Resuscitation, and Emergency Medicine*, 18 (October 7, 2010): 52.

Wampler, D. A., Shumaker, J., Manifold, C., S. Bolleter, and J. Frandsen. "Humeral Intraosseous Access Success Rate in Adult Out-of-Hospital Cardiac Arrest." *Annals of Emergency Medicine*, 56, no. 3, Suppl. (September 2010): S88–S89.

Head Trauma and Traumatic Brain Injury

David E. Manthey, MD, FAAEM, FACEP
Shin Tsuruoka, MD
Roy L. Alson, PhD, MD, FACEP

Trauma Cranico	Traumatismo Craneal	Traumatisme Crânien
Urazy czaszkowo-mózgowe	Schädel Hirn Trauma	Ozljede glave
إصابات الرأس	trauma glave	Poškodbe glave
Koponya-Agy-sérülés		

(Ambulance photo © Pierre Landry, Fotolia, LLC)

Key Terms

Objectives

Upon successful completion of this chapter, you should be able to:

1. Describe the anatomy of the head and brain.
2. Describe the pathophysiology of traumatic brain injury.
3. Explain the difference between primary and secondary brain injury.
4. Describe the mechanisms for the development of secondary brain injury.
5. Describe the assessment of the patient with a head injury.
6. Describe the prehospital management of the patient with a traumatic brain injury.
7. Recognize and describe the management of the cerebral herniation syndrome.
8. Identify potential problems in the management of the patient with a traumatic brain injury.

Chapter Overview

Head injury or, more specifically, traumatic brain injury (TBI), is a major cause of death and disability in multiple-trauma patients worldwide. Of all multiple-system trauma patients, 40% have a central nervous system (CNS) injury. Those patients have a death rate twice as high (35% versus 17%) as that of patients with no CNS injuries. Traumatic brain injuries account for an estimated 25% of all trauma deaths and up to one-half of all motor-vehicle fatalities. Worldwide, the cost of TBI is staggering in terms of lives lost, families destroyed, and money spent for care. Prevention remains the most effective treatment. EMS personnel can help reduce this major epidemic by encouraging the use of helmets in sports and work and restraint devices in vehicles.

As an emergency care provider, you may encounter head injuries that can range from the trivial to the immediately life threatening. By recognizing injuries that need immediate intervention and providing transport to the appropriate facility, you can significantly improve the chances for a patient to have a good outcome. Not every injury to the head results in a traumatic brain injury. Some may only involve the scalp, skull, or face. An injury above the clavicle should prompt the emergency care provider to look for TBI.

Because it is not possible to perform a field clearance of the cervical spine in a patient with altered mental status, you must always assume that a serious head injury is accompanied by an injury to the cervical spine and spinal cord and provide appropriate spinal motion restriction (SMR), as described elsewhere in this text. (See Chapter 12.)

Beginning with the third edition of this text, material included in this chapter has been based on the recommendations of the Brain Trauma Foundation (BTF; a multidisciplinary organization dedicated to improving care of TBI victims by use of evidence-based treatment).

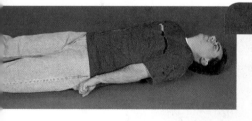

Case Presentation

You are the lead emergency care provider in an ALS ambulance transporting a seriously injured motorcyclist to a trauma center. Primary and rapid trauma surveys identified the life-threatening external hemorrhage in the area of the left knee, now controlled by tourniquet. Findings on exam indicating possible head, chest, and abdominal injuries and concern for possible spine injury occasioned by lack of movement in the lower extremities. Due to respiratory compromise, the patient was intubated, and a right tension pneumothorax was decompressed. The patient now shows decerebrate posturing to noxious stimuli. After treating the patient for shock, you reassess him. He continues to posture to noxious stimuli, his airway patent, breathing now considerably slower (6 to 8 and assisted), his

pulse rate is now below 80, and his BP is 88/40, SaO_2 is 95, and $ETCO_2$ is 38. Arrival time to the trauma center is now six to eight minutes. Neurologic exam shows no movement of lower extremities to noxious stimulation. His right pupil is now dilated and nonresponsive.

Before proceeding, consider the following questions: What do you suspect is happening to the patient? What are possible reasons for the continued decreased responsiveness? Will an ITLS Ongoing Exam reveal anything? Did you ever check a finger-stick blood sugar? Keep these questions in mind as you read through the chapter. Then, at the end of the chapter, find out how the emergency care providers managed this patient.

Anatomy of the Head

To most effectively manage the head-injured patient, one must understand the basic anatomy and physiology of the head and brain. The head (excluding the face and facial structures) includes the following (Figure 10-1):

- Scalp
- Skull
- Fibrous coverings of the brain (meninges: dura mater, arachnoid mater, pia mater)
- Brain tissue
- Cerebrospinal fluid
- Vascular compartments

The cutaneous tissue covering the skull, referred to as scalp, is very vascular and therefore bleeds freely when lacerated. The skull itself is a closed box. The rigid and unyielding bony skull protects the brain from injury. It also contributes to sev-

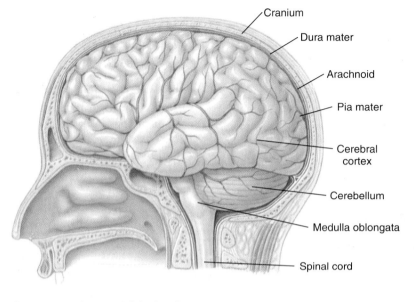

Figure 10-1 Anatomy of the head.

eral injury mechanisms in head trauma. The temporal bone (temple) is quite thin and easily fractured, as are portions of the base of the skull. The fibrous coverings of the brain are inside the skull and include the dura mater ("tough mother"), which covers the entire brain; the thinner pia arachnoid (called simply the *arachnoid*), which lies underneath the dura and in which are suspended both arteries and veins; and the very thin pia mater ("soft mother"), which lies underneath the arachnoid and is adherent to the surface of the brain. The cerebrospinal fluid (CSF) is found between the arachnoid and pia mater.

Because the brain "floats" inside the cerebrospinal fluid and is anchored at its base, there is greater movement at the top of the brain than at the base. On impact, the brain is able to move within the skull and can strike bony prominences within the cranial cavity. (This is the "third collision" described in mechanisms of injury in Chapter 1.)

The intracranial volume is composed of the brain, the CSF, and the blood in the blood vessels, which completely fill the cranial cavity. Thus, any increase in one of the components is at the expense of the other two. This concept (the **Monro-Kellie Doctrine**) is of great importance in the pathophysiology of head trauma. Following injury, the brain will swell. Because of the fixed space within rigid skull, as the brain tissue swells, it takes up more volume of the skull. Initially, with the brain swelling, blood and CSF volumes inside the skull decrease and compensate for the rise in pressure. As brain swelling continues, however, compensation fails, and intracranial pressure (ICP) begins to rise. As the ICP increases, the amount of blood that can enter the skull and perfuse the brain decreases, leading to further brain injury. As the ICP continues to rise, the only significant opening through which the pressure can be released is the foramen magnum at the base of the skull. A significant rise in ICP can cause the brain to herniate through the foramen magnum with devastating effects.

Cerebrospinal fluid (also called *spinal fluid*) is a nutrient fluid that bathes the brain and spinal cord. Spinal fluid is continually created within the ventricles of the brain at a rate of 0.33 mL/minute. The arachnoid granulations protruding into the superior sagittal sinus are the major site of absorption of spinal fluid. Anything obstructing the flow of spinal fluid, such as traumatic blood in the ventricles or subarachnoid space, will cause an accumulation of spinal fluid within the brain (hydrocephalus) and an increase in ICP.

PEARLS

Cervical-Spine Injury

Always treat as if there is a cervical-spine injury in the head-injured patient.

Monro-Kellie Doctrine: states that the contents of the skull—brain, blood, and CSF—are at a fixed volume and a change in volume of one is compensated by a decrease in the other two.

Pathophysiology of Head Trauma

Head injuries are either open or closed, depending on whether or not the brain is exposed. Brain injury also can be divided into two components, primary and secondary.

Primary and Secondary Brain Injuries

primary brain injury: the immediate damage to the brain tissue that is the direct result of an injury force.

Primary brain injury is the immediate damage to the brain tissue that is the direct result of the injury force and is essentially fixed at the time of injury. Little can be done to change the injury after it has occurred. Primary brain injury is better managed by prevention, using measures such as the use of occupant restraint systems in autos; the use of helmets in sports, work, and cycling; and firearms education.

Most closed head primary injuries occur either as a result of external forces applied against the exterior of the skull or from movement of the brain inside the skull. In deceleration injuries, the head usually strikes an object such as the windshield of an automobile, which causes a sudden deceleration of the skull. The brain continues to move forward, impacting first against the skull in the original direction of motion ("third" collision of a motor-vehicle collision) and then rebounding to hit the opposite side of the inner surface of the skull (a "fourth" collision). Thus, injuries may occur to the brain in the area of original impact ("**coup**") or on the opposite side ("**contracoup**"). The interior base of the skull is rough (Figure 10-2), and movement of the brain over this area may cause various degrees of injury to the brain tissue or to blood vessels supporting the brain.

coup: an injury to the brain in the area of original impact.

contracoup: an injury to the brain on the opposite side of the original impact.

secondary brain injury: an injury to the brain that is the result of hypoxia and/or decreased perfusion of brain tissue after a primary injury.

Secondary brain injury is the result of hypoxia and/or decreased perfusion of brain tissue. Good prehospital care can help prevent the development of secondary brain injury. In response to the primary insult, swelling can cause a decrease in perfusion. As a consequence of other injuries, hypoxia or hypotension may occur with either insult damaging to brain tissue. Bruising or injury of the brain results in vasodilatation with increased blood flow to the injured area Because there is no extra space inside the skull, swelling of the injured area or newly formed intracerebral hematoma

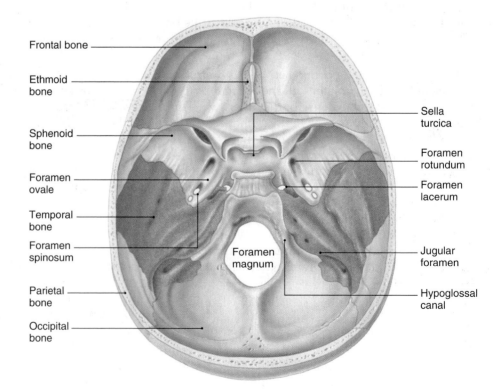

Figure 10-2 The rough inner base of the skull.

increases intracerebral pressure, and this leads to a decreased cerebral blood flow that causes further brain injury. The increase in cerebral water (edema) does not occur immediately, but develops over hours. Early efforts to prevent the accumulation of edema and to maintain perfusion of the brain can be life saving.

The brain normally adjusts its own blood flow in response to metabolic needs. The autoregulation of blood flow is adjusted based on the level of carbon dioxide (CO_2) in the blood. The normal level of CO_2 is 35 to 45 mm Hg. An increase in the level of CO_2 (hypoventilation) promotes vasodilatation of vessels supplying the brain, whereas lowering the level of CO_2 (hyperventilation) causes vasoconstriction and decreases blood flow to the brain. In the past, swelling was believed to be worsened if there was increased blood flow to the injured brain. Therefore, hyperventilation was recommended to prevent the swelling and the associated increase in ICP associated due to the swelling of the brain. This increased pressure would in turn decrease blood flow to the brain, adding insult to injury.

Research has shown that hyperventilation actually has only a slight effect on brain swelling, but causes a significant decrease in cerebral perfusion from that same vasoconstriction, resulting in cerebral hypoxia. Thus, both hyperventilation and hypoventilation can cause cerebral ischemia and increased mortality in the TBI patient. Maintaining normal ventilation (not hyperventilation) with high-flow oxygen at a rate of about one breath every 6 to 8 seconds (8 to 10 per minute) to maintain an end-tidal CO_2 (ETCO$_2$) of 35–45 is very important. Prophylactic hyperventilation for TBI is no longer recommended.

Intracranial Pressure

Brain tissue, cerebrospinal fluid, and blood reside within the skull and fibrous coverings of the brain. An increase in the volume of any one of those components must be at the expense of the other two because the adult skull (a rigid box) cannot expand. Although there is some displacement volume of cerebrospinal fluid and venous blood, it accounts for little space and cannot offset rapid brain swelling. Blood supply will be decreased by increased ICP, and because the brain requires a constant supply of blood (oxygen and glucose) to survive, brain swelling can be rapidly catastrophic.

The pressure of the brain and contents within the skull is termed **intracranial pressure (ICP)**. ICP is considered dangerous when it rises above 15 mm Hg; cerebral herniation may occur at pressures above 25 mm Hg. The net pressure gradient causing blood flow through the brain is termed the **cerebral perfusion pressure (CPP)**. Its value is obtained by subtracting the intracranial (intracerebral) pressure from the **mean arterial blood pressure (MAP)**.

$$MAP = Diastolic\ BP + 1/3\ (Systolic\ BP - Diastolic\ BP)$$

$$CPP = MAP - ICP$$

If the brain swells or if bleeding occurs inside the skull, ICP increases, and the perfusion pressure decreases, resulting in cerebral ischemia (hypoxia). If the swelling of the brain is severe enough, the ICP equals the MAP, and blood flow to the brain ceases. In the late stage, hypertension, bradycardia, and irregular respiration known as **Cushing's reflex** occurs, which is associated with markedly elevated ICP and herniation. When the ICP increases, the systemic blood pressure increases to try to preserve blood flow to the brain. The body senses the rise in systemic blood pressure, and this triggers a drop in the pulse rate as the body tries to lower the systemic blood pressure. With severe injury or ischemia, the pressure within the skull continues in an upward spiral until a critical point at which the ICP approaches the MAP, and there is no cerebral perfusion. All vital signs deteriorate, and the patient dies. Because CPP depends on both the arterial pressure and the ICP, hypotension also will have a devastating effect if the ICP is high.

intracranial pressure (ICP): the pressure of the brain and contents within the skull.

cerebral perfusion pressure (CPP): the net pressure gradient causing blood flow through the brain.

mean arterial blood pressure (MAP): the sum of the diastolic blood pressure plus one-third of the pulse pressure (systolic blood pressure minus the diastolic blood pressure).

Cushing's reflex: a reflex in which the body responds to markedly elevated ICP by raising both the diastolic and systolic blood pressure, reduction of heart rate, and irregular respiration. Also called *Cushing's response*, this happens late in the course of the head injury.

cerebral herniation syndrome: a critical syndrome in which swelling of the brain forces portions of the brain tissue down through the opening at the base of the skull squeezing the brainstem and causing coma, and eventually death. Signs include dilatation of pupils, contralateral paralysis, elevated blood pressure, and bradycardia.

PEARLS
Cerebral Herniation Syndrome

A patient who, after correction of hypoxia and hypotension, shows rapid progression of brain injury (e.g., unresponsive with dilated pupil; decerebrate posturing; or drop in GCS score of > 2 with an initial GCS score of < 9) should be transported rapidly to a trauma center capable of managing severe TBI patients. This is the only situation in which hyperventilation is still indicated. Hyperventilation, although known to cause ischemia, may decrease brain swelling temporarily. Although a desperate measure, this might buy enough time to get the patient to surgery that might be life saving. Call ahead so that a neurosurgeon can be available and the operating room prepared by the time you arrive at the hospital.

As stated earlier, the injured brain loses the ability to autoregulate blood flow. In this situation perfusion of the brain is directly dependent on arterial blood pressure. You must maintain a CPP of at least 60 mm Hg (see earlier formula), which requires maintaining a systolic blood pressure of at least 100 mm Hg in the patient with TBI. Hypotension due to TBI is rare, occurring in about 5% of patients with isolated severe TBI (GCS of < 9). A patient with a significant TBI who is hypotensive is bleeding from somewhere or has a cord injury causing spinal shock. Stopping the hemorrhage and restoring perfusion is important. Overly aggressive attempts to maintain CPP above 70 mm Hg with fluids may lead to the development of the adult respiratory distress syndrome (ARDS). However, this does not happen immediately. Pressors such as dopamine may also be helpful in maintaining perfusion. Remember, hypotension and the associated poor perfusion is devastating to the injured brain.

Cerebral Herniation Syndrome

When the brain swells or intracranial hemorrhage occurs, particularly after a blow to the head, a sudden rise in ICP may occur. This may force portions of the brain downward, through the tentorium cerebelli. This leads to obstruction of the flow of cerebrospinal fluid and applies significant pressure to the brainstem, resulting in **cerebral herniation syndrome**. The classic findings of this life-threatening situation are a decreasing level of consciousness (LOC) that rapidly progresses to coma, dilation of the pupil and an outward–downward deviation of the eye on the side of the injury, paralysis of the arm and leg on the side opposite the injury, or decerebrate posturing (arms and legs extended). As the cerebral herniation is occurring, the vital signs frequently reveal increased blood pressure and bradycardia (Cushing's reflex). The patient may soon cease all movement, stop breathing, and die. This syndrome often follows an acute epidural or subdural hemorrhage.

If these signs are developing in a TBI patient, cerebral herniation is imminent, and aggressive therapy is needed. As noted earlier, hyperventilation will decrease the size of the blood vessels in the brain and briefly decrease ICP. In this situation the danger of immediate herniation outweighs the risk of cerebral ischemia that can follow hyperventilation. The cerebral herniation syndrome is the only situation in which hyperventilation is still indicated. (You must ventilate every three seconds [20/minute] for adults, every two and one-half seconds [25/minute] for children older than one year, and every two seconds [30/minute] for infants younger than one year.) If you have waveform capnography, attempt to keep the ETCO$_2$ at about 30 to 35 mm Hg.

To simplify knowing when to hyperventilate in the field, the clinical signs of cerebral herniation in the patient who has had hypoxemia and hypotension corrected are any one (or more) of the following:

- TBI patient with a Glasgow Coma Scale (GCS) score < 9 with extensor posturing (decerebrate posturing)
- TBI patient with a GCS score < 9 with asymmetric (or bilateral), dilated, or nonreactive pupils
- TBI patient with an initial GCS score < 9, who then drops his or her GCS by more than two points

For the preceding, "asymmetric pupils" means 1 mm (or more) difference in the size of one pupil, "fixed" means no response (<1 mm) to bright light. Bilateral dilated and fixed pupils usually are a sign of brainstem injury and are associated with greater than 90% mortality. A unilateral dilated and fixed pupil has been associated with good recovery in up to 54% of patients. Remember that hypoxemia, orbital trauma, drugs, lightning strike, and hypothermia also affect pupillary reaction, so take this into account before beginning hyperventilation. Flaccid paralysis usually means spinal-cord injury. If the patient has signs of herniation (as listed earlier) and the signs resolve with hyperventilation, you should discontinue the hyperventilation. (See Table 10-1.)

Table 10-1: Normal Ventilation Rates and Hyperventilation Rates		
Age Group	**Normal Ventilation Rate**	**Hyperventilation Rate**
Adult	8–10 breaths/minute (ETCO$_2$ 35–45)	20 breaths/minute (ETCO$_2$ about 30–35)
Children	15 breaths/minute (ETCO$_2$ 35–45)	25 breaths/minute (ETCO$_2$ about 30–35)
Infants	20 breaths/minute (ETCO$_2$ 35–45)	30 breaths/minute (ETCO$_2$ about 30–35)

As this text goes to press, there is emerging data from studies that suggest prehospital hyperventilation may be detrimental, even when herniation is present. The Arizona EPIC-TBI project reports that because it is very difficult to identify herniation without a CT scan, some patients in the field receive hyperventilation when not necessary, which can cause harm. The EPIC guidelines stress maintaining cerebral perfusion (systolic blood pressure > 110 mm Hg), keeping ETCO$_2$ at 35 mm Hg, and keeping blood glucose above 70 mg/dL.

ITLS guidelines, as of the date of publication of this edition, continue to follow the BTF recommendations, including mild hyperventilation in the presence of cerebral herniation. ITLS has, since the previous edition, advocated maintaining systolic blood pressure of at least 110 mm Hg in the TBI patient to ensure adequate perfusion, which is higher than the BTF guidelines but consistent with those put forth by Arizona EPIC. As more data becomes available these recommendations will be updated and made available on the ITLS Website.

Head Injuries

The head is made up of the face, scalp, skull, and brain. Serious injuries can occur to any one or all. The head is the heaviest part of a young child's body, so children involved in falls or other deceleration trauma frequently strike their head.

Facial Injuries

The soft tissue of the face is very vascular. Facial wounds can range from minor contusions, abrasions, and lacerations to wounds that can be fatal from airway compromise or hemorrhagic shock. Most bleeding can be controlled by direct pressure, but some hemorrhage from the nose or pharynx can be life threatening and impossible to control in the prehospital setting.

Nasal fractures are the most common fractures of facial bones and rarely are associated with severe hemorrhage. Fractures of the bones of the face and jaw are common, and the greatest danger is airway compromise caused by swelling and bleeding or loss of facial stability.

Injuries to the eyes are not life threatening but can be severely disabling. Treatment of eye trauma in the field should be gentle irrigation with normal saline if needed for chemicals and then application of an eye shield. If there is a possible open globe, characterized by an irregularly shaped pupil, do not irrigate. Cover with an eye shield. Do not allow any pressure on the globe itself to prevent extrusion of the eye contents.

Scalp Wounds

The scalp is highly vascular and often bleeds briskly when lacerated. Because many of the small blood vessels are suspended in an inelastic matrix of supporting tissue, the normal protective vasospasm that would limit bleeding is inhibited, which may lead to prolonged bleeding and significant blood loss. Though an uncommon cause of shock in an adult, a child may develop shock from a briskly bleeding scalp wound, due to a smaller blood volume.

PEARLS
Shock

Any unexplained shock in a patient with head injury is hypovolemic until proven otherwise. Treat hypotension.

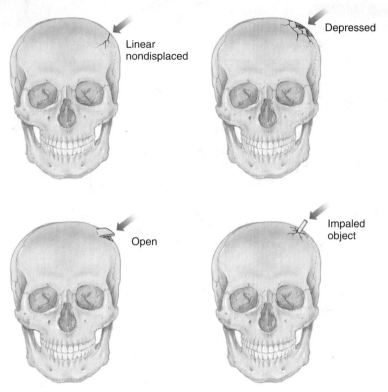

Figure 10-3 Types of skull fractures.

As a general rule, if you have an adult patient who is in shock, look for a cause other than the scalp wound, such as internal bleeding. Most bleeding from the scalp can be easily controlled in the field with direct pressure if your exam reveals no unstable fractures under the wound.

Skull Injuries

Skull injuries can be linear nondisplaced fractures, depressed fractures, or compound fractures (Figure 10-3). Suspect an underlying skull fracture in adults who have a large contusion or darkened swelling of the scalp. There is very little that can be done for skull fractures in the field except to avoid placing direct pressure on an obvious depressed or compound skull fracture. The real concern is that the amount of force that can cause a skull fracture may cause a brain injury.

Open skull fractures should have the wound dressed, but avoid excess pressure when controlling bleeding. Penetrating objects in the skull should be secured in place (not removed) and the patient transported immediately. Gunshot wounds to the head often have brain injury from the bullet and the bone fragments

Consider child abuse when you find a child with a head injury and no clear explanation of the cause. Suspect possible abuse if the story about the injury is inconsistent with the injury or the responsible adult suggests the child performed an activity that a child of this age is not physically capable of performing. Pay particular attention to the setting from which you rescued the child. Request police or social service assistance if the circumstances are suspicious for child abuse.

Brain Injuries

There are multiple types of injuries to the brain and associated blood vessels. They are discussed in this section, beginning with the least severe and progressing through to life-threatening injuries.

Concussion

A concussion implies no structural injury to the brain that can be demonstrated by current imaging techniques. There is a brief disruption of neural function that often results in loss of consciousness, but many people will have a concussion without a loss of consciousness.

Classically, there is a history of trauma to the head with a variable period of unconsciousness or confusion and then a return to normal consciousness. There may be amnesia following the injury. The amnesia usually extends to some point before the injury (retrograde short-term amnesia), so often the patient will not remember the events leading to the injury. Short-term memory is often affected, and the patient may repeat questions over and over as if the injured person has not been paying attention to your answers. Patients also may report dizziness, headache, ringing in the ears, or nausea.

Concussion is not a benign injury. Long-term effects of concussion, although variable, can be devastating to the individual, especially if a patient has had multiple episodes, such as seen in athletes involved in contact sports, such as boxers, soccer or football players, and rugby players. Any person who sustains a concussion while playing sports or other activities should not be allowed to return to that activity that day and should not resume playing until cleared by a physician. Better protective equipment can reduce the occurrence of concussion. Additional information and guidelines for post-concussive assessment and return to play are available from the U.S. Centers for Disease Control and the American Academy of Neurology websites.

Cerebral Contusion

A patient with cerebral contusion (bruised brain tissue) will have a history of prolonged unconsciousness or serious alteration in level of consciousness (profound confusion, persistent amnesia, abnormal behavior, for example). Brain swelling may be rapid and severe. The patient may have focal neurologic signs (weakness, speech problems) and appear to have suffered a cerebrovascular accident (stroke). Depending on the location of the cerebral contusion, the patient may have personality changes such as inappropriate or rude behavior or agitation.

Subarachnoid Hemorrhage

Blood can enter the subarachnoid space as a result either of trauma or a spontaneous hemorrhage. Traumatic subarachnoid hemorrhage rarely occurs alone. Often there is an associated subdural hematoma or cerebral contusion. The subarachnoid blood causes irritation that results in intravascular fluid "leaking" into the brain and causing more edema as well as spasm of the small arteries, which can reduce cerebral perfusion. Severe headache, coma, and vomiting are common findings. Patients may have significant brain swelling and may develop cerebral herniation syndrome.

Diffuse Axonal Injury

Diffuse axonal injury is the most common type of injury following severe blunt head trauma. The brain is injured so diffusely that there is generalized edema. Usually, there is no evidence of a structural lesion such as a hematoma on cerebral computerized tomography (CAT scan). In most cases the patient presents unconscious, due to disruption of nerve fibers between cortex and brainstem, with no focal motor deficits.

Anoxic Brain Injury

Injuries to the brain from lack of oxygen (such as from cardiac arrest, airway obstruction, near-drowning) affect the brain in a serious fashion. Following an anoxic episode, perfusion of the cortex is interrupted because of spasm that develops in the small cerebral arteries. After four to six minutes of anoxia, restoring oxygenation and blood pressure will not restore perfusion of the cortex (**no-reflow phenomenon**), and there will be continuing anoxic injury to the brain cells, and irreversible damage almost always occurs.

no-reflow phenomenon: the inability of restoring oxygenation and blood pressure to restore perfusion to the cortex after an anoxic episode of 4 to 6 minutes or more.

Hypothermia seems to protect against this phenomenon, and there have been reported cases of hypothermic patients being resuscitated after almost an hour of anoxia. Many patients undergoing planned neurosurgical procedures will have hypothermia induced to help protect the brain. Recent research following medical cardiac arrest shows improved neurologic outcome when resuscitated patients are treated with controlled hypothermia. This has yet to be established in the head-injured trauma patient. Induction of hypothermia does take time. Current research is directed toward finding medications that either reverse the persistent postanoxic arterial spasm or protect against the anoxic injury to the cells.

Intracranial Hemorrhage

Hemorrhage can occur between the skull and dura (the fibrous covering of the brain), between the dura and the arachnoid, or directly in the brain tissue.

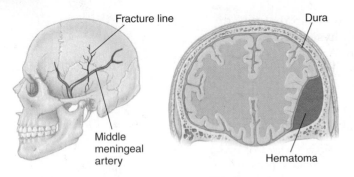

Figure 10-4 Acute epidural hematoma. This hemorrhage may follow injury to the extradural arteries. The blood collects between the fibrous dura and the periosteum.

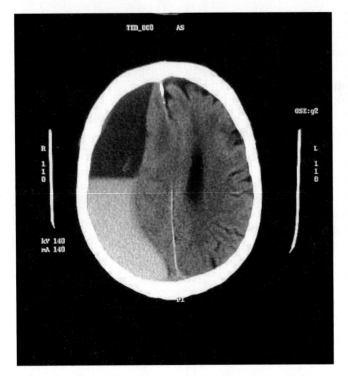

Figure 10-5 Acute subdural hematoma. This usually occurs following the rupture of dural veins. Blood collects and often severely compresses the brain. *(Photo courtesy of Roy Alson, MD)*

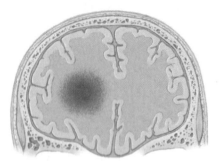

Figure 10-6 Intracerebral hemorrhage.

Acute Epidural Hematoma An acute epidural hematoma is most often caused by a tear in the middle meningeal artery that runs along the inside of the skull in the temporal region. The arterial injury is often caused by a linear skull fracture in the temporal or parietal region (Figure 10-4). Because the bleeding is usually arterial (although it may be venous from one of the dural sinuses), the bleeding and rise in ICP can occur rapidly, and death may occur quickly.

Symptoms of an acute epidural hematoma include a history of head trauma with initial loss of consciousness often followed by a period during which the patient is conscious and coherent (the "lucid interval"). After a period of a few minutes to several hours, the patient will develop signs of increasing ICP (vomiting, headache, altered mental status), lapse into unconsciousness, and develop body paralysis on the side opposite the head injury (see the earlier section on cerebral herniation syndrome). There is often a dilated and fixed (no response to bright light) pupil on the side of the head injury. The signs are usually followed rapidly by death. The classic example is the boxer who is knocked unconscious, wakes up, and is allowed to go home, only to be found dead in bed the next morning. The "lucid interval" suggests that the brain does not have a serious structural injury, so surgical removal of the blood and ligation of the ruptured blood vessel before herniation occurs often allows for full neurologic recovery. Be aware that not every epidural patient will show this lucid interval. Careful observation for the other signs of an epidural hematoma, mentioned earlier, is critical so this life-threatening injury is not missed.

Acute Subdural Hematoma This is the result of bleeding from bridging veins and/or from arteries complicated with brain contusion (Figure 10-5). In the case of bleeding from veins, ICP increases more slowly, and the diagnosis often is not apparent until hours or days after the injury. If the bleeding is from arteries associated with a brain contusion, the symptoms will develop earlier.

The signs and symptoms include headache, fluctuations in the level of consciousness, and focal neurologic signs (such as weakness of one extremity or one side of the body, altered deep tendon reflexes, and slurred speech). Because of underlying brain tissue injury, prognosis is often poor. Mortality is very high (60% to 90%) in patients who are comatose when found. Use of anticoagulants increases the risk of subdural bleeding.

Always suspect a subdural hematoma in an alcoholic with any degree of altered mental status following a fall. Elderly patients and those taking anticoagulants are also at high risk for this injury and may not show signs and symptoms until many days after injury.

Intracerebral Hemorrhage Intracerebral hemorrhage is bleeding within the brain tissue (Figure 10-6). Traumatic intracerebral hemorrhage may result from blunt or penetrating injuries of the head. Unfortunately, surgery often is not helpful. The signs and symptoms depend on the regions involved and the degree of injury. They occur in patterns similar to those that accompany a stroke. Spontaneous hemorrhages of this type may be seen in patients with severe hypertension. Alteration in the level of consciousness is commonly seen, though awake patients may complain of headache and vomiting.

Evaluation of the Traumatic Brain Injury Patient

Determining the exact type of TBI or hemorrhage cannot be done in the field because it requires imaging techniques such as a CAT scan. It is more important that you recognize the presence of a brain injury and be ready to provide supportive measures while transporting the patient to the appropriate facility. TBI patients can be difficult to manage because they often are uncooperative and may be under the influence of alcohol or drugs. As an emergency care provider, you must pay extraordinary attention to detail and never lose your patience with an uncooperative patient.

ITLS Primary Survey

Remember that every trauma patient is initially evaluated in the same sequence (Figure 10-7).

Scene Size-up

The results of the scene size-up will begin to determine if you have a load-and-go patient. Dangerous generalized mechanisms (motor-vehicle collision, fall from a height) will require a complete examination (rapid trauma survey). Dangerous focused mechanisms (hit in the head with a baseball bat) will allow you to "focus" your exam (ABCs, with head, neck, and neurologic exams) rather than having to perform a complete exam.

Initial Assessment

The goals of the initial assessment are to determine the priority of the patient and to find immediate life threats. The initial assessment in the head-trauma patient is used to determine quickly if the patient is brain injured and, if so, if the patient's condition is deteriorating. Obviously, a patient with a history and physical examination that indicate a loss of consciousness following a lucid period post injury (possible epidural hematoma) should be transported with more urgency than one who is alert and oriented after being knocked out (possible concussion). It is very important that all observations be recorded (but do not interrupt patient care to do this) because later treatment is often dictated by detection of the deterioration of clinical stability.

All patients with head or facial trauma and an *altered level of consciousness* should be assumed to have a cervical-spine injury until proven otherwise. Because of the altered level of consciousness, it is often not possible to clear the cervical spine until after arrival at the hospital. Restriction of cervical-spine movement should accompany airway and breathing management. Evaluation for TBI is begun as you obtain your initial level of consciousness by speaking to the patient.

During the initial assessment your neurologic exam is limited to level of consciousness and any obvious paralysis. Level of consciousness is the most sensitive indicator of brain function. Initially, the AVPU (alert, responds to verbal stimuli, responds to pain, and unresponsive) method is adequate. (See Chapter 2.) If there is a history of trauma to the head, or if the initial exam reveals an altered mental status, then the rapid trauma survey will include a more complete neurologic exam. A decrease in the level of consciousness is an early indicator of a brain injury or rising ICP.

Control of the airway cannot be overemphasized. The supine, restrained, and unconscious patient is prone to airway obstruction from the tongue, blood, vomit, or other secretions. Vomiting is very common within the first hour following a head injury. Suction should be immediately available.

PEARLS
Altered Mental Status

Remember that hypoglycemia, hypoxia, cardiac dysrhythmias, and drugs can cause altered mental status. When narcotic abuse is a possibility, administer naloxone (Narcan®) to any patient with altered mental status. Monitor the heart and oxygenation, and check the blood glucose level on all patients with altered mental status. If you cannot perform a glucose determination but suspect hypoglycemia (diabetics and alcoholics), give glucose or thiamine and glucose.

Figure 10-7 The ITLS Primary Survey.

ITLS PRIMARY SURVEY

SCENE SIZE-UP
Standard Precautions Hazards, Number of Patients, Need for additional resources, **Mechanism of Injury**

INITIAL ASSESSMENT
GENERAL IMPRESSION
Age, Sex, Weight, General Appearance, Position, Purposeful Movement, Obvious Injuries, Skin Color
Life-threatening Bleeding

LOC
A-V-P-U
Chief Complaint/Symptoms

AIRWAY
(WITH C-SPINE CONTROL)
Snoring, Gurgling, Stridor; Silence

BREATHING
Present? Rate, Depth, Effort

CIRCULATION
Radial/Carotid Present? Rate, Rhythm, Quality
Skin Color, Temperature, Moisture; Capillary Refill
Has bleeding been controlled?

RAPID TRAUMA SURVEY
HEAD and NECK
Wounds?
Neck Vein distention? Tracheal Deviation?

CHEST
Asymmetry (Paradoxical Motion?), Contusions, Penetrations, Tenderness, Instability, Crepitation
Breath Sounds
Present? Equal? (If unequal: percussion)
Heart Tones

ABDOMEN
Contusions, Penetration/Evisceration; Tenderness, Rigidity, Distension

PELVIS
Tenderness, Instability, Crepitation

LOWER/UPPER EXTREMITIES
Obvious Swelling, Deformity
Motor and Sensory

POSTERIOR
Obvious wounds, Tenderness, Deformity

If radial pulse present:
VITAL SIGNS
Measured Pulse, Breathing, Blood Pressure

If altered mental status: Brief Neurologic exam
PUPILS
Size? Reactive? **Equal?**

GLASGOW COMA SCALE
Eyes, Voice, Motor

Protect the airway of the unconscious patient who has no gag reflex by endotracheal intubation or by placement of an oral or nasal airway and frequent suctioning. Perform endotracheal intubation of the unconscious head-injured patient as rapidly and smoothly as possible to avoid patient agitation, straining, and breath-holding, which may contribute to elevated ICP. Use of intravenous lidocaine when intubating head-injured patients is no longer recommended. Head-injured patients may seize from their injury (if hypoxic) or have their teeth and jaws clenched, making intubation difficult. Attempting to force an artificial airway into such a patient may cause additional injury.

Drug-assisted intubation (DAI) or use of nasotracheal intubation should be considered in this situation, if permitted under local protocols. Before beginning intubation, ventilate (do not hyperventilate) with high-flow oxygen. (See Chapters 4 and 5.) Do not allow the TBI patient to become hypoxic. Even one brief episode of hypoxia can increase mortality. Be aware that DAI of TBI patients in the field has been reported to increase mortality. This is thought to be due to the patient becoming hypoxic during the intubation attempt. If you can adequately manage the patient's airway noninvasively and transport times are short, consider deferring intubation until arrival at the hospital.

As stated earlier, it is important to note the patient's basic neurologic status prior to DAI because the medications given can prevent a complete neurologic assessment in the hospital.

Rapid Trauma Survey

Perform a rapid trauma survey on all patients who have an abnormal level of consciousness. (See Chapter 2.)

Head When the initial assessment is completed, perform a rapid trauma survey guided by the mechanism of injury. Begin with the scalp and quickly, but carefully, examine for obvious injuries such as lacerations or depressed or open skull fractures. The size of a laceration is often misjudged because of the difficulty in assessment through hair matted with blood. Feel the scalp gently for obvious unstable areas of the skull. If none are present, you may safely apply a pressure dressing or hold direct pressure on a bandage to stop scalp bleeding.

A basilar skull fracture may be indicated by any of the following: bleeding from the ear or nose, clear or serosanguineous fluid running from the nose or ear, swelling and/or discoloration behind the ear (Battle's sign), and swelling and discoloration around both eyes (raccoon eyes; Figure 10-8). Raccoon eyes are a sign of anterior

drug-assisted intubation (DAI): the administration of a sedative and paralytic agent to improve the ability to intubate a patient. This is also called *rapid sequence intubation (RSI)*.

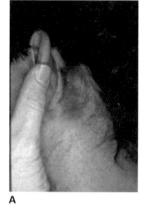

A

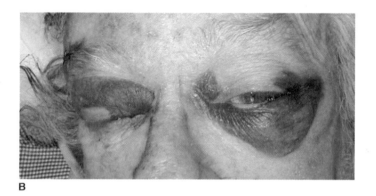

B

Figure 10-8a Battle's sign—evidence of a posterior basilar skull fracture. *(Photo courtesy of Roy Alson, MD)*

Figure 10-8b Raccoon eyes—evidence of an anterior basilar skull fracture. *(Photo courtesy of Roy Alson, MD)*

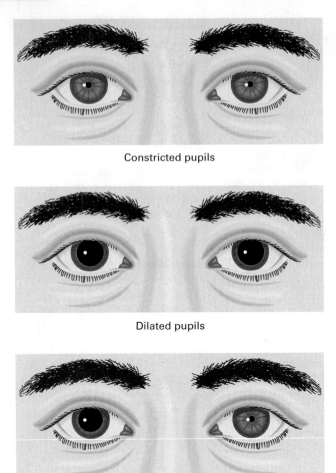

Constricted pupils

Dilated pupils

Unequal pupils

Figure 10-9 Examination of pupils.

basilar skull fracture that may go through the thin cribriform plate in the upper nasal cavity and allow spinal fluid and blood to leak out. Raccoon eyes with or without drainage from the nose are relative contraindications to inserting a nasogastric tube or nasotracheal intubation. The tube can go through the fractured cribriform plate and into the brain.

Pupils The pupils (Figure 10-9) are controlled in part by the third cranial nerve. This nerve takes a long course through the skull and is easily compressed by brain swelling and thus may be affected by increasing ICP. Following a head injury, if both pupils are dilated and do not react to light, the patient probably has a brainstem injury, and the prognosis is grim. If the pupils are dilated but still react to light, the injury is often still reversible, so every effort should be made to transport the patient quickly to a facility capable of treating a traumatic brain injury. A unilaterally dilated pupil that remains reactive to light may be the earliest sign of cerebral herniation. The development of a unilaterally dilated, nonreactive pupil ("blown pupil") while you are observing the comatose patient is an extreme emergency and mandates rapid transport. Also consider initiating hyperventilation. Other causes of dilated pupils that may or may not react to light include hypothermia, lightning strike, anoxia, optic nerve injury, drug effect, or direct trauma to the eye. Fixed and dilated pupils signify increased ICP only in patients with a decreased level of consciousness. If the patient has a normal level of consciousness, the dilated pupil is not from head injury (more likely due to eye trauma or drugs such as atropine).

Fluttering eyelids are often seen with emotional disorders. Slow lid closure (like a curtain falling) is usually caused by brain injury or effect of toxins (such as alcohol or other sedatives). Testing for a blink response (corneal reflex) by touching the cornea with the edge of a gauze pad or cotton swab, or by applying overly noxious stimuli to a patient to test for response to pain, are techniques that are unreliable and do not contribute to prehospital assessment.

Extremities Note sensation and motor function in the extremities. Can patients feel you touch their hands and feet? Can they wiggle their fingers and toes? If patients are unconscious, note their response to pain. If they withdraw or localize to the pinching of the fingers and toes, they have grossly intact sensation and motor function. This usually indicates that there is normal or only minimally impaired cortical function.

Both decorticate posturing or rigidity (arms flexed, legs extended) and decerebrate posturing or rigidity (arms and legs extended) are ominous signs of deep cerebral hemispheric or upper brainstem injury (Figure 10-10). Decerebrate posturing is worse and usually signifies cerebral herniation. It is one of the indications for hyperventilation. Flaccid paralysis usually denotes spinal-cord injury.

Neurologic Exam To apply the revised trauma score and other field triage scoring systems, you should be familiar with the Glasgow Coma Scale score (GCS). It is simple, is easy to use, and has good prognostic value for eventual outcome (Table 10-2). In the TBI patient, a Glasgow Coma Scale score of 8 or less is considered evidence of a severe

Figure 10-10 Decorticate (A) and decerebrate (B) posturing.

Table 10-2: Glasgow Coma Scale

Eye Opening	Points	Verbal Response	Points	Motor Response	Points
Spontaneous	4	Oriented	5	Obeys commands	6
To voice	3	Confused	4	Localizes pain	5
To pain	2	Inappropriate words	3	Withdraws	4
None	1	Incomprehensible sounds	2	Abnormal flexion	3*
		Silent	1	Abnormal extension	2**
				No movement	1

* Decorticate posturing to pain.

** Decerebrate posturing to pain.

brain injury. The GCS score determined in the field serves as the baseline for the patient; be sure to record it. You should note that early GCS assessment may not reflect the severity of the head injury itself because systemic causes (hypoxia, hypotension, hypoglycemia, alcohol, and so on) may cause altered mental status. Evaluation after the correction of those factors represents the severity of brain damage correctly. Record the score for each part of the GCS, not just the total score. You also should perform a finger-stick glucose on all patients with altered mental status.

Vital Signs Vital signs should be obtained by another team member while you are performing the exam. Vital signs are extremely important in following the course of a patient with head trauma. Most important, they can indicate changes in ICP (Table 10-3). Observe and record vital signs at the end of the ITLS Primary Survey, during the detailed exam, and each time you perform the ITLS Ongoing Exam. In the patient with TBI, look for the following:

- *Respiration.* Increasing ICP causes the respiratory rate to increase, decrease, and/or become irregular. Unusual respiratory patterns may reflect the level of brain or brainstem injury. Just before death, the patient may develop a rapid, noisy respiratory pattern called *central neurogenic hyperventilation.* Because respiration is affected by so many factors (such as fear, emotional disorders, chest injuries, hypoxia, spinal-cord injuries, diabetes), it is not as useful an indicator as are the other vital signs in monitoring the course of head injury. Abnormal respiratory patterns may indicate a chest injury or other problem that could lead to hypoxia if untreated.

Table 10-3: Comparison of Vital Signs in Shock and Head Injury

	Shock	Head Injury with Increased Intracranial Pressure
Level of consciousness	Decreased	Decreased
Respiration	Increased	Varies but frequently decreased
Pulse	Increased	Decreased
Blood pressure	Decreased	Increased
Pulse pressure	Narrows	Widens

- *Pulse.* Increasing ICP causes the pulse rate to decrease. However, this is a late sign. Tachycardia may be a sign of shock or pain.
- *Blood pressure.* Increasing ICP causes increased blood pressure. This hypertension is usually associated with a widening of the pulse pressure (systolic minus diastolic pressure). Other causes of hypertension include fear and pain. Hypotension in the presence of a head injury is usually caused by hemorrhagic or neurogenic shock and should be treated as if caused by hemorrhage. It is very rate to have hypotension due solely to a TBI. Keep in mind that the injured brain does not tolerate hypotension. A single instance of hypotension (90 mm Hg systolic) in an adult with a brain injury may increase the mortality rate by 150%. The increase in mortality rate for hypotension and a severe TBI is even worse in children. Give IV fluids to maintain a blood pressure of at least 110 to 120 mm Hg systolic in the adult patient with a severe head injury (GCS 8 or less), even if the patient has associated penetrating trauma with hemorrhage. As noted earlier, the goal is to maintain CPP above 60 mm Hg, as recommended by the BTF. Children with severe TBI should have their blood pressure maintained at the normal range for their age.

History Begin obtaining the history before and continue during the rapid trauma survey. It is essential to obtain as thorough a history about the event as possible. The circumstances of the head injury may be extremely important for patient management and may be of prognostic importance to the ultimate outcome. Pay particular attention to reports of near-drowning, electrocution, lightning strike, drug abuse, smoke inhalation, hypothermia, and seizures. Always inquire about the patient's behavior from the time of the head injury until the time of your arrival. Try to obtain the past medical history. Nontraumatic events also can cause an alteration in the LOC. A blood glucose should always be checked in patients with altered mental status.

ITLS Secondary Survey

Suspected TBI patients with altered mental status are load-and-go situations. The ITLS Secondary Survey will be done during transport (or not at all, if a short transport). (See Chapter 2.)

ITLS Ongoing Exam

Each time you perform the ITLS Ongoing Exam, record the level of consciousness, the pupil size and reaction to light, the Glasgow Coma Scale score, and the development (or improvement) of focal weakness or paralysis. This, along with the vital signs, provides enough information to monitor the condition of the brain-injured patient. Decisions on the management of the TBI patient are based on the changes in all the parameters of the physical and neurologic examination. You are establishing the baseline from which later judgments must be made. Record your observations.

Management of the TBI Patient

Your job is to prevent secondary brain injury. It is extremely important to make a rapid assessment and then transport the patient to a facility capable of managing TBI. Appropriate triage of the patient to facilities capable of managing TBI can have a significant impact on the outcome of the patient. The important points of management in the prehospital phase are listed here.

BTF guidelines are classified as follows:

- Level I recommendations, supported by Class I scientific evidence (formerly called *Standards*)
- Level II recommendations, supported by Class II scientific evidence (formerly called *Guidelines*)
- Level III recommendations, supported by Class III scientific evidence (formerly called *Options*)

PEARLS
Seizures

Seizures in TBI patients are usually caused by hypoxia. If the patient has an open airway and you are already ventilating with 100% oxygen, you may be ordered to administer IV medication to control the seizures. Seizures should always cause you to recheck the airway, ventilation, and oxygenation of your patient.

PEARLS
Hyperventilation

Emergency care providers tend to assist respiration at too fast a rate. Use of an $ETCO_2$ monitor can prevent this.

Procedure

Managing the Head-Trauma Patient

1. Secure the airway, and provide good oxygenation. The injured brain does not tolerate hypoxia, so every TBI patient should receive 100% oxygen. If possible, monitor the oxygen saturation with a pulse oximeter. Do not allow the SaO_2 to become less than 90% (Level II). It is best to maintain a level about 95%.

   Maintain good ventilation (not hyperventilation) with high-flow oxygen at a rate of about one breath every 6 to 8 seconds (8 to 10 breaths per minute). Studies have found that emergency medical providers tend to hyperventilate the critical patient without realizing it. You can prevent this if you have an $ETCO_2$ monitor. Try to keep the CO_2 between 35 and 45 mm Hg.

   Endotracheal intubation is still recommended for adults if the airway cannot be maintained or if you cannot maintain adequate oxygenation with supplemental oxygen. There is no reason to routinely intubate patients who are maintaining their airway and have normal oxygen saturation. Some studies have found a decreased survival rate for TBI patients who have been intubated in the field. Possible causes of this are unrecognized hypoxemia, unrecognized hyperventilation, or unrecognized esophageal intubation. Use of capnography will prevent those problems. (See Chapter 5.) BTF guidelines recommend capnography, pulse oximetry, and blood pressure monitoring as critical monitoring procedures for all intubated TBI patients (Level III).

   There is no evidence to support out-of-hospital endotracheal intubation over bag-valve-mask ventilation of pediatric patients with TBI (Level II).

   Because TBI patients are prone to vomiting, be prepared to log roll the motion-restricted patient and to suction the oropharynx, particularly if an endotracheal tube has not been placed. Try to avoid use of antiemetics because some may decrease the level of consciousness.

2. Apply spinal motion restriction based on the mechanism of injury as the status of the spine cannot be clinically assessed in a head-injured patient with altered mental status. (See Chapter 12.) When possible, elevate the head of the stretcher to help reduce ICP.

3. Agitated and combative patients fighting against restraints or ventilations can raise their ICP, as well as place themselves at risk for further cervical-spine injury. Consider sedation in this situation, though be aware that sedation will complicate the neurologic evaluation of your patient.

   Careful use of benzodiazepines can decrease agitation without dropping blood pressure. An added benefit to the use of benzodiazepines is that they prevent seizures. Seizure prophylaxis in the head-injured patient should be initiated on the recommendation of medical direction. Other agents suitable for use include phenytoin. Do not use barbiturates because they can cause hypotension.

4. Record baseline observations. Record vital signs (describe rate and pattern of breathing), the level of consciousness, the pupils (size and reaction to light), the Glasgow Coma Scale score, and the development (or improvement) of focal weakness or paralysis. If the patient develops hypotension, suspect hemorrhage or spinal-cord injury. Every patient with altered mental status should have a finger-stick glucose checked and recorded.

5. Continuously monitor the observations listed in step 4. Record them every five minutes.

6. Insert two large-bore IV catheters. Fluid resuscitation (crystalloid) in patients with TBI should be administered to avoid hypotension and/or limit hypotension to the shortest duration possible (Level II). In the past it was thought that fluids should be limited in head-injured patients. It has been found that the danger of increasing brain swelling by giving fluids is much less than the danger of allowing the patient to be hypotensive.

   Hyperventilation is recommended for use in treating the patient with signs of cerebral herniation after correcting hypotension or hypoxia (Level III).

   If you have capnography available, try to maintain the $ETCO_2$ level at about 35 to 40 mm Hg. If you have to hyperventilate the patient, keep the $ETCO_2$ between 30 and 35 mm Hg. Further research is needed on the utility of hypertonic saline solutions over current crystalloids for treatment of hypotension in TBI patients. Routine administration of steroids for TBI has not been shown to improve outcomes.

Case Presentation (continued)

You are the lead emergency care provider in an ALS ambulance transporting a seriously injured motorcyclist to a trauma center. The patient has had a tension pneumothorax decompressed and is intubated for respiratory difficulty. You perform an ITLS Ongoing Exam and find no further hemorrhage from the leg and a change in vital signs as noted here. As part of the ongoing exam, you repeat the neurologic exam, which still shows decerebrate posturing of the upper extremities. Spontaneous respirations are irregular and slow (they are being assisted at about 8/minute) and the pulse now below 80. Other vital signs are BP of 88/40, SaO_2 of 95, $ETCO_2$ of 38, and GCS-3. You look in the "window of the brain." The right pupil is now fixed and dilated. You are concerned about possible cerebral herniation, given the fixed pupil and bradycardia. You instruct your partner to increase his ventilatory rate to 12 per minute and aim for an $ETCO_2$ of 30 to 35 mm Hg. You also open the IV lines to achieve a systolic BP of > 100 mm Hg. You then call the trauma center back with the report of the patient's deterioration. They report they will have a neurosurgeon respond to the trauma room.

Classically, herniation syndrome is characterized by hypertension, bradycardia, and irregular respirations, but the other injuries of this patient prevent their manifestation. The patient is in hemorrhagic shock and should be tachycardic, so the normalization of the heart rate is likely an inappropriate bradycardia. Furthermore, the possible spinal-cord injury would also block the autonomic response (tachycardia) to hemorrhagic shock. The hypotension from the traumatic blood loss along with spinal shock will worsen this patient's cerebral ischemia, so management of hypoxemia and poor perfusion are key components in the prehospital care of the severe brain trauma.

In follow-up of this call, you are notified by the trauma center that a cerebral CAT scan showed a right-sided subdural hematoma with midline shift (herniation), along with cerebral contusion. The neurosurgeon along with the trauma team was able to successfully decompress this patient's hematoma after the patient's shock had been stabilized. Imaging of the spine showed a compression fracture of the first thoracic vertebrae with retropulsion of fragments into the spinal cord. This was surgically repaired, and the patient began moving lower extremities.

Summary

Traumatic brain injury is a serious complication of trauma. To give your patient the best chance of recovery, you should be familiar with the important anatomy of the head and central nervous system and understand how trauma to the various areas presents clinically. The most important steps in the management of the head-injured patient are rapid assessment, good airway management, prevention of hypotension, rapid transport to a trauma center, and frequent ITLS Ongoing Exams. Implementation of BTF guidelines leads to significant improvement in outcome of patients with severe head injury. In no other area of trauma care is the recording of repeated assessments so important to future management decisions.

Bibliography

Badjatia, N., N. Carney, T. J. Crocco, M. E. Fallat. H. M. Hennes, A. S. Jagoda. S. Jernigan, P. B. Letarte, E. B. Lerner, T. M. Moriarty, et al. "Guidelines for Prehospital Management of Traumatic Brain Injury 2nd Edition." *Prehospital Emergency Care* 12, Suppl. 1 (2008): S1–S52.

Brain Trauma Foundation, American Association of Neurological Surgeons/College of Neurological Surgeons, Joint Section on Neurotrauma and Critical Care. "Guidelines for the Management of Severe Head Injury, 3rd Edition." *Journal of Neurotrauma* 24, Suppl. 1 (2007).

Chestnut, R. M., L. F. Marshall, M. R. Klauber, B. A. Blunt, N. Baldwin, H. M. Esenbert, J. A. Jane, A. Marmarou, and M. A. Foulkes. "The Role of Secondary Brain Injury in Determining Outcome from Severe Head Injury." *Journal of Trauma* 34, no. 2 (February 1993): 216–22.

Davis, D. P., D. B. Hoyt, M. Ochs, D. Fortlage, T. Holbrook, L. K. Marshall, and P. Rosen. "The Effect of Paramedic Rapid Sequence Intubation on Outcome in Patients with Severe Traumatic Brain Injury." *Journal of Trauma—Injury, Infection, and Critical Care* 54, no. 3 (March 2003): 444–53.

Davis, D. P., J. V. Dunford, J. C. Poste, M. Ochs, T. Holbrook, D. Fortlage, M. J. Size, F. Kennedy, and D. B. Hoyt. "The Impact of Hypoxia and Hyperventilation on Outcome After Paramedic Rapid Sequence Intubation of Severely Head-Injured Patients." *Journal of Trauma* 57, no. 1 (July 2004): 1–8.

Davis, D. P., J. V. Dunford, M. Ochs, K. Park, and D. B. Hoyt. "The Use of Quantitative End-Tidal Capnometry to Avoid Inadvertent Severe Hyperventilation in Patients with Head Injury After Paramedic Rapid Sequence Intubation." *Journal of Trauma—Injury, Infection, and Critical Care* 56, no. 4 (April 2004): 808–14.

Franschman, G., S. M. Peerdeman, S. Greuters, J. Vieveen, A. C. Brinkman, H. M. Christiaans, E. J. Toor, G. N. Jukema, S. A. Loer, C. Boer, and ALARM-TBI Investigators. "Prehospital Endotracheal Intubation in Patients with Severe Traumatic Brain Injury: Guidelines versus Reality." *Resuscitation* 80, no. 10 (October 2009): 1147–51.

Langlois, J. A., W. Rutland-Brown, and M. A. Wald. "The Epidemiology and Impact of Traumatic Brain Injury: A Brief Overview." *Journal of Head Trauma Rehabilitation* 21, no. 5 (September–October 2006): 375–78.

McCrory, P., W. Meeuwisse, K. Johnston, J. Dvorak, M. Aubry, M. Molloy, and R. Cantu. "Consensus Statement on Concussion in Sport: The 3rd International Conference on Concussion in Sports held in Zurich, November 2008." *British Journal of Sports Medicine* 43, Suppl. 1 (May 2009): i76–90.

Pigula, F. A., S. L. Wald, S. R. Shackford, and D. W. Vane. "The Effect of Hypotension and Hypoxia on Children with Severe Head Injuries." *Journal of Pediatric Surgery* 28, no. 3 (March 1993): 310–16.

Stolz, U., K. Denninghoff, D. Spaite, et al. "Association Between Lowest Prehospital Systolic Blood Pressure and Non-Mortality Outcomes in Major Traumatic Brain Injury: Is There a 'Hypotension' Threshold?" *Prehospital Emergency Care* 19, no. 1 (January–March 2015): 143.

Wang, H. E., A. B. Peitzman, L. D. Cassidy, P. D. Adelson, and D. M. Yealy. "Out-of-Hospital Endotracheal Intubation and Outcome After Traumatic Brain Injury." *Annals of Emergency Medicine* 44, no. 5 (November 2004): 439–50.

Get more information about this course by calling
ITLS International at 888-495-4875
(outside the United States call +1-630-495-6442) or visit

www.itrauma.org

11

Spinal Trauma and Patient-Centered Spinal Motion Restriction

James J. Augustine, MD, FACEP

Trauma Spinale	Traumatismo Raquídeo	Traumatisme Médullaire
Urazy kręgosłupa	Wirbelsäulentrauma	Ozljede kralježnice
إصابات العمود الفقري	trauma kičme	Poškodbe hrbtenjače Gerincsérülés

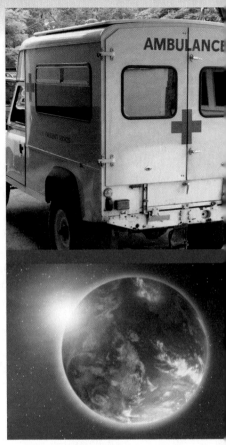

Key Terms

Emergency Rescue, *p. 218*
neutral alignment, *p. 219*
paresthesia, *p. 216*
primary spinal-cord injury, *p. 216*
rapid extrication, *p. 218*
secondary spinal-cord injury, *p. 216*
spinal column, *p. 212*
spinal cord, *p. 213*

Objectives

Upon successful completion of this chapter, you should be able to:

1. Explain the normal anatomy and physiology of the spinal column and spinal cord.
2. Define spinal motion restriction (SMR) and its relationship to patient safety.
3. Describe elements of injury, history, and assessment that may assist in determining which patients will benefit from spinal motion restriction (SMR).
4. Describe at least one mechanism of injury for which spinal motion restriction (SMR) can cause a significant decrease in survival.
5. Explain the difference between Emergency Rescue and rapid extrication techniques, and describe the appropriate utilization of each.
6. Using the clinical evaluation, differentiate neurogenic shock from hemorrhagic shock.

Chapter Overview

Spinal-cord injury is a devastating and life-threatening result of modern trauma. In the United States it is likely that one million patients have injuries each year that will require emergency care providers to consider the risk of spine injury. Fortunately, only about 2% of those injuries actually injure the spinal column, and most are stable and not associated with spinal-cord injury. The management of trauma patients requires continuous vigilance for injuries to the spinal column and to the spinal cord and expedient treatment for the complications of those injuries.

This chapter reviews the process of evaluating the injured patient and providing appropriate treatment, transportation to the hospital, and protection from problems that will have lifelong implications. Spinal-cord damage represents an injury that may not be obvious upon initial evaluation, but requires EMS management to prevent further damage. This preventive care is called *spinal motion restriction (SMR)* and includes techniques and equipment that help to minimize movement of the spine. It most accurately defines the process used in the field because in certain patients, the spine cannot be completely immobilized.

As outlined in the chapter, there is a significant change in the application of spinal motion restriction (SMR) to trauma patients based on recent literature and guidance from trauma leaders. Emergency care providers must skillfully assess the mechanism of injury and the patient to provide a structured assessment and in packaging, treating, and transporting patients with known or potential spinal-cord injuries.

Case Presentation

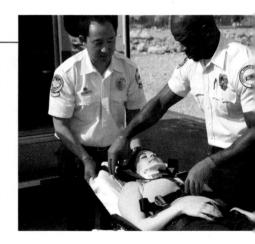

You are a paramedic on the third ambulance dispatched to the scene of a multiple-vehicle collision, involving a truck, a motorcycle, and a sedan. The additional ambulances were requested by the first arriving ambulance. The second arriving ambulance crew is directed to the sedan with several passengers, and the initial crew passes on the following information about the occupants of the sedan to the second crew: The patients are an elderly couple, with the man in the driver's seat alert, talking normally, and complaining of left arm and left ankle pain. Pointing to the motorcycle, he tells you, "He just swerved into me, flew over the hood right into the windshield in front of me. Ripped my side mirror off as he fell past me!" His wife says, "I'm okay. Just take care of my husband and our granddaughter." The crew of the second ambulance finds an infant in a car seat, both of which have been thrown onto the floor. As they carefully lift the seat and baby, the baby begins to cry.

You and your partner are sent to check on the driver of the truck, who is walking around and complaining of a stiff neck. As you approach the truck driver, your partner is asked by the second ambulance crew to help them at the sedan and to check on the female front seat passenger, while the second crew assesses the baby in the back of the car. Your partner notices the damaged windshield on the passenger side of the car and a woman holding the back of her neck.

Before proceeding, consider these questions: Is this a high-risk or low-risk mechanism for spine injury in the truck driver? Are there clues from the scene that help guide you to find possible injuries in the female front-seat passenger? Does the age of the victims influence the assessment for spine injury? What are the indications for active spinal motion restriction? Keep these questions in mind as you read through the chapter. Then, at the end of the chapter, find out how the emergency care providers managed these patients.

Evolution of Spinal Motion Restriction (SMR)

Its Relationship to Patient Safety

Since reports of spine injury began 50 years ago, emergency care providers have performed a highly ritualized immobilization of patients on hard boards, using straps and tape to provide a firm attachment of the patient to the board. This has been done despite research that clearly shows a very low incidence of unstable injuries, the low likelihood of significant complications related to this positioning, and incredible discomfort caused to patients. For certain groups of patients, such as those with penetrating injuries to the torso, immobilization on a long board is associated with higher levels of mortality.

The recognition of the dangers of overimmobilization has resulted in an attempt to identify patients who will benefit from this procedure and the publication of papers that encourage a much more limited use of the procedure with patients at highest risk of an unstable injury that can worsen during emergency treatment and transportation. The document summarizing this advocacy for selective use of immobilization was released jointly at the beginning of 2013 by the American College of Surgeons Committee on Trauma and the National Association of EMS Physicians. Shortly before that text went to press, the American College of Emergency Physicians released their position paper on the topic, strongly recommending SMR be applied only when there is a clinical indication, not simply based on mechanism of injury.

One study was done on an international cohort of patients that shows limited use of spinal motion restriction results in better patient outcomes. Combined with the studies showing higher mortality in patients with penetrating trauma when standard immobilization was done, many emergency care providers have sought to change the process of packaging for trauma patients, particularly related to spinal motion restriction.

EMS systems have modified the injury protocols to reduce the use of spinal motion restriction and to use tools that only restrict the area of the spine at risk for bony or soft-tissue injury. These protocols are based on patient-centered immobilization, for the comfort of the patient, and to reduce the risks of secondary injury from full restriction on a rigid board. In applying the protocols that reduce the use of full spinal motion restriction, emergency care providers must apply the process at a time coordinated among EMS providers, emergency department personnel, and surgeons who participate in the regional systems of trauma care.

Patient-Specific and Appropriate Spinal Motion Restriction

The selective use of spinal motion restriction in prehospital care, with patient-centered immobilization, is based on the following principles.

- Acute spine injuries that are unstable and have not already caused irreversible damage are the primary reason to place a patient on a rigid board. These situations are extraordinarily rare.
- Patients who have spinal-column injuries are more common. The vast majority are already stable due to bony fragments forming an immovable complex, swelling in the surrounding tissues, spasm of nearby muscles, and the patient's own ability to recognize injury and associated pain, particularly with movement.
- Injuries to the spinal column, even if they are unstable, are adequately stabilized with a simple process at the site of the injury and do not require spinal motion restriction of the entire spine

- Spine injury can occur at multiple sites in high-speed and impact mechanisms of injury, particularly if associated with head injury and an altered level of consciousness. Those victims will be most safely extricated and transported with full spinal motion restriction.
- Patients on spine boards report an increase of pain over time on the board. Many patients are at risk for significant and life-threatening complications of spinal motion restriction, including respiratory insufficiency, aspiration, skin breakdown, vomiting, and loss of airway.

Based on the mechanism of trauma, patient-centered immobilization is to be applied using protocols that account for the principles noted earlier.

On arrival at the scene, as information is being gathered, it is appropriate to ask the patient to place and maintain his or her head and neck in a neutral position. Patients with high-velocity or high-impact injuries and those who are unconscious should be placed or maintained in a neutral position and prepared for spinal motion restriction of the entire spine. Failing to prevent a spine injury that causes disability of the patient is among the greatest concerns of emergency care providers. These types of injuries are almost always in patients who are already complaining about pain or loss of function, or who are unconscious.

The patient complaining of pain along the spinal column should be examined and prepared for packaging of the area of the spine that is uncomfortable. Devices that reduce movement during prehospital treatment and transportation should not produce pain and should not distract any injury already present in the spinal column. The use of a comfortably firm, high-friction surface is rational, as is a surface that will dissipate energy during transport and movement. A vacuum mattress or the pad on a stretcher is ideal for this purpose, with straps applied to maintain the patient on the surface should collision or rapid change in direction of the transport vehicle occur. The patient should have his or her airway in a position where it can be protected and where respiratory effort is minimized. For many larger patients, an upright position is the position of choice.

Rigid boards may be very useful to move the patient for short distances away from the emergency scene or in vertical movement of the patient out of a structure. The patient then may be transferred from the rigid board to the stretcher pad or mattress for transportation.

For the many patients who have neck pain related to an injury event, cervical-spine motion restriction with a short board or a cervical immobilization device may be utilized. Vehicle damage can predict those at highest risk for cervical-spine injury and for injuries to the thoracic and lumbar spine and who will need complete spinal motion restriction. Cervical-spine motion restriction can be performed with lateral supports for the head being the most important element of care. A well-fitted anterior neck support will prevent gross flexion of the head should a sudden movement occur.

Cervical collars decrease visible motion of the head and neck and provide immediate feedback to the patient that the emergency care providers want to minimize any gross movements of the cervical spine. The collars do transfer movement to the ends of the device, and in unstable cervical injuries they can cause the injured segments to distract. Tight collars can compromise the airway, increase intracranial pressure, and decrease blood flow to the brain. Therefore, many patients have a collar placed during initial extrication and later removed when the patient is placed on a rigid board with lateral cervical supports.

Lower-risk patients can have cervical motion restriction provided with a collar appropriate for the patient. There are many different collar configurations, divided into one- and two-piece designs, with features that can restrict motion higher or lower on the back, posterior scalp, and chest wall. None of the collar designs have proved to be any more effective in patient-oriented outcomes, so choice of a device should be based on patient comfort. With a collar in place, the patient can be in a position of comfort for further treatment and transport, again without compromising the airway or respiratory effort.

Patients with injuries to the thoracic area of the spine generally have injuries that are mechanically stable and best treated by placing the patient in a position of comfort that allows safe treatment and transportation. These patients may be very uncomfortable when placed on a rigid backboard and, if the victim is elderly, may have skin breakdown in a short period of time.

Patients with lumbar spine injuries can again be placed in a position of comfort on a stretcher pad or mattress and have the pelvis strapped to provide stability during transportation. Patients with isolated low-back injuries often express a preference on how their lower back can be positioned to reduce pain and how they wish to have their legs flexed or extended. Some injured patients will request placement on a rigid board, as long as they have some support to the tissue surfaces of the low back and buttocks.

Multiple studies, including those from the combat zones, have documented the increased mortality of patients with penetrating trauma who have complete spinal immobilization. A number of surgical groups have written statements that support limited spinal motion restriction except for the very rare patient who has a neurologic deficit or wound to the spinal area that is noted on prehospital evaluation. These patients require protocols that prioritize airway protection, optimize ventilation, protect from vomiting and aspiration, and require short prehospital times.

Complete spinal motion restriction is important for the multiple-trauma patient, as well as victims of high-impact and high-velocity events. Unconscious trauma patients have a much higher incidence of spine injury and should be packaged on a long board to prevent movement of the spinal column during initial treatment and transportation. Patients with neurologic deficits should have them assessed carefully to determine if time and immobilization are preventing any further deterioration. If the spine is already deformed, it should be immobilized in the position found.

Summary of Patient-Centered Spinal Motion Restriction

Selective patient spine immobilization protocols have been developed and studied. Recent literature provides even greater support for use of limited spinal motion restriction to improve patient comfort and the outcomes of a larger number of adult and pediatric trauma patients. Children with significant head injuries are very difficult to evaluate in the prehospital environment, and it is wise for EMS providers to immobilize them while maintaining the airway and treating other traumatic injuries.

Not all trauma patients must be treated with complete spinal immobilization during prehospital treatment and transport. Many patients do not have spine injuries and therefore do not require any intervention for spinal motion restriction. All patients who are being transported must be safe during movement in the vehicle, so securing them to an ambulance stretcher is mandatory. Trauma patients must have consideration of airway, respiratory function, and perfusion, and those are priority areas. For the conscious patient, selective immobilization will allow emergency care to be more comfortable for the patient and reduce injuries that result from strapping patients onto rigid boards.

The Normal Spinal Column and Cord
Spinal Column

It is important to differentiate the **spinal column** from the spinal cord. The spinal column is a bony tube composed of 33 vertebrae (Figure 11-1). It supports the body in an upright position, allows the use of our extremities, and protects the delicate spinal cord. The column's 33 vertebrae are identified by their location: 7 cervical

spinal column: the 33 vertebrae that house and protect the spinal cord.

(the C-spine), 12 thoracic (the T-spine), 5 lumbar (the L-spine), and the remainder fused together as the posterior portion of the pelvis (5 sacral and 4 coccygeal). The vertebrae are numbered in each section, from the head down to the pelvis. The third cervical vertebra from the head is designated C3, the sixth is called C6, and so forth. The thoracic vertebrae are T1 through T12, and each attaches to one of the 12 pairs of ribs. The lumbar vertebrae are numbered L1 through L5, with L5 being the last vertebra above the pelvis.

The vertebrae are each separated by a fibrous disc that acts as a shock absorber. The alignment is maintained by strong ligaments between the vertebrae and by muscles that run along the length of the bony column from head to pelvis. (Those are the muscles strained when one lifts improperly.) The spinal column is aligned in a gentle S-curve that is most prominent at the C5–C6 and T12–L1 levels in adults, making those areas the most susceptible to injury.

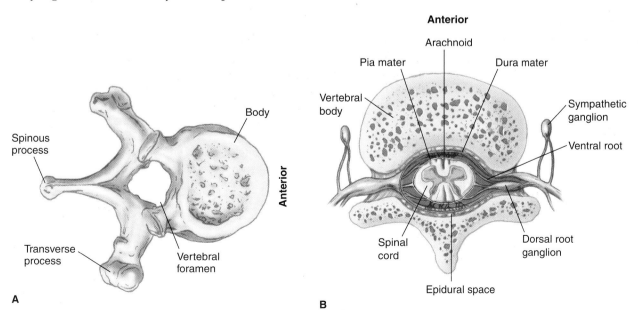

Figure 11-1 Anatomy of the spinal column.

Spinal Cord

The **spinal cord** is an electrical conduit that serves as an extension of the brainstem. It is continuous down to the level of the first lumbar vertebra and at that point separates into nerves. The cord is 10 mm to 13 mm in diameter and is suspended in the middle of the vertebral foramen (Figure 11-2). The cord is soft and flexible like a cotton rope and is surrounded and bathed by cerebrospinal fluid along its entire length. The fluid and the flexibility provide some protection to the cord from injury.

The cord is composed of specific bundles of nerve tracts that are arranged in a predictable manner, much as a rope is composed of individual strands of fiber. The spinal cord passes down the vertebral canal and gives off pairs of nerve roots that exit at each vertebral level (Figure 11-3). The roots lie next to the intervertebral discs and the lateral part of the vertebrae, making the nerve roots susceptible to injury when trauma occurs in these areas (Figure 11-4). The nerve roots carry sensory signals from the body to the spinal cord and then to the brain.

spinal cord: an electrical conduit composed of specific bundles of nerve tracts. It connects the brain to the muscles and organs of the body.

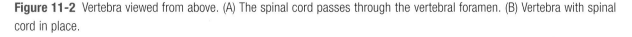

Figure 11-2 Vertebra viewed from above. (A) The spinal cord passes through the vertebral foramen. (B) Vertebra with spinal cord in place.

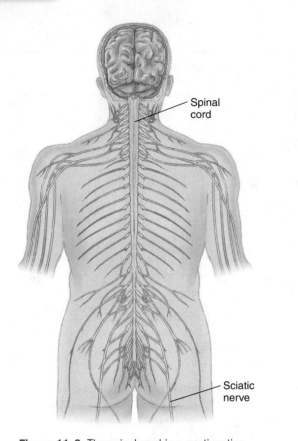

Figure 11-3 The spinal cord is a continuation of the central nervous system outside the skull.

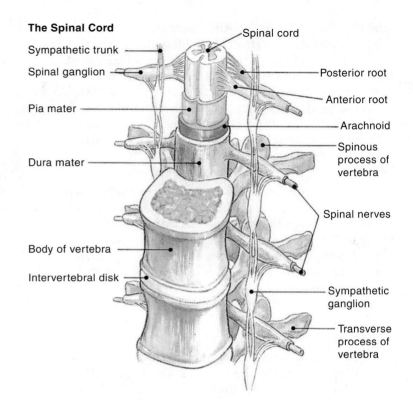

Figure 11-4 Relationship of the spinal cord to the vertebrae. Note how the nerve roots exit between the vertebrae.

The roots also carry signals from the brain to specific muscles, causing them to move. Those signals pass back and forth rapidly, and some are strong enough to cause actions on their own, called reflexes. This reflex system can be demonstrated by tapping the patella tendon below the knee, causing the lower leg to jerk. If you accidentally put your finger on a hot burner, your reflex system causes your hand to move even before your brain receives the warning message. Strong signals also can overwhelm the spinal cord's ability to keep signals moving separately to the brain. This is why a trauma patient with a fractured hip may complain of knee pain or a patient with a ruptured spleen may complain of shoulder pain.

The integrity of spinal-cord function is tested by motor, sensory, and reflex functions. The level of sensory loss is most accurate for predicting the level of spinal-cord injury. Muscle strength is another function that is easy to assess in the conscious patient. Reflexes are helpful for distinguishing complete from partial spinal-cord injuries, but are best left for hospital assessment. The spinal cord is also an integrating center for the autonomic nervous system, which assists in controlling heart rate, blood vessel tone, and blood flow to the skin. Injury to this component of the spinal cord results in neurogenic shock (commonly called spinal shock), which is discussed later.

Spine Injury

A normal healthy spinal column can be severely stressed and maintain its integrity without damage to the spinal cord. However, certain mechanisms of trauma can overcome the protective properties, injuring the spinal column and cord. The most common mechanisms are hyperextension, hyperflexion, compression, and rotation. Less commonly, lateral stress or distraction will injure the cord. Those mechanisms and their subsequent injuries are illustrated in Table 11-1.

Table 11-1: Mechanisms of Blunt Spine injury

Description		Examples
Hyperextension (excessive posterior movement of the head or neck)		Face into windshield in MVC Elderly person falling to the floor Football tackler Dive into shallow water
Hyperflexion (excessive anterior movement of head onto chest)		Rider thrown off horse or motorcycle Dive into shallow water
Compression (weight of head or pelvis driven into stationary neck or torso)		Dive into shallow water Fall of greater than 10 to 20 feet onto head or legs
Rotation (excessive rotation of the torso or head and neck, moving one side of the spinal column against the other)		Rollover MVC Motorcycle crash
Lateral Stress (direct lateral force on spinal column, typically shearing one level of cord from another)		"T-bone" MVC Fall
Distraction (excessive stretching of column and cord)		Hanging Child inappropriately wearing shoulder belt around neck Snowmobile or motorcycle under rope or wire

Mechanisms of Blunt Spinal-Column Injury

The head is a relatively large ball perched on top of the neck. Sudden movement of the head or trunk will produce stresses that can damage the bony or connective tissue components of the spinal column. Injury to the spinal column is similar to injury to any other bone in the body. It requires a significant amount of force, unless there is a pre-existing weakness or defect in the bone. For that reason, the elderly and those with severe arthritis are at higher risk for spine injuries.

Like other bone injuries, pain is the most common symptom, but it may be unnoticed by the patient, especially if the patient has other very painful injuries. At the site of a bone injury, local muscle spasm may occur. Injury to individual nerve roots can result from bony spinal-column injury, with resulting localized pain, paralysis, or sensory loss. Therefore, signs that indicate spine injury include back pain, tenderness along the spinal column, pain with movement of the back, obvious deformity or wounds of the back, paralysis, weakness, or **paresthesia** (tingling or burning feeling to the skin).

Fortunately, spinal-column injury can occur without injuring the spinal cord. In the cervical spine region it is much more common to have cord injury associated with column injury, with almost 40% of column injuries also having cord damage. The converse is also possible, in that cord injuries can occur in the absence of obvious spinal column damage. This is particularly true in children and is referred to as *spinal-cord injury without radiographic abnormality (SCIWORA)*.

Pathophysiology of Spinal-Cord Injury

Spinal-cord injury results in a defective signal-conducting function, presenting as a loss of motor function and reflexes, loss or change in sensation, or neurogenic shock. The delicate structure of the spinal cord's nerve tracts makes it very sensitive to any form of trauma. What is termed **primary spinal-cord injury** occurs at the time of the trauma itself. Primary spinal-cord injury results from the cord being cut, torn, or crushed or by its blood supply being cut off. The damage is usually irreversible despite the best trauma care. **Secondary spinal-cord injury** occurs from poor perfusion, generalized hypoxemia, injury to blood vessels, swelling, compression of the cord from surrounding hemorrhage, or injury to the cord from movement of an unstable spinal column. Emergency efforts are directed at preventing secondary spinal-cord injury through attention to the ABCs, medications, and careful packaging of the patient.

Neurogenic Shock

Injury to the cervical or thoracic spinal cord can produce high-space shock. (See Chapter 8.) Neurogenic shock results from the malfunction of the autonomic nervous system in regulating blood vessel tone and cardiac output. Classically, neurogenic shock in the injured patient results in hypotension, with normal skin color and temperature and an inappropriately slow heart rate in contrast to the tachycardia normally seen with hypovolemic shock.

In the healthy patient, blood pressure is maintained by the controlled release of catecholamines (epinephrine and norepinephrine) from the adrenal glands. Sensors in the aortic and carotid arteries monitor the blood pressure. Catecholamines cause constriction of the blood vessels, increase the heart rate, increase the strength of heart contractions, and stimulate sweat glands. The brain and spinal cord signal the adrenal glands to release catecholamines to keep the blood pressure in the normal range. In pure hemorrhagic shock, those sensors detect the hypovolemic state and compensate by constricting the blood vessels and speeding the heart rate. The high levels of catecholamines cause pale skin, tachycardia, and sweating.

The mechanism of shock from spinal-cord injury is just the opposite. There is no significant blood loss, but the injury to the spinal cord destroys the ability of the brain to regulate the release of catecholamines from the adrenals (no messages reach the adrenals), so no catecholamines are released. When the levels of catecholamines drop, the blood vessels dilate, causing the blood to pool. This drop in preload causes

paresthesia: abnormal sensation; a "tingling" or "burning" sensation.

primary spinal-cord injury: injury to the spinal cord that occurs at the time of the trauma itself. This injury results from the cord being cut, torn, or crushed, or by its blood supply being cut off.

secondary spinal-cord injury: injury to the spinal cord that occurs from hypotension, generalized hypoxia, injury to blood vessels, swelling, compression of the cord from surrounding hemorrhage, or injury to the cord from movement of a damaged and unstable spinal column.

PEARLS
High-Space Shock

Injury to the spinal cord can produce high-space shock, with the patient experiencing hypotension, normal skin color and temperature, and an inappropriately slow heart rate.

the blood pressure to fall. The brain cannot correct this because it cannot get the message to the adrenal glands.

The patient with neurogenic shock cannot show the signs of pale skin, tachycardia, and sweating because the cord injury prevents release of catecholamines. Intra-abdominal injury is difficult to evaluate because the patient with neurogenic shock usually has a spinal-cord injury above the level of the abdomen, so there is no sensation in the abdomen. The multiple-trauma patient may have both neurogenic shock and hemorrhagic shock. Neurogenic shock is a diagnosis of exclusion, after all other potential causes of shock have been ruled out. In the prehospital setting, neurogenic shock is treated in the same way as hemorrhagic shock. (See Chapter 8.)

Assessment of the Trauma Patient
Assessing for Possible Spine Injury

All trauma patients are evaluated in the same manner using the ITLS Primary Survey, of which evaluation of spinal-cord function is a part. Clues to spinal-cord injury are given in Table 11-2. Parts of the neurologic exam are performed during the ITLS Primary Survey, and the remainder of the neurologic exam is performed during the ITLS Secondary Survey. This is frequently done after the patient is loaded into the ambulance.

Focused Evaluation of the Spinal Cord

All unconscious trauma patients should be treated as if they have spine injuries. Conscious and cooperative patients can be assessed for potential spine injury by asking about pain, numbness, unusual sensations, and ability to move. Trauma patients who report new symptoms of weakness or numbness of arms or legs must be

PEARLS
Motor and Sensory Function

Perform brief motor and sensory checks in the upper and lower extremities before and after moving any patient.

Table 11-2: Clues to Spinal-Cord Injury Revealed During Patient Assessment
Mechanism of Injury
Blunt trauma above the clavicle
Diving accident
Motor-vehicle or bicycle crash
Fall
Stabbing or impalement anywhere near the spinal column
Shooting or blast injury to the torso
Any violent injury with forces that could act on the spinal column or cord
Patient Complaints
Neck or back pain
Numbness or tingling
Loss of movement or weakness
Signs Revealed During Assessment
Pain on movement of back or spinal column
Obvious deformity of back or spinal column
Guarding against movement of back
Loss of sensation
Weak or flaccid muscles
Loss of bladder or bowel control
Erection of the penis (priapism)
Neurogenic shock

assumed to have spine injuries and treated as such. The examination of the patient includes these elements:

- *Pain.* The patient may be aware of pain in an area around the spine and of blunt or penetrating injuries near the spine.
- *Numbness.* Emergency care providers should examine the suspected area and report any areas where the patient reports no feeling or where the patient does not feel the emergency care provider touching the area.
- *Tenderness.* Emergency care providers should examine the suspected area and report any associated pain with touching or movement of the area around the spine.
- *Painful movement.* If the patient tries to move the area of potential injury, the pain may increase. In patients with potential spine injuries, it is not necessary for emergency care providers to have the patient move the spinal area.
- *Deformity.* Deformity is rare, although there may be an abnormal bend or bony prominence.
- *Lacerations, holes, or skin wounds such as bruises.* Patients with injuries in the area of the spine may have wounds in the back or abdomen.
- *Paralysis.* The patient is unable to move or hold a part of the body against gravity.

The patient who requires extrication is a special situation. Before beginning extrication, emergency care providers should check sensory and motor function in the hands and feet and document the findings later in the written report. Not only does this pre-extrication neurologic exam give an indication of spine injury, but it also provides documentation on whether or not there was loss of function before extrication. Sadly, there are a few reports of patients who have claimed that their spine injuries were caused by their emergency care providers. In patients who require **Emergency Rescue** and in some of the patients needing **rapid extrication** (see following), there will not be sufficient time to perform a pre-extrication neurologic exam.

The ITLS Primary Survey must be time efficient. If the conscious patient can move his fingers and toes, the motor nerves are intact. Anything less than normal sensation (tingling or decreased sensation) is suspicious for cord injury. The unconscious patient may withdraw from a pinch of the fingers and toes. If so, the patient has demonstrated intact motor and sensory nerves and thus an intact cord. All unconscious trauma patients should be placed in SMR. Flaccid paralysis and no reflexes or withdrawal, even in the unconscious head-injury patient, usually means spinal-cord injury. Document those important findings. (The neurologic exam is described in more detail in Chapters 2 and 10.)

Management of the Trauma Patient
Minimizing Spinal Movement

Two types of situations require modification of the usual SMR. The patient who is in immediate danger of death in a hostile environment or in an immediate life-threatening position in a structure or vehicle may require Emergency Rescue. An example would be the patient who is in a motor-vehicle collision and the auto is on fire. In some cases even a few seconds can mean the difference between life and death, and emergency care providers are justified in saving the patient in any way possible. This is called Emergency Rescue. Any time this manner of rescue is used, document the reason, and notify the staff at the emergency department where the patient is transported.

Some examples of situations that might require emergency rescue are when scene size-up identifies a condition that could immediately endanger you or the patient, such as:

- Fire or immediate danger of fire or explosion
- Hostile environment, gunfire, or the presence of other weapons
- Danger of being carried away by rapidly moving water

Emergency Rescue: the immediate removal, without use of SMR, of a patient from an immediately life-threatening situation.

rapid extrication: the rapid removal of a patient from a dangerous position or situation using modified SMR.

PEARLS
Emergency Rescue

Emergency Rescue is reserved for those situations in which there is immediate (within seconds) environmental threat to the life of the victim and/or emergency care responder. Patients should be moved to a safe area in a manner that places the emergency care responder at the least risk.

Rapid extrication should be considered for patients whose medical conditions or situations require fast intervention (1 or 2 minutes—but not seconds) to prevent death.

- Structure in immediate danger of collapse
- Continuing immediately life-threatening toxic exposure

The second situation that requires modification of usual SMR is for patients whose ITLS Primary Survey indicates a critical degree of ongoing danger that requires an intervention within one or two minutes. Indications for rapid extrication are the following:

- Airway obstruction that cannot be relieved by a modified jaw-thrust maneuver or a finger sweep
- Cardiac or respiratory arrest
- Chest or airway injuries requiring ventilation or assisted ventilation
- Deep shock or bleeding that cannot be controlled

Rapid extrication requires multiple emergency care providers who remove the patient along the long axis of the body, using their hands to minimize movement of the spine. (See skills in Chapter 12.) When the rapid extrication technique is used, the written report should be carefully reviewed to ensure appropriate documentation of the technique and its indication.

The most easily applied and readily available method of cervical motion restriction is with the emergency care provider's hands or knees. Hands should be placed to stabilize the neck in **neutral alignment** to the long axis of the spinal column (Figure 11-5). "Pulling traction" is not a prehospital option, and the term *traction* is not an appropriate description for motion restriction of the spine. Traction usually results in further instability of any spinal-column injury. The correct approach is stabilization, with no pulling on the neck. When packaging the body on a backboard, the neutral in-line position allows the most room for the spinal cord, so that is the optimal position for SMR.

Emergency care providers can place an appropriately sized cervical collar on the patient as airway assessment is being done. The one- or two-piece collars are not definitive devices for restricting cervical-spine motion, but should be used only as a reminder that SMR is necessary and to prevent gross neck movement. The emergency care provider's hands can be removed only when the patient (head and body) has been secured on a backboard with an attached head motion restriction device.

For the conscious patient, having the head and neck in a position of comfort is a good guideline. Adequate strapping must secure the head, torso, and upper legs to the backboard. Inadequate strapping will torque the neck against the body if the patient moves, rolls, or is dropped or rotated.

Placing and strapping a patient on the board effectively eliminates the patient's ability to protect the airway. Once a patient is secured to a rigid board, an emergency care provider must be present and capable of rolling the board if the patient begins to vomit or loses his airway. This rule continues in effect in the emergency department, where an emergency department staff person must assume responsibility for airway protection.

Definitive SMR occurs when the body is strapped securely to the stretcher (or board with cushions, blanket, or towel rolls), maintaining the head, cervical spine, torso, and pelvis in line. Sandbags are not useful in the field for this purpose. When applied properly, such devices allow removal of the front portion of the cervical collar and observation of the neck, as in the patient with open neck wounds.

Some patients (frightened children and patients with altered mental status) will struggle so violently that they defeat any attempts to eliminate movement of the spine. There may be no good solution to this. Always carefully document those situations in which the patient refuses to cooperate with SMR.

Elderly patients whose necks have a natural flexed posture will require posterior padding. This is accomplished with the head pad on a cervical motion restriction device or the padding used with many backboard devices. Because their heads are proportionately larger, children usually require padding under the shoulders to prevent neck flexion on the backboard.

PEARLS
Traction

Do not apply traction to the head and neck. Maintain in-line stabilization of the head, neck, and spine.

neutral alignment: aligning the patient according to the baseline physiologic spinal position.

PEARLS
Protecting the Airway

A patient in spinal motion restriction is at risk for aspiration and other problems. You are responsible for checking and maintaining the airway.

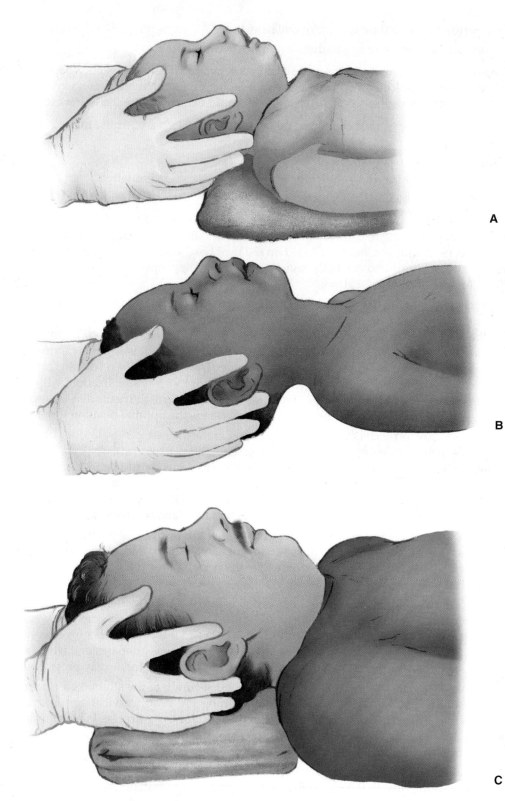

Figure 11-5 Neutral spinal positioning for infant, child, and adult patients. (A) Due to the large heads of younger children, you may need to raise the shoulders with padding. (B) In older children, obtain neutral positioning with shoulders and head on a flat surface. (C) With adults, elevate the head one to two inches.

Spinal Motion Restriction in the Trauma Patient

Spinal motion restriction (SMR) is not indicated in every trauma patient. SMR should be applied appropriately to a patient who has indicators that they may have sustained or are high risk for spine injuries or who cannot be adequately assessed clinically due to an altered level of consciousness. Emergency care providers should apply the appropriate guideline in these situations (see Figure 11-6, Decision Tree, for spinal motion restriction) and apply a cervical collar if needed. Spinal motion restriction is accomplished when the trauma patient is appropriately secured to the rigid backboard, a mattress, or stretcher pad. *SMR can be accomplished without the patient being on a long spine board.*

The long rigid board is primarily an extrication device designed to move a patient to a transport stretcher. Having the patient remain on the board for prolonged periods can produce discomfort, pressure sores, and respiratory compromise. Patients should be removed from the long spine board when it is safe and practical to do so to minimize negative occurrences.

Immobilization onto a long backboard is not indicated in penetrating wounds of torso, neck, or head unless there is clinical evidence of a spine injury.

Research points out that crews should not apply any neck traction or allow the cervical collar or device to purposely, accidentally, or unintentionally extend the neck upward during application, adjustment, or tightening. This is particularly true for severe multiple-trauma patients, who could have very unstable injuries to the spinal column. In those patients, traction would pull the spinal cord apart or worsen an existing injury.

In certain situations, once the patient is packaged onto the backboard, the board and patient might have to be rolled up onto the side (Figure 11-7). Careful strapping can prevent lateral movement of the spine in this situation, but use of the vacuum backboard is far superior. Women who are more than 20 weeks pregnant should always be transported with the backboard tilted 20 to 30 degrees to the patient's left side to keep the uterus off the inferior vena cava.

Patients with airway problems who are not intubated are better transported on their side. This is especially critical when there is uncontrolled bleeding into the airway or if there is massive face or neck trauma. In those situations gravity helps drain fluids out of the airway and could prevent aspiration if the patient vomits. Because of the danger of vomiting and aspiration, unconscious patients who are not intubated should be transported tilted to the side. Once patients are placed on a backboard in SMR, they might not be able to clear their airway should they begin to vomit. Therefore, an emergency care provider should remain with them at all times.

The Log Roll

The log-roll technique is used for moving a patient onto a backboard. It is commonly used because it is easy to perform with a minimum number of emergency care providers. As yet, no technique has been devised that maintains complete spinal immobilization while moving a patient onto a backboard. When properly performed, the log-roll technique minimizes movement of the spinal column as safely and efficiently as any other technique for moving a patient onto the backboard.

The log-roll technique moves the spinal column as a single unit with the head and pelvis. It can be performed on patients lying either prone or supine. Using three or more emergency care providers—controlled by the provider at the patient's head—the patient (with her arms at her side) is rolled onto her uninjured side, a board is slid underneath her, and the patient is rolled faceup onto the board. The log-roll technique is then completed when the patient's chest, pelvis, and head are secured to the board.

The log roll may be modified for patients with painful arm, leg, and chest wounds who need to be rolled onto their uninjured side. The side to which you turn the

Initial Assessment of Spinal Injury
Clinical Criteria

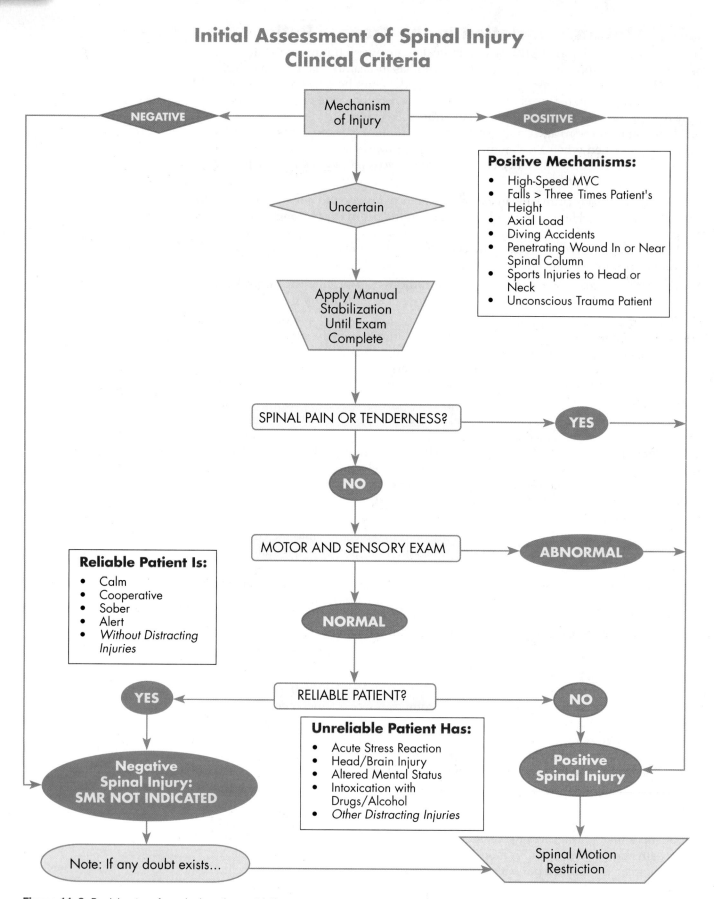

Figure 11-6 Decision tree for spinal motion restriction. *(Reprinted by permission of Peter Goth, MD)*

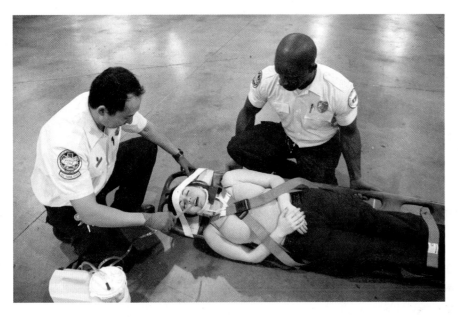

Figure 11-7 Patient on backboard turned on side.

patient during the log-roll procedure is not critical and can be changed in situations in which you can only place the backboard on one side of the patient.

The log-roll technique is useful for most trauma patients, but for patients with an unstable fractured pelvis, rolling their weight onto the pelvis could aggravate the injury. If the pelvic fracture appears stable, the log roll should be carefully performed, turning the patient onto the uninjured side (if it can be identified). Patients with obviously unstable pelvic fractures should not be log rolled, but should be lifted carefully onto a board by four or more emergency care providers. The scoop stretcher also could be used to move patients with unstable pelvic fractures onto the backboard. At least one model of scoop stretcher can be used in place of a backboard.

Spinal Motion Restriction Devices

A wide range of devices that provide SMR for injured patients is available in the marketplace (Figure 11-8). No device has yet been proven to excel over all others, and no device will ever be produced that can be used to provide SMR for all patients. No device is better than the crew using it. Training with the available tools is the most critical factor in providing good patient care.

Complications of Spinal Motion Restriction

There are complications of strapping a patient to a board. The patient will be uncomfortable and will often complain of head and low back pain that is directly related to being strapped onto the hard backboard. The head and airway are in a fixed position, which can produce airway compromise and aspiration if the patient vomits. Obese patients and those with congestive heart failure can suffer life-threatening hypoxia. On a rigid board there is uneven skin pressure that can result in pressure sores. Lifting the patient and the board can cause injuries to rescue personnel. SMR should be applied appropriately to those who will most likely benefit, and it should be avoided if not necessary.

Airway Intervention

When the emergency care provider performs SMR in any manner, the patient loses some of her ability to maintain her own airway. As mentioned earlier, the emergency care provider must then assume this responsibility until the patient has a controlled airway or has the spinal column cleared in the emergency department and is released

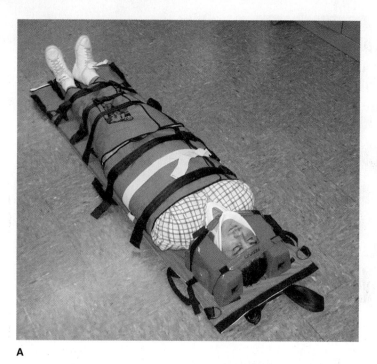

A

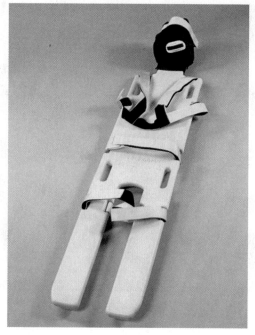

B

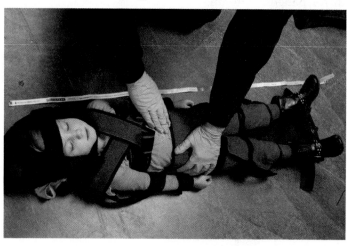

C

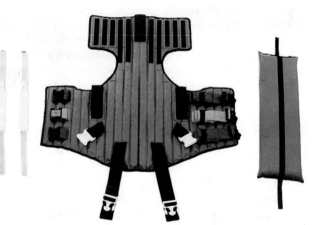

D

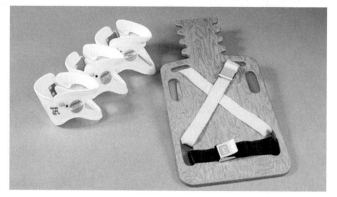

E

Figure 11-8 (A) Reeves™ sleeve; (B) Miller body splint; (C) pediatric SMR device; (D) Kendrick extrication device; and (E) short backboard.

from the motion-restricting equipment (Figure 11-9). This is particularly critical in children, who have a greater potential for vomiting and aspiration after a traumatic injury.

Airway manipulation in the trauma patient requires careful application. Current research indicates that any airway intervention will cause some movement of the spinal column, but it is likely that movement will not worsen any injury that is present. Obtaining and controlling an airway is clearly a priority compared to the small risk of a spine injury. In-line manual stabilization is the most effective manner for minimizing this movement.

Nasotracheal and orotracheal intubations or a cricothyrotomy all induce some bony movement. The ITLS Primary Survey should include manual stabilization followed by the use of the airway control method you are most skilled at performing. When weighing the risks and benefits of each airway procedure, recall that the risk of dying with an uncontrolled airway is greater than the risk of inducing spinal-cord damage using a careful approach to intubation.

Special Spinal Motion Restriction Situations

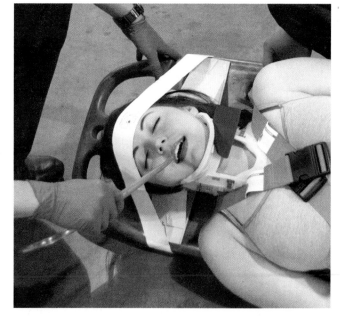

Figure 11-9 Suctioning of airway while secured on a backboard.

Emergency care providers must stabilize the spinal column of all patients who sustain major trauma. In some patients (see following), traditional techniques must be modified to provide safe and effective SMR.

Closed-Space Rescues

Closed-space rescues are performed in a manner appropriate for the clinical condition of the patient. The only general rules that can be applied to these rescues are to prevent gross spinal movement and to move patients in line with the long axis of the body (Figure 11-10). Safety of the emergency care provider is of prime importance in

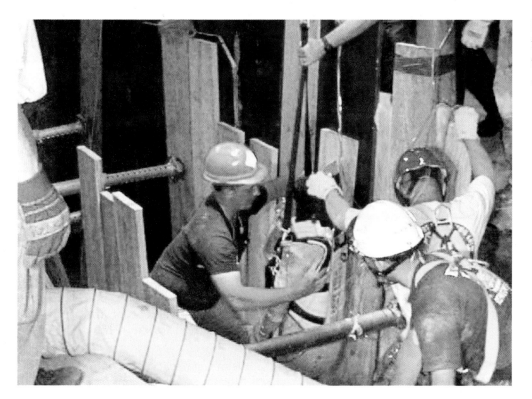

Figure 11-10 Patient entrapped in trench cave-in being lifted out along the long axis of the body. *(Photo courtesy of Roy Alson, MD)*

all closed-space rescues. Asphyxia, toxic gases, and structure collapse are dangers of closed-space rescue and may require the use of Emergency Rescue. Emergency care providers should never enter a closed space unless properly trained, equipped (air pack, safety line, and so on), and sure of scene safety.

Water Emergencies

Water rescues are performed by moving the patient in line, thereby preventing gross spinal movement. When the emergency care providers are in a stable position for performing SMR, the backboard is floated under the patient, and the patient is then secured and removed from the water (Scan 11-1). Safety of both emergency care providers and patients is of paramount importance. Emergency care providers should not attempt to rescue victims in hazardous situations such as deep or swift water.

Prone, Seated, and Standing Patients

Prone, seated, and standing patients are stabilized in a manner that minimizes spinal column movement, ending with the patient in the conventional supine position. (See Chapter 12 for techniques.)

- Prone patients are either log rolled onto a backboard, with careful coordination between the emergency care providers performing it, or moved using a scoop stretcher
- Seated patients may be stabilized using short backboards if they have an indication for SMR. Used appropriately, short backboards can provide initial stabilization of the cervical and thoracic spine and can be used to transfer the patient onto a long backboard for transfer to the transport stretcher or directly to the transport stretcher
- Standing patients will rarely need to be placed on a spine board, especially if they are ambulatory on the scene. If a standing patient has an indication for SMR, he or she may be placed against the long board while upright and secured. The board is then gently lowered to the supine position. The patient is then moved to the transport stretcher and then removed from the long spine board.

Pediatric Patients

It is best to provide initial SMR of the pediatric patient with the emergency care provider's hands, and then use cushions or towel rolls to help secure the child on an appropriate board or device. Some pediatric trauma specialists suggest padding beneath the back and shoulders on the board in a child under the age of 3 years. (See Figures 11-5 and 11-11.) Those children normally have a relatively large head that flexes the neck when placed on a straight board. Padding under the back and shoulders will prevent this flexion and also make the child more comfortable.

Children who are involved in a motor-vehicle collision while restrained in a child safety seat but have no apparent injuries may be packaged in the safety seat for transport to the hospital. If there is a consideration of spine injuries, which would be very rare, emergency care providers can use towel or blanket rolls to secure the child in the safety seat and then belt the seat into the ambulance (Figure 11-12). The technique minimizes movement of the child and provides a secure method for child transport in the ambulance.

When the child is in a car seat that is damaged, or in a built-in child-restraint seat that cannot be removed,

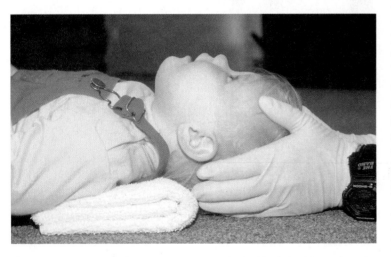

Figure 11-11 Most children require padding under back and shoulders to keep the cervical spine in a neutral position. *(Photo courtesy of Bob Page, MEd, NRP, CCP, NCEE)*

SCAN 11-1 Water Rescue

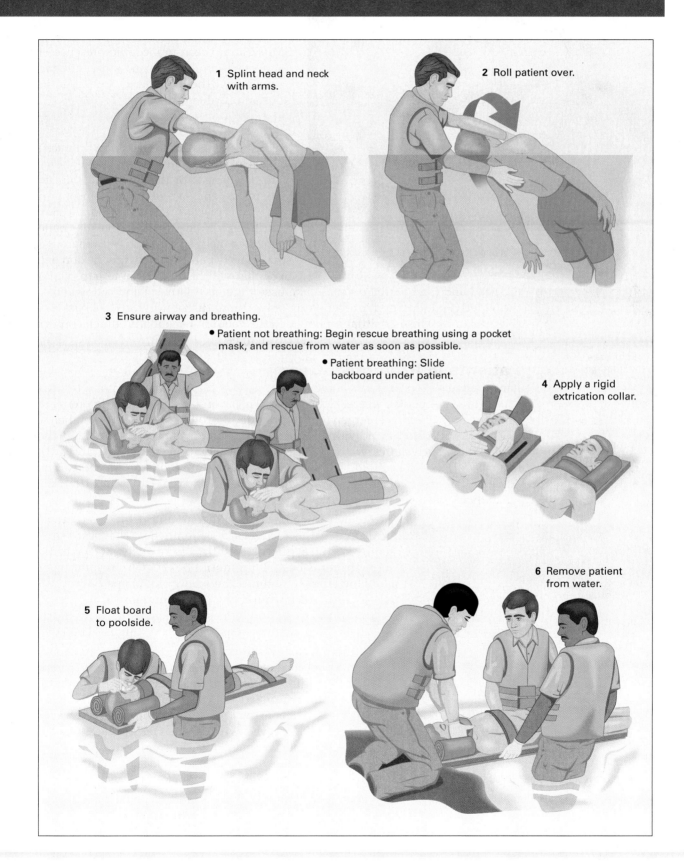

1 Splint head and neck with arms.

2 Roll patient over.

3 Ensure airway and breathing.

• Patient not breathing: Begin rescue breathing using a pocket mask, and rescue from water as soon as possible.

• Patient breathing: Slide backboard under patient.

4 Apply a rigid extrication collar.

5 Float board to poolside.

6 Remove patient from water.

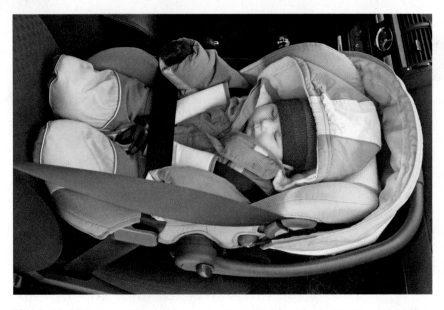

Figure 11-12 Infant secured in car seat. *(Photo courtesy of Andrey Kekyalyaynen/Alamy)*

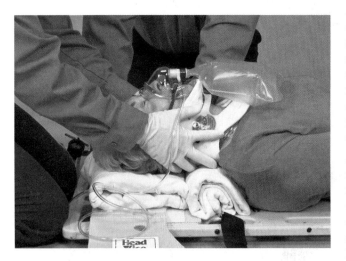

Figure 11-13 Additional padding, such as rolled blankets or towels behind the head, may be needed to keep the head in a neutral, in-line position.

the child must be removed for SMR. Children in such situations will have to be carefully extricated onto a backboard or another pediatric SMR device, using manual stabilization. For the child who is frightened and struggling, there may be no good way to obtain SMR. Careful reassurance, the presence of a comforting family member, and gentle management will help prevent more complications and further struggling.

Elderly Patients

Elderly patients require flexibility in packaging techniques. Many elderly patients have arthritic changes of the spine and thin, frail skin. Such patients will be very uncomfortable when placed on a backboard. Some arthritic spines are so rigid that the patient cannot be laid straight on the board, and some elderly patients have rigid flexion of the neck that will result in a large gap between the head and the board. You can make use of towels, blankets, and pillows to pad the elderly patient and prevent movement and discomfort on the backboard (Figure 11-13). This is a situation in which the vacuum backboard (which conforms to the shape of the patient) works very well. (See Figure 11-7.)

Patients in Protective Gear

Large helmets used in sports and cycling must be removed at some point to permit complete assessment and care. Helmets used in various sports present different management problems for emergency care providers. Football and ice hockey helmets are custom fitted to the individual. When special circumstances exist in the prehospital setting, such as respiratory distress or an inability to access the airway, the helmet will need to be removed. The 2015 updated guidelines from the National Athletic Trainers Association recommend helmet and pad removal prior to transport, when there is a suspected unstable spine injury.

Athletic helmet design will generally allow easy airway access once the face guard is removed. The best way to remove a face guard is with a screwdriver. (A cordless screwdriver is best.) One should be on every response vehicle. However, sometimes the screw slot strips out, and the face guard will have to be cut off. Commercial devices can do this, but cost 10 to 20 times as much as plain anvil pruning shears, which are just as satisfactory (Figure 11-14).

The athlete wearing shoulder pads usually has his neck in a neutral position when on the backboard with the helmet in place. If the helmet is removed, padding must be inserted under the head to keep the neck from extending (Figure 11-15). After arrival at the emergency facility, the cervical spine can be x-rayed with the helmet in place. Once the spine is evaluated, the helmet can be removed by stabilizing head and neck, removing cheek pads, releasing the air inflation system, and then sliding the helmet off in the usual manner.

For emergency care providers, field removal of an athletic helmet is best performed in coordination with the athletic

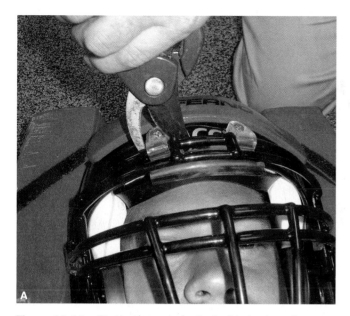

Figure 11-14a The face guard of a football helmet can be removed with a screwdriver or pruning shears. *(Photo courtesy of Jeff Hinshaw, MS, PA-C, NREMT-P)*

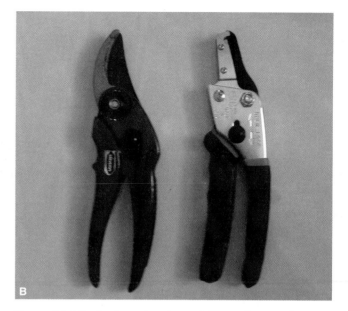

Figure 11-14b Anvil pruning shears (left) or a face mask extractor (right) can be used to remove a football helmet face guard. *(Photo courtesy of Jeff Hinshaw, MS, PA-C, NREMT-P)*

trainer and should be considered in certain patient care situations. Recently released guidelines from the National Athletic Trainers Association recommend helmet and pad removal prior to transport, when there is a suspected unstable spine injury. The four main reasons to consider field athletic helmet removal are

- Face mask cannot be removed in a timely fashion
- Airway cannot be controlled due to the design of the helmet and chin strap
- Helmet and chin straps do not hold the head securely
- Helmet prevents stabilization for transport in an appropriate position

When removing an athletic helmet, it is imperative to cut the chin strap and not attempt to unsnap or unbuckle the device.

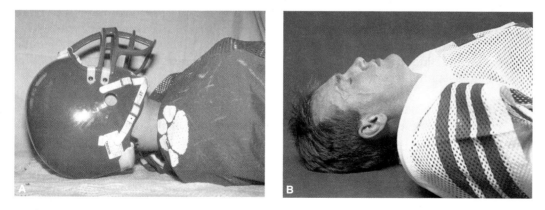

Figure 11-15 (A) Patients with shoulder pads and helmets are usually best immobilized with the helmet in place. The spine is maintained in a neutral position with a minimum of movement. *(Photo courtesy of Bob Page, MEd, NRP, CCP, NCEE)* (B) Patients with shoulder pads must have padding under the head to maintain a neutral position if the helmet is removed.

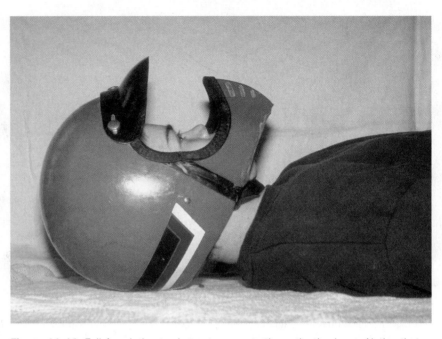

Figure 11-16 Full-face helmets obstruct access to the patient's airway. Notice that the helmet flexes the neck in a patient who is not wearing shoulder pads. *(Photo courtesy of Bob Page, MEd, NRP, CCP, NCEE)*

Football shoulder pad removal is often linked to helmet removal in the athletic setting. Not only is this done routinely with helmet removal, but it is also done when faced with the inability to maintain neutral cervical-spine alignment (often due to ill-fitting shoulder pads), when you are unable to secure the athlete to the stretcher or spine board, and when you need access to the chest for resuscitation efforts. Most shoulder pads can be removed by cutting the axillary straps and the laces on the front of the appliance, opening the appliance from the core outward (like a clam shell), and sliding the appliance out from under the athlete.

In contrast, motorcycle helmets are usually removed in the prehospital setting. The removal technique is modified to accommodate the different designs. Motorcycle helmets often are designed with a continuous solid face guard that limits airway access. Those helmets are not custom designed and frequently are poorly fitted to the patient. Their large size will usually produce significant neck flexion if left in place when the patient is positioned on a backboard (Figure 11-16). The motorcycle helmet can make it difficult to stabilize the neck in a neutral position, obstruct access to the airway, and hide injuries to the head or neck. It should be removed in the prehospital setting, using the techniques described in Chapter 12.

Very Large or Obese Patients

Very large or obese patients might not fit appropriately in standard equipment. EMS systems should have available appropriate equipment to care for the bariatric patient. In the absence of such resources, emergency care providers may improvise, such as using sheets of plywood with head cushions or towel rolls to stabilize the spine. This should be done with caution because the weight capacity and safety of such improvised equipment may not be known.

Any immobilized large patient should have the head elevated to prevent respiratory compromise. Larger patients who do not have spine injuries should be transported in an upright position, which is typically the position of comfort. In cold climates, patients in bulky warm clothing will need to be snugly secured to prevent excessive movement.

Patients with Neck Wounds

Patients with penetrating and disfiguring wounds of the neck or lower face must be continually observed, particularly for airway loss. Cervical collars should not be used because they will prevent continued examination of the wound site and could compromise the airway in wounds with expanding hematomas or subcutaneous air. If the mandible is fractured, the collar might again cause airway compromise. Therefore, for patients with such injuries, it may be wise to avoid collars and use instead manual stabilization and head cushion devices or blanket rolls for cervical motion restriction, if clinically indicated.

Case Presentation (continued)

You are on the third ALS ambulance dispatched to a multiple-vehicle collision. The first arriving unit has transported the motorcyclist. You are asked to check on the driver of the overturned truck, who extricated himself and is standing, talking to a police officer.

All emergency care providers have donned personal protective equipment (PPE). The Fire Department has informed you that all hazards are controlled. You approach the truck driver from his front and ask him not to move his head. You note that he is ambulatory and says he is alright. He says his neck is stiff. Because he is speaking, answering questions, and walking, you conclude that his primary survey is intact. He has no pain on palpation of his cervical spine or the paraspinal muscles, and he has been ranging his neck without problems before you reached him to start your assessment. At this point you conclude he does not require spinal motion restriction, and you begin your secondary assessment, which is remarkable only for some abrasions. At this point the driver states he does not wish to go to the hospital, and you begin to discuss refusal of care with him.

Your partner, who has been assessing the female patient in the front passenger seat of the sedan, now asks you to help. She has a damaged windshield in front of her. Your partner has placed her in manual spinal motion restriction. She reports some tingling in her arms. She speaks in full sentences, denies shortness of breath or chest pain. No reported loss of consciousness. Primary survey shows intact airway and no evidence of chest or abdominal

trauma. Secondary survey shows a contusion on top of her head. She has tenderness to palpation of the midportion of her cervical spine. No focal neurologic deficits except for tingling in both her arms and weakness of her grips compared to lower extremity strength. Vital signs are pulse of 75, blood pressure is 166/96, and her respirations are 14. Her pupils are equal and reactive.

Given the mechanism of injury and the exam findings, this patient is at risk for a significant spine injury, and you and your partner decide to place her into spinal motion restriction. A correctly sized cervical collar is applied, and with the assistance of the fire department she is placed onto a long spine board for extrication from the vehicle and onto the ambulance stretcher. Once in the ambulance, given the short distance to the trauma center, it is decided not to remove her from the long spine board and to secure her to the ambulance stretcher. While performing the log roll (as described in Chapter 12), the remainder of her spine is palpated, and no tenderness is noted. She is placed on a nasal cannula. Reassessment en route remains unchanged.

Subsequently, evaluation at the trauma center showed spinal-cord contusion upon MRI but no fractures of the spinal column. She recovered from her injury uneventfully.

Because the child, who was in a child seat was thrown to the floor, there is a risk for injury. The discussion of the management of this child is at the end of the pediatric trauma chapter.

Summary

Spinal-cord injury is a devastating consequence of trauma. Patient-centered care allows emergency care responders to use appropriate methods to provide spinal motion restriction to persons at risk for a spine injury. Unstable or incomplete damage to the spinal column or cord is not completely predictable. Therefore, trauma patients who are unconscious or who have any dangerous mechanism of injury affecting the head, neck, or trunk should have SMR. Less severely injured and cooperative patients can be packaged and transported with less-restrictive devices, such as a cervical collar. Special trauma cases may require special spinal motion restriction (SMR) techniques. Once SMR is performed, the patient loses some ability to control his airway, so EMS providers must be prepared at all times to intervene should the patient become compromised.

Bibliography

ACEP Board of Directors. "EMS Management of Patients with Potential Spinal Injury," Practice Management Policy Statement adopted January, 2015. Accessed March 1, 2015, at http://www.acep.org/Physician-Resources/Policies/Policy-Statements/EMS-Management-of-Patients-with-Potential-Spinal-Injury

Anderson, R. C., P. Kan, M. Vanaman, J. Rubsam, K. W. Hansen, E. R. Scaife, and D. L. Brockmeyer. "Utility of a Cervical Spine Clearance Protocol After Trauma in Children Between 0 and 3 Years of Age." *Journal of Neurosurgery Pediatrics* 5, no. 3 (March 2010): 292–96.

Augustine, J. "Failure on the Board." *Emergency Medical Services* 33, no. 5 (2004): 52–53.

Ben-Galim, P., N. Dreiangel, K. L. Mattox, C. A. Reitman, S. B. Kalantar, and J. A. Hipp. "Extrication Collars Can Result in Abnormal Separation Between Vertebrae in the Presence of a Dissociative Injury." *Journal of Trauma and Acute Care Surgery* 88, no. 1 (August 2010): 447–50.

Bernhard, M., A. Gries, P. Kremer, and B. W. Böttiger. "Spinal Cord Injury (SCI): Prehospital Management." *Resuscitation* 66, no. 2 (August 2005): 127–39.

Burton, J. H., M. G. Dunn, N. R. Harmon, T. A. Hermanson, and J. R. Bradshaw. "A Statewide Prehospital Emergency Medical Service Selective Patient Spine Immobilization Protocol." *Journal of Trauma* 61, no. 1 (July 2006): 161–67.

Cordell, W. H., J. C. Hollingsworth, M. L. Olinger, S. J. Stroman, and D. R. Nelson. "Pain and Tissue-Interface Pressures During Spine-Board Immobilization." *Annals of Emergency Medicine* 26, no. 1 (July 1995): 31–36.

DeVivo, M. J. "Epidemiology of Traumatic Spinal Cord Injury." In *Spinal Cord Medicine,* edited by S. Kirshblum D. I. Campagnolo, and J. A. DeLisa, 69–81. Baltimore, MD: Lippincott Williams & Wilkins, 2002.

DeVivo, M. J., B. K. Go, and A. B. Jackson. "Overview of the National Spinal Cord Injury Statistical Center Database." *Journal of Spinal Cord Medicine* 25, no. 4 (Winter 2002): 335–38.

Domeier, R. M., R. A. Swor, R. W. Evans, J. B. Hancock, W. Fales, J. Krohmer, S. M. Frederiksen, E. J. Rivera-Rivera, and M. A. Schork. "Multicenter Prospective Validation of Prehospital Clinical Spinal Clearance Criteria." *Journal of Trauma* 53, no. 4 (October 2002): 744–50.

Dunn, T. M., A. Dalton, T. Dorfman, and W. W. Dunn. "Are Emergency Medical Technician–Basics Able to Use a Selective Immobilization of the Cervical Spine Protocol? A Preliminary Report." *Prehospital Emergency Care* 8, no. 2 (April–June 2004): 207–11.

Ehrlich, P. F., C. Wee, R. Drongowski, and A. R. Rana. "Canadian C-Spine Rule and the National Emergency X-Radiography Utilization Low-Risk Criteria for C-Spine Radiography in Young Trauma Patients." *Journal of Pediatric Surgery* 44, no. 5 (May 2009): 987–91.

Farrington, J. D. "Death in a Ditch." *Bulletin of the American College of Surgeons* 52, no. 3 (1967): 121.

Farrington, J. D. "Extrication of Victims: Surgical Principles." *Journal of Trauma* 8, no. 4 (1968): 493–512.

Garton, H. J., and M. R. Hammer. "Detection of Pediatric Cervical Spine Injury." *Neurosurgery* 62, no. 3 (March 2008): 700–708.

Hauswald, M., G. Ong, D. Tandberg, and Z. Omar. "Out-of-Hospital Spinal Immobilization: Its Effect on Neurological Injury." *Academic Emergency Medicine* 5, no. 3 (March 1998): 214–19.

Hauswald, M. "A Re-conceptualization of Acute Spinal Care." *Emergency Medicine Journal* 30, no. 9 (September 2013): 720–23.

Haut, E. R., B. T. Kalish, D. T. Efron, A. H. Haider, K. A. Stevens, A. N. Kieninger, E. E. Cornwell 3rd, and D. C. Chang. "Spine Immobilization in Penetrating Trauma: More Harm Than Good?" *Journal of Trauma* 68, no. 1 (January 2010): 115–21.

Hoffman, J. R., W. R. Mower, A. B. Wolfson, K. H. Todd, and M. I. Zucker. "Validity of a Set of Clinical Criteria to Rule Out Injury to the Cervical Spine in Patients with Blunt Trauma: National Emergency X-Radiography Utilization Study Group." *New England Journal of Medicine* 343, no. 2 (July 13, 2000): 94–99.

Hutchings, L., O. Atijosan, C. Burgess, and K. Willett. "Developing a Spinal Clearance Protocol for Unconscious Pediatric Trauma Patients." *Journal of Trauma* 67, no. 4 (October 2009): 681–86.

Katz, J. S., C. O. Oluigbo, C. C. Wilkinson, S. McNatt, and M. H. Handler. "Prevalence of Cervical Spine Injury in Infants with Head Trauma." *Journal of Neurosurgery Pediatrics* 5, no. 5 (May 2010): 470–73.

Kossuth, L. C. "The Removal of Injured Personnel from Wrecked Vehicles." *Journal of Trauma* 5, no. 6 (1965): 703–8.

Kossuth, L. C. "The Initial Movement of the Injured." *Military Medicine* 132, no. 1 (1967): 18–21.

Krell, J. M., M. S. McCoy, P. J. Sparto, G. L. Fisher, W. A. Stoy, and D. P. Hostler. "Comparison of the Ferno Scoop Stretcher with the Long Backboard for Spinal Immobilization." *Prehospital Emergency Care* 10, no. 1 (January–March 2006): 46–51.

Kwan, I., and F. Bunn. "Effects of Prehospital Spinal Immobilization: A Systematic Review of Randomized Trials on Healthy Subjects." *Prehospital and Disaster Medicine* 20, no. 1 (January–February 2005): 47–53.

Kwan, I., F. Bunn, and I. G. Roberts. "Spinal Immobilisation for Trauma Patients (Review)." *Cochrane Library* (2008): 1–19.

Manoach, S., and L. Paladino. "Manual In-Line Stabilization for Acute Airway Management of Suspected Cervical Spine Injury: Historical Review and Current Questions." *Annals of Emergency Medicine* 50, no. 3 (September 2007): 236–45.

Milby, A. H., C. H. Halpern, W. Guo, and S. C. Stein. "Prevalence of Cervical Spinal Injury in Trauma." *Neurosurgical Focus* 25, no. 5 (2008): E10.

National Athletic Trainers Association. "Executive Summary: Appropriate Care of the Spine Injured Athlete." Available on the NATA Web site. Last reviewed June 28, 2015. Accessed July 18, 2015, at http://www.nata.org/access-read/public/cosensus-statements

National Association of EMS Physicians and the American College of Surgeons Committee on Trauma. "EMS Spinal Precautions and the Use of the Long Backboard." *Prehospital Emergency Care* 17, no. 3 (July–September 2013): 392–93.

Pieretti-Vanmarcke, R., G. C. Velmahos, M. L. Nance, S. Islam, R. A. Falcone Jr., P. W. Wales, et al. "Clinical Clearance of the Cervical Spine in Blunt Trauma Patients Younger than 3 Years: A Multi-Center Study of the American Association for the Surgery of Trauma." *Journal of Trauma* 67 no. 3 (September 2009): 543–50.

Rhee, P., E. J. Kuncir, L. Johnson, C. Brown, G. Velmahos, M. Martin, D. Wang, A. Salim, J. Doucet, S. Kennedy, and D. Demetriades. "Cervical Spine Injury Is Highly Dependent on the Mechanism of Injury Following Blunt and Penetrating Assault." *Journal of Trauma* 61, no. 5 (November 2006): 1166–70.

Sochor, M., S. Althoff, D. Bose, R. Maio, and P. Deflorio. "Glass Intact Assures Safe Cervical Spine Protocol." *Journal of Emergency Medicine* 44, no. 3 (March 2013): 631–36.

Stroh, G., and D. Braude. "Can an Out-of-Hospital Cervical Spine Clearance Protocol Identify All Patients with Injuries? An Argument for Selective Immobilization." *Annals of Emergency Medicine* 37, no. 6 (June 2001): 609–15.

Theodore, N., M. N. Hadley, B. Aarabi, S. S. Dhall, D. E. Gelb, R. J. Hurlbert, C. J. Rozzelle, T. C. Ryken, and B. C. Walters. "Prehospital Cervical Spinal Immobilization After Trauma." *Neurosurgery* 72, no. 3, Suppl. 2 (March 2013): 22–34.

Theodore, N., B. Aarabi, S. S. Dhall, D. E. Gelb, R. J. Hurlbert, C. J. Rozzelle, T. C. Ryken, B. C. Walters, and M. N. Hadley. "Transportation of Patients with Acute Traumatic Cervical Spine Injuries." *Neurosurgery* 72 no. 3, Suppl. 2 (March 2013): 35–39.

Vanderlan, W. B., B. E. Tew, and N. E. McSwain, Jr. "Increased Risk of Death with Cervical Spine Immobilisation in Penetrating Cervical Trauma." *Injury* 40, no. 8 (August 2009): 880–83.

Get more information about this course by calling
ITLS International at 888-495-4875
(outside the United States call +1-630-495-6442) or visit

www.itrauma.org

Spine Management Skills

S. Robert Seitz, MEd, RN, NRP
Darby L. Copeland, EdD, RN, NRP

Trauma Spinale

Urazy kręgosłupa

إصابات العمود الفقري

Gerincsérülés

Traumatismo Raquídeo

Wirbelsäulentrauma

trauma kičme

Traumatisme Médullaire

Ozljede kralježnice

Poškodbe hrbtenjače

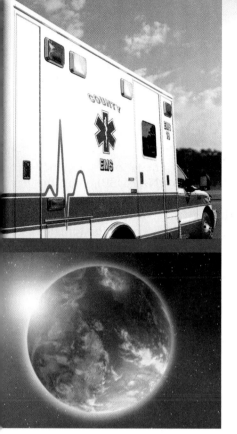

(Ambulance photo courtesy of Cheryl Casey,
Shutterstock.com)

Objectives

Upon successful completion of this chapter, you should be able to:

1. Describe the essential components of a spinal motion-restriction (SMR) system.
2. Describe the goals and principles of SMR.
3. Explain when to use SMR.
4. Explain when to perform an Emergency Rescue and a rapid extrication.
5. Perform SMR with a short extrication device.
6. Log roll a patient onto a long backboard.
7. Properly secure a patient to a long backboard.
8. Transfer a patient using a scoop stretcher
9. Stabilize a patient's head and neck when a neutral position cannot be safely attained.
10. Perform a rapid extrication.
11. Explain when helmets should and should not be removed from injured patients.
12. Properly remove a motorcycle helmet.

Essential Components of a Spinal Motion Restriction System

All trauma patients are evaluated in the same manner, using the ITLS Primary Survey, which includes a brief neurologic assessment. Traditionally, the prehospital management of trauma patients has equated the use of a long backboard with the provision of SMR. Studies suggest that not all trauma patients must be treated with spinal motion restriction and that every patient does not need to be strapped onto a rigid backboard.

In addition, the published positions of the American College of Emergency Physicians, the National Association of EMS Physicians (NAEMSP), and the American College of Surgeons (ACS) agree that the benefit of long backboard immobilization is largely unproven, and its utilization during transport should be judicious so that the potential benefits outweigh the risks. Based on current literature, the Faculty of Prehospital Care of the Royal College of Surgeons of Edinburgh (UK) consensus group also published two consensus statements related to SMR that are in alignment with the preceding positions.

Given that the backboard is primarily used as a transfer device, patients who are placed on a backboard or other rigid device should be removed as expeditiously as possible. When the backboard is used as part of an SMR procedure, it along with other components serve to restrict body movement. The additional essential components necessary to perform full spinal motion restriction (SMR) system are

- *Cervical collar.* Though cervical collars do not immobilize the neck, they provide some support and can serve to remind the patient to keep the neck still. Several types are available.
- *Straps.* Strapping systems are used to secure the patient's body to the backboard to restrict movement of the spinal column. The straps should be positioned to decrease patient movement from side to side and from sliding up and down on the backboard. Several different systems are available.
- *Head motion-restriction device.* These devices attach to the backboard and are used to restrict movement of the patient's head after the patient's body has been strapped to the backboard. When the head motion-restriction device has been applied, the cervical collar may be removed if necessary. There are several different types of the devices.
- *Airway management kit.* When you strap someone's body and head to a board, you must assume responsibility for his or her airway. You must have the airway kit immediately available, and you must have the skills to use it. Airway management is a priority consideration with SMR. So, airway management skills and equipment are necessary components.

Principles of SMR

The goal of spinal motion restriction (SMR) is to reduce or prevent secondary injury to the spine during transport. SMR should be applied appropriately to those patients who may have sustained or are at high risk for spine injuries and cannot be adequately assessed clinically for the presence of such injuries. Where indicated, maintenance of in-line spinal alignment when moving the patient and appropriately securing him or her to the transport stretcher remains a critical component of spinal motion restriction.

Patients whose cervical spine has been cleared by a physician or advanced practice clinician in the emergency department or who do not meet SMR requirements and are being transferred between facilities for additional care do not need to be placed or remain on a long backboard during the transfer. If it is necessary to remove a patient from a long backboard, either the traditional log roll or lift-and-slide technique should be used. The decision to utilize one method opposed to the other should be made based on the situation and with guidance from your local medical direction. Note that current research suggests the lift-and-slide technique reduces the motion between C5 and C6. Perform these moves as follows (Scan 12-1):

- *Log roll.* One team member manually maintains the cervical spine while one at the shoulders, one at the hips, and one at the legs log roll the patient 90 degrees. Once the patient is on his or her side, the backboard is slid away to the side of the patient. The patient is then log rolled back to the supine position.

- *Lift-and-slide technique.* One team member manually maintains the cervical spine, while additional team members align on both sides of the long backboard at the shoulders, hips, and legs and lift the patient four inches. While the patient is lifted, another team member slides the backboard out from the foot end of the patient. The patient is then slowly lowered to a supine position.

SCAN 12-1 Patient Removal from Backboard

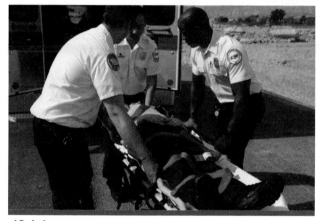

12-1-1 Utilize the appropriate number of resources to ensure patient safety. Lock the stretcher in place, and position the backboard slightly to the left or right side of the stretcher.

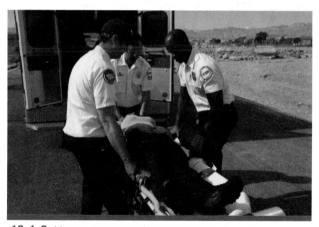

12-1-2 Have a team member manage the head in a neutral position and unstrap the patient from the backboard.

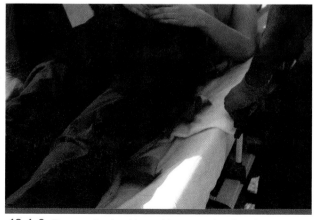

12-1-3 Prepare the backboard by removing the straps or securing them under the backboard.

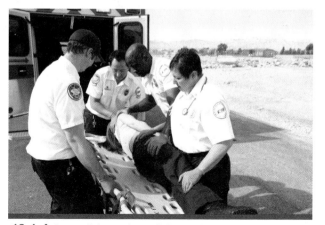

12-1-4 Log roll the patient off the backboard onto the stretcher. Inspect the patient's posterior surface as needed during transfer to the stretcher.

(continued)

SCAN 12-1 Patient Removal from Backboard (*continued*)

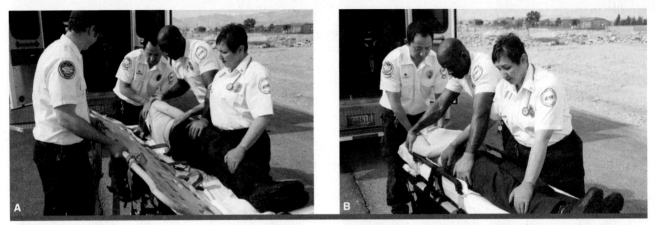

12-1-5 (A) Remove the backboard from under the patient and (B) roll the patient back onto the center of the stretcher.

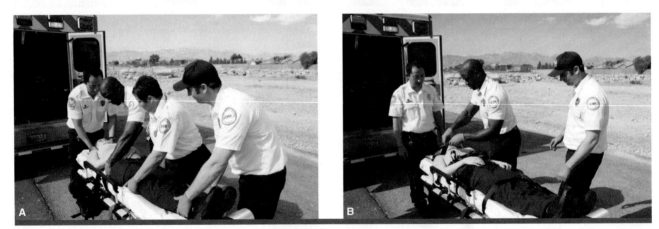

12-1-6 (A) Reposition the patient as needed and (B) secure him or her to stretcher.

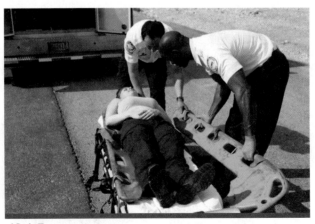

12-1-7 When limited resources exist, the use of a scoop stretcher may be the preferred method of transferring the patient to the stretcher.

The principles of SMR are

- SMR should be applied only to those patients in whom there are clinical indicators or in whom it is not possible to assess for spine injury and have a high risk mechanism of injury (see following).
- Stabilization of the spine must be done so the patient is in the anatomical (neutral) position. Padding is frequently required to achieve this position.
- Straps should be placed over stable bony structures. Avoid placing straps over the neck, navel, and knees.
- Patients placed in SMR are at risk for airway problems and should be monitored by an emergency care provider at all times.

Applying the principles of SMR helps the emergency care provider adapt to the various situations in which patients are found. Understand that SMR precautions are taken to minimize the potential of secondary trauma during the prehospital phase of a patient encounter. Though SMR decreases the patient's risk for such injury, studies have demonstrated that prolonged time on a long backboard can be detrimental to the patient and can impair respiratory effort, increase the risk of aspiration, or result in pressure sores. Strapping the patient to a backboard "as a precaution" may not be best for the patient.

Applying SMR
Patients Requiring SMR

Appropriately applied SMR should be considered for patients who fit the following criteria (Figure 12-1):

- Spinal deformity, pain, or tenderness
- Blunt trauma and altered level of consciousness
- High-energy mechanism of injury with drug or alcohol intoxication
- Focal neurologic complaint

In addition, SMR should be applied to patients who cannot be adequately assessed clinically for the presence of such injuries.

Patients requiring SMR must have the procedure completed before they are moved in any way. In the case of an automobile collision, you must stabilize the spine before removing the patient from the wreckage. More patient movement is involved in extrication than at any other time, so you must carefully stabilize the neck and spine before beginning extrication. If SMR is indicated, stabilize the spine, do not pull on it. Except in situations requiring Emergency Rescue or rapid extrication, always try to document pulse, motor function, and sensation in the extremities before and after you move the patient.

Any patient who has the clinical indications to be placed in SMR, as listed earlier, should have an appropriate-size cervical collar placed to reduce motion of the cervical spine. Scan 12-2 illustrates the placement of a cervical collar.

SMR with a Short Extrication Device

A short extrication device is used for patients who are in a position that does not permit use of the long backboard (such as in a motor vehicle). There are several different devices of this type. Some have strapping mechanisms different from the one explained here. Become familiar with your equipment before employing it in an emergency. (See Scan 12-3 for directions on how to apply one type of short extrication device.)

PEARLS
The Short Extrication Device

- When placing the straps around the legs on a male patient, be careful not to compress the genitals with the straps.
- Do not use the device as a "handle" to move the patient. Move patient and device as a unit. Many short extrication devices come with built-in handles. For safety purposes these are not to be used alone to move a patient.
- You may need to modify your strapping techniques, depending on injuries.

Initial Assessment of Spinal Injury
Clinical Criteria

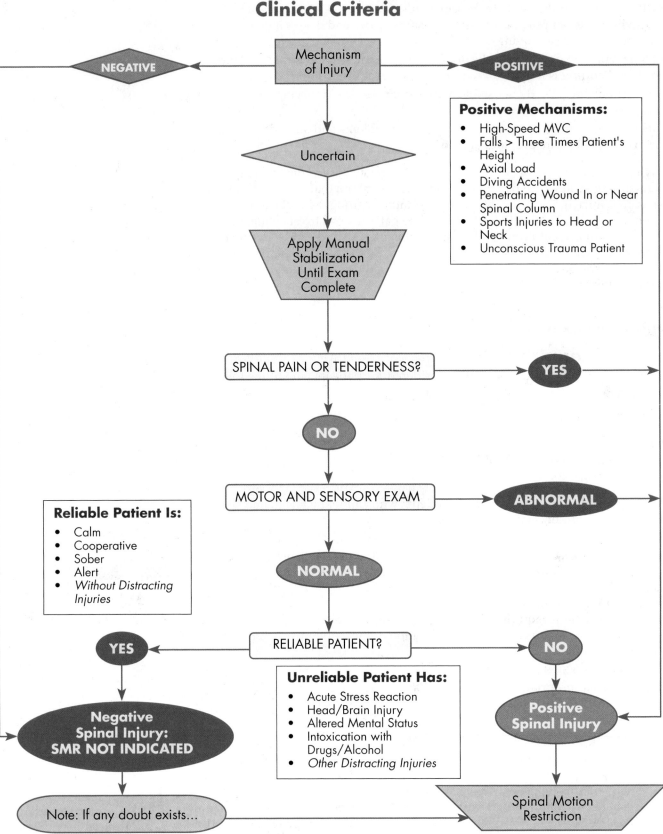

Figure 12-1 Decision tree for spinal motion restriction. *(Reprinted by permission of Peter Goth, MD)*

SCAN 12-2 Cervical Collar Placement

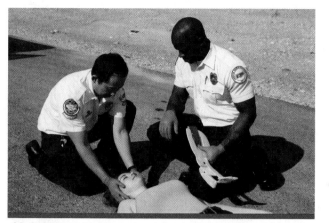

12-2-1 Establish manual stabilization by holding the head between the two hands of emergency care provider 1. Application of the semirigid cervical collar is best accomplished when the patient is in a supine position. If necessary, emergency care provider 1 may attempt to reposition the head if the patient is unresponsive and not in a midline neutral position.

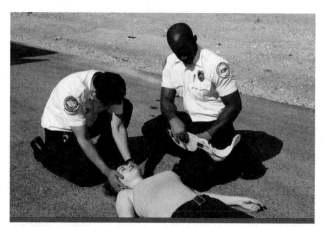

12-2-2 Emergency care provider 2 measures the patient to identify an appropriate size semirigid collar. Although the angle of the mandible and the trapezius are the most common anatomical points for measuring the size of the collar needed, providers must refer to the individual manufacturer instructions for application.

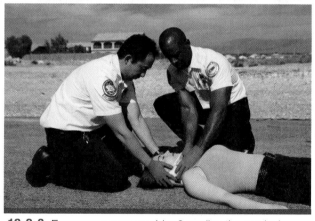

12-2-3 Emergency care provider 2 applies the cervical collar and secures in place.

Emergency Rescue and Rapid Extrication

Patients left inside vehicles following a collision are usually stabilized on a short extrication device and then transferred onto a long backboard. Although this is the best way to extricate anyone with a possible spine injury, there are certain situations in which a more rapid method must be used.

Note: International Trauma Life Support (ITLS) offers a one-day course called "Access" on basic extrication from motor vehicles using basic hand tools. Call 888-495-4857 for information (international call +1-630-495-6442).

Situations Requiring Emergency Rescue

Emergency Rescue is used only in situations in which the patient's life is in immediate danger because of environmental hazards. In some of those situations you may

SCAN 12-3 Applying a Kendrick Extrication Device

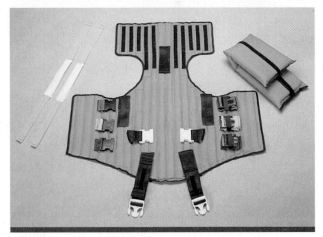

12-3-1 The Ferno Kendrick Extrication Device (KED).
(©Ferno Corporation)

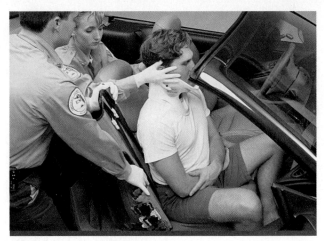

12-3-2 After a cervical collar has been applied, slip the KED behind the patient and center it.

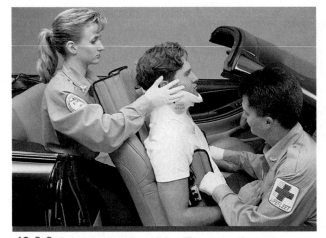

12-3-3 Properly align the device. Then wrap the vest around the patient's torso.

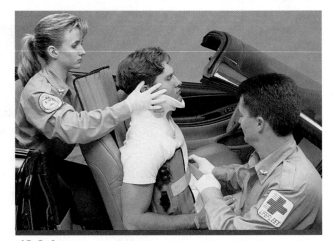

12-3-4 When the device is tucked well up into the armpits, secure the chest straps.

not have time to use any technique other than pulling the patient to safety. This is an example of "desperate situations demanding desperate measures." Use good judgment. Do not sacrifice your life in a dangerous situation. Whenever you use this procedure, it should be noted in the written report, and you should be prepared to justify your actions at a review by your medical director.

Perform an Emergency Rescue if the scene size-up identifies a condition that could immediately (within seconds) endanger you or the patient, such as (Figure 12-2):

- Fire or immediate danger of fire or explosion
- Hostile environment, gunfire, or other weapons

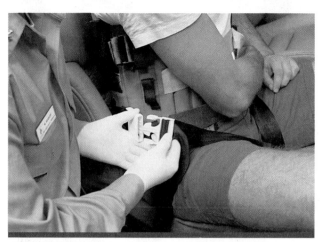

12-3-5 Bring each leg strap around the ipsilateral (same side) leg and back to the buckle on the same side. Fasten snugly.

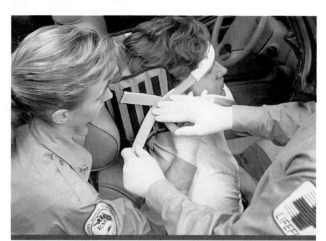

12-3-6 Secure the patient's head with the Velcro head straps. Apply padding as needed to maintain a neutral position.

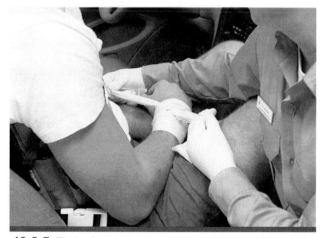

12-3-7 Tie the hands together or secure arms and hands to side of patient with straps.

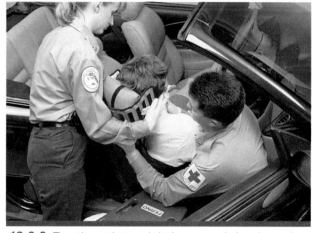

12-3-8 Turn the patient and device as a unit then lower the patient onto a long backboard. Loosen the leg straps, and allow the legs to extend out flat. Finally, secure the patient and device to the backboard.

- Danger of being carried away by rapidly moving water
- Structure in immediate danger of collapse
- Continuing and immediate life-threatening toxic exposure

Situations Requiring Rapid Extrication

You should perform a rapid extrication (Scan 12-4) if your ITLS Primary Survey of a patient identifies a critical degree of ongoing danger that requires an intervention within one to two minutes. In such a situation, you must act immediately and rapidly, but you still can stabilize the patient to some degree as you

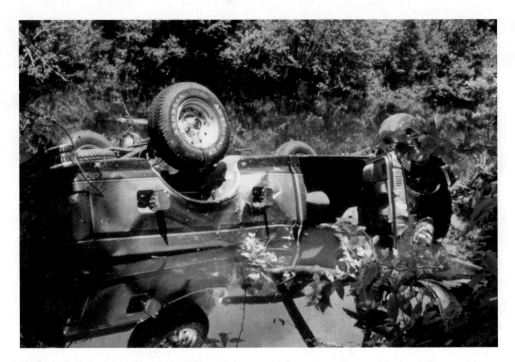

Figure 12-2 Example of a situation in which you may have to perform an Emergency Rescue. *(Photo courtesy of Bonnie Meneely, EMT-P)*

extricate him or her. Example situations that may require rapid extrication are as follows:

- Airway obstruction that you cannot relieve by a jaw-thrust maneuver or a finger sweep
- Cardiac or respiratory arrest
- Chest or airway injuries requiring ventilation or assisted ventilation
- Late shock or bleeding that you cannot control

SMR with the Long Backboard

The traditional way to apply SMR to a patient with a suspected spine injury is to secure him from head to toe to a long backboard. Log rolling the patient onto the backboard must be accomplished in a careful, coordinated way that protects him from any further injury.

See Scan 12-5 for log rolling a supine patient onto a long backboard. In contrast, the prone patient most commonly has his head turned to one side. In that case, emergency care providers will need to bring the head into neutral alignment. This can be done in one of three ways:

- Just before the log roll, bring the patient's head into the neutral position (nose down).
- During the log roll, gradually bring the patient's head into a neutral position.
- Keep the head turned in the direction the body is moving during the log roll. Upon completion of the log roll, bring the head into a neutral position.

The status of the airway in a prone patient is critical for decisions about the order in which a log roll is performed. There are three clinical situations that dictate how to proceed. The first is for the patient who is not breathing or who is in severe respiratory difficulty. He must be log rolled immediately so you can manage the airway. Unless the backboard is already positioned, you must log roll the patient, manage

SCAN 12-4 Rapid Extrication

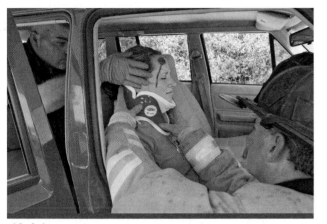

12-4-1 Stabilize the neck and perform the initial assessment. Apply a semirigid extrication collar.

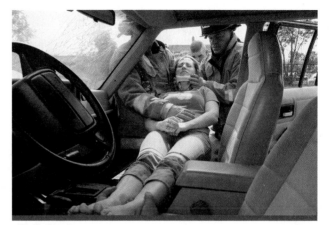

12-4-2 A second emergency care provider stands beside the open door of the vehicle and takes over control of the cervical spine. Slide the long backboard onto the seat and slightly under the patient. Carefully supporting the neck, torso, and legs, the emergency care providers turn the patient.

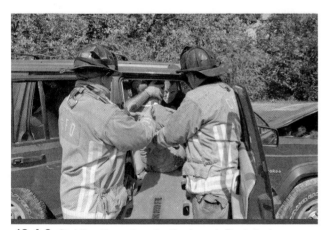

12-4-3 Stabilize the cot under the board. Begin to lower the patient onto the board.

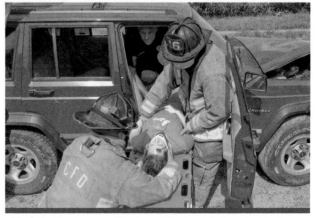

12-4-4 The legs are lifted, and the back is lowered to the backboard. Carefully slide the patient to the full length of the backboard. The patient is immediately moved away from the vehicle and into the ambulance, if available. Secure the patient to the backboard as soon as possible.

the airway, and then transfer the patient to the backboard (in a second log-rolling step) when ready to transport.

The second clinical situation occurs when a patient with profuse bleeding of the mouth or nose must not be turned to the supine position. Profuse upper airway bleeding in a supine patient is a guarantee of aspiration. This patient will have to have careful SMR and be transported prone or on his side, allowing gravity to help keep the airway clear. The vacuum backboard could be very useful in this situation. (See Chapter 11, Figure 11-7.)

The third clinical situation occurs when the patient with an adequate airway and respiration must be log rolled directly onto a backboard.

SCAN 12-5 Log Rolling a Supine Patient onto a Long Backboard

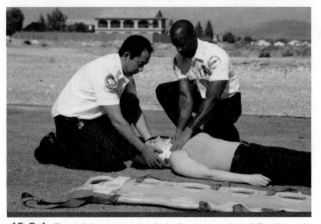

12-5-1 Establish and maintain in-line manual stabilization while applying a semirigid cervical collar.

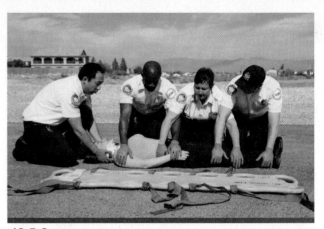

12-5-2 With the long board positioned beside the patient, emergency care providers 2, 3, and 4 assume their positions at the patient's side opposite the board, leaving space to roll the patient toward them.

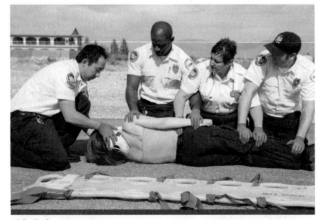

12-5-3 Emergency care provider 1 or emergency care provider 2 may direct the other team members to roll the patient as a unit onto the side toward the emergency care providers.

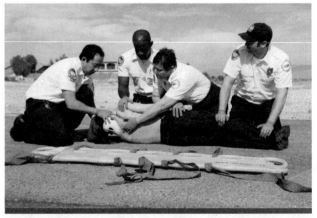

12-5-4 After assessing the patient's posterior surface from occiput to heels, the emergency care provider at the waist reaches over, grasps the backboard, and pulls it into position against the patient. This also can be done by a fifth emergency care provider. Emergency care provider 1 or emergency care provider 2 instructs the emergency care providers to roll the patient onto the backboard.

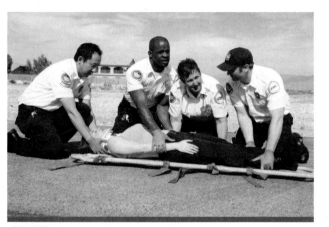

12-5-5 Position the patient midline on the backboard, and secure the patient's body to the board with straps. Manage the extremities and hands appropriately so as not to allow uncontrolled movement.

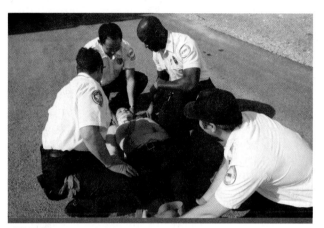

12-5-6 Use a head/cervical immobilization device to secure the patient's head to the backboard after securing the body and extremities.

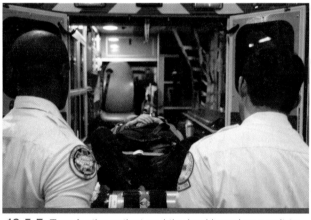

12-5-7 Transfer the patient and the backboard as a unit to the stretcher and proceed to loading the patient into the ambulance.

Procedure

Log Rolling the Prone Patient with an Adequate Airway onto a Long Backboard

1. Emergency care provider 1 stabilizes the neck. When placing his hands on the patient's head and neck, the emergency care provider's thumbs always point toward the patient's face (Figure 12-3). This prevents having the emergency care provider's arms crossed when the patient is log rolled. An initial assessment and exam of the backside is done. Then a semirigid extrication collar should be applied.

2. The patient is placed with his legs extended in the normal manner and his arms (palms inward) extended by his sides. The patient will be rolled up on one arm, with that arm acting as a splint for the body.

3. The long backboard is positioned next to the patient's body on the side of the first emergency care provider's lower hand. (If the first emergency care provider's lower hand is on the patient's right side, the backboard is placed on the patient's right side.) If the patient's arm next to the backboard is the one injured, carefully raise it above the patient's head so he does not roll on the injured arm.

4. Emergency care providers 2 and 3 kneel at the patient's side opposite the board.

5. Emergency care provider 2 is positioned at the midchest area. Emergency care provider 3 should be beside the patient's upper legs.

6. Emergency care provider 2 grasps the shoulder and the hip. Usually, it is possible to grasp the patient's clothing (if not too loose) to help with the roll.

7. Emergency care provider 3 grasps the hip (holding the near arm in place) and the lower legs (holding them together).

8. When everyone is ready, emergency care provider 1 or emergency care provider 2 gives the order to log roll the patient.

9. Emergency care providers 2 and 3 roll the patient away from them and onto his side. The patient's arms are kept locked to his side to maintain a splinting effect. The head, shoulders, and pelvis are kept in line during the roll.

10. The backboard is now positioned next to the patient and held at a 30- to 45-degree angle by emergency care provider 4. If there are only three emergency care providers, the board is pulled into place by emergency care provider 2 or 3. The board is left flat in this case.

11. When everyone is ready, emergency care provider at the head gives the order to roll the patient onto the backboard. This is accomplished by keeping the head, shoulders, and pelvis in line.

12. The ITLS Primary Survey should now be completed.

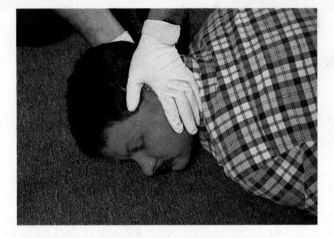

Figure 12-3 When stabilizing the neck of the prone (or supine) patient, your thumbs should always point toward the face (not the occiput). This prevents having your arms crossed when the patient is rolled over.

Special Considerations

The patient with chest or abdominal injuries should be log rolled onto his uninjured side. Do it quickly so lung expansion is not compromised. In the case of a patient with injuries to the lower extremities, position emergency care provider 2 at the feet of the patient to provide in-line support to the injured leg during the log roll. Again, try to roll the patient onto the uninjured side. In general, the side to which you turn a patient during a log roll is not critical and can be changed in situations where you can only place the backboard on one side of the patient.

Though the log-roll technique is useful for most trauma patients, it could aggravate a fractured pelvis. If the pelvic fracture appears stable, the log roll should be carefully performed, turning the patient onto the uninjured side (if this can be identified). Patients with obviously unstable pelvic fractures should not be log rolled but instead should be lifted carefully onto a board using four or more emergency care providers.

The scoop stretcher is another device that could help move the patient onto the backboard when specific injuries complicate log rolling. Some newer scoop stretchers have been found to provide equal or superior stabilization when compared to the long backboard, and may be used in place of a long backboard to transfer or as part of the SMR procedure.

Scan 12-6 outlines the application of the scoop stretcher as a transfer board. If it is being used as part of the SMR procedure, manual stabilization of the head along with application of a cervical collar should occur prior to initiating placement onto the scoop stretcher.

Another device that can be used for SMR is the vacuum mattress. More commonly used in Europe, these devices have a lower risk of pressure sores and better patient comfort (Figure 12-4).

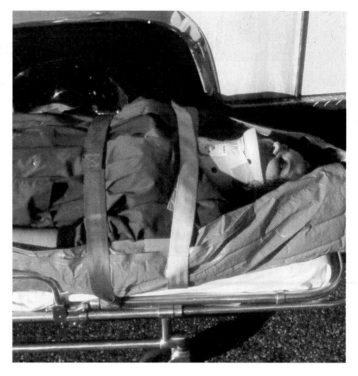

Figure 12-4 A vacuum mattress.

Securing the Patient to the Backboard

There are several different methods of securing the patient to the long backboard using straps. As with all equipment, you should become familiar with your strapping system before using it in an emergency situation.

Two examples of commercial devices for full-body immobilization are the Reeves sleeve and the Miller body splint. The Reeves sleeve is a heavy-duty sleeve into which a standard backboard will slide. Attached to this sleeve are the following:

- Head motion-restriction device
- Heavy vinyl-coated nylon panels that go over the chest and abdomen and are secured with seat-belt-type straps and quick-release connectors
- Two full-length leg panels to secure the lower extremities
- Straps to hold the arms in place
- Six handles for carrying the patient
- Metal rings (2,500-pound strength) for lifting the patient by rope

When the patient is in the Reeves sleeve, he remains immobilized when lifted horizontally, vertically, or even carried on his side (like a suitcase; Figure 12-5).

The Miller body splint is a combination backboard, head immobilizer, and body immobilizer. (See Chapter 11, Figure 11-6b.) Like the Reeves sleeve, it does an excellent job of SMR with a minimum of time and effort.

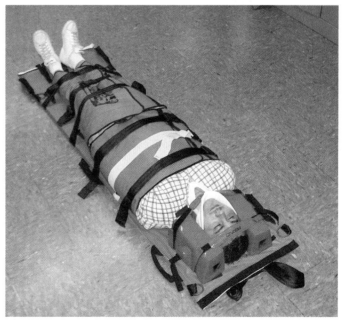

Figure 12-5 Reeves sleeve as an optional motion restriction/confined space extrication device. Patient's arms are enclosed within the panels and straps.

SCAN 12-6 Application of the Scoop Stretcher

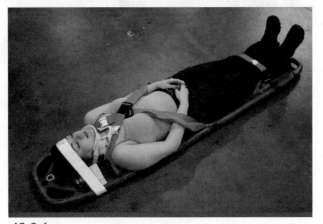

12-6-1 Placement of the head immobilization device and head restraint strap occurs following securing the patient to the scoop stretcher.

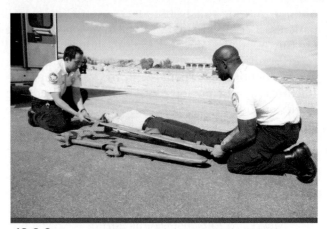

12-6-2 Separate the scoop stretcher into two halves.

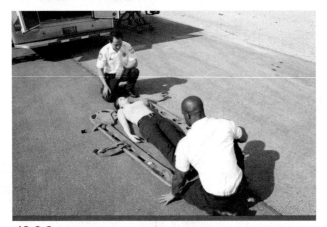

12-6-3 Place on either side of the patient, being careful not to pass the scoop stretcher directly over the patient.

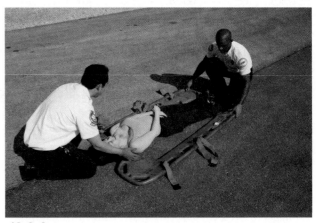

12-6-4 Adjust height of scoop halves to match, ensuring the head and heals will be positioned within the scoop area.

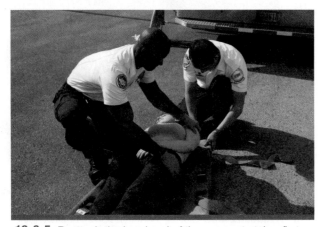

12-6-5 Reattach the head end of the scoop stretcher first. This may require repositioning the patient's shoulder.

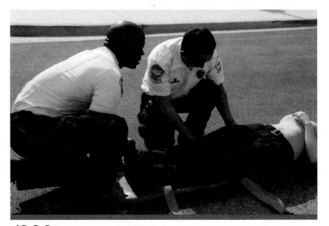

12-6-6 Carefully close the foot end of the scoop stretcher so as to not pinch the patient's posterior tissue, and reattach.

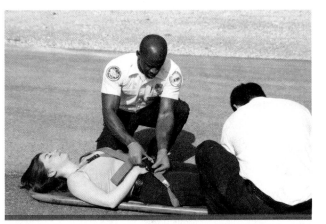

12-6-7 Secure the patient to the scoop stretcher utilizing an appropriate number of straps to ensure patient safety while moving.

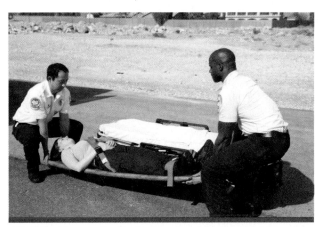

12-6-8 After confirming the head and foot ends of the scoop stretcher are locked together, transfer of the patient may now occur.

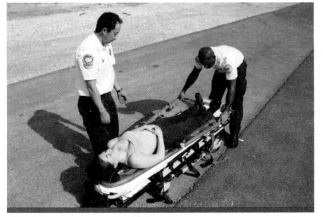

12-6-9 Removal of the patient from the scoop stretcher is completed by reversing steps of application.

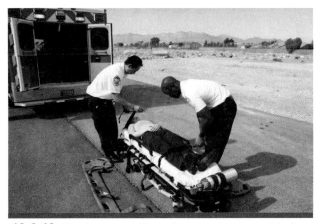

12-6-10 Once removed, the patient may be secured to the stretcher.

Special Considerations for the Head and Neck

Stabilizing the head and neck in a neutral position sometimes cannot be accomplished safely. If the head or neck is held in an angulated position and the patient complains of pain upon any attempt to straighten it, you should stabilize it in the position found. The same is true of the unconscious patient whose neck is held to one side and does not easily straighten with a gentle attempt. The use of a commercially available head motion-restriction device that permits cervical collar application in other than a midline position of the head may be considered, or the use of a blanket roll carefully taped to stabilize the head and neck in the position found is warranted.

Helmet Management

Motorcycle helmet management for a trauma patient is shown in Scans 12-7 and 12-8. The primary reason to remove the helmet is to permit management of the airway, especially in those helmets designed with integral face guards. In the supine position the motorcycle helmet will cause flexion of the neck and make SMR difficult.

PEARLS
Protective Equipment

- Patients wearing both helmets and shoulder pads usually can have their spines maintained in a more neutral position by leaving the helmet in place and padding and taping the helmet to the backboard.

- Patients wearing helmets but no shoulder pads usually can have their spines maintained in a more neutral position by removing the helmet.

- Face guards on helmets can be removed with screwdrivers or pruning shears.

- Full-face motorcycle-type helmets must be removed to evaluate and manage the airway.

SCAN 12-7 Removing a Motorcycle Helmet

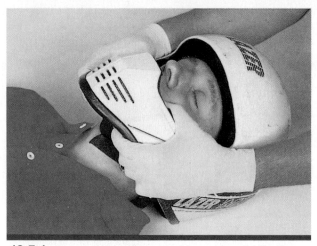

12-7-1 One emergency care provider applies stabilization by placing hands on each side of the helmet with fingers on the patient's mandible. This prevents slippage if the strap is loose.

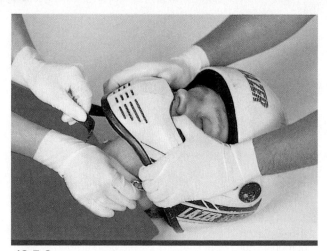

12-7-2 A second emergency care provider loosens the strap at the D-rings while stabilization is maintained.

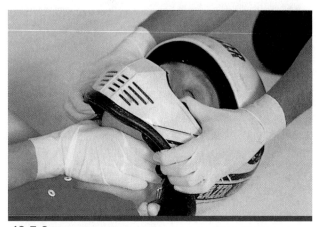

12-7-3 The second emergency care provider places one hand on the mandible at the angle, thumb on one side, long and index fingers on the other.

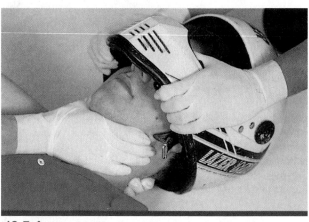

12-7-4 With the other hand, the second emergency care provider holds the occipital region. This maneuver transfers the stabilization responsibility to the second emergency care provider. The emergency care provider at the top removes the helmet in two steps, allowing the second emergency care provider to readjust his hand position under the occipital region. Three factors should be kept in mind: (a) The helmet is egg-shaped and therefore must be expanded laterally to clear the head. (b) If the helmet provides full facial coverage, glasses must be removed first. (c) If the helmet provides full facial coverage, the nose will prevent removal. To clear the nose, the helmet must be tilted back and raised over it.

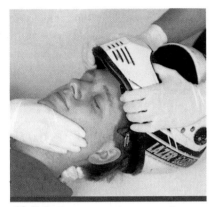

12-7-5 Throughout the removal process, the second emergency care provider maintains in-line stabilization from below to prevent head tilt.

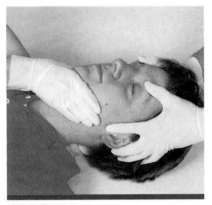

12-7-6 After the helmet has been removed, the emergency care provider at the top replaces his hands on either side of the patient's head with his palms over the ears, taking over stabilization.

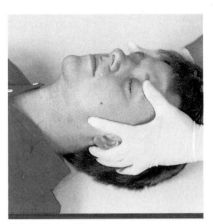

12-7-7 Stabilization is maintained from above until SMR is completed.

SCAN 12-8 Alternative Procedure for Removing a Motorcycle Helmet

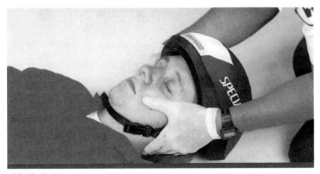

12-8-1 Apply steady stabilization in neutral position.

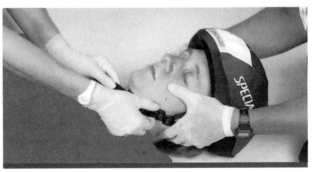

12-8-2 Remove the chin strap.

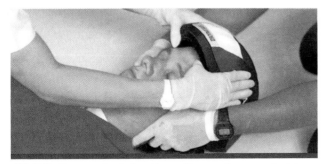

12-8-3 Remove the helmet by pulling gently on each side.

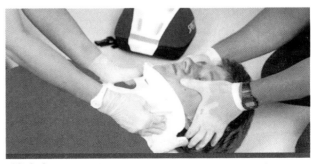

12-8-4 Apply a suitable cervical collar, and secure the patient to a long backboard as warranted.

Bibliography

Horodyski, M., B. P. Conrad, G. Del Rossi, C. P. DiPaola, and G. R. Rechtine 2nd. "Removing a Patient from the Spine Board: Is the Lift and Slide Safer Than the Log Roll?" *Journal of Trauma* 70, no. 5 (May 2011): 1282–85.

Johnson, D. R., M. Hauswald, and C. Stockhoff. "Comparison of a Vacuum Splint Device to Rigid Backboard for Spinal Immobilization." *American Journal of Emergency Medicine* 14, no. 4 (July 1996): 369–72.

Kleiner, D. M., A. Pollak, and C. McAdam. "Helmet Hazards. Do's and Don'ts of Football Helmet Removal." *Journal of Emergency Medical Services (JEMS)* 26, no. 7 (July 2001): 36–44, 46–48.

Krell, J. M., M. S. McCoy, P. J. Sparto, G. L. Fisher, W. A. Stoy, and D. P. Hostler. "Comparison of the Ferno Scoop Stretcher with the Long Backboard for Spinal Immobilization." *Prehospital Emergency Care* 10, no. 1 (January–March 2006): 46–51.

Rozzelle, C. J., B. Aarabi, S. S. Dhall, D. E. Gelb, R. J. Hurlbert, T. C. Ryken, N. Theodore, B. C. Walters, and M. N. Hadley. "Management of Pediatric Cervical Spine and Spinal Cord Injuries." *Neurosurgery* 72, Suppl. 2 (March 2013): 205–26.

Theodore, N., M. N. Hadley, B. Aarabi, S. S. Dhall, D. E. Gelb, R. J. Hurlbert, C. J. Rozzelle, T. C. Ryken, and B. C. Walters. "Prehospital Cervical Spinal Immobilization After Trauma." *Neurosurgery* 72, Suppl. 2 (March 2013): 22–34.

Abdominal Trauma

Ingrid Bloom, MD
Melissa White, MD, MPH
Arthur H. Yancey II, MD, MPH, FACEP

Trauma Addominale	Traumatismo Abdominal	Traumatisme Abdominal
Urazy brzucha	Ozljede trbuha	إصابات البطن
abdominalna trauma	Poškodbe trebuha	Hasi sérülés

(Ambulance photo courtesy of J. van der Wolf, Shutterstock.com)

Key Terms

evisceration, *p. 259*
intrathoracic abdomen, *p. 257*
peritoneum, *p. 259*
retroperitoneal abdomen, *p. 257*
seat-belt sign, *p. 259*
true abdomen, *p. 257*

Objectives

Upon successful completion of this chapter, you should be able to:

1. Identify the basic anatomy of the abdomen, and explain how abdominal and chest injuries may be related.
2. Differentiate between blunt and penetrating injuries, and identify characteristic complications associated with each.
3. Describe the treatment required for the patient with protruding viscera.
4. Describe how to identify and stabilize a pelvic fracture, why this is important, and contraindications.
5. Relate how injuries apparent on the exterior of the abdomen reflect possible damaged underlying structures.
6. Describe the findings indicating possible intra-abdominal injuries based on history, physical examination, and mechanism of injury (MOI).
7. List the critical interventions for patients with abdominal injuries.

Chapter Overview

Injury to the abdomen can be a difficult condition to evaluate in the hospital setting. In the field it can be even more challenging. Nevertheless, because intra-abdominal injury is one of the major causes of preventable traumatic death, the possibility of intra-abdominal injury must be recognized, addressed, and documented immediately. Penetrating abdominal injuries usually need immediate surgical attention. Blunt injuries (contact sports, motor-vehicle collisions, assault) may be more subtle, but potentially just as deadly.

Whether caused by blunt or penetrating trauma, an abdominal injury can result in life-threatening problems such as hemorrhage and infection. Hemorrhage has immediate consequences, so you must be vigilant in assessing the signs and symptoms of shock in all patients with abdominal injury. Infection, which presents late, may be just as lethal, but does not require field intervention beyond prevention of gross contamination.

The role of any emergency care provider in the management of abdominal trauma has been the subject of some controversy. Studies in the mid-1980s demonstrated that appropriate and timely intervention by well-trained Paramedics could improve the hemodynamic status of critically injured patients who have wounds to the abdomen. Subsequent studies have suggested that pneumatic antishock garment (PASG) application and/or vigorous intravenous (IV) fluid resuscitation in the prehospital setting may do more harm than good for patients who have penetrating abdominal injuries. (See Chapter 8.) For blunt trauma, the effects of aggressive fluid resuscitation are less defined.

In the field, rapid patient assessment and early treatment of shock, followed by prompt and safe transport to definitive care, are critical aspects in the management of the patient with abdominal trauma.

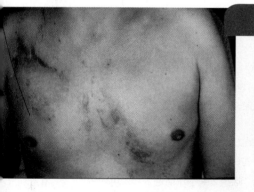

Case Presentation

As fire services are finishing up at the scene of a truck collision and the police are getting ready to re-open the highway, the Incident Commander contacts EMS dispatch and requests an ambulance to the scene, routine response. The truck driver who after the incident had no complaints of injuries and declined EMS transport, is now complaining of midabdominal pain. When he raised his shirt, he noticed bruising on his chest and abdomen. He also reports passing blood when he urinated. You have just left the hospital, where you had transported the motorcyclist injured in the same incident, and you now return to the scene.

Before proceeding, consider these questions: What elements in the history and mechanism of injury (MOI) indicate possible internal injuries? What critical signs would you search for in your primary and secondary surveys? Does this patient require spinal motion restriction (SMR)? What treatment should you provide? Keep these questions in mind as you read through the chapter. Then, at the end of the chapter, find out how the emergency care providers managed this patient.

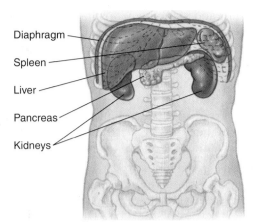

Figure 13-1 Intrathoracic abdomen.

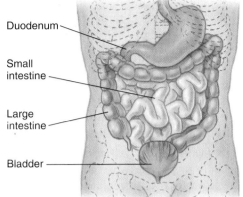

Figure 13-2 True abdomen.

Anatomy of the Abdomen

The abdomen is traditionally divided into three regions: the **intrathoracic abdomen** (Figure 13-1), the **true abdomen** (Figure 13-2), and the **retroperitoneal abdomen** (Figure 13-3).

Although hemorrhage in the true abdomen may cause the anterior abdominal wall to become distended, hemorrhage severe enough to cause shock can occur in the retroperitoneal space without this dramatic sign. Because of its location away from the anterior body surface, injuries here are difficult to evaluate in the field. The iliac blood vessels and their branches, located in the pelvic portion of the retroperitoneal abdomen, may be damaged by abdominal trauma or pelvic fracture. Injury to this vasculature may cause serious hemorrhage with minimal localized or external symptoms.

Types of Abdominal Injuries

Injuries to the abdomen are usually categorized as blunt or penetrating trauma, but a combination of the two also can occur. Blunt trauma is the most common mechanism of abdominal injury and has relatively high mortality rates of 10% to 30%. The reason is likely related to the frequency of accompanying injuries to the head, chest, pelvis, and/or an extremity in as many as 70% of motor-vehicle collision victims.

Blunt abdominal injury may be from direct compression of the abdomen against a fixed object with resulting tears or subcapsular hematomas involving the solid organs, especially the spleen and liver. Injury also may arise from deceleration forces, with tearing of organs and their blood vessels at fixed areas within the abdominal region. This is particularly true of the liver and the renal arteries. Hollow organs (typically small intestine) may rupture due to increased intraluminal pressures.

The patient who has suffered blunt trauma may have no pain and little external evidence of injury, which may give a false sense of security. Patients with multiple lower rib fractures are notorious for having severe intra-abdominal injuries without significant abdominal pain. The severe pain from the rib fractures becomes a distracting injury for the less noticeable abdominal pain. As a result, the patient may have a poor outcome because abdominal injuries are not recognized.

intrathoracic abdomen: the part of the abdomen located under a thin sheet of muscle, called the *diaphragm*, and enclosed by the lower ribs; contains the liver, gallbladder, spleen, stomach, and transverse colon.

true abdomen: the part of the abdomen from the lower ribs and including the pelvis but anterior to the retroperitoneum; contains the large and small intestines, a portion of the liver, and the bladder. In a female, the uterus, fallopian tubes, and ovaries are also part of the true abdomen.

retroperitoneal abdomen: the part of the abdomen behind the thoracic and true portions of the abdomen, separated from the other abdominal regions by a thin retroperitoneal membrane; includes the kidneys, ureters, pancreas, posterior duodenum, ascending and descending colon, abdominal aorta, and the inferior vena cava.

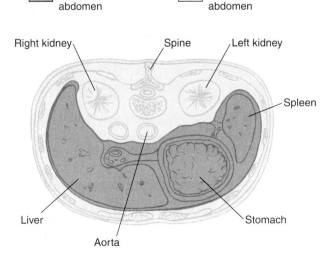

Figure 13-3 Retroperitoneal abdomen.

PEARLS
Abdominal Injury

When the mechanisms of trauma or associated injuries, such as lower rib fractures or gluteal penetrating wounds, suggest possible intra-abdominal injury, do not be fooled by the patient's lack of abdominal pain or tenderness. Be prepared to treat hypovolemic shock from occult intra-abdominal bleeding.

The patient who has sustained blunt trauma to the abdomen and has abdominal pain and/or tenderness probably has serious abdominal injuries and is likely to develop shock quickly (even if vital signs are initially normal). Load and go, and prepare to treat the development of hemorrhagic shock en route to the hospital.

Most penetrating injuries are caused by gunshot and stabbing. Gunshot wounds to the abdomen may include direct trauma to an organ and vasculature through penetration from the bullet, its fragments, or the energy transmitted from the bullet's mass and velocity. This is known as cavitation. (See Chapter 1.)

As a general rule, most patients with gunshot wounds to the abdomen will require definitive treatment in the operating room and should be taken to a trauma center. These patients have mortality rates between 5% and 15% because of a greater incidence of injury to abdominal viscera from the higher energy imparted to the intra-abdominal organs than that imparted by stab wounds. (See Chapter 1.)

The mortality rate from abdominal stab wounds is relatively low (1% to 2%). Unless the knife penetrates a major vessel or organ, such as the liver or spleen, the patient may not initially appear to be in shock at the scene. However, some patients can develop life-threatening peritonitis over the next few hours or days. Those wounds need to be carefully evaluated in the emergency department because approximately one-third of stab-wound patients require surgery for intra-abdominal bleeding or perforation of a viscus with spilling of gastrointestinal contents, leading to peritonitis.

Because the path of the penetrating object might not be readily apparent from the wound location, any penetrating wound of the chest could also have penetrated the abdomen and vice versa. The course of a bullet may pass through numerous structures in different body locations. Inspection of the patient's entire posterior surface is necessary because penetrating trauma in the gluteal area (iliac crests to the gluteal folds, including the rectum) is associated with as many as 50% of significant intra-abdominal injuries.

Assessment and Stabilization
Scene Size-up

One can glean important information from the scene by noting the circumstances surrounding the patient's injury. An accurate but rapid size-up of the scene will usually guide the emergency care provider to the possibility of intra-abdominal trauma. For example, do circumstances on the scene suggest that the victim has fallen from a height or been hit by a passing vehicle? Has there been an explosion that could have hurled the victim against immobile objects or transmitted blast pressure to organs inside the abdomen? Has the victim of an automobile crash had the shoulder strap under the arm rather than over the shoulder? Or was the lap belt worn too high over the unprotected, soft true abdomen instead of correctly across the bony pelvis? Many of these clues can be found at the scene.

If the patient was involved in a motor-vehicle crash, during scene size-up, quickly observe the damage to the vehicle, such as passenger compartment intrusion, airbag deployment, broken windows, bent steering wheel/steering column, and location of occupants. If the patient needs to be extricated, note the location of the safety belts. Although they certainly save lives, safety belts incorrectly worn can cause blunt abdominal injuries by compressing the intra-abdominal organs against the spine. Remember that for the same reason, lap belt-only restraints, especially in the adolescent age group, may predispose the passenger to intra-abdominal injuries in a motor-vehicle crash.

The patient who is stabbed or shot may be able to give some idea of the size of the weapon used and its trajectory. With gunshot wounds, it is also important to know (if possible) the caliber, the range from which the gun was fired, and the number of rounds fired. A bystander or the police may be able to provide such information. On arrival at the hospital (optimally, a trauma center), be sure to report any mechanism that suggests abdominal injury. However, while at the scene, it is important not to spend a great deal of time attempting to obtain a history. The major cause of preventable mortality in abdominal trauma is delayed diagnosis and treatment.

Patient Assessment

As in treating any injured patient, the patient with an injured abdomen should first undergo the ITLS Primary Survey. During the rapid trauma survey, the essence of the prehospital abdominal exam is rapid visualization and palpation of both the chest and abdomen. Quickly inspect the chest and abdomen for deformities, contusions, abrasions, punctures, **evisceration**, and distention.

evisceration: the protruding of intestinal organs through a wound.

The chest is only one thin muscle sheet (the diaphragm) away from the abdominal cavity. Abdominal organs are enclosed within the lower ribs, thus injury to both chest and abdomen is not uncommon. Blunt or penetrating injuries to the chest from about the nipple line (fourth or fifth rib) down should lead to concern for the possibility of both chest and abdominal injuries. Rib fractures may suggest hepatic, splenic, and diaphragmatic trauma. Splenic injury may present with referred left posterior shoulder pain (*Kehr's sign*), and a liver injury may present with referred right posterior shoulder pain. The presence of a **seat-belt sign**, which is a large bruise or abrasion across the abdomen, is indicative of intra-abdominal injury in approximately 25% of cases.

seat-belt sign: a bruise or abrasion across the abdomen from an improperly positioned lap belt. It can be a clue to blunt intra-abdominal injury.

Observation of the abdomen may reveal periumbilical bruising (*Cullen's sign*), raising suspicion for retroperitoneal hemorrhage, but be mindful that this finding usually takes several hours to develop. Palpate the patient's abdomen for distention, tenderness, or rigidity. Distention of the abdomen should be interpreted as a sign of severe intra-abdominal trauma with likely hemorrhage. Tenderness or guarding over the abdominal wall, especially away from wounds, is also usually a sign of intra-abdominal injury. If tenderness or guarding is present in the prehospital setting, there is usually significant extravascular, or free, blood in the abdomen from hemorrhage, causing irritation of the **peritoneum**. This is an indication that shock may be imminent. (See Chapter 8.) Pelvic fractures frequently result in hemorrhagic shock. Gentle palpation of the iliac crests (pelvic wings) and pubis of the pelvis may reveal signs associated with fractures, including tenderness, bony crepitation, or instability. Note: The pelvis should not be compressed, as this can cause clot dislodgement or possible worsening of a fracture, nor should more than one emergency care provider palpate the pelvis for instability. The perineum (genitalia and buttocks) should be visualized for bruising or hemorrhage during the ITLS Secondary Survey.

peritoneum: a thin serous membrane that lines the abdominal cavity and covers the organs of the abdomen.

Auscultation of the abdomen in the field usually does not offer reliable information. Abdominal wounds should never be probed with a finger or an instrument. *If clothing must be removed to visualize injury, try to preserve important potential legal evidence by cutting around (rather than through) areas that have signs of possible penetration.*

Stabilization

Interventions should follow priorities established by the ITLS Primary Survey. They should proceed in the same order in which assessment occurred: (A) airway, (B) breathing, and (C) circulation. (This sequence changes to CABC if there is obvious severe uncontrolled external hemorrhage.) For the patient in whom only intra-abdominal injury is suspected, give supplemental oxygen by the most appropriate method, and be sure breathing is adequate before dealing with the circulatory issue of shock or potential shock.

The patient should be readied for immediate transport with appropriate spinal motion restriction, if indicated. Of note, penetrating trauma to the abdomen or chest with no signs of neurologic deficit does not require immobilization of the spine.

Time to definitive care at the trauma center is critical. Unnecessary intervention on scene should be avoided. Once en route to an appropriate trauma center, establish two large-bore IV lines of normal saline. If the patient's blood pressure drops below 90 mm Hg systolic with signs of shock, then the IV fluids should be titrated to maintain the systolic blood pressure at 80 to 90 mm Hg. (See Chapter 8.) However, keep in mind that overly aggressive fluid resuscitation might dislodge protective clots and/or dilute clotting factors, both of which lead to worsening hemorrhage.

SCAN 13-1 Caring for an Evisceration

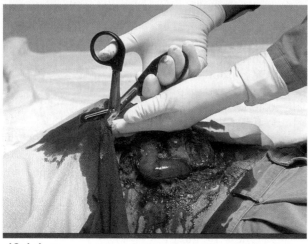

13-1-1 Remove clothing to fully expose the abdominal wound.

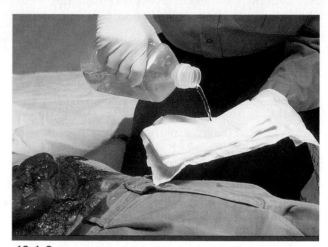

13-1-2 Cover the wound with a sterile gauze dressing soaked with normal saline.

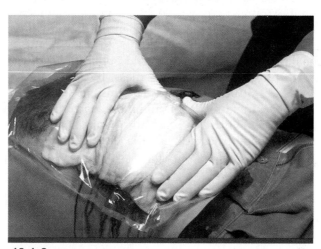

13-1-3 Cover the moistened sterile dressing with an occlusive dressing (such as plastic wrap) to prevent evaporative drying.

Gently cover any organ or viscera protruding from a wound with gauze moistened with saline or water. If long transport time is anticipated, also apply over the gauze a nonadherent material, such as plastic wrap or aluminum foil, to prevent drying of the applied gauze and underlying intestines (Scan 13-1). If the intestines are allowed to dry, they may become irreversibly damaged. Do not push abdominal contents protruding from a wound back into the abdomen. Similarly, if a foreign body (such as a knife or glass shard) is impaled in the abdomen, do not attempt to remove or manipulate it because it may precipitate uncontrollable hemorrhage. Carefully stabilize the object in place without moving it. (Pregnant patients deserve the special considerations addressed in Chapter 19.)

Although difficult to assess for, if a pelvic fracture resulting from high-energy blunt trauma (motor-vehicle collision) is suspected on prehospital exam, a pelvic binder (or circumferential bed sheet) can be placed to help stabilize and allow clot formation en route, which can help to minimize further blood loss into the retroperitoneum. The potential space into which the patient can bleed is reduced. If using a sheet, it should be folded to a width of 8 to 12 inches (20 to 30 cm) and centered over the greater trochanters, positioned beneath the patient, then crossed anteriorly before pulling tightly and tying the ends into a knot. Avoid wrinkles, and do not pull too tightly. Be sure to re-examine the patient's neurovascular status distally. If pelvic fracture is suspected, but the patient has sustained a low-energy injury or one due to a lateral force, pelvic binding should be avoided because applying pressure could cause further injury (especially if the patient has weak bones due to osteoporosis, for example).

Areas of Current Study

Deciding which patient(s) should be taken to a local community hospital and which should be taken directly to a trauma center can be a difficult decision, with only a patient history, scene size-up, and patient assessment to guide it. Better tools are needed to distinguish between patients who have injuries that are neither severe nor time-critical and will remain stable, and those who have a significant mechanism and/or signs of injury who appear stable initially, but are at risk for decompensation or subsequently do decompensate, requiring emergent transfer to a trauma center. Diagnostic tools and the procedures to use them that are quickly performed on scene or en route in the ambulance would advance field triage immensely because they have the potential to predict which apparently stable patients might deteriorate. Current studies using abdominal ultrasound in the field show some promise.

Focused assessment with sonography in trauma (FAST) is an ultrasound scan and triage tool routinely used in the emergency department to assess patients presenting with blunt abdominal trauma. A potential benefit of FAST exam use in the prehospital setting is accelerated diagnosis of intraperitoneal hemorrhage from blunt abdominal trauma. A study on the feasibility of a real-time mobile telesonography system found that it can perform point-of-care ultrasound and transmit real-time data obtained in a prehospital setting to experts in the hospital. The use of the FAST exam in the prehospital setting may allow patients with blunt abdominal trauma to be triaged to a higher acuity level. By alerting emergency departments with the transmission of ultrasound images, trauma centers could be better prepared to allocate resources in anticipation of the patient's arrival. An early diagnosis in the prehospital setting may also give the physician knowledge enough to prioritize relevant treatment. Though the adoption of this novel telesonography system may lead to improved management of trauma patients in the prehospital setting, the degree to which its use would be a productive use of health resources in terms of training and equipment remains unclear. Ultrasound in the prehospital setting is becoming more common in European systems, especially as size and cost of units have decreased in the past few years. Studies have shown ultrasound can also be used to help detect the presence of pneumothoracies, tamponade, and endotracheal tube position in the field, as well as help with IV access and to assess for cardiac activity during management of cardiac arrest.

Management of abdominal trauma in the field not only focuses on rapid transport to an appropriate facility, but also on the identification of internal bleeding. Exsanguination is a common cause of death in trauma patients. If a patient has sustained an abdominal injury that is causing hemorrhage, there are few helpful prehospital management options. Because tranexamic acid (TXA) reduces bleeding in patients undergoing elective surgery, investigators in two different studies sought to evaluate the use of this drug to help with clotting in trauma patients. Based on the Clinical Randomisation of an Antifibrinolytic in Significant Haemorrhage (CRASH-2) trial, researchers found the importance of using TXA in bleeding trauma patients. The effectiveness and safety of early administration of TXA was investigated, and it was discovered to be associated with a decrease in mortality, but unlikely to benefit the patient if treated beyond three hours after the time of initial injury. It seems crucial that this drug is given within three hours after onset of injury. If given later, outcomes are worse. The Military

Application of Tranexamic Acid in Trauma Emergency Resuscitation (MATTER) study showed that with use of TXA after combat injury, a decrease in total blood product needed as well as an increase in survival was demonstrated, especially among patients requiring massive transfusion. (Please see Chapter 8 for further discussion on the management of internal hemorrhage.)

Lactate has been shown to be a biochemical marker of developing shock. Newer systems to measure lactate levels at the bedside have been developed and are proving useful to identifying patients in shock before clinical symptoms develop. This may be another clue to ongoing internal hemorrhage, which would be an indication to transport directly to a trauma center or other facility capable of managing internal trauma.

Prompt diagnosis and treatment of patients with abdominal trauma is considered essential in the successful management of the trauma patient. Continued study of these and other innovative prehospital diagnostics and treatment options is needed.

Case Presentation (continued)

You arrive back at the scene and are met by the patient at the Incident Commander's car. The patient is ambulatory, in no acute distress, speaking in full sentences, and answering questions appropriately. His ITLS Primary Survey was noted to be intact. The patient complains of lower midabdominal pain, left shoulder pain, and some nausea and reports a second episode of gross hematuria. On exam his neck is found to be nontender. His chest is clear with some anterior bruising noted. Breath sounds are equal. Palpation of his abdomen produces tenderness where his contusion is noted, but he also complains of left upper quadrant pain on palpation. Vital signs show a pulse rate of 110, blood pressure of 130/88, and respirations are 10 and unlabored. He reports only a history of hypothyroidism but states two months ago he developed a DVT (deep vein thrombosis) in his right leg and is taking warfarin for prevention of another clot. While getting onto the stretcher, he has an episode of vomiting, but no blood is noted.

You establish a peripheral IV while en route to the hospital. You administer ondansetron, 4 mg IV. Because of his continued pain, you also administer 4 mg morphine sulfate IV per protocol.

The ITLS Ongoing Survey shows no changes en route to the hospital. Subsequent evaluation in the emergency department shows the patient has a small splenic hematoma and a bladder contusion from the seat belt. Both the hematuria and the subcapsular hematoma are likely related to his use of anticoagulants for his prior DVT. He was managed nonoperatively and discharged the following day. This case illustrates that intra-abdominal injury can sometimes be delayed in presentation.

Summary

Effective prehospital management of the patient who has abdominal trauma entails the following:

- Scene size-up for MOIs and pertinent history from the patient and/or witnesses
- Rapid patient assessment
- Rapid transport to the appropriate hospital (optimally, a trauma center)
- IV lines, pelvic binding, and other interventions as needed (usually performed en route)

The enemies of the abdominal trauma patient are bleeding and time elapsed from injury until hemostasis from optimal emergency and surgical care. If on-scene delays can be minimized, this will help to maximize the patient's chances for survival.

Bibliography

Aprahamian, C., B. M. Thompson, J. B. Towne, and J. C. Darin. "The Effect of a Paramedic System on Mortality of Major Open Intra-abdominal Vascular Trauma." *Journal of Trauma* 23, no. 8 (August 1983): 687–90.

Bickell, W. H., M. J. Wall Jr., P. E. Pepe, R. R. Martin, V. F. Ginger, M. K. Allen, and K. L. Mattox. "Immediate Versus Delayed Fluid Resuscitation for Hypotensive Patients with Penetrating Torso Injuries." *New England Journal of Medicine* 331, no. 17 (October 1994): 1105–09.

Brooke, M., J. Walton, and D. Scutt. "Paramedic Application of Ultrasound in the Management of Patients in the Prehospital Setting: A Review of the Literature." *Emergency Medicine Journal* 27, no. 9 (September 2010): 702–7.

Collopy, K. T., and G. Friese. "Abdominal Trauma: A Review of Prehospital Assessment and Management of Blunt and Penetrating Abdominal Trauma." *EMS Magazine* 39, no. 3 (March 2010): 62-66, 68–69.

Heegaard, W., D. Hildebrandt, D. Spear, K. Chason, B. Nelson, and J. Ho. "Prehospital Ultrasound by Paramedics: Results of Field Trial." *Academic Emergency Medicine* 17, no. 6 (June 2010): 624–30.

Hoyer, H. X., S. Vogl, U. Schiemann, A. Haug, E. Stolpe, and T. Michalski. "Prehospital Ultrasound in Emergency Medicine: Incidence, Feasibility, Indications, and Diagnoses." *European Journal of Emergency Medicine* 17, no. 5 (October 2010): 254–59.

Jansen, T. C., J. van Bommel, P. G. Mulder, J. H. Rommes, S. J. M. Schieveld, and J. Bakker. "The Prognostic Value of Blood Lactate Levels Relative to That of Vital Signs in the Prehospital Setting: A Pilot Study." *Critical Care* 12, no. 6 (2008): R160–66.

Korner, M., M. M. Krotz, C. Degenhart, K. J. Pfeifer, M. F. Reiser, and U. Linsenmaier. "Current Role of Emergency Ultrasound in Patients with Major Trauma." *Radiographics* 28 no. 1 (January–February 2008): 225–42.

Legome, E. L., S. M. Keim, and J. P. Salomone. "Blunt Abdominal Trauma." *Medscape* website, updated August 19, 2014. Accessed January, 2015, at http://emedicine.medscape.com/article/821995-overview.

Martin, R. S., and J. W. Meredith. "Management of Acute Trauma." In *Sabiston Textbook of Surgery: The Biological Basic of Modern Surgical Practice*. 19th ed. Philadelphia: Saunders, 2011.

Melville, S., and D. Melville. "Abdominal Trauma." In *Current Diagnosis and Treatment Emergency Medicine*. 7th ed. New York: McGraw-Hill, 2011.

Morrison, J. J., J. J. Dubose, T. E. Rasmussen, and M. J. Midwinter. "Military Application of Tranexamic Acid in Trauma Emergency Resuscitation (MATTERs) Study." *Archives of Surgery* 147, no. 2 (February 2012): 113–19.

Newgard, C. D., et al. 2005. "Steering Wheel Deformity and Serious Thoracic or Abdominal Injury Among Drivers and Passengers Involved in Motor Vehicle Crashes." *Annals of Emergency Medicine* 45 (January 2005): 43–50.

Ogedegbe, C., H. Morchel, V. Hazelwood, W. F. Chaplin, and J. Feldman. "Development and Evaluation of a Novel, Real Time Mobile Telesonography System in Management of Patients with Abdominal Trauma: Study Protocol." *BMC Emergency Medicine* 12, no. 19 (December 2012): 12–19.

Pepe, P. E., V. N. Mosesso, and J. L. Falk. "Prehospital Fluid Resuscitation of the Patient with Major Trauma." *Prehospital Emergency Care* 6, no. 1 (January–March 2002): 81–91.

Rajab, T. K., W. J. Weaver, and J. M. Havens. "Videos in Clinical Medicine: Technique for Temporary Pelvic Stabilization After Trauma." *New England Journal of Medicine* 369, no. 17 (October 24, 2013): 369.

Roberts, I., H. Shakur, T. Coats, B. Hunt, E. Balogun, L. Barnetson, L. Cook, T. Kawahara, P. Perel, D. Prieto-Merino, M. Ramos, J. Cairns, and C. Guerriero. "The CRASH-2 Trial: A Randomised Controlled Trial and Economic Evaluation of the Effects of Tranexamic Acid on Death, Vascular Occlusive Events, and Transfusion Requirement in Bleeding Trauma Patients." *Health Technology Assessment* 17, no. 10 (March 2013): 1–79.

Scalea, T. M., and S. A. Boswell. "Abdominal Injuries." In *Tintinalli's Emergency Medicine: A Comprehensive Study Guide.* 6th ed. New York: McGraw-Hill, 2004.

Scott, I., K. Porter, C. Laird, I. Greaves, and M. Bloch. 2013. "The Prehospital Management of Pelvic Fractures: Initial Consensus Statement." *Emergency Medicine Journal* 30, no. 12 (December 2013): 1070–72.

Smith, J. "Focused Assessment with Sonography in Trauma (FAST): Should Its Role Be Reconsidered?" *Postgraduate Medical Journal* 86, no. 1015 (May 2010): 285–91.

Strode, C. A., B. J. Ruba, R. T. Gerhardt, J. R. Bulgrin, and S. Y. Boyd. "Wireless and Satellite Transmission of Prehospital Focused Abdominal Sonography for Trauma." *Prehospital Emergency Care* 7, no. 3 (July–September 2003): 375–79.

Taylor, J., K. McLaughlin, A. McRae, E. Lang, and A. Anton. "Use of Prehospital Ultrasound in North America: A Survey of Emergency Medical Services Medical Directors." *BMC Emergency Medicine* 14, no. 6 (March 2014). doi:10.1186/1471-227X-14-6

Todd, S. R. "Critical Concepts in Abdominal Injury." *Critical Care Clinics* 20 (January 2004): 119–34.

van Beest, P. A., P. J. Mulder, S. B. Oetomo, B. van den Broek, M. A. Kuiper, and P. E. Spronk. "Measurement of Lactate in a Prehospital Setting Is Related to Outcome." *European Journal of Emergency Medicine* 16, no. 6 (December 2009): 318–22.

Get more information about this course by calling
ITLS International at 888-495-4875
(outside the United States call +1-630-495-6442) or visit

www.itrauma.org

Extremity Trauma

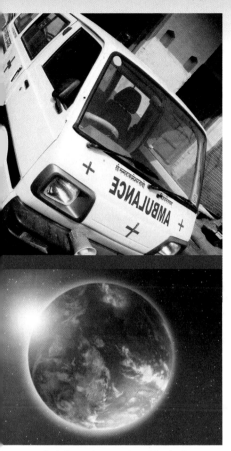

Sabina Braithwaite, MD, MPH, FACEP
S. Robert Seitz, MEd, RN, NREMT-P

Trauma alle Estremità   Traumatismo de Extremidades   Traumatisme d'extrémité

Obrażenia kończyn   Extremitäten Trauma   Ozljede ekstremiteta

إصابات الأطراف   trauma ekstremiteta   Poškodbe okončin

Végtagsérülés

(Ambulance photo courtesy of Regien Paassen, Shutterstock.com)

Key Terms

amputation, *p. 269*
closed fracture, *p. 267*
compartment syndrome, *p. 270*
crepitation, *p. 273*
impaled object, *p. 270*
joint dislocation, *p. 268*
neurovascular injury, *p. 266*
open-book pelvic fracture, *p. 280*
open fracture, *p. 267*
sprain, *p. 270*
strain, *p. 270*

Objectives

Upon successful completion of this chapter, you should be able to:

1. Prioritize extremity trauma in the assessment and management of life-threatening injuries.
2. Discuss the major immediate and short-term complications and treatment of the following extremity injuries: amputations, crush injuries, dislocations, fractures, impaled objects, neurovascular injuries, open wounds, and sprains and strains.
3. Discuss the pathophysiology of compartment syndrome and which extremity injuries are most likely to develop this complication.
4. Describe the potential amount of blood loss from pelvic and femur fractures.
5. Discuss major mechanisms of injury, associated injuries, potential complications, and management of injuries to the following: clavicle and shoulder, elbow, forearm and wrist, hand, pelvis, hip, femur, knee, tibia and fibula (including ankle), and foot.

Chapter Overview

Emergency care providers should never allow a deformed or injured extremity to divert their attention from more life-threatening injuries that may also be present. Extremity injuries often have a dramatic appearance that can be seen as you approach the patient. Such injuries may be disabling and can occasionally be life threatening. But do not be distracted by those injuries. It is important to remember that the movement of air through the airway, the mechanics of breathing, the maintenance of circulating blood volume, and the appropriate treatment of shock must always come before fracture or dislocation management.

Hemorrhagic shock is a potential danger with major musculoskeletal injuries. Lacerations of arteries or fractures of the pelvis or femur can cause major bleeding. Unfortunately, that bleeding is often internal and may not be detectable upon physical examination until enough blood is lost for the patient to develop signs and symptoms of shock. (See Chapter 8.) Injuries to the nerves or the blood vessels that serve the hands and feet are common complications of fractures and dislocations. Such injuries cause the loss of function or sensation, which is included in the term *neurovascular compromise*, or **neurovascular injury**. Thus, evaluation of pulses, motor function, and sensation (PMS) distal to fractures is a very important component of the evaluation of the injured patient.

neurovascular injury: an injury that involves nerves and blood vessels. Also called *neurovascular compromise*.

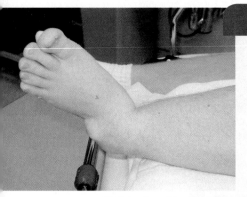

(Photo courtesy of Roy Alson, MD)

Case Presentation

Your EMS service has responded to a major-road traffic collision involving a truck, car, and motorcyclist. You are an emergency care provider on the second unit dispatched to the scene. The motorcyclist was critically injured and has already been transported to the hospital by the time you arrive. Hazards already controlled, the fire service officer directs you toward the sedan that was in the collision and has damage down the driver's side and a cracked windshield. The lead emergency care provider on your unit goes to assess the elderly woman who was the passenger in the front of the car and directs you to assess the driver. You note an older gentleman with a cervical collar that was placed by fire department personnel. He is cradling his left arm, is complaining of shoulder pain, and tells you he also has pain in his left ankle. You see that the airbag deployed during the incident and the windshield is cracked on the passenger side. The driver states he tried to stand but could not due to ankle pain.

Before proceeding, consider these questions: What should the emergency care provider do? What injuries should he suspect? What additional injuries might also have occurred? How should he assess and treat this patient? Keep these questions in mind as you read through the chapter. Then, at the end of the chapter, find out how the emergency care providers managed this patient.

Injuries to Extremities
Fractures

A fracture may be open, with the broken end of the bone still protruding or having once protruded through the skin, or it may be closed, with no communication to the outside (Figure 14-1). Fractured bone ends are extremely sharp and can cut the tissues that surround the bone. Because nerves, veins, and arteries frequently travel

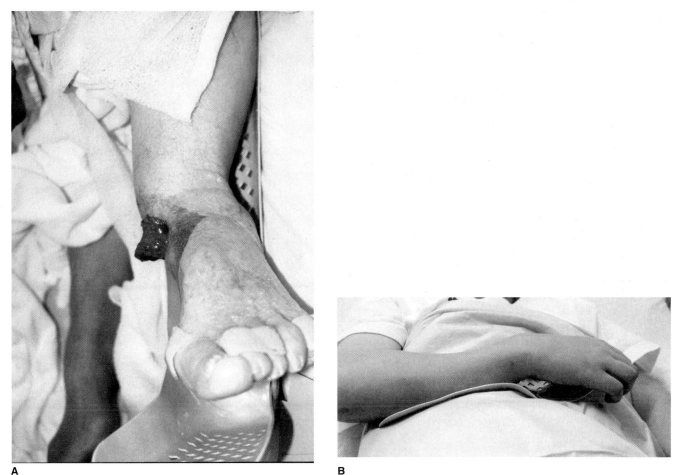

A   B

Figure 14-1 (A) Open ankle fracture. (B) Closed forearm fracture. (This is a good example of a Colles' fracture of the wrist, which can result from a fall on an outstretched hand.) *(Photos courtesy of Roy Alson, MD)*

either near the bone, generally across the flexor side of joints, or very near the skin (hands and feet), they are easily injured. Such neurovascular injuries may be due to direct injury from bone fragments, or the injuries may be indirect, from pressure due to swelling or hematoma following a fracture

A **closed fracture** can be just as dangerous as an **open fracture** because injured soft tissues often bleed profusely. It is important to remember that any break in the skin near a fractured bone may be considered an opening for contamination. All broken bones bleed, and a closed fracture of one femur can cause the loss of one to two liters (two to four units) of blood. Thus, bilateral femur fractures can cause life-threatening hemorrhage (Figure 14-2).

A fractured pelvis can cause extensive bleeding into the abdomen or the retroperitoneal space. An unstable pelvis is usually fractured in at least two places and may have caused more than one liter of associated blood loss (two units of blood). Depending on the location of the pelvic fracture, there may be associated injury to the urinary tract, bladder, or bowel. Posterior pelvic fractures or fracture-dislocations, which may include the sacroiliac joints, can damage the large pelvic blood vessels and result in massive retroperitoneal or intra-abdominal hemorrhage. Because of the significant force needed to fracture the pelvis, one-third of all patients with pelvic fractures have associated intra-abdominal injuries. Remember, multiple fractures can cause life-threatening hemorrhage without any external blood loss.

closed fracture: a break in a bone in which there is no break in the continuity of the overlying skin.

open fracture: a broken bone in which a piece of the bone is protruding or has protruded through the overlying skin.

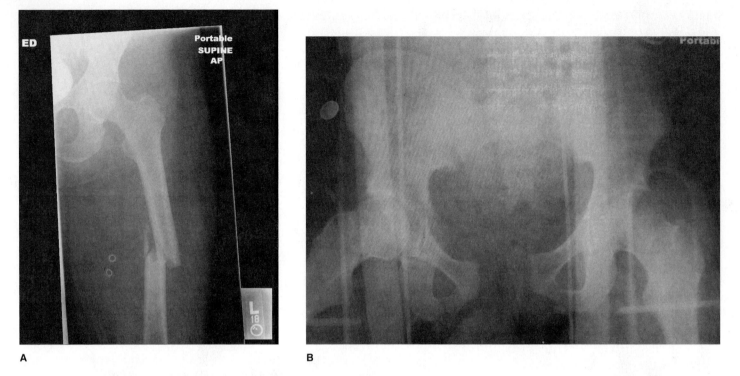

A

B

Figure 14-2 Internal blood loss from fractures. (A) May lose up to two units of blood from closed femur fracture. *(Photo © E.M. Singletary, MD)* (B) May lose two units up to complete blood volume in closed pelvic fractures. This pelvic fracture, although usually a closed fracture, is called an "open-book" fracture because the pelvic symphysis is pulled apart like an open book. *(Photo courtesy of Sabina Braithwaite, MD)*

joint dislocation: a complete disruption of a joint with total loss of contact between the joint's articular surfaces.

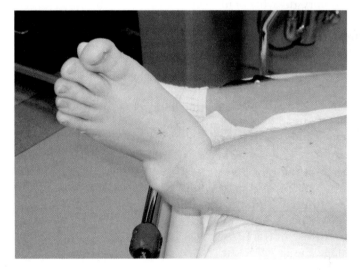

Figure 14-3 Ankle dislocation and fracture. Note tenting of the skin, which can become necrotic if the ankle is not promptly reduced. *(Photo courtesy of Roy Alson, MD)*

Open fractures add the dangers of wound contamination and subsequent infection to the risk of external hemorrhage. If protruding bone ends are pulled back into the skin when the limb is splinted, bacteria-contaminated debris will be introduced into the wound. Infection from such debris may slow or prevent healing of the bone. Be sure to notify the receiving hospital if there is a possibility of the fracture being open because the wound may be hidden by splints and dressings applied to stabilize the fracture.

Generally, fractures are quite painful. Once you have fully assessed and stabilized the patient, your management should include splinting of the fracture not only to avoid further injury, but also for patient comfort. Control of pain is an important part of emergency care. Unless there is a specific contraindication such as hypotension, you also should provide analgesic medication if your protocols and the patient's situation allow.

Dislocations

A **joint dislocation** is an extremely painful injury. It is generally easy to identify because normal joint anatomy is significantly distorted (Figure 14-3). Although major joint dislocations are not life threatening, they are still true emergencies because of the neurovascular compromise that can lead to significant disability and even amputation if not recognized and treated promptly. Because of this, it is critical to assess for pulses, motor function, and sensation (PMS) distal to major joint dislocations; to reassess following splinting, reduction, or movement; and to document your findings.

Ordinarily, dislocations and fractures should be splinted in the position in which they are found with adequate padding and stabilization. As with fractures, pain management should be considered for patients with dislocations, if that option is available. There are certain exceptions to the general rule of splinting injuries in the position found, including when loss of distal pulse is noted. In that case, especially if you have a long transport time to the appropriate hospital, gentle traction should be applied in an effort to bring the injured extremity into a more anatomic position and restore the distal pulse. Ideally, this should occur after administration of analgesics and/or sedation for the patient.

Open Wounds

If the initial assessment (C-ABC) of the ITLS Primary Survey shows exsanguinating bleeding, apply a tourniquet to the affected extremity immediately. Most bleeding can be controlled with direct pressure or pressure dressings. It is important to apply direct manual pressure on the site of the bleeding, not just the area of injury. However, if the patient has severe bleeding from an extremity injury and you cannot stop the bleeding with pressure dressings, you should not hesitate to use a tourniquet. If you have bleeding that cannot be stopped with pressure or with a tourniquet, such as injuries to the axilla, neck, or groin, you should use a hemostatic dressing or one of the newer junctional tourniquets, if available. (See Chapter 15.)

When used correctly, hemostatic agents or dressings in conjunction with direct pressure or tourniquets can be effective in stopping bleeding from penetration and laceration-type injuries. Note that hemostatic agents are not to be used in open abdominal or chest wounds, and some agents may require modification of the shape of the dressing to conform to the irregular shape of a wound. Patients with severe hemorrhage should be transported immediately after the ITLS Primary Survey. With obvious life-threatening hemorrhage, the order of the initial assessment changes to CABC (control bleeding, airway, breathing, and circulation). (See Chapter 2.) It is very rare for a tourniquet not to control severe bleeding. Consider application of a second tourniquet in this situation. Do not take the first tourniquet down to reapply.

For an open wound from a fracture, where bleeding is controlled, carefully cover it with a moist sterile dressing and bandage. Gross contamination, such as leaves or gravel, should be removed from the wound if possible. For patients with very long transport times, such as for a wilderness rescue, consider irrigation of the wound to remove smaller pieces of contamination, based on consultation with medical direction and local protocols. Perform this irrigation in the same manner you would irrigate a chemically contaminated eye.

Amputations

An **amputation** is a disabling and sometimes life-threatening injury that may present as a partial or complete loss of the body part. Although an amputation has the potential for massive hemorrhage, usually the bleeding can be controlled with direct pressure applied to the stump. The stump should be covered with a damp sterile dressing and an elastic wrap that will apply uniform, reasonable pressure across the entire stump. If life-threatening bleeding cannot be controlled with direct pressure, a tourniquet should be applied (Figure 14-4). A tourniquet can be life saving with this type of injury, when the proximal extremity is involved.

Make an effort to find the amputated part and bring it to the hospital with the patient. However, do so only as long as the patient is stable and there is no significant delay in transporting the patient. Bringing the amputated part is sometimes a neglected detail that can have serious future implications for the patient. It is difficult to determine in the field whether an amputated part can be replanted, revascularized, or used

amputation: an open injury caused by the cutting or tearing away of a limb, body part, or organ.

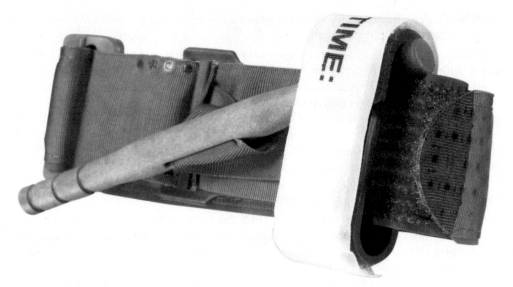

Figure 14-4 Combat application tourniquet (CAT). *(Photo courtesy of 2010 North American Rescue, LLC)*

for tissue grafting as part of the amputation repair. So, it is important to transport the amputated parts even if replantation seems impossible. Note, for example, that digits have been successfully replanted many hours following injury.

Small amputated parts should be rinsed off, wrapped in saline-moistened sterile gauze, and placed in a plastic bag (Figure 14-5). Label the bag with the patient's name, date, time the amputation happened, and time the part was wrapped and cooled. If ice is available, place the sealed bag in a larger bag or container containing ice and water. *Never* immerse the amputated part in water or saline or use ice directly on the amputated part, and never use dry ice. Cooling the part slows the chemical processes and will increase the part's viable time for replantation. Patients with amputations should be transported directly to a facility that has the ability to perform replantations when possible.

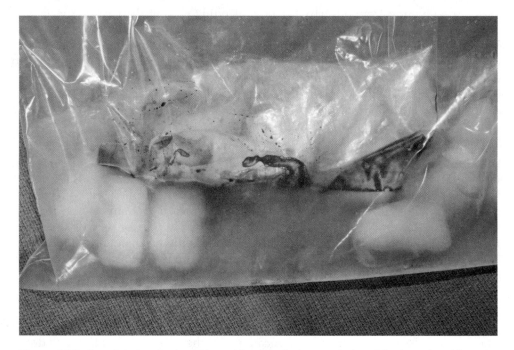

Figure 14-5 Amputated parts should be put in a plastic bag, sealed, and the bag placed in water that contains a few ice cubes. *(Photo courtesy of Stanley Cooper, EMT-P)*

Neurovascular Injuries

The nerves and major blood vessels generally run beside each other, usually in the flexor area of the major joints. They may be injured together, and loss of circulation or sensation can be due to disruption, swelling, or compression by bone fragments or hematomas. Foreign bodies or broken bone ends may well impinge on delicate structures and cause them to malfunction. Always check for distal pulses, motor function, and sensation before and after any extremity manipulation, application of a splint, or traction.

If there is loss of sensation or circulation in an extremity, the patient should be promptly transported to a hospital with emergency orthopedic care available. If extremity position is causing the deficit, you may or may not be able to correct it in the field. Generally, it is best to splint the injured limb in the position found if transport time is not prolonged. If splinting or traction has caused the deficit, then the splint or traction should be removed or repositioned until pulse is restored.

Sprains and Strains

A **sprain** is a stretching or tearing of ligaments of a joint because of a sudden twist. It will cause pain and swelling. In the field, sprains cannot be differentiated from a fracture, so they should be splinted as if they were fractures.

A **strain** is a stretching or tearing of a muscle or musculotendinous unit that will cause pain, and often, it will cause swelling. The injured limb should be splinted for comfort. Strains can usually (but not always) be differentiated from a fracture, but by splinting, you have protected the patient even if a fracture is present. Application of ice, if available, can reduce the swelling.

Impaled Objects

Do not remove objects impaled in extremities. The skin is a pivot point in these situations, and any motion of the **impaled object** outside the body is translated or magnified within the tissues, where the end of the object inside the body can lacerate or cause additional harm to sensitive structures. So, secure the object in place with bulky padding. Then transport the patient.

Note: Objects that obstruct the airway, such as those impaled in the neck or the cheek of the face, are exceptions and must be removed or the patient could die from airway loss or hypoxia. Removal of the object could cause severe hemorrhage, and careful pressure plus hemostatic agents may be needed to control it. Impaled objects in the cheek can be safely removed because you can apply pressure from both inside and outside the wound.

Compartment Syndrome

The extremities contain muscles and other structures surrounded by tough membranes, known as *fascia*. These membranes do not stretch, but instead create multiple closed spaces known as *compartments*. Crush injuries, as well as closed (and some open) fractures can cause bleeding and swelling. When this bleeding or swelling is contained within the muscle by the fascia, pressure in the compartments can rise. This results in what is called **compartment syndrome**.

Lower leg injuries have the greatest risk of developing compartment syndrome, although it can occur in the forearm, thigh, hand, and foot as well. As the injured area swells, pressure compresses all the structures within the compartment, including arteries, veins, nerves, and muscle. At a certain point, the pressure prevents venous return. Then, as pressure continues to increase, it cuts off arterial circulation. The nerves also are compromised by the effect of the pressure and the lack of blood flow.

Because these processes take some time, compartment syndrome does not present immediately, but tends to develop over several hours following the initial injury. It is very important if performing a transfer of a trauma patient between medical

---

PEARLS
Sprains and Strains

In the field, sprains cannot be differentiated from fractures. Treat them as though they were fractures. Strain injuries can usually be differentiated from factures, but may be splinted for comfort.

sprain: a sudden twist of a joint with stretching or tearing of ligaments.

strain: a stretching or partial tearing of a muscle or musculotendinous unit.

impaled object: an injury in which an object is embedded in the body tissue.

compartment syndrome: a condition in which increased tissue pressure in a muscle compartment results in decreased blood flow, leading to tissue hypoxia and possible muscle, nerve, and vessel impairment, and which can be permanent if the cells die.

facilities to perform the ITLS Ongoing Exam and assess distal neurovascular function. Elevation of the injured extremity and application of ice can be used to manage suspected compartment syndrome in the field. Adequate control of pain is an important part of care of compartment syndrome.

Late signs and symptoms of compartment syndrome are the "Five Ps": pain, pallor, pulselessness, paresthesia, and paralysis. The early symptoms are usually pain, typically described as pain out of proportion to the injury, and paresthesia (numbness and tingling). Treatment of compartment syndrome requires emergent surgical compartment decompression by a fasciotomy. As with shock, a high degree of suspicion is important. One should consider this diagnosis before the later symptoms develop and likely result in permanent damage.

Crush Injury and Crush Syndrome

Crushing injuries result from application of external force on the body. Crush injuries to the torso can cause traumatic asphyxia and death. Crush injuries to the extremities can cause direct damage to the tissues, especially muscles, and compromise circulation. The injured tissues swell, further decreasing perfusion. Because of poor perfusion and a lack of oxygen delivery, the tissues switch to anaerobic metabolism, which results in the buildup of toxic metabolites such as lactic acid. In addition, the damaged cells can leak potassium and myoglobin, a protein, from muscle. Most extremities can tolerate up to four hours of ischemia due to compromised flow before cell death occurs, though tissue injury can happen in as little as an hour of circulatory compromise.

When circulation is restored, those toxic products are carried throughout the body and affect many organ systems. This is known as crush syndrome. The heart pumps less effectively due to the acidosis and hyperkalemia, and the myoglobin, as it is filtered by the kidney, causes acute renal failure. Crush syndrome is a significant problem in earthquakes and other types of structural collapse events.

Management of crush syndrome is directed toward management of immediate life threats as identified in the ITLS Primary Survey followed by fluid resuscitation. The goal is to maintain urine output at 0.5 to 1.0 mL/kg body weight per hour. Alkalinization of the urine by administering intravenous sodium bicarbonate is believed to increase excretion of myoglobin and reduce risk of renal failure. If possible, fluid administration should begin before the patient is pulled from the collapsed structure.

Assessment and Management
Scene Size-up and History

When assessing the patient with extremity trauma, it is especially important to get a history because the mechanism of injury may not be apparent in your scene size-up. The mechanism of injury and your assessment of the extremity may give you important clues to the potential severity of the injury. If there are enough emergency care providers, one can obtain the history while you are performing the ITLS Primary Survey. If additional help is not available, you should *not* attempt to obtain a detailed history until you have assessed the status of the patient's airway, breathing, and circulation. For the conscious patient, obtain most of the history at the end of the ITLS Primary Survey.

Foot injuries from long jumps (falls landing on the feet) often have lumbar-spine injuries associated with them. Any injury to the knee, when the patient is in the sitting position, can have associated injuries to the hip. Similarly, hip injuries can refer pain to the knee. So the knee and the hip are intimately connected and must be evaluated together rather than separately.

Falls onto the wrist frequently injure the elbow, and so the wrist and elbow must be evaluated together. The same is true of the ankle and the proximal fibula of the outside of the lower leg. Shoulder pain may be from the joint itself or may be due to injury to the neck, chest, or even abdomen.

Fractures of the pelvis, which require a high-energy impact, are often associated with very large amounts of blood loss. Whenever a fracture in the pelvis is identified, shock must be suspected and proper treatment begun immediately.

Assessment

During the ITLS Primary Survey, focus on identifying immediate life threats as well as obvious fractures to the pelvis and large bones of the extremities. You should also find and control major external bleeding from the extremities.

During the ITLS Secondary Survey, quickly assess the full length of each extremity, looking for deformity, contusions, abrasions, penetrations, burns, tenderness, lacerations, and swelling (DCAP-BTLS). Feel for instability and **crepitation**. (See Chapters 2 and 3.) Check the joints for pain and spontaneous movement if there is no obvious deformity or pain. Check and record distal pulses, motor function, and sensation. Pulse location may be marked with a pen to identify the area where the distal pulse is best felt (Figure 14-6).

Crepitation or grating of bone ends is a definite sign of fracture. Once identified, the bone ends should be stabilized to prevent further soft-tissue injury. Checking for crepitation should be done very gently, especially when checking the pelvis, to avoid further injuries.

Management of Extremity Injuries

Proper management of fractures and dislocations will decrease the incidence of pain, disability, and serious complications. Treatment in the prehospital setting is directed at proper immobilization of the injured part by the use of an appropriate splint and

crepitation: the sound or feel of broken fragments of bone grinding against each other.

PEARLS
Priorities

- First assess and treat the ABCs and do not be distracted by obvious extremity trauma.

- Exsanguinating hemorrhage is the exception to the preceding point (follow CABC rather than ABC), but you must not forget to assess airway and breathing.

- Be alert to the mechanism of injury so that you know what fractures to suspect and so that you can predict possible complications.

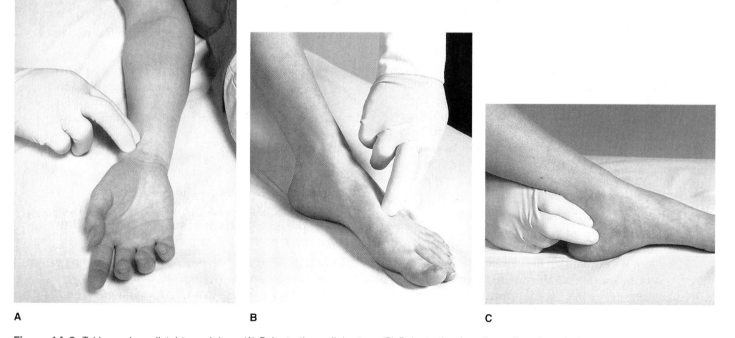

A   **B**   **C**

Figure 14-6 Taking pulses distal to an injury: (A) Palpate the radial artery. (B) Palpate the dorsalis pedis pulse. (C) Palpate the posterior tibial pulse. *(Photos courtesy of Michal Heron)*

padding. Pain control with appropriate analgesics is another major component of the care of injured extremities.

Purpose of Splinting

The objective of splinting is to prevent motion of the broken bone ends. The nerves that cause the most pain in a fractured extremity lie next to the bone. The broken bone can injure the nerves, causing very deep, severe pain. Splinting not only decreases pain, but also limits further damage to muscles, nerves, and blood vessels by preventing further motion of the broken bone ends.

When to Splint

There is no simple rule for splinting that determines the precise sequence to follow in every patient. For the multiple-trauma patient, extremity fractures can be temporarily stabilized by careful packaging on the long backboard for patients who require a load-and-go approach, with short transport times. This does not mean that you should *not* identify and protect extremity fractures. After priorities such as hemorrhage control and airway and shock management have been addressed and the patient has been packaged on the transport stretcher, perform additional splinting en route to the hospital. It is never appropriate to spend time splinting a limb to prevent disability when that time may be needed to save the patient's life. Conversely, if the patient appears to be stable, extremity fractures should be splinted before moving the patient for all the reasons noted earlier.

PEARLS
The Golden Period

- Do not waste the Golden Period. Be cautious but be rapid, and prioritize life over limb.
- Splint at an appropriate time. The axial skeleton is splinted after the ITLS Primary Survey. If a critical situation exists, extremities should be splinted en route if time allows.

PEARLS
Pulses, Motor Function, Sensation

Always assess and record distal pulses, motor response, and sensation initially and after any manipulation, particularly splinting.

Procedure

Rules of Splinting

1. You must adequately expose the injured part. Clothing should be removed, preferably by cutting it off, to allow adequate assessment of the injury and proper immobilization.

2. Check and record distal pulses, motor function, and sensation before and after splinting. To check motor function distal to the fracture, ask the conscious patient to wiggle his fingers and toes, or you can observe motion in an unconscious patient when a painful stimulus is applied. Pulses may be marked with a pen to identify where they were palpated.

3. If the extremity is severely angulated, pulses are absent, and you have a long transport to the appropriate hospital, apply gentle traction in an attempt to straighten the extremity (Figure 14-7). If you encounter significant resistance, splint the extremity in the position found. When you are attempting to straighten an extremity, it is very important to be honest with yourself with regard to resistance. It takes very little force to lacerate the wall of a vessel or to interrupt the blood supply to a large nerve. If the appropriate hospital is near, it is probably best to splint in the position found.

4. Open wounds should be covered with a moist sterile dressing before you apply the splint. Whenever possible, splints should be applied on the side of the extremity away from any open wounds. At the hospital, notify the staff of any open wounds.

5. Use a splint that will immobilize one joint above and one joint below the injury site.

6. Pad the splint well. This is particularly true if there is any skin defect or if bony prominences might press against a hard splint and cause additional pain or injury to the skin.

7. Do not attempt to push bone ends back under the skin. If you apply traction and the bone end retracts back into the wound, do not increase the amount of traction. Do not try to pull the bone ends back out. It is important to be sure to notify the receiving physician that the bone ends were visible. Carefully cover bone ends with moist

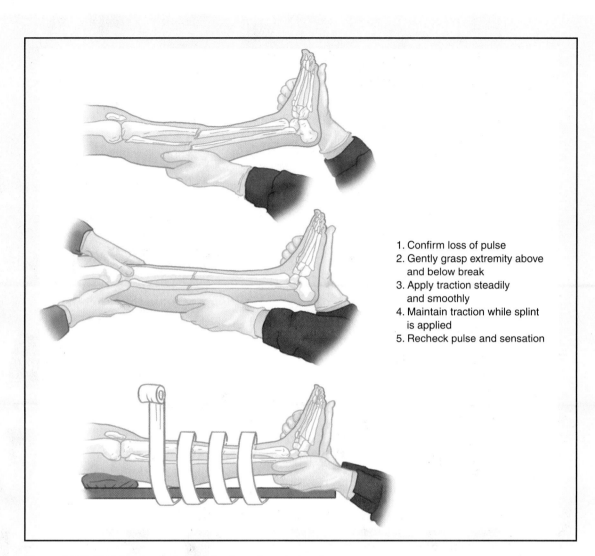

1. Confirm loss of pulse
2. Gently grasp extremity above and below break
3. Apply traction steadily and smoothly
4. Maintain traction while splint is applied
5. Recheck pulse and sensation

Figure 14-7 Straightening angulated fractures to restore pulses.

sterile bandages. If transport is prolonged, this will help improve bone healing.

8. In a life-threatening situation, injuries may be splinted while the patient is being transported.

When the patient appears stable, splint fractures or deformities before moving him or her.

9. If in doubt, splint a possible injury.

Types of Splints

For examples of splinting extremities, please see Figure 14-8.

Rigid Splints Rigid splints can be made from many different materials. They can be made of cardboard, hard plastic, metal, or wood. The type of splint that is made rigid by evacuating air from a moldable splint (vacuum splint) is also classified as a rigid splint. Rigid splints should be well padded over bony prominences and should always immobilize one joint above and one joint below the fracture.

Soft Splints Soft splints include pillows, sling and swath-type splints, and air splints. Pillows make good splints for injuries to the ankle or foot, providing immobilization

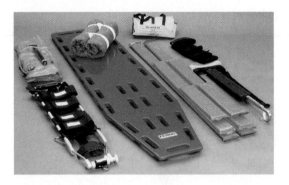

Figure 14-8a Splinting materials.

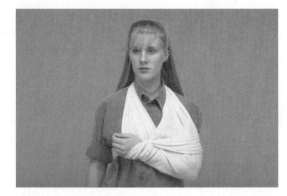

Figure 14-8b Sling and swathe.

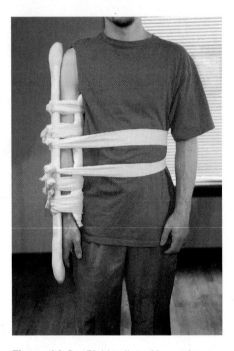

Figure 14-8c Rigid splint with swathes.

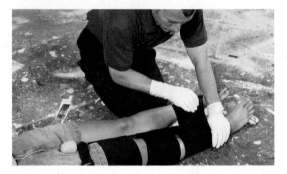

Figure 14-8d Traction splint.

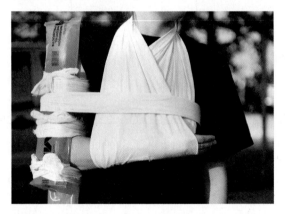

Figure 14-8f Fixation or rigid splint with a sling and swathe.

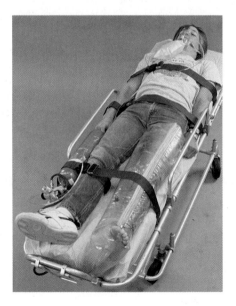

Figure 14-8e Air splint.

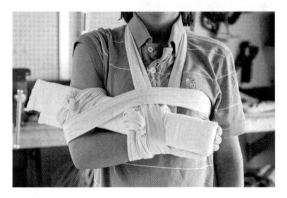

Figure 14-8g Injured elbow immobilized in a bent position.

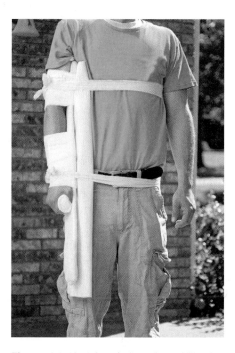

Figure 14-8h Injured elbow immobilized in a straight position.

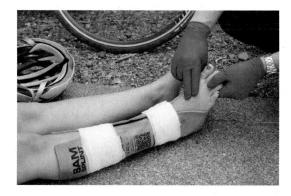

Figure 14-8j Immobilization of an injury to lower leg with SAM splint.

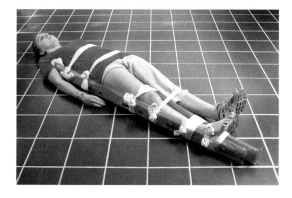

Figure 14-8l A high femur fracture immobilized in a fixation splint.

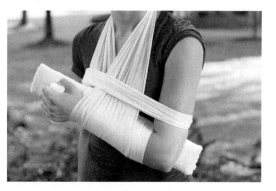

Figure 14-8i Immobilization of an injury to the forearm, wrist, or hand.

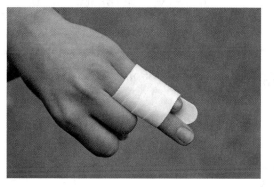

Figure 14-8k A tongue depressor used as a splint and then taped to an adjoining finger for stabilization.

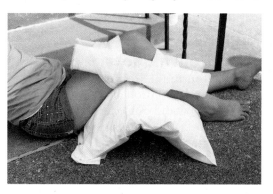

Figure 14-8m A splinted knee.

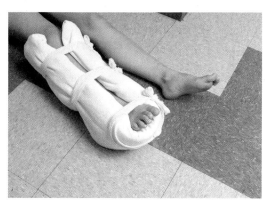

Figure 14-8n Blanket roll splint of the ankle and foot.

as well as padding to the injured area. Used with a sling and a swathe, they are useful for stabilizing a dislocated shoulder.

The sling and swathe are excellent for immobilizing injuries to the clavicle, shoulder, upper arm, elbow, and sometimes the forearm. They utilize the chest wall as a solid foundation and splint the arm against it. Some shoulder injuries cannot be brought close to the chest wall without applying significant force. In those instances, pillows are used to bridge the gap between the chest wall and the upper arm.

Air splints may be useful for fractures of the lower arm and lower leg. They are light and easily carried. They provide compression, which helps to slow bleeding. Disadvantages include increasing pressure as the temperature rises or the altitude increases, inability to monitor distal pulses, and potential pain with removal. They should not be used on angulated fractures because they apply straightening pressure as they are inflated.

To apply an air splint it must be inflated by mouth or by pump (never by compressed air) until it provides good support, yet is still able to be dented easily with slight pressure from a fingertip. When using air splints, you must frequently check the pressure to be sure the splint is not getting too tight or too loose. (They often leak.)

Traction Splints The traction splint is designed to stabilize fractures of the midfemur. They should not be used in hip fractures or if there is more than one fracture in the lower extremity. The traction splint holds the fracture immobile by application of a steady pull on the ankle while applying countertraction to the ischium and the groin. This steady traction overcomes the tendency of the very strong thigh muscles to spasm. If traction is not applied, the pain worsens because the bone ends tend to impact or override. Traction also prevents free motion of the ends of the femur, which could lacerate the femoral nerve, artery, or vein.

There are many designs and types of splints available to apply traction to the lower extremity (Figure 14-9). Several of them are reviewed in Chapter 15. As with other splints, traction splints must be carefully padded and applied with care to prevent excessive pressure on the soft tissues around the pelvis.

PEARLS
Shock

Be prepared for hemorrhagic shock when there is a pelvic or femur fracture.

Tourniquets

Tourniquets have returned to common use in both the military and tactical settings for uncontrollable extremity hemorrhage. They have been shown to improve survival and outcomes in those settings and are regaining acceptance in civilian use as well. Tourniquet use has been shown to be life saving in patients with shock due to massive blood loss from extremity injuries, allowing for circulatory resuscitation. There is a potential for ischemic injury if a tourniquet is left on too long, but that risk must be balanced against the tourniquet's ability to stop life-threatening hemorrhage. Ideally, tourniquets should not be used for longer than two to four hours. Complications can increase if left on longer. The ability to salvage the injured limb also decreases with long periods of ischemia (no blood flow).

Recommended indications for tourniquet use include significant extremity bleeding together with other ITLS Primary Survey issues (such as the need for airway or breathing intervention or shock), hostile environment, a mass-casualty event, or the inability to manage bleeding with pressure dressings. In general, you should not remove a tourniquet you have placed for the indications noted.

Follow the specific guidelines for the commercial tourniquet you are using. One of the most important factors is to ensure that all providers are aware that a tourniquet has been applied to the patient. One method is to write "TK" and the time of application on the patient's forehead. Never cover a tourniquet. Commercial tourniquets are preferable to improvised tourniquets because their design better distributes the pressure and limits damage to the tissues. Once you have placed a tourniquet, you should expedite transport to the trauma center.

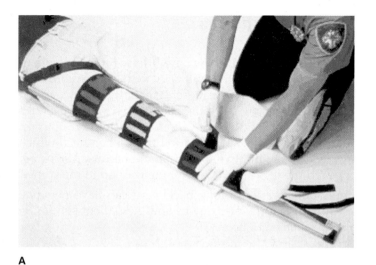

A

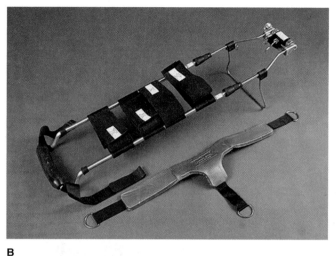

B

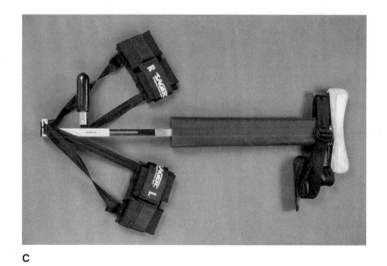

C

Figure 14-9 (A) Kendrick traction device. *(Photo courtesy of Eduardo Romero Hicks, MD)* (B) Hare traction splint. (C) Sager traction splint. Caution: Traction splints should not be used if pelvic fracture is suspected.

Hemostatic Agents

For bleeding that is uncontrollable with direct pressure or the use of tourniquets, hemostatic agents have demonstrated the ability to reduce or stop bleeding through the promotion of clot formation. The form of hemostatic agent available (dressing, powder, packets, and so on) depends on the specific product used. Regardless, direct application and pressure to the source of the bleeding vessel, not just the area of the wound, is required to maximize effectiveness of hemostatic agents. Powder agents are more difficult to use versus impregnated gauze or dressing. There have been reports of increased systemic thrombus formation with use of powdered agents.

Direct pressure should be maintained for a minimum of four minutes or until bleeding is controlled. Following cessation of bleeding, the application of a pressure dressing or gauze to the wound is recommended. To maximize effectiveness, it is recommended that prior to using a hemostatic agent, EMS personnel should become familiar with and follow the application instructions for each type of product used in practice.

Management of Specific Injuries
Spine Injuries

Spine injuries are covered in Chapters 11 and 12. They are briefly included here to remind you that when there are findings to suggest an injury to the spinal cord, spinal motion restriction (SMR) must be used to prevent permanent disability or even death. In the most urgent cases, careful packaging of the patient on a long backboard can provide adequate splinting for a number of different extremity injuries. Remember that certain mechanisms of injury, such as a fall from a height in which the patient lands on both feet, can cause lumbar-spine fracture because forces are transmitted from the heels through the legs and pelvis, all the way up to the spine.

Remember that prolonged immobilization on a long backboard can have negative effects on the patient. The backboard is a transfer device and the patient should be removed as soon as it is safe and practical to do so.

Pelvis Injuries

It is practical to include injuries to the pelvis with extremities because they are frequently associated. Pelvic injuries are usually caused by motor-vehicle collisions or by severe trauma such as falls from heights. They are identified by instability or pain in response to gentle pressure on the iliac crests, hips, and pubis during the ITLS Primary Survey. There is always the potential for serious hemorrhage in pelvic fractures, so shock should be expected, and the patient must be rapidly transported (load and go). Presence of a pelvic fracture suggests that the patient has sustained a high-force injury.

Internal bleeding from unstable pelvic fractures can be decreased by circumferential stabilization of the pelvis. Slings made from sheets have been used in the past for stabilization, but there are now several commercially available devices that provide more consistent stabilization (Figure 14-10). Pelvic stabilization is most beneficial in an **open-book pelvic fracture** (Figure 14-2b) and decreases the need for blood transfusion. Pelvic slings should be applied such that their compressive force is at the level of the greater trochanters and not the iliac crests.

Any patient with a pelvic injury should be evaluated for spine injuries. If SMR is indicated, the vacuum mattress is useful because it is much more comfortable than the hard backboard.

open-book pelvic fracture: a severe pelvic fracture in which the symphysis is torn apart and the anterior pelvis is "opened" like a book. This is frequently associated with disruption of both sacroiliac joints.

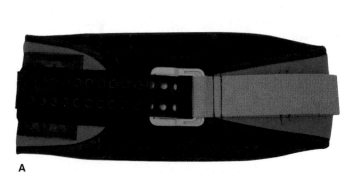

A

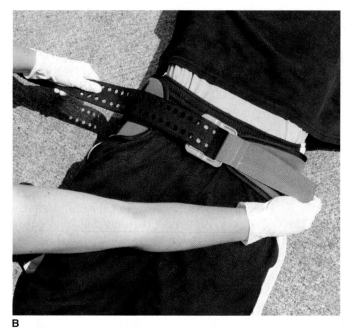

B

Figure 14-10 (A) Commercial pelvic sling device. (B) Pelvic sling applied. *(Photos courtesy of SAM Splint)*

Log rolling a patient with an unstable pelvic fracture can aggravate the injury. Adequate assistance and a tool such as the scoop stretcher are useful to move patients to the ambulance stretcher because they will limit motion of the fractured pelvis and associated pain. As mentioned in Chapter 2, some of the new, more rigid scoop stretchers provide SMR equal to a backboard (Figure 14-11).

Femur Injuries

Femur fractures may have associated open wounds, and if so, they must be presumed to be open fractures. There is a lot of muscle tissue surrounding the femur, and when spasm develops after a femur fracture, it can cause the bone ends to override, causing more muscle damage, bleeding, potential nerve damage, and significant pain. Because of this, traction splints are usually used to stabilize midshaft femur fractures and limit additional injury and pain. As mentioned earlier, the large size of the thigh muscle can hide one to two liters of blood loss with each femur fracture. Bilateral femur fractures can be associated with a loss of up to 50% of the circulating blood volume.

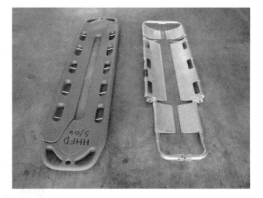

Figure 14-11 The scoop stretcher has been found to provide spinal stabilization equal to a backboard. *(Photo courtesy of Leon Charpentier, EMT-P; and Ferno Washington, Inc.)*

Hip Injuries

Hip fractures are most often in the narrow "neck" of the femur, where strong ligaments occasionally allow this type of fracture to bear weight. The ligaments are very strong, and there is very little movement of the bone ends in the most frequent type of hip fracture. You must consider hip fractures in any elderly person who fell and now has pain in the knee, hip, or pelvic region. A geriatric patient who fell and cannot bear weight should be assumed to have a pelvic or hip fracture. The affected leg will often (but not always) be externally rotated and shortened. In the geriatric patient, fracture pain may be well tolerated and sometimes even ignored or denied. In general, the tissues in the elderly patient are more delicate, and less force is required to disrupt a given structure. Remember that isolated knee pain may well be coming from damage to the hip. Do not use a traction splint for a hip fracture.

The hip may be dislocated either posteriorly or anteriorly. Posterior hip dislocations are most common and can result when the knee is struck by a dashboard, forcing the relatively loose, relaxed hip out of the posterior side of its cup in the pelvis (Figure 14-12). Thus, any patient in a severe automobile crash with a knee injury must have the hip examined very carefully. Posterior hip dislocation is an orthopedic emergency and requires reduction as soon as possible to prevent sciatic nerve injury or necrosis of the femoral head due to interrupted blood supply. Patients with prosthetic hips can dislocate a hip without large forces being applied.

The posteriorly dislocated hip usually is flexed, and the patient will not be able to tolerate having the leg straightened. The leg will almost invariably be rotated toward the midline. A posterior hip dislocation should be supported in the most comfortable position by the use of pillows and by splinting to the uninjured leg (Figure 14-13).

An anterior hip dislocation is rare because of the complex mechanism required to produce it. The patient with an anterior hip dislocation will present with external rotation of the affected leg, much like a fractured hip, except you may not be able to bring the leg forward in line with the body. It may be very difficult to place this person in the supine position on a backboard or on the stretcher in the ambulance. Whereas the posterior hip dislocation puts pressure on the sciatic nerve, the anterior hip dislocation puts pressure on the femoral artery and vein. If the vein has collapsed, a clot can form distally, producing a large pulmonary embolus as soon as the hip is reduced.

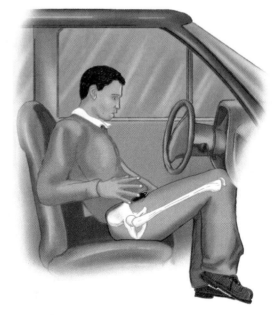

Figure 14-12 Mechanism of posterior dislocation of the hip, "down and under."

Figure 14-13 Splinting posterior dislocation of the hip. *(Photo courtesy of Louis B. Mallory, MBA, REMT-P)*

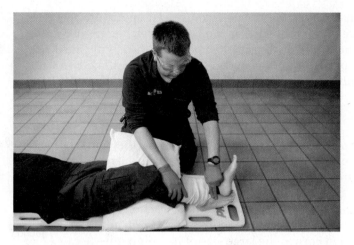

Knee Injuries

Fractures or dislocations of the knee (Figure 14-14) are quite serious because the blood vessels and nerves that cross the knee joint are often injured if the joint is in an abnormal position. There is no way to know whether a fracture exists in an abnormally positioned knee and, in either case, the decision must be based on the circulation and neurologic function distally in the foot.

A significant number of knee dislocations have associated artery and nerve injury. It is important to restore the circulation below the knee as quickly as possible and to transport the patient rapidly to definitive care to avoid devastating complications such as amputation. Because of this, prompt reduction of knee dislocation is very important. If there is loss of pulse or sensation, apply gentle traction by hand. Traction must be applied along the long axis of the leg. If there is resistance to straightening the knee, splint it in the most comfortable position and transport the patient rapidly. Knee dislocation is an orthopedic emergency.

Do not confuse knee joint dislocation with patellar dislocation. The patella can dislocate to the side, and the affected leg will be held slightly flexed at the knee. You can easily see that the patella is out of place. Although painful, this is not a serious injury and should simply be splinted with a pillow under the knee and the patient taken to the emergency department. Straightening the leg often reduces the patella dislocation, and often the patient will spontaneously reduce this injury prior to your arrival.

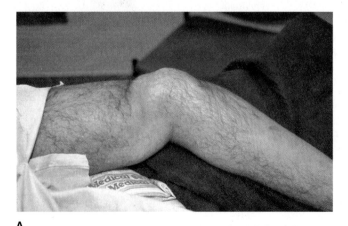

A

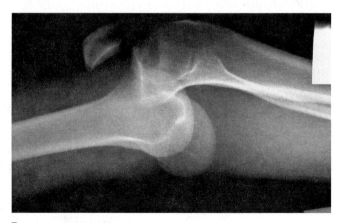

B

Figure 14-14 Knee dislocation. (A) Presentation of a knee dislocation. (B) X-ray of the dislocation. *(Photos © Edward T. Dickinson, MD)*

Tibia and Fibula Injuries

Fractures of the lower leg are common injuries. Over time, swelling and internal hemorrhage can cause compartment syndrome. It is rarely possible for patients to bear weight on fractures of the tibia, but fractures of the distal fibula can be mistaken for sprains. Fractures of the lower leg and ankle may be splinted with a rigid splint, an air splint, or a pillow. As with other fractures, it is important to dress any wound, pad any exposed bone ends under a splint, and manage the patient's pain. A dislocation of the ankle may require a gentle attempt at reduction if there is loss of circulation in the foot and you have a very long transport. Elevate the extremity to reduce risk of developing compartment syndrome

Clavicle Injuries

The clavicle is the most frequently fractured bone in the body, with injury most common in the middle third of the bone. Clavicular injuries rarely cause major complications (Figure 14-15). Occasionally, there may be associated injuries to the subclavian blood vessels or to the nerves of the arm. You should carefully assess a patient with a clavicle fracture for other, more significant, chest wall injuries. This injury is best immobilized with a sling and swathe.

Shoulder Injuries

Most shoulder injuries are not life threatening, but because of the force required, they may be associated with severe injuries of the chest or neck. Many shoulder injuries are dislocations or separations of the shoulder from the clavicle and may appear as a defect at the upper outer portion of the shoulder. The upper humerus is fractured with some degree of frequency, however. The radial nerve travels quite closely

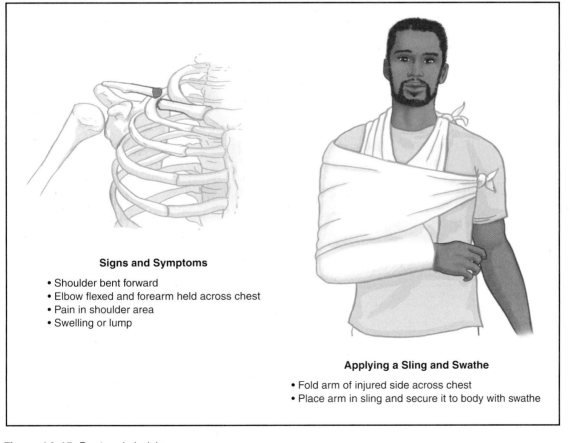

Signs and Symptoms

- Shoulder bent forward
- Elbow flexed and forearm held across chest
- Pain in shoulder area
- Swelling or lump

Applying a Sling and Swathe

- Fold arm of injured side across chest
- Place arm in sling and secure it to body with swathe

Figure 14-15 Fractured clavicle.

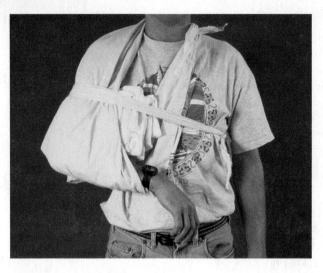

Figure 14-16 Dislocated shoulder.

around the humerus and may be injured in humeral fractures. Injury to the radial nerve results in an inability of the patient to lift the hand (wrist drop).

Dislocated shoulders are very painful and quite often require a pillow between the arm and body to hold the upper arm in the most comfortable position. Shoulders that are held in abnormal positions should never be forced into a more anatomic alignment (Figure 14-16). Scapular fractures may refer pain to the shoulder joint itself. Because considerable force is required to fracture the scapula, if you suspect it, carefully evaluate the patient for other chest injuries such as rib fractures and pulmonary contusion.

Elbow Injuries

It may be difficult to see the difference between a fracture and a dislocation. Both can be serious because of the danger of damage to the vessels and nerves that run across the flexor surface of the elbow. The most common mechanism of injury is a fall onto an outstretched arm, fracturing the radial head. Elbow injuries should always be splinted in the most comfortable position and the distal function clearly evaluated (Figure 14-17). Never attempt to straighten or apply traction to an elbow injury due to the complexity of the anatomy. Transport these patients promptly.

Forearm and Wrist Injuries

Fractures to the forearm and wrist are very common (Figure 14-18). Like elbow injuries, a common mechanism is a fall onto an outstretched arm. Usually, such a fracture

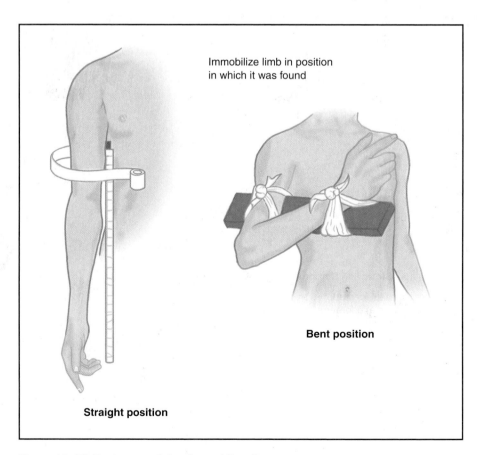

Immobilize limb in position in which it was found

Bent position

Straight position

Figure 14-17 Fractures or dislocations of the elbow.

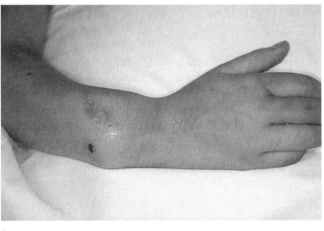

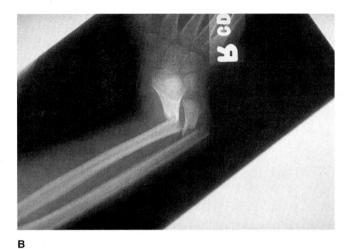

A   **B**

Figure 14-18 Presentation of a forearm fracture. (A) A fracture will often present with deformity. (B) An x-ray of the fracture.

is best immobilized with a rigid splint or an air splint (Figure 14-19). If a rigid splint is used, a roll of gauze in the hand will allow the hand and arm to be splinted in the position of function, which is often the most comfortable. Forearm fractures also put the patient at risk for compartment syndrome, so monitor closely.

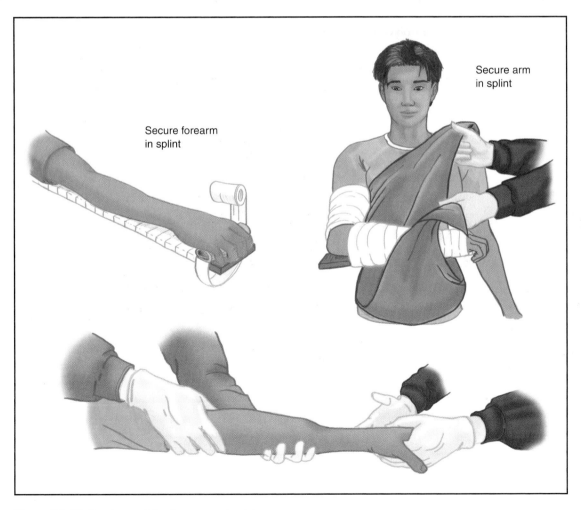

Secure arm in splint

Secure forearm in splint

Figure 14-19 Fractures of the forearm and wrist.

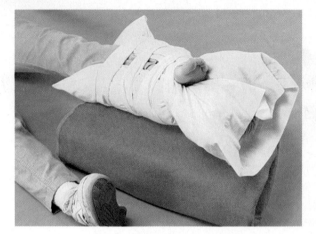

Figure 14-20 Pillow splinting an injured foot.

Hand or Foot Injuries

Many industrial accidents involving the hand or the foot produce multiple open fractures and avulsions. The injuries are often gruesome in appearance but are seldom associated with life-threatening bleeding. A pillow may be used very effectively to support them (Figure 14-20). An alternative method of dressing the hand is to insert a roll of gauze in the palm, then arrange the fingers and thumb in their position of function. The entire hand is then wrapped as though it were a ball inside a very large and bulky dressing (Figure 14-21).

Crush Injuries

Performing frequent ongoing assessments and close monitoring of vital signs is required for patients with a crush injury. To effectively address the toxins released and reduce the risk of developing crush syndrome, aggressive hydration with normal saline is required. Avoid Ringer's lactate because it contains potassium. In addition, alkalizing agents such as sodium bicarbonate and osmotic diuretics such as mannitol can increase urine flow through the kidneys and reduce the risk of renal failure. The addition of sodium bicarbonate (3 × 50 mEq ampules) to a one liter bag of 5% dextrose (D_5W) will make a nearly isotonic solution.

Initial administration of sodium bicarbonate should be at 1 mEq/kg bolus followed by an infusion of 0.25 mEq/kg body weight per hour of the solution described earlier. If administration of fluids or medications prior to releasing the entrapped body area is not possible, consider application of a tourniquet proximal to the injury site on the extremity. Although application of the tourniquet will reduce systemic toxin release, crush syndrome will continue to develop. Early contact with medical direction or the receiving trauma facility is recommended for all patients who have experienced a crush injury.

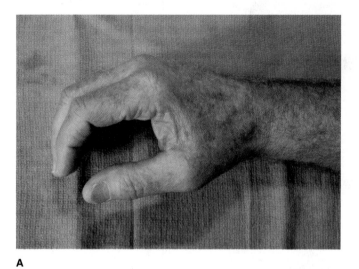

A

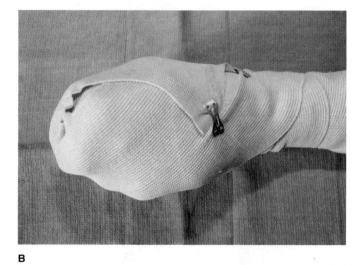

B

Figure 14-21 (A) Hand in position of function. (B) Hand dressing. *(Photos courtesy of Stanley Cooper, EMT-P)*

Case Presentation *(continued)*

The emergency care provider performs an initial assessment on the driver, which reveals an alert elderly male, who is anxious about his wife, not to mention his soon-to-arrive daughter, but without respiratory distress, and with a strong radial pulse of 96. His color is good, his head and neck are unremarkable, his chest is unmarked and his breath sounds clear and equal. His abdomen is soft and nontender and his pelvis apparently stable. His left ankle is swollen and rotated inward. The provider removes the shoes and finds pedal pulses are present in both feet. The patient's left wrist is swollen, and his distal radius and ulna are tender to palpation. His left radial pulse is difficult to palpate, but his capillary refill time (CRT) is less than two seconds and sensation is intact.

You decide that with no loss of consciousness, a normal neurological exam, and no neck pain that SMR is not needed. The emergency care provider splints the left arm from above the elbow to the hand, leaving only the fingers exposed, and adds a sling and swath. He then pillow-splints the left ankle. After re-checking distal circulation and finding pedal pulses present and capillary refill time in the fingers unchanged, the patient is placed on a stretcher to transfer him to the ambulance, where he will be placed on the squad bench with his left foot elevated. The other providers have been caring for the female passenger and after she is loaded into the ambulance, they depart for the hospital.

Summary

Although usually not life threatening, extremity injuries can be disabling. These injuries can be more dramatic than more serious internal injuries, but do not let them distract you from following the usual steps of the ITLS Primary Survey. Keep in mind that unstable pelvic fractures and femur fractures can be associated with life-threatening internal bleeding, so patients with these injuries are in the load-and-go category. Both of these injuries are considered high-force injuries.

Proper splinting is important to protect the injured extremity from further injury. Dislocations of elbows, hips, and knees require careful splinting and rapid reduction to prevent severe disability. They are frequently load-and-go situations, not because they are life threatening, but because they are limb threatening. Assessment of the neurovascular function distal to the injury should always be performed and the fracture or dislocation realigned if there is as loss of pulses distal. A high index of suspicion and early intervention for crush injuries are paramount to reducing the harmful effects of crush syndrome.

Bibliography

Abarbanell, N. R. "Prehospital Midthigh Trauma and Traction Splint Use: Recommendations for Treatment Protocols." *American Journal of Emergency Medicine* 19, no. 2 (March 2001): 137–40.

Baek, S. M., and S. S. Kim. "Successful Digital Replantation After 42 Hours of Warm Ischemia." *Journal of Reconstructive Microsurgery* 8, no. 6 (November 1992): 455–58.

Brown, D. M., and J. Worley. "Experience with Chitosan Dressings in a Civilian EMS System." *Journal of Emergency Medicine* 37, no. 1 (2009): 1–7.

Bledsoe, B. E., R. S. Porter, and R. A. Cherry. *Paramedic Care: Principles and Practice*, 4th ed. Vol. 7, 223-75. Upper Saddle River, NJ: Pearson Education, 2012.

Bledsoe, B., and D. Barnes. "Traction Splint: An EMS Relic?" *Journal of Emergency Medical Services (JEMS)* 29, no. 8 (August 2004): 64–69.

Brodie, S., T. J. Hodgetts, J. Ollerton, J. McLeod, P. Lambert, and P. Mahoney. "Tourniquet Use in Combat Trauma: UK Military Experience." *Journal of the Royal Army Medical Corps* 153, no. 4 (December 2007): 310–13.

Centers for Disease Control and Prevention. "CDC Offers Primer on Blast Injury." *Journal of the American Medical Association (JAMA)* 309, no. 20 (2013): 2088.

Chudnofsky, C. R. "Splinting Techniques." In *Clinical Procedures in Emergency Medicine,* 6th ed., edited by J.R. Roberts, 999-1027. Philadelphia: Saunders, 2013.

Committee on Trauma, American College of Surgeons. "Musculoskeletal Trauma." In *Advanced Trauma Life Support,* 9th ed., 206–223. Chicago: American College of Surgeons, 2012.

Cross, D. A., and J. Baskerville. "Comparison of Perceived Pain with Different Immobilization Techniques." *Prehospital Emergency Care* 5, no. 3 (July–September 2001): 270–74.

Dayan, L., C. Zinmann, S. Stahl, and D. Norman. "Complications Associated with Prolonged Tourniquet Application on the Battlefield." *Military Medicine* 173, no. 1 (January 2008): 63–66.

Demetriades, D., M. Karaiskakis, K. Toutouzas, K. Alo, G. Velmahos, and L. Chan. "Pelvic Fractures: Epidemiology and Predictors of Associated Abdominal Injuries and Outcomes." *Journal of the American College of Surgeons* 195, no. 1 (July 2002): 1–10.

Dischinger, P. C., K. M. Read, J. A. Kufera, T. J. Kerns, C. A. Burch, N. Jawed, and S. M. Ho. "Consequences and Costs of Lower Extremity Injuries." *Annual Proceedings of the Association for the Advancement of Automotive Medicine* 48 (2004): 339–53.

Doyle, G. S., and P. P. Taillac. "Tourniquets: A Review of Current Use with Proposals for Expanded Prehospital Use." *Prehospital Emergency Care* 12, no. 2 (April–June 2008): 241–56.

Friese, G., and G. LaMay. " Emergency Stabilization of Unstable Pelvic Fractures." *Emergency Medical Services* 34, no. 5 (May 2005): 65, 67–71.

Granville-Chapman, J., and J. N. Midwinter. "Pre-hospital Haemostatic Dressings: A Systemic Review." *Injury* 42, no. 5 (2011): 447–559.

Greaves, I., K. Porter, and J. E. Smith. "Consensus Statement on the Early Management of Crush Injury and Prevention of Crush Syndrome." *Journal of the Royal Army Medical Corps* 149, no. 4 (December 2003): 255–59.

Heightman, A. "Out of Sight, Out of Mind: A Dangerous Practice." *Journal of Emergency Medical Services (JEMS)* 31, no. 7 (2006): 14–17.

Krell, J. M., M. S. McCoy, P. J. Sparto, G. L. Fisher, W. A. Stoy, and D. P. Hostler. "Comparison of the Ferno Scoop Stretcher with the Long Backboard for Spinal Immobilization." *Prehospital Emergency Care* 10, no. 1 (January–March 2006): 46–51.

Lee, C., K. M. Porter, and T. J. Hodgett. "Tourniquet Use in the Civilian Prehospital Setting." *Emergency Medicine Journal* 24, no. 8 (August 2007): 584–87.

Sever, M. S., R. Vanholder, and N. Lameire. "Management of Crush-Related Injuries After Disasters." *New England Journal of Medicine* 354, no. 10 (March 9, 2006): 1052–63.

Walters, T. J., and R. I. Mabry. "Issues Related to the Use of Tourniquets on the Battlefield." *Military Medicine* 170, no. 9 (September 2005): 770–75.

Wedmore, I., J. G. McManus, A. E. Pusateri, and J. E. Holcomb. "A Special Report on the Chitosan-Based Hemostatic Dressing: Experience in Current Combat Operations." *Journal of Trauma* 60, no. 3 (March 2006): 655–58.

Get more information about this course by calling
ITLS International at 888-495-4875
(outside the United States call +1-630-495-6442) or visit

www.itrauma.org

Extremity Trauma Skills

S. Robert Seitz, MEd, RN, NRP
Darby L. Copeland, EdD, RN, NRP

Trauma alle Estremità	Traumatismo de Extremidades
Traumatisme d'extrémité	Obrażenia kończyn Extremitäten Trauma
Ozljede ekstremiteta	إصابات الأطراف trauma ekstremiteta
Poškodbe okončin	Végtagsérülés

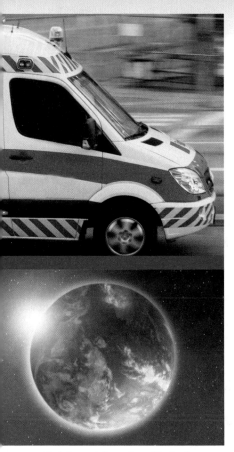

(Ambulance photo courtesy of Regien Paassen, Shutterstock.com)

Objectives

Upon successful completion of this chapter, you should be able to:

1. Explain when to use a traction splint.
2. Describe the complications of using a traction splint.
3. Apply the most common traction splints: Hare splint, Sager splint, and Thomas splint.
4. Demonstrate pelvic stabilization techniques.
5. Explain the use of and demonstrate the application of tourniquets on a mannequin model.
6. Explain the use of and demonstrate the application of hemostatic agents on a mannequin model.

Traction Splints

Traction splints are designed to immobilize fractures of the femur. They are not useful for fractures of the hip, knee, or lower leg. Applying firm traction to a fractured or dislocated knee may tear the blood vessels behind the knee. If there appears to be a pelvic fracture, do not use a traction splint because it can cause further damage to the pelvis. Fractures below the midthigh that are not angulated or severely shortened may be immobilized with rigid or air splints.

A traction splint works by applying linear forces along the bone to keep ends immobilized. A padded device is first applied to the back of the pelvis (ischium) or to the groin, and a hitching device is applied to the ankle. The splint then applies countertraction until the limb is straight and well immobilized. Apply the splint to the pelvis and groin very carefully to prevent excessive pressure on the genitalia. Also use care when attaching the hitching device to the foot and ankle so as not to interfere with circulation. Because you must always check distal pulses when you finish splinting, remember to remove the patient's shoe before attaching the hitching device.

In every case at least two people are needed to apply traction. One must hold steady, gentle traction on the foot and leg while the other applies the splint. When dealing with load-and-go situations, do not apply the splint until critical life-saving interventions have been completed and the patient is in the ambulance en route to the hospital (unless the ambulance has not arrived).

Use caution when the patient is placed on the transport stretcher (or backboard, if clinically indicated). If the splint extends beyond the end of the stretcher, be very careful when moving the patient and when closing the ambulance door so that you do not hit the splint and cause movement in the fracture site.

Multiple types and models of traction splints are available today. The application of three different types is described in the sections that follow.

Procedure

Applying a Thomas Traction Splint (Half-Ring Splint)

The Thomas splint was used exclusively prior to the advent of modern traction devices. During World War I, its use decreased the mortality rate for battlefield femur fractures from 80% to 40%. At that time it was considered one of the greatest advancements in medical care. It is still used in some countries and in the absence of other options. Of note, gunshot wounds were the major cause of femur fractures during World War I, which by definition are open fractures. The traction splint often caused bone ends to retract back under the skin and in the preantibiotic era, infections were very common. Despite that, the mortality from femur fractures dropped significantly following the introduction of the Thomas splint.

To apply a Thomas traction splint, follow these steps (Scan 15-1):

1. Have your partner support the leg and maintain gentle traction, while you cut away the clothing and remove the shoe and sock to check pulse, motor function, and sensation at the foot.

2. Position the splint under the injured leg. The ring goes down, and the short side of the splint goes to the inside of the leg. Slide the ring snugly up under the hip, where it will be pressed against the ischial tuberosity.

3. Attach the top ring strap.

4. Apply padding to the foot and ankle.

5. Apply the traction hitch around the foot and ankle.

6. Maintain gentle traction by hand.

7. Attach the traction hitch to the end of the splint.

8. Increase traction by Spanish windlass action, using a stick or several tongue depressors.

9. Position two support straps above the knee and two below the knee. Do not place straps over fracture site.

10. Release manual traction, and reassess pulse, motor function, and sensation.

11. Support the end of the splint so that there is no pressure on the heel.

SCAN 15-1 Applying a Thomas Traction Splint

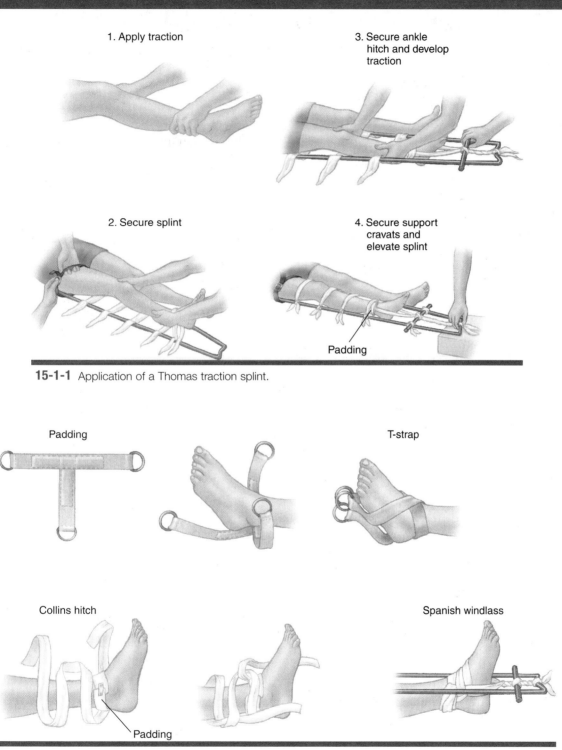

1. Apply traction

2. Secure splint

3. Secure ankle hitch and develop traction

4. Secure support cravats and elevate splint

Padding

15-1-1 Application of a Thomas traction splint.

Padding

T-strap

Collins hitch

Padding

Spanish windlass

15-1-2 Application of the traction hitch to the ankle.

Procedure

Applying a Hare® Traction Splint

The Hare traction splint is the modern version of the Thomas splint. To apply the Hare® traction splint, follow these steps (Scan 15-2):

1. Position the patient on the backboard or stretcher.

2. Have your partner support the leg and maintain gentle traction, while you cut away the clothing and remove the shoe and sock to check pulse, motor function, and sensation at the foot.

3. Using the uninjured leg as a guide, pull the splint out to the correct length.

4. Position the splint under the injured leg. The ring goes down, and the short side goes to the inside of the leg. Slide the ring up snugly under the hip against the ischial tuberosity.

5. Attach the ischial strap.

6. Apply the padded traction hitch to the ankle and foot.

7. Attach the traction hitch to the windlass by way of the S-hook.

8. Turn the ratchet until the correct tension is applied.

9. Reassess pulses, motor function, and sensation of the leg.

10. Position and attach two support straps above the knee and two below the knee. Do not place over fracture site.

11. Release manual traction, and recheck pulse, motor function, and sensation.

12. To release mechanical traction (when too tight or when removing the splint), pull the ratchet knob outward and then slowly turn to loosen.

Procedure

Applying a Sager® Traction Splint

The Sager traction splint is different from the two splints already described in several ways. It works by providing countertraction against the pubic ramus and the ischial tuberosity medial to the shaft of the femur; thus, it does not go under the leg. The hip does not have to be slightly flexed, as with the Hare® splint, because the Sager® splint is lighter and more compact. You also can splint both legs with one splint, if needed.

The current Sager® traction splints are significantly improved over older models and may represent the state of the art in traction splints. To apply one, follow these steps (Scan 15-3):

1. Position the patient on a long backboard or stretcher.

2. Have your partner support the leg and maintain gentle traction, while you cut away the clothing and remove the shoe and sock to check the pulse, motor function, and sensation at the foot.

3. Using the uninjured leg as a guide, pull the splint out to the correct length.

4. Position the splint to the inside of the injured leg with the padded bar fitted snugly against the pelvis in the groin. Attach the strap to the thigh. The splint can be used on the outside of the leg, using the strap to maintain traction against the pubic ramus. Be very careful not to catch the genitals under the bar (or strap).

5. While your partner maintains gentle manual traction, attach the padded hitch to the foot and ankle.

6. Extend the splint until the correct tension is obtained.

7. Apply the elastic straps to secure the leg to the splint. Do not place them over the fracture site.

8. Release manual traction, and recheck pulse, motor function, and sensation.

SCAN 15-2 Applying a Hare® Traction Splint

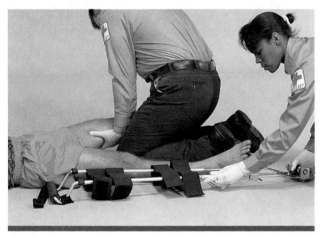

15-2-1 Assess distal pulse, motor function, and sensation.

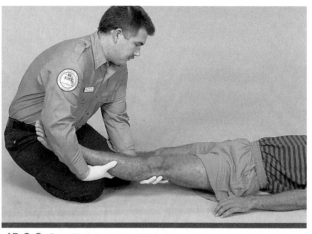

15-2-2 Stabilize the injured leg by applying manual traction.

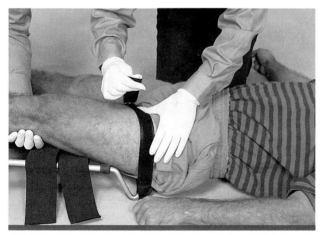

15-2-3 Adjust the splint for proper length.

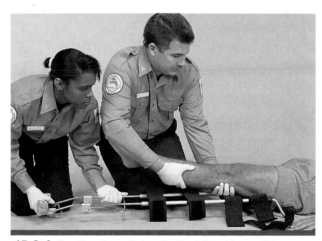

15-2-4 Position the splint under the injured leg until the ischial pad rests against the bony prominence of the buttocks. Once the splint is in position, raise the heel stand.

15-2-5 Attach the ischial strap over the groin and thigh.

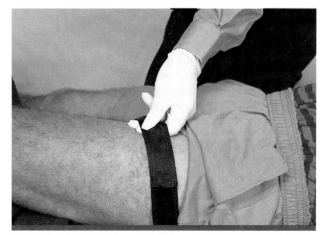

15-2-6 Make sure the ischial strap is snug but not tight enough to reduce distal circulation.

(continued)

SCAN 15-2 Applying a Hare® Traction Splint (*continued*)

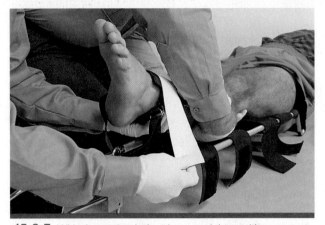

15-2-7 With the patient's foot in an upright position, secure the ankle hitch.

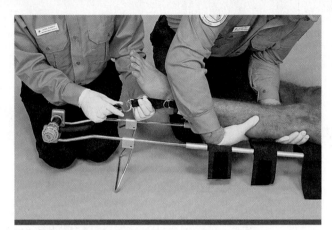

15-2-8 Attach the S-hook to the D-ring, and apply mechanical traction. Full traction is achieved when the mechanical traction is equal to the manual traction and the pain and muscle spasms are reduced. In an unresponsive patient, adjust the traction until the injured leg is the same length as the uninjured leg.

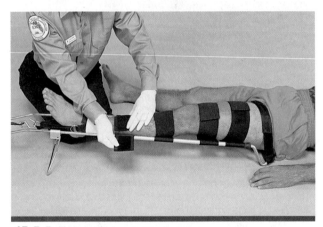

15-2-9 Fasten the leg support straps.

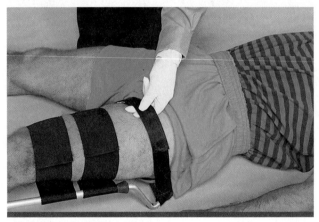

15-2-10 Reevaluate the ischial strap and ankle hitch to ensure that both are securely fastened.

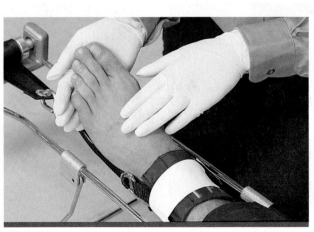

15-2-11 Reassess distal pulse, motor function, and sensation.

SCAN 15-3 Applying a Sager® Traction Splint

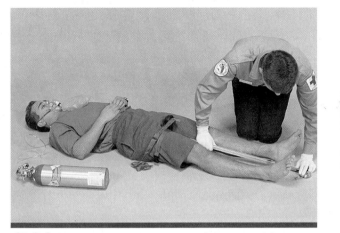

15-3-1 Place the splint along the medial aspect of the injured leg. Adjust it so that it extends about four inches beyond the heel.

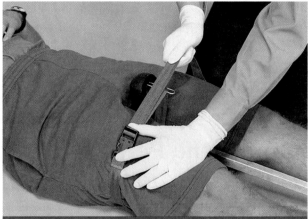

15-3-2 Secure the strap to the thigh. Caution: The Sager® splint should not be used if pelvic fracture is suspected.

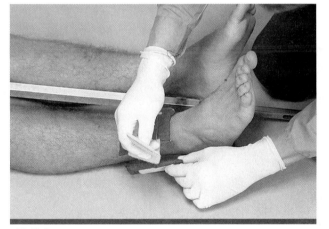

15-3-3 Apply the ankle hitch, and attach it to the splint.

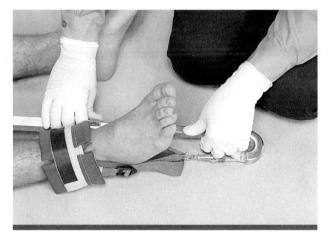

15-3-4 Apply traction by extending the splint. Adjust the splint to 10% of the patient's body weight or up to 15 lb (7 kg) per extremity being immobilized.

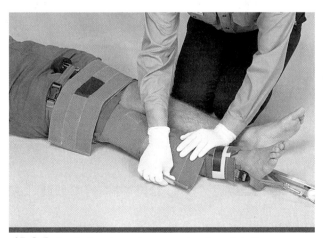

15-3-5 Apply the straps to secure leg to splint. Reassess distal pulse, motor function, and sensation.

Pelvic Stabilization Techniques

Pelvic fractures involve either the iliac crest or the pelvic ring. Fractures to the iliac crest indicate that the patient was subjected to major force and is at risk for serious abdominal trauma. However, the fractures themselves are not as life threatening as fractures of the pelvic ring, which have a much higher blood loss. In either case, the actual technique for stabilizing the fracture is the same and may be accomplished by either of two common approaches (described here).

Procedure

Stabilizing the Pelvis with a Sheet or Blanket

1. Place a sheet or blanket horizontally on the lower half of the backboard prior to moving the patient.

2. Use a scoop stretcher, if available, to move the patient onto the ambulance stretcher or backboard (if clinically indicated), placing the pelvis onto a sheet or blanket. If a scoop stretcher is not available, log roll the patient as gently and quickly as possible onto the sheet or blanket.

3. Tie two diagonal corners of the sheet or blanket together with a knot at the hip on one side. Repeat with the remaining two corners, tying the knot on the opposite hip. In each case, gently and smoothly increase the tension until firm support is provided for the pelvis (Figure 15-1).

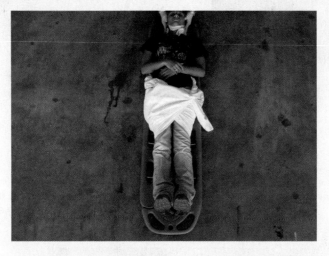

Figure 15-1 Manual stabilization of unstable pelvic fracture using a sheet. *(Courtesy of Leon Charpentier, EMT-P)*

Procedure

Stabilizing the Pelvis with a Commercial Device

1. Open the device and place it horizontally on the lower half of the backboard prior to moving the patient.

2. Use a scoop stretcher, if available, to move the patient onto the ambulance stretcher or backboard (if clinically indicated), placing the pelvis

onto a sheet or blanket. If a scoop stretcher is not available, log roll the patient as gently and quickly as possible onto the sheet or blanket.

3. Tighten the device as the manufacturer recommends. Gently and smoothly increase the tension until firm support is provided for the pelvis (Figure 15-2). It is important to remember that the compressive forces need to be applied at the level of the greater trochanters of the femur (hip level) and not at the iliac wings.

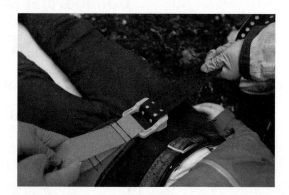

Figure 15-2 Stabilization of an unstable pelvic fracture using a commercial device. *(Courtesy of SAM Medical Products)*

Bleeding

The immediate control of massive, life-threatening bleeding from external injuries is vital to the survival and recovery of the trauma patient. Although varying definitions of massive bleeding exist, it may be identified by bleeding that cannot be controlled by the conventional method of direct pressure. During your approach to the patient and as part of your ITLS Primary Survey, assess for life-threatening bleeding. If it is present and you are unable to immediately control it with direct pressure, do not delay applying a tourniquet to the bleeding extremity.

Direct pressure is widely accepted as a standard of practice for the control of all levels of injury severity. However, scientific research that quantifies the applicability and efficacy of this technique has been very limited. In the past, basic and advanced-level provider education presented various methodologies to control external bleeding, including direct pressure, elevation of an extremity in conjunction with direct pressure, packing with fingertips, or sterile gauze and direct pressure over pressure points. Pressure points are not effective in controlling hemorrhage.

Currently, if direct pressure is unsuccessful, the recommendation is to immediately apply a tourniquet, if control of bleeding is in a location where the tourniquet may be applied. If a tourniquet cannot be applied, a hemostatic dressing along with direct pressure should be utilized immediately. All methods of controlling hemorrhage serve to restrict blood flow and augment the body's response to blood loss, which includes vascular constriction, platelet aggregation, and coagulation.

Application of Tourniquets

Injuries to extremities, such as avulsions, amputations, and lacerations, with bleeding that is not quickly controlled by direct pressure meet the criteria for the application of a tourniquet. Tourniquets provide circumferential compression to the vascular structures just proximal to the wound, inhibiting distal blood flow. Data accumulated during recent conflicts and civilian incidents show marked improvement in survival for wounded soldiers who had prompt application of tourniquets.

Commercial Devices

The ideal tourniquet occludes the injured arteries effectively, is easy to use, and is lightweight, compact, and of rugged construction. Key elements of the tourniquet design must address the width of the occluding strap/pneumatic band and its ability to overcome soft-tissue resistance to compression. The combination of appropriate mechanical assistance and width designs of two inches or greater appears to provide adequate soft-tissue compression and stop bleeding at lower pressures, decreasing tissue damage and discomfort at the tourniquet site. The issue of expense is applicable to EMS, and thus the addition of cost consideration is appropriate to this list. It should be noted that compared to commercially available devices, most improvised tourniquets are not wide enough nor do they have sufficient mechanical force to compress the artery.

Multiple types of tourniquet devices are now commercially available. Relatively low cost and easy to use, many military units now include tourniquets as part of the basic kit carried by all personnel. Some studies have shown some designs to be more effective than others. It is recommended that all agencies within a system use the same model of device to reduce confusion and improve speed of application. Application of two types of tourniquets is described next.

The Combat Application Tourniquet® (CAT) is manufactured by Composite Resources and designed with a self-adherent Velcro band, friction adaptor buckle, and a windlass rod and clip (Figure 15-3). The self-adherent Velcro band is reportedly made from a nonstretch material long enough for application on large and obese extremities. The surface area width is sufficient for distributing the application of pressure circumferentially around an extremity.

Application of the CAT is accomplished by feeding the Velcro band around an extremity and inserting the free-running end through the buckle. Insertion into the buckle locks the band in place on the extremity. Turning the windlass rod creates circumferential tightening and is locked into place with the clip and secured with a small strap after bleeding has been controlled. A location on the top of the windlass strap is available to note the time of application. Included is an independent internal band and clip that permit one-handed or self-application.

The Emergency and Military Tourniquet® (EMT) by Delfi Medical (Figure 15-4) is a pneumatic-based device with an inflatable bladder and a hand bulb inflator permanently attached to the bladder by way of a flexible hose. A twist-type air release valve is included between the hand bulb inflator and the bladder to allow deflation of the

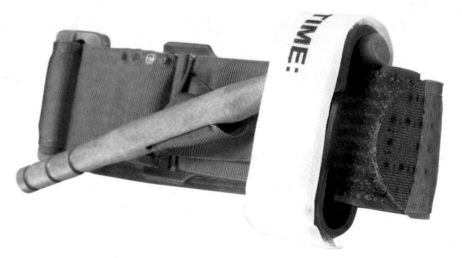

Figure 15-3 Combat Application Tourniquet® (CAT). (© 2010 North American Rescue, LLC)

bladder. The clamp secures a portion of the bladder around the limb and seals the bladder across its width, such that the portion of the bladder surrounding the limb inflates, and the remaining portion of the bladder does not inflate. This Delfi tourniquet is available in one size and able to encircle a 3- to 34-inch circumference around an extremity. A blood pressure cuff may be used in exactly the same way.

Both the CAT and EMT tourniquets advocate use of minimal pressure to control bleeding and include mechanisms for increasing and decreasing the pressure exerted by the devices. In the absence of a purpose-designed tourniquet, a blood pressure cuff may be used, though it must be monitored closely because it can lose effectiveness if the pressure in the cuff drops.

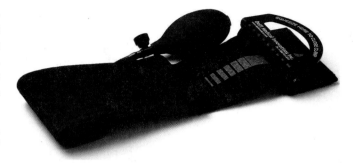

Figure 15-4 The Emergency and Military Tourniquet® (EMT). *(Courtesy of Delphi Medical Innovations, Inc.)*

Procedure

Applying a Tourniquet

Regardless of the device used, the following procedure may be employed for hemorrhage that cannot be controlled with conventional methods of direct pressure and is anatomically appropriate to tourniquet application:

1. Identify massive extremity bleeding caused by avulsions, amputations, and lacerations.

2. If not immediately life threatening, attempt direct pressure to control bleeding. If the patient appears to be exsanguinating or if you are unable to control bleeding quickly with direct pressure, proceed immediately to application of tourniquet.

3. Position tourniquet proximal to the source of bleeding, avoiding application over any joints on the extremity.

4. Secure the tourniquet in place, and apply circumferential pressure by a method recommended by the tourniquet manufacturer.

5. Tighten the tourniquet until bleeding stops.

6. Secure the tourniquet in place.

7. Note the time of application. Because all medical providers look at the patient's face, some advocate marking the patient's forehead with the time of tourniquet placement.

8. Do not cover the tourniquet.

9. Frequently reassess for bleeding. Increase tourniquet pressure as needed.

10. Contact receiving facility, and notify them of the application of a tourniquet.

The use of a tourniquet is not a benign procedure. Application of a tourniquet can cause extreme pain and discomfort at and distal to the site of application. When appropriate, the use of analgesic medications to decrease pain should be considered. Complications such as inappropriate positioning and device malfunction can occur. In addition, necrosis to the muscle at and distal to the application, compartment syndrome, and nerve palsy are all possible. Ischemic time (time without blood perfusion) before permanent damage can be up to four hours at room temperature. Ideally, to prevent these secondary injuries, efforts should be made to limit the time the tourniquet is in place to two to four hours. Unless extreme circumstances exist where delivery to definitive care is delayed, the removal of a tourniquet or reperfusion of an extremity following tourniquet application should be carried out only on orders of medical direction.

Massive bleeding in the groin and axilla presents a special challenge to the emergency care provider. The vessels in these regions are very large, and it is extremely difficult to apply a tourniquet to this area. Recently, several manufacturers have developed "junctional tourniquets" (Sam® Junctional Tourniquet; Abdominal, Aortic, and Junctional Tourniquet® [AAJT] are examples). Junctional tourniquets and others are being used currently, and the results are very encouraging, especially when used along with hemostatic agents, which are discussed in the next section.

Use of Hemostatic Agents

For injuries where the control of massive bleeding is not successful with direct pressure and the use of a tourniquet, or where the application of a tourniquet is not possible, such as at the neck, axilla, or groin, the use of a hemostatic agent in combination with direct pressure is warranted as an additional resource to control bleeding. Laboratory studies and field trials conducted by the U.S. military and limited research completed by EMS agencies indicate hemostatic agents have benefit when used in conjunction with existing methods of bleeding control.

Hemostatic Agent Types

This is a technology that is rapidly changing, and there are many competing hemostatic products. Various chitosan, mineral, and nonmineral-based hemostatic agents are currently available to EMS personnel. Product names such as Celox™, QuikClot Combat Gauze®, HemCon®, and TraumaDex™ promote clotting (with different degrees of effectiveness) through various mechanisms of action. Most hemostatic agents are available in powder, granular, or bandage form. The U.S. military is currently using QuikClot Combat Gauze.

Common to each currently approved hemostatic agent regardless of application form is the requirement to make direct contact with the primary source of bleeding and for the emergency care provider to exert external compression directly to the source of bleeding. Clotting time based on blood vessel type, size, and level of exsanguination presenting may vary, with two minutes of direct pressure required to facilitate cessation of bleeding. These agents are not to be used for internal bleeding. Some of the powder-based agents may have a higher rate of thromboembolic events later in the course of care.

Hemostatic Agent Application

The following procedure may be used for hemorrhage that cannot be controlled with conventional methods of direct pressure, when the injury is anatomically inappropriate for the application of a tourniquet, or when bleeding does not stop following direct pressure and tourniquet application.

Procedure

Applying a Hemostatic Agent

1. Identify massive bleeding caused by avulsions, amputations, or lacerations.

2. Attempt direct pressure to control bleeding. If you are unable to facilitate rapid cessation of bleeding, proceed immediately to application of tourniquet for anatomically appropriate locations.

3. If bleeding is not controlled or in an area where a tourniquet cannot be applied, apply a hemostatic agent directly to the source of the bleeding.

4. With fingertip pressure and a 4 × 4 or trauma dressing, compress the wound and hemostatic agent for at least two minutes. Failure to apply

pressure directly to the source of the bleeding may delay or prevent cessation of bleeding.

5. While leaving the 4 × 4 or trauma dressing in place, evaluate for cessation of bleeding. If bleeding has stopped, dress the wound as appropriate.

6. If bleeding continues, remove the 4 × 4 or trauma dressing and reapply the hemostatic agent and 4 × 4 or trauma dressing. Confirm direct pressure is being placed on the source of bleeding.

Complications include ineffectiveness of the hemostatic agent, continued bleeding (recognized and unrecognized), and tissue damage secondary to the type of hemostatic agent used. Any bleeding that cannot be controlled must be considered life threatening. Do not delay transportation for reapplication of tourniquets or hemostatic agents. Immediately package and transport the patient upon completion of the rapid survey, and continue interventions en route to definitive care.

Bibliography

Acheson, E. M., B. S. Kheirabadi, R. M. Deguzman, E. J. Dick, and J. B. Holcomb. "Comparison of Hemorrhage Control Agents Applied to Lethal Extremity Arterial Hemorrhages in Swine." *Journal of Trauma* 59, no. 4 (October 2005): 865–75.

Adams, D. B., and C. W. Schwab. "Twenty-One-Year Experience with Land Mine Injuries." *Journal of Trauma* 28, Suppl. 1 (January 1988): S159–S162.

Alam, H. B., G. B. Uy, D. Miller, E. Koustova, T. Hancock, R. Inocencio, D. Anderson, O. Llorente, and P. Rhee. "Comparative Analysis of Hemostatic Agents in a Swine Model of Lethal Groin Injury." *Journal of Trauma* 54, no. 6 (June 2003): 1077–82.

Alam, H. B., D. Burris, J. A. DaCorta, and P. Rhee. "Hemorrhage Control in the Battlefield: Role of New Hemostatic Agents." *Military Medicine* 170, no. 1 (January 2005): 63–69.

Bledsoe, B., R. Porter, and R. Cherry. *Paramedic Care: Principles and Practices,* 4th ed., 87–120. Upper Saddle River, NJ: Pearson, 2012.

Brown, M., M. R. Daya, and J. A. Worley. "Experience with Chitosan Dressings in a Civilian EMS System." *Journal of Emergency Medicine* 37, no. 1 (July 2009): 1–7.

Carr, M. E., Jr. "Monitoring of Hemostasis in Combat Trauma Patients." *Military Medicine* 169, Suppl. 12 (December 2004): 11–15.

Jackson, M. R., S. A. Friedman, A. J. Carter, V. Bayer, J. R. Burge, M. J. MacPhee, W. N. Drohan, and B. M. Alving. "Hemostatic Efficacy of a Fibrin Sealant Based on Topical Agent in a Femoral Artery Injury Model: A Randomized, Blinded, Placebo-Controlled Study." *Journal of Vascular Surgery* 26, no. 2 (August 1997): 274–80.

Kheirabadi, B. S., E. M. Acheson, R. M. Deguzman, J. L. Sondeen, K. L. Ryan, A. P. Delgado, E. J. Dick, and J. B. Holcomb. "Efficacy of Two Advanced Dressings in an Aortic Hemorrhage Model in Swine." *Journal of Trauma* 59, no. 1 (July 2005): 25–35.

King, R. B., D. Filips, S. Blitz, and S. Logsetty. "Evaluation of Possible Tourniquet Systems for Use in the Canadian Forces." *Journal of Trauma* 60, no. 5 (May 2006): 1061–71.

Kragh, J. F. Jr., T. J. Walters, D. G. Baer, C. J. Fox, C. E. Wade, J. Salinas, and J. B. Holcomb. "Practical Use of Emergency Tourniquets to Stop Bleeding in Major Limb Trauma." *Journal of Trauma* 64, Suppl. 2 (February 2008): S38–S50.

Lawton, G., J. Granville-Chapman, and P. J. Parker. "Novel Heamostatic Dressings." *Journal of the Royal Army Medical Corps* 155, no. 4 (December 2009): 309–14.

Lee, C., K. M. Porter, and T. J. Hodgetts. "Tourniquet Use in the Civilian Prehospital Setting." *Emergency Medicine Journal* 24, no. 8 (August 2007): 584–87.

Naimer, S. A., M. Tanami, A. Malichi, and D. Moryosef. "Control of Traumatic Wound Bleeding by Compression with a Compact Elastic Adhesive Dressing." *Military Medicine* 171, no. 7 (July 2006): 644–47.

Neuffer, M. C., J. McDivitt, D. Rose, K. King, C. C. Cloonan, and J. S. Vayer. "Hemostatic Dressings for the First Responder: A Review." *Military Medicine* 169, no. 9 (September 2004): 716–20.

Payne, E. K., D. Berry, and R. Seitz. "Educating the Educator: Use of Advanced Bleeding Control Mechanisms in Athletic Training: A Shift in the Thought Process of Prehospital Care–Part 2: Hemostatic Agents." *Athletic Training Education Journal* 9, no. 4 (October–December 2014): 193–201.

Pusateri, A. E., J. B. Holcomb, B. S. Kheirabadi, H. B. Alam, C. E. Wade, and K. L. Ryan. "Making Sense of the Preclinical Literature on Advanced Hemostatic Products." *Journal of Trauma* 60, no. 3 (March 2006): 674–82.

Walters, T. J., and M. C. Mabry. "Issues Related to the Use of Tourniquets on the Battlefield." *Military Medicine* 170, no. 9 (September 2005): 770–75.

Walters, T. J., J. C. Wernke, D. S. Kauvar, J. G. McManus, J. B. Holcomb, and D. G. Baer. "Effectiveness of Self-Applied Tourniquets in Human Volunteers." *Prehospital Emergency Care* 9, no. 4 (October 2005): 416–22.

Ward, K. R., M. H. Tiba, W. H. Holbert, C. R. Blocher, G. T. Draucker, E. K. Proffitt, G. L. Bowlin, R. R. Ivatury, and R. F. Diegelmann. "Comparison of a New Hemostatic Agent to Current Combat Hemostatic Agents in a Swine Model of Lethal Extremity Arterial Hemorrhage." *Journal of Trauma* 63, no. 2 (August 2007): 276–84.

Wedmore, I., J. G. McManus, A. E. Pusateri, and J. E. Holcomb. "A Special Report on the Chitosan-Based Hemostatic Dressing: Experience in Current Combat Operations." *Journal of Trauma* 60, no. 3 (March 2006): 655–58.

Wenke, J. C., T. J. Walters, D. J. Greydanus, A. E. Pusateri, and V. A. Convertino. "Physiological Evaluation of the U.S. Army One-Handed Tourniquet." *Military Medicine* 170, no. 9 (September 2005): 776–81.

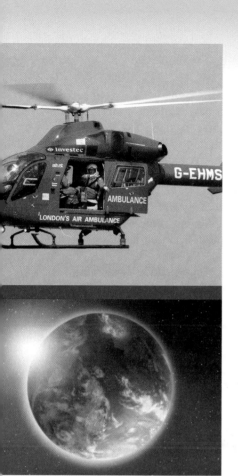

(Ambulance photo courtesy of Paul Drabot, Shutterstock.com)

16

Burns

Roy L. Alson, PhD, MD, FACEP, FAAEM

| Ustioni | Quemaduras | Brûlures | Oparzenia | Verbrennungen |
| Opekline | الحروق | opekotine | Opekline | Égés |

Key Terms

burn depth, *p. 306*
carbon monoxide poisoning, *p. 313*
chemical injury, *p. 315*
electrical injury, *p. 318*
heat-inhalation injury, *p. 313*
lightning injury, *p. 319*
rhabdomyolysis, *p. 319*
radiation injury, *p. 321*
rule of nines, *p. 307*
smoke-inhalation injury, *p. 315*
thermal injury, *p. 314*

Objectives

Upon successful completion of this chapter, you should be able to:

1. Identify the basic anatomy of the skin, including
   a. Epidermal and dermal layers
   b. Structures found within
2. List the basic functions of the skin.
3. Describe types of burns as a function of burn depth.
4. Estimate depth of burn based on skin appearance.
5. Estimate extent of burn using the rule of nines.
6. Identify complications and describe the initial management of:
   a. Thermal burns
   b. Chemical burns
   c. Electrical burns
7. List situations and physical signs that:
   a. Indicate thermal airway or inhalation injury
   b. Suggest carbon monoxide poisoning
8. Discuss how carbon monoxide causes hypoxia.
9. Describe the initial treatment for carbon monoxide poisoning.
10. Identify which patients may require transport to a burn center.

Chapter Overview

According to the American Burn Association, there are over 1 million burn injuries per year in the United States, resulting in more than 4,500 deaths. The World Health Organization (WHO) reports that there are over a quarter of a million deaths worldwide from burns, many of them in developing countries. Burns are a major public health problem worldwide. Many who survive their burns are left severely disabled and/or disfigured. Although the number of those killed or injured has decreased in the last 40 years, particularly in North America due to the use of smoke detectors and the improvements in burn care, burn injury is still a major problem. Applying the basic principles taught in this book can help decrease death, disability, and disfigurement from burn injuries. Because the rescue of burn patients can be extremely dangerous, following the rules of scene safety is extremely important. Multiple agents (Table 16-1) can cause burn injuries, but in general, pathologic damage to the skin is similar no matter what the cause. Specific differences among the types of burns will be discussed in later sections.

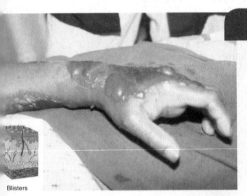

Blisters

(Photo courtesy of Roy Alson, MD)

Case Presentation

You are the senior emergency care provider on an ambulance dispatched along with the fire department to a reported grill fire with injuries at a residence. On arrival, the fire officer informs you that there are two injured persons. The fire has been extinguished. The injured were part of a group attending a party at the residence. The grill was not heating fast enough, and one of the guests threw a cup of gasoline onto the grill to get it to burn faster. There was a large flash of flame. The person who threw the cup of gasoline, which did spill on his shirt, sustained burns to arms, chest, and face. A second person who was close to the grill has some burns to the face.

Before proceeding, consider these questions: What critical signs are you looking for? What are your treatment priorities? How would you triage these patients? Keep these questions in mind as you read through the chapter. Then, at the end of the chapter, find out how the emergency care providers managed these patients.

Anatomy and Pathophysiology
The Skin

The largest organ of the body, the skin, is made up of two layers. The outer layer, which we can see on the surface, is called the *epidermis*. It serves as a barrier between the environment and the body. Underneath the thin epidermis is a thick layer of collagen connective tissue called the *dermis*. This layer contains the important sensory nerves and also the support structures such as the hair follicles, sweat glands, and oil glands (Figure 16-1).

Table 16-1: Types of Burn injuries
• Thermal: flame, scald, steam
• Electrical
• Chemical
• Radiation

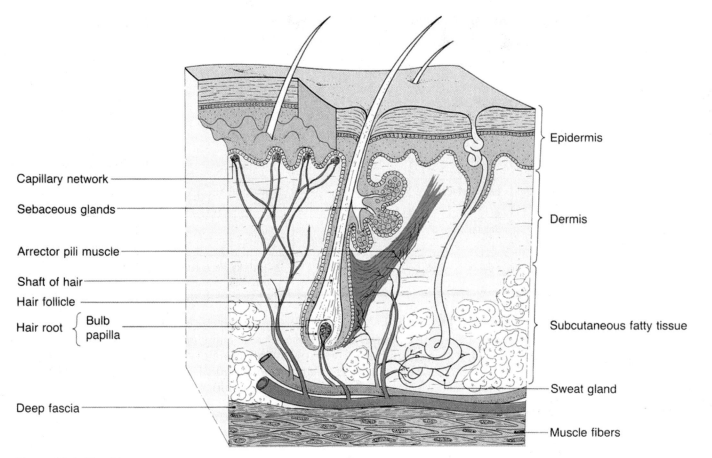

Figure 16-1 The skin.

The skin has many important functions, which include acting as a mechanical and protective barrier between the body and the outside world, sealing fluids inside, and preventing bacteria and other microorganisms from readily entering the body.

The skin is also a vital sensory organ that provides input to the brain on general and specific environmental data and serves a primary role in temperature regulation. Damage to the skin renders it unable to carry out these functions and puts the body at risk for serious problems.

Burn damage occurs when heat or caustic chemicals come in contact with the skin and damage its chemical and cellular components. In addition to actual tissue injury, the body's inflammatory response can cause additional injury or increase the severity of a burn. The portions of the skin that are necrosed by the thermal insult are referred to as the *zone of coagulation* and have suffered irreversible injury. Surrounding this area is a *zone of stasis*, where blood flow is compromised and tissues will die if blood flow is not restored. This condition is seen in the deeper areas of partial-thickness burns and is helped by good burn care and fluid resuscitation. Surrounding the zone of stasis is the *zone of hyperemia*, where there is increased blood flow to the tissues as a result of the actions of inflammatory mediators released by damaged skin.

Classifying Burns by Depth

Burns are characterized, based on the depth of tissue damage and skin response, as superficial (first degree), partial thickness (second degree), or full thickness (third

Table 16-2: Characteristics of Various Depths of Burns

	Superficial (First Degree)	Partial Thickness (Second Degree)	Full Thickness (Third Degree)
Cause	Sun or minor flash	Hot liquids, flashes, or flame	Chemicals, electricity, flame, hot metals
Skin color	Red	Mottled red	Pearly white and/or charred, translucent and parchment-like
Skin surface	Dry with no blisters	Blisters with weeping	Dry with thrombosed blood vessels
Sensation	Painful	Painful	Anesthetic with peripheral pain
Healing	3–6 days	2–4 weeks, depending on depth	Requires skin grafting

burn depth: a classification of severity of burns by how deep the skin is burned. In order of worsening injury: superficial burns (first degree), partial-thickness burns (second degree), and full-thickness burns (third degree).

degree). Superficial burns result in minor tissue damage to the outer epidermal layer only, but do cause an intense and painful inflammatory response. The most common injury of this type is "sunburn." Although no medical treatment is usually required, various medications can be prescribed that significantly speed healing and reduce the painful inflammatory response.

Partial-thickness burns cause damage through the epidermis and into a variable depth of the dermis. Such injuries will heal (usually without scarring) because the cells lining the deeper portions of the hair follicles and sweat glands will multiply and grow new skin for healing. Antibiotic creams or various specialized types of dressings are routinely used to treat these burns, and therefore, appropriate medical evaluation and care should be provided for patients with these injuries. Emergency care of partial-thickness burns involves cooling the burn and covering it with a clean dry dressing.

Full-thickness burns cause damage to all layers of the epidermis and dermis. No more skin cell layers are left, so healing by regrowth of epidermal cells is impossible. All full-thickness burns leave scars that later may contract and limit motion of the burned extremity (or restrict movement of the chest wall). Deeper full-thickness burns usually result in skin protein becoming denatured and hard, forming a firm, leather-like covering that is referred to as *eschar*.

Characteristics of burns are listed in Table 16-2. Depth levels and examples are shown in Figures 16-2, 16-3, and 16-4.

Determining the Severity of Burns

The body's normal inflammatory response to a burn injury can result in progressive tissue damage for a day or two following the injury, which may well result in an increase in **burn depth**. Any condition that either reduces circulation (shock) to this damaged tissue or by itself causes further tissue damage will lead to burn progression with increasing burn depth. Because of this process of burn progression, it is not essential to determine exactly the burn depth in the field.

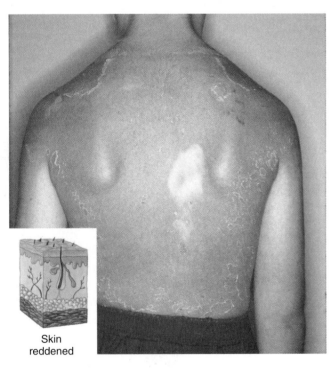

Skin
reddened

Figure 16-2 Superficial (first-degree) burn.

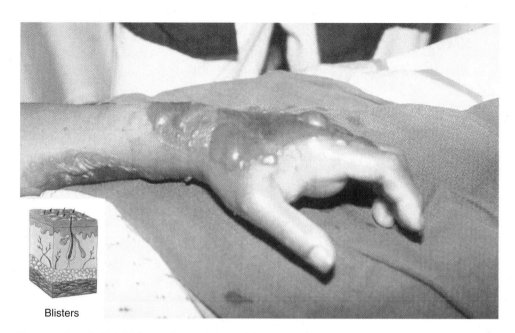

Figure 16-3 Partial-thickness (second-degree) burn. *(Photo courtesy of Roy Alson, MD)*

You should, however, be able to clearly discern between superficial and deep burns. Because the decision to transport to a burn center is based on both depth and extent of the burn, you also should be able to estimate the amount of body surface involved in the burn.

Burn size is best estimated in the field using the **rule of nines** (Figure 16-5). In the rule of nines, the body is divided into areas that are either 9% or 18% of the total body surface, and by roughly drawing in the burned areas, the extent can be estimated. Only partial-thickness and full-thickness burns are used for this calculation.

rule of nines: a method of estimating the body surface area burned by a division of the body into regions, each of which represents approximately 9% of the total surface area, plus 1% for the genital area.

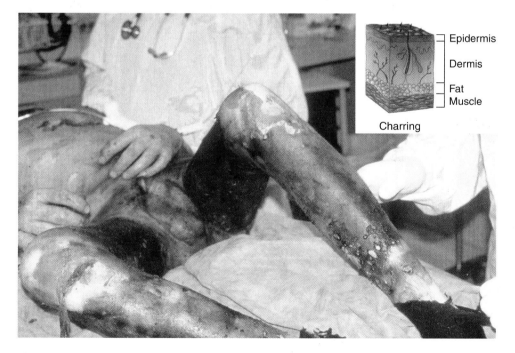

Figure 16-4 Full-thickness (third-degree) burn. *(Photo courtesy of Roy Alson, MD)*

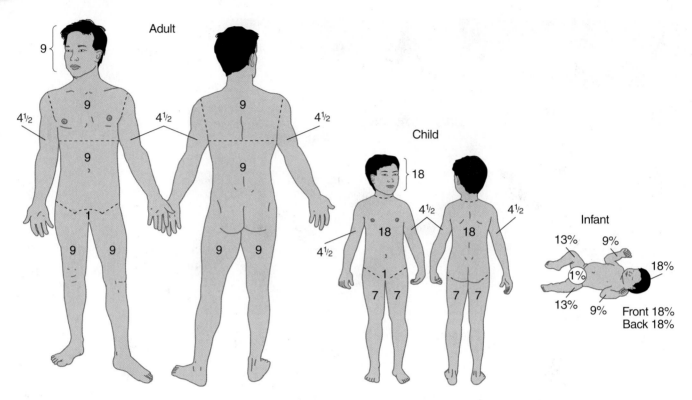

Figure 16-5 The rule of nines.

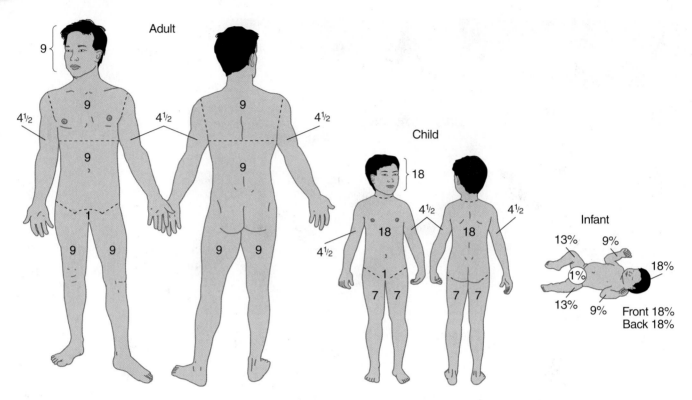

Figure 16-6 Areas in which small burns are more serious: Partial- or full-degree burns in these areas (shaded portions) should be treated in the hospital.

In small children there are some differences in body size proportions, so a *Lund and Browder chart* is helpful (Table 16-3).

For smaller or irregular burns, the size can be estimated using the entire palmar surface (including the fingers) of the patient's hand, which is very close to 1% of the total body surface area. Even small burns can be serious if they involve certain parts of the body that affect function or appearance (Figure 16-6).

Initial care that is directed specifically toward the burn should concentrate on limiting any progression of the burn depth and extent.

Patient Assessment and Management

Evaluation of the burn patient is often complicated by the dramatic nature of the injuries. You can easily be overwhelmed by the extent of such injuries. You must remember that even patients with major burns rarely expire in the initial post-burn period from the burn injury. Death in the immediate post-burn period is a consequence of associated trauma or conditions such as airway compromise or smoke inhalation. A careful, systematic approach to patient evaluation will allow you to identify and manage critical life-threatening problems and to improve patient outcome.

The ITLS Primary and Secondary Surveys should follow the standard format described in Chapter 2.

ITLS Primary Survey
Scene Size-up

The steps for assessing a major burn patient are the same as for any other major trauma patient. Begin by performing a scene size-up as outlined in Chapter 1, with an emphasis on your own safety. After the size-up is completed, your next priority is to remove the patient to a safe area away from the source of the burn.

Table 16-3: Lund and Browder Chart

Area	Age (Years) 0–1	1–4	5–9	10–15	Adults	% 2°	% 3°	% Total
Head	19	17	13	10	7			
Neck	2	2	2	2	2			
Ant. Trunk	13	17	13	13	13			
Post. Trunk	13	13	13	13	13			
R. Buttock	2 ½	2 ½	2 ½	2 ½	2 ½			
L. Buttock	2 ½	2 ½	2 ½	2 ½	2 ½			
Genitalia	1	1	1	1	1			
R.U. Arm	4	4	4	4	4			
L.U. Arm	4	4	4	4	4			
R.L. Arm	3	3	3	3	3			
L.L. Arm	3	3	3	3	3			
R. Hand	2 ½	2 ½	2 ½	2 ½	2 ½			
L. Hand	2 ½	2 ½	2 ½	2 ½	2 ½			
R. Thigh	5 ½	6 ½	8 ½	8 ½	9 ½			
L. Thigh	5 ½	6 ½	8 ½	8 ½	9 ½			
R. Leg	5	5	5 ½	6	7			
L. Leg	5	5	5 ½	6	7			
R. Foot	3 ½	3 ½	3 ½	3 ½	3 ½			
L. Foot	3 ½	3 ½	3 ½	3 ½	3 ½			
					Total			

Weight _____

Height _____

Adapted from Lund, C. C., and N. C. Browder. "The Estimation of Areas of Burns," Surgery, Gynaecology, Obstetrics, Vol. 79 (1944): pp. 352–58.

There are specific and significant dangers in removing the burn source in all types of burn injuries. As a structure fire progresses, there is a point at which flashover occurs. Flashover is the sudden explosion into flame of everything in the room, with the temperature rising instantaneously to over 3,600°F (2,000°C). There is often little warning before this happens. Thus, rescue of patients from burning buildings takes priority over all other treatment.

Remember also that fire consumes oxygen and produces large quantities of toxic products and smoke. Personnel making entry to carry out rescue should wear breathing apparatus or risk becoming victims themselves. Extrication of the patient from the burn source is usually the responsibility of fire department personnel rather than EMS personnel. As an emergency care provider, your responsibility should begin when the patient is delivered to you in a safe place, unless you are a trained firefighter.

Chemicals are not always easy to detect, either on patients or on objects in the environment. Rescuers have suffered severe chemical burns because of the failure to note

PEARLS
Assessment

Treat burn patients as trauma patients: ITLS Primary Survey, critical interventions, transport decision, ITLS Secondary Survey, and ITLS Ongoing Exam.

PEARLS
Safety

- Maintain appropriate safety when removing patients from the source of a burn injury.
- Remember that dealing with hazardous materials requires proper training and equipment. You must always use the appropriate personal protective equipment.

sources of toxic and caustic chemicals and to use the appropriate personal protective equipment (PPE). Special training in hazardous materials management is recommended for all rescuers so that they can recognize such dangers.

Electricity, even at household voltages, is exceptionally dangerous, as is the handling of high-voltage wires. Specialized training, knowledge, and equipment are required to appropriately deal with these situations, and you should not attempt to remove wires unless specifically trained and equipped to do so. Even objects commonly believed to be safe, such as wooden sticks, manila rope, and firefighter's gloves, may not be protective and may result in electrocution. If at all possible, the source of electricity should be turned off before any attempt at rescue is made.

Initial Assessment

Burn patients differ from other trauma patients in that the burning process must be halted immediately upon removal of the patient from the source of the burn. This is best done with a quick irrigation of the burn with room-temperature tap water. Any source of clean water can be used, but do not use cold water. Irrigate for only a minute or two so that the patient does not become hypothermic. This can be done by another emergency care provider while the team leader begins the ITLS Primary Survey.

People do not actually die rapidly from burn injuries. Early burn deaths are usually the result of airway compromise, smoke inhalation, or associated trauma. Death from shock due to fluid loss from the burn will not be seen for many hours (or days), and sepsis usually takes days to develop. Burn victims may also sustain multiple trauma from falls or other mechanisms. Hemorrhagic shock will develop rapidly compared to burn shock, so that management of the patient's blunt or penetrating trauma using ITLS guidelines is very important. Even though the burn is highly visible and makes an intense impression at the scene, other than stopping the burn process, care of the burn itself has a lower priority than airway management. You should perform an initial assessment as soon as the burn victim is in a safe area.

Begin by assessing level of consciousness, while securing the cervical spine if indicated. Assess the airway. If the patient is hoarse or exhibits stridor, protecting the airway is an immediate concern. Assessment of breathing, circulation, and control of major hemorrhage is then carried out.

Rapid Trauma Survey

Based on findings from the scene size-up and the initial assessment, a rapid trauma survey or focused exam is then performed, a baseline set of vital signs is obtained, and if possible, a SAMPLE history is obtained. At this point a determination is made on the need for immediate transport and critical interventions. Critical problems in the burn patient that require immediate intervention include airway compromise, altered level of consciousness, or the presence of major injuries in addition to the burn. Clues from the mechanism of injury that point to critical problems include a history of being confined in a closed space with the fire or smoke, electrical burns, chemical exposure, falls from a height, or other major blunt force trauma. Oxygen at 12 to 15 L/minute by nonrebreather mask (or endotracheal tube if indicated) should be initiated as soon as possible for all major burn patients.

The rapid trauma survey of the burn patient is directed toward identification of causes of breathing and circulatory compromise. In addition to clues from the mechanism of injury, findings that should alert the responder to potential airway problems are the presence of facial and scalp burns, sooty sputum, and singed nasal hair and eyebrows. Examine the oral cavity, and look for soot, swelling, or erythema (redness). Ask the patient to speak. A hoarse voice, stridor, or persistent cough suggests involvement of deeper airway structures and is an indication for aggressive airway management. Auscultate the chest. Wheezing or rales should alert you to the presence of lower airway injury from inhalation. Examine burned areas and check

PEARLS
Airway Compromise

Early deaths from burns are rarely due to burn injury but due to airway compromise. Perform frequent exams of the airway, and be prepared to secure it with an endotracheal tube or other method.

PEARLS
Inhalation Injury

- Any type of burn can have some degree of inhalation injury.
- Remember that a history of smoke exposure in a closed space is the best predictor of smoke inhalation or other airway injuries.

for distal pulses. Based on the initial assessment and the mechanism of injury, a search for associated injuries should be the focus of the rapid trauma survey.

In your assessment of the burn patient, note and record the type of burn mechanism and the particular circumstances such as entrapment, explosion, mechanisms for other possible injuries, smoke exposure, chemical/electrical details, and so forth. An appropriate past medical history should also be documented in writing. If the patient is unable to speak, ask other witnesses and/or fire personnel about the circumstances of the injury.

ITLS Secondary Survey

Perform a standard ITLS Secondary Survey on stable patients. This survey should include an evaluation of the burn, estimating the depth based on appearance, and also estimating the burn size. Those findings are important in determining the level of medical care that is appropriate for the burn victim.

Patient Management

Once the immediate life threats have been addressed, you should attend to the burn wound itself. As mentioned earlier, try to limit burn wound progression as much as possible. Rapid cooling early in the course of a surface burn injury can help limit this progression. Following removal from the source of the burn, the skin and clothing are still hot, and this heat continues to injure the tissues, causing an increase in burn depth and seriousness of the injury. Cooling halts this process and, if done appropriately, is beneficial. Cooling should be done with tap water or any source of clean room-temperature water, but it should be undertaken for no more than 5 to 10 minutes. Cooling for longer periods of time can induce hypothermia and subsequent shock. Do not use ice or ice water because this may induce hypothermia.

Following the brief period of cooling, manage the burn by covering the patient with clean, dry sheets and blankets to keep the patient warm and to prevent hypothermia. It is not necessary to have sterile sheets. Usually, nothing other than a clean sheet should be put on the burn, but antimicrobial sheets (Acticoat™ or Silverlon®) can be used if you have transport times of an hour or more. The patient should be covered even when the environment is not cold because damaged skin loses temperature regulation capacity.

Patients should never be transported on wet sheets, wet towels, or wet clothing, and ice is absolutely contraindicated. Ice will worsen the injury because it causes vasoconstriction and thus reduces the blood supply to already damaged tissue. Cooling the burn wound improperly can cause hypothermia and additional tissue damage and could be worse than not cooling the burn at all. Initial management of chemical and electrical burn injuries will be described later in this chapter in the sections on those injuries.

During the evaluation of the extent of the burn injury, you should remove the patient's loose clothing and jewelry. Cut around burned clothing that is adherent, but do not try to pull the clothing off the skin. Intravenous (IV) line insertion is rarely needed on scene during initial care unless delay in transport to a hospital is unavoidable. It takes hours for burn shock to develop. Therefore, the only reason to initiate IV therapy on scene is if other factors indicate a need for fluid volume or medication administration. Attempting to start IV therapy on scene in major burn patients is often difficult and routinely delays initial transport and arrival at the hospital. IV or intraosseous (IO) access should be established during transport.

Normal saline in large volumes can lead to hyperchloremia. If available, lactated Ringer's solution is preferred for fluid resuscitation in major burns. Colloid containing fluids are generally not be used in the prehospital setting.

Burn wounds hurt. This is obvious to anyone who has sustained even a minor burn. Administration of pain medication, in the field setting, to the multiple-trauma patient has long been a controversial and debated topic. The biggest risk of using analgesics was thought to be a masking of associated trauma and also central nervous system or

PEARLS
Cooling

Early after the burn event, properly cool the surface thermal injury with room temperature water, but do not cause hypothermia.

PEARLS
Fluid Resuscitation

Initiation of fluid resuscitation on scene is not as important as management of other potential life threats. Most burn injuries do not require large fluid volumes in the prehospital phase unless there is a long transport time.

Table 16-4: Injuries That Benefit from Care at a Burn Center
• Partial-thickness burns greater than 10% total body surface area (TBSA)
• Burns that involve the face, hands, feet, genitalia, perineum, or major joints
• Third-degree burns in any age group
• Electrical burns, including lightning injury
• Chemical burns
• Inhalation injury
• Burn injury in patients with pre-existing medical disorders that could complicate management, prolong recovery, or affect mortality
• Any patients with burns and concomitant trauma (such as fractures) in which the burn injury poses the greatest risk of morbidity or mortality. In such cases, if the trauma poses the greater immediate risk, the patient may be initially stabilized in a trauma center before being transferred to a burn unit. Physician judgment will be necessary in such situations and should be in concert with the regional medical direction plan and triage protocols.
• Burned children in hospitals without qualified personnel or equipment for the care of children
• Burn injury in patients who will require special social, emotional, or long-term rehabilitative intervention

Source: Committee on Trauma, American College of Surgeons. Guidelines for the Operations of Burn Units: Resources for Optimal Care of the Injured Patient. Chicago: American College of Surgeons, 2006.

cardiovascular depression associated with the use of pain medications. In reality, these have not been problematic. In the major burn patient, with or without coexisting trauma and especially with long transport times, administration of analgesics in appropriate dosages will improve patient comfort. Therefore, control of the patient's pain using pain control protocols or after consultation with medical direction is an essential component of burn care.

All but the most minor of burn injuries should be evaluated at the hospital. There are now available specialized forms of therapy that offer specific advantages in the treatment of superficial, partial-thickness, and full-thickness burns. Partial-thickness burns can become infected and progress to full-thickness burns because of poor care. The sooner specialized burn therapy can be initiated, the more rapid and satisfactory the results will be.

Table 16-4 lists conditions that would benefit from care at a burn center. Based on available local resources and protocols, it may be appropriate to bypass a local facility and transport these patients directly to the burn center.

Special Problems in Burn Management

The following sections review management of specific types of burns based on the injury mechanism. Be aware that more than one type of burn can be present in a patient. For example, a high-voltage electrical burn injury may also produce flame burns due to ignition of the patient's clothing.

Circumferential Burns

Full-thickness burns result in the formation of an eschar that is tough and unyielding. If the full-thickness burn is circumferential to an extremity, as the burn edema develops in the extremity, the eschar can act like a tourniquet and result in loss of circulation to that extremity. Thus, all extremity burns should undergo regular pulse checks. Though not a prehospital procedure, consideration should be given to the performance of an escharotomy at the hospital prior to transfer to a burn center. If the chest is the site of the circumferential burn, the eschar may limit chest excursion during respiration and lead to hypoxia. Intubation and escharotomy can prevent hypoventilation in this situation.

Flash Burns

Flash burns are virtually always superficial or partial-thickness burns. A flash burn occurs when there is some type of explosion, but no sustained fire. The single heat wave traveling out from the explosion results in such short patient/heat contact that full-thickness burns almost never occur. Only areas directly exposed to the true heat wave will be injured. Typically, face and hands are involved. An example of this type of burn is seen when someone pours gasoline on a charcoal fire to get it to heat up faster. In situations of possible flash explosion risk, you should always wear proper protective clothing and avoid entry into explosive environments. Other injuries (fractures, internal injuries, blast chest injuries, and so on) may occur as a result of an explosion.

Inhalation Injuries

Inhalation injuries account for more than half of the 4,500 plus burn-related deaths in the United States each year. Inhalation injuries are classified as carbon monoxide poisoning, **heat-inhalation injury**, or smoke (toxic) inhalation injury. Most frequently, inhalation injuries occur when a patient is injured in a confined space or is trapped; however, even victims of fires in open spaces may have inhalation injuries. Flash explosions (no fire) practically never cause inhalation injuries.

heat-inhalation injury: thermal burns of the upper airway caused by inhaling flame or hot gases. The lower airways are usually not affected because of efficient cooling by moist mucous membranes.

Carbon Monoxide Poisoning   **Carbon monoxide poisoning** and asphyxiation are by far the most common causes of early death associated with burn injury. When any material burns, oxygen in the air is consumed, and the fire environment should be considered to be an oxygen-deprived environment. Carbon monoxide is a by-product of combustion and is one of the numerous chemicals in common smoke. It is present in high concentrations in auto exhaust fumes and fumes from some types of home space heaters. Because it is colorless, odorless, and tasteless, its presence is virtually impossible to detect without special instruments.

carbon monoxide poisoning: a type of inhalation injury from inhalation of the colorless, odorless, and tasteless gas, carbon monoxide. Carbon monoxide binds to the hemoglobin molecule and prevents oxygenation of the cells of the body.

Carbon monoxide binds to hemoglobin (257 times stronger than oxygen), resulting in the hemoglobin being unable to transport oxygen. Patients quickly become hypoxic even in the presence of low concentrations of carbon monoxide. An alteration in level of consciousness is the predominant sign of this hypoxia (Table 16-5). A cherry-red skin color or cyanosis is rarely present as a result of carbon monoxide poisoning and, therefore, cannot be used in the assessment of patients for carbon monoxide poisoning.

Pulse oximetry will remain normal to high in the presence of carbon monoxide and cannot be used to assess patients for carbon monoxide poisoning. Some newer model pulse oximeters (Figure 16-7) can specifically measure carboxyhemoglobin levels and, if available, should be used on all those who have the possibility of exposure to carbon monoxide. Death usually occurs because of either cerebral or myocardial ischemia or myocardial infarction due to progressive cardiac hypoxia.

Table 16-5: Symptoms Associated with Increasing Levels of Carboxyhemoglobin Binding

Carboxyhemoglobin Level	Symptoms
20%	Headache common, throbbing in nature; shortness of breath on exertion
30%	Headache present; altered central nervous system function with disturbed judgment; irritability, dizziness, decreased vision
40% to 50%	Marked central nervous system alteration with confusion, collapse; also fainting with exertion
60% to 70%	Convulsions; unconsciousness; apnea with prolonged exposure
80%	Rapidly fatal

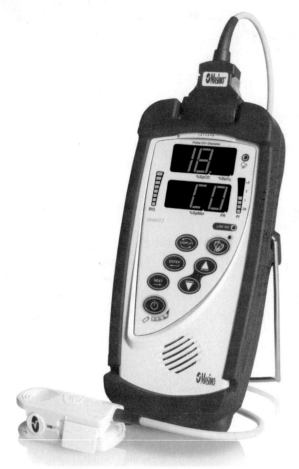

Figure 16-7 Example of a carbon monoxide monitor. *(Images of the Masimo Rad-57 Pulse CO-Oximeter are ©2011 Masimo Corporation. All rights reserved. Masimo, Rad-57, Pulse CO-Oximeter, and SpCO are trademarks or registered trademarks of Masimo Corporation)*

thermal injury: injury to the skin caused by heat from flame, hot liquids, hot gases, or hot solids.

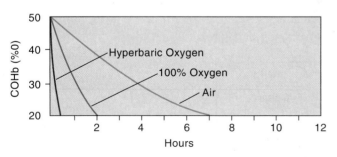

Figure 16-8 Decay curve for disappearance of carboxyhemoglobin from 50% lethal level to 20% acceptable level in air, 1 atm. O_2 (100% oxygen) and 2.5 atm. O_2 (hyperbaric oxygen—100% at 2.5 atmospheres).

Treat patients suspected of having carbon monoxide poisoning with high-flow oxygen by mask. If such a patient loses consciousness, begin advanced life support with intubation and ventilation using 100% oxygen. If a patient is simply removed from the source of the carbon monoxide and allowed to breathe fresh air, it takes up to seven hours to reduce the carbon monoxide/hemoglobin complex to a safe level. Having the patient breathe 100% oxygen decreases this time to about 90 to 120 minutes, and use of hyperbaric oxygen (100% oxygen at 2.5 atmospheres) will decrease this time to about 30 minutes (Figure 16-8).

All suspected cases of carbon monoxide poisoning or toxic inhalation should be transported to an appropriate hospital. The decision to transport the patient to a hyperbaric chamber should be made in consultation with medical direction.

Cyanide and Smoke Inhalation In the modern world, many items in homes and businesses are made of plastics. When combusted, many of them give off toxic gases, which can cause significant pulmonary injury. Among the toxic components in smoke is hydrogen cyanide. It is highly toxic and causes cellular hypoxia by preventing the cell from using oxygen to generate energy to function. Studies of smoke inhalation victims have shown elevated levels of cyanide in some cases.

Opinions regarding empirical treatment of smoke inhalation victims for cyanide poisoning still vary. Several studies suggest that patients who do not respond rapidly to treatment for hypoxia and carbon monoxide poisoning should be treated for cyanide exposure. The current recommended agent for such treatment is IV hydroxocobalamin (Cyanokit®), which combines with cyanide to form nontoxic cyanocobalamin (vitamin B_{12}). Hydroxocobalamin is easier and safer to use in the prehospital setting than the previous "Lilly" or "Pasadena" cyanide antidote kits. This is an area of burn management that is continuing to evolve as more research is conducted.

Heat-Inhalation Injuries Heat-inhalation injuries are confined to the upper airway because breathing in flame and hot gases does not result in heat transport down to the lung tissue itself. The water vapor in the air in the tracheal–bronchial tree effectively absorbs this heat. Steam inhalation is the exception to this rule because steam is superheated water vapor. A second exception to this rule is if the patient has inhaled a flammable gas that then ignites and causes **thermal injury** to the level of the alveoli (example: a painter in a closed space where the paint fumes are ignited by a spark).

As a result of the heat injury, tissue swelling occurs just as it does with surface burns. The vocal cords themselves do not swell because they are dense fibrous bands of connective tissue. However, the loose mucosa in the supraglottic area (the hypopharynx) is where the swelling occurs, and it can easily progress to complete airway obstruction and death (Figure 16-9). There is usually some time between the injury and the development of airway edema, so loss of airway due to direct thermal injury is rare in the initial prehospital phase. However, be aware that once the swelling begins, the airway can obstruct rapidly. Development of a hoarse voice or stridor is an indication for immediate protection of the airway by endotracheal intubation. Aggressive fluid resuscitation can hasten this swelling.

During secondary transport to a burn center, the risk of airway swelling can become significant and can cause airway obstruction as volume-resuscitation IV fluids are being administered. For this reason, patients with airway burns

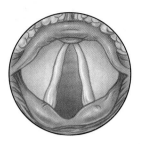 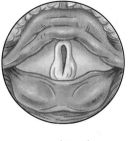 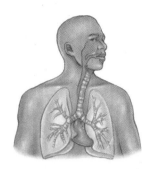

Figure 16-9 Heat inhalation can cause complete airway obstruction by swelling of the hypopharynx: left side—normal anatomy; right side—swelling proximal to cords.

- Burns of the face
- Singed eyebrows or nasal hair
- Burns in the mouth
- Carbonaceous (sooty) sputum
- History of being confined in a closed space while being burned
- Exposure to steam

Figure 16-10 Danger signs of upper airway burns.

should be sedated and intubated before a transfer. It is much easier to electively intubate a patient in the emergency department than do a crash intubation in the back of an ambulance.

Figure 16-10 lists signs that should alert you to the danger of your patient having upper airway burns. Swollen lips indicate the presence of thermal injury at the airway entrance, and hoarseness (indicating altered air flow through the larynx area) is a warning of early airway swelling. Stridor (high-pitched inspiratory breathing and/or a seal-bark cough) indicates severe airway swelling with pending airway obstruction and represents an immediate emergency. The only appropriate treatment is airway stabilization, preferably via nasotracheal intubation or by paralysis and drug-assisted intubation (DAI). This procedure may be far more difficult than under other routine circumstances because of significant anatomic alterations due to swelling.

In addition, because of irritation of inflamed damaged tissue, lethal laryngospasm may occur when the endotracheal tube first touches the laryngeal area. Therefore, this procedure is best undertaken in a hospital emergency department and should be done in the field only when absolutely necessary. Consider contacting medical direction. You should be prepared to perform a surgical airway in these patients if you are unable to intubate.

Smoke Inhalation Injuries **Smoke-inhalation injury** (Figure 16-11) is the result of inhaled toxic chemicals that cause structural damage to lung cells. Smoke may contain hundreds of toxic chemicals that damage the delicate alveolar cells. Smoke from plastic and synthetic products is the most damaging. Tissue destruction in the bronchi and alveoli may take hours to days. However, because the toxic products in the smoke are very irritating, they can precipitate bronchospasm or coronary artery spasm in susceptible individuals. Treat bronchospasm with inhaled beta agonists (albuterol) and oxygen.

Chemical Burns

Thousands of different types of chemicals can cause burn injuries. Chemicals may not only injure the skin, but they also can be absorbed into the body and cause internal organ failure (especially liver and kidney damage). Volatile forms of chemicals may be inhaled and cause lung tissue damage with subsequent severe life-threatening respiratory failure. The effects of the chemical agents on the other organ systems, such as the lung or liver, may not be immediately apparent after exposure.

A **chemical injury** frequently is deceiving in that initial skin changes may be minimal even when the injury is severe. This could lead to secondary contamination of rescuers. Minimal burns on the patient may not be obvious. As a result, you can get the chemicals on your own skin unless appropriate precautions are taken.

Factors that lead to tissue damage include chemical concentration; amount, manner, and duration of skin contact; and the mechanism of action of the chemical agent. The pathological process causing the

smoke-inhalation injury: injury to the lungs or other body organs from inhalation of toxic gases found in smoke.

PEARLS
Chemical Burns

Chemical injuries, in general, require prolonged and copious irrigation.

chemical injury: injury to the skin or other body organs from exposure to caustic or toxic chemicals.

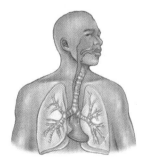

- Victims exposed to smoke in an enclosed place
- Victims who were unconscious while exposed to smoke or fire
- Victims with a cough after being exposed to smoke or fire
- Victims short of breath after being exposed to smoke or fire
- Victims with chest pain after being exposed to smoke or fire

Figure 16-11 Patients in whom you should suspect smoke inhalation.

tissue damage continues until the chemical is either consumed in the damage process, detoxified by the body, or physically removed. Attempts at inactivation with specific neutralizing chemicals are dangerous because the process of neutralization may generate other chemical reactions (heat) that may worsen the injury. Therefore, you should aim treatment at chemical removal by following these four steps.

Procedure

Removing the Source of Chemical Burns

1. Wear appropriate protective gloves, eyewear, and respiratory protection if needed. In some situations you will need to wear a chemical protective suit as well.

2. Remove all the patient's clothing. Place in plastic bags to limit further contact.

3. Flush chemicals off the body by irrigating copiously with any source of available clean water or other irrigant. If dry chemicals are on the skin, they should first be thoroughly brushed off before performing copious irrigation. Remember: The solution to pollution is dilution.

4. Remove any retained agent adhering to the skin by any appropriate physical means such as wiping or gentle scraping. Follow this with further irrigation (Figures 16-12 and 16-13).

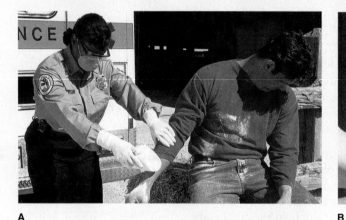

A

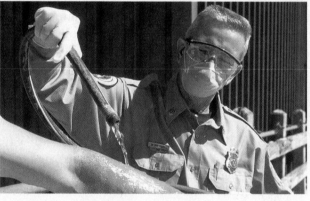

B

Figure 16-12 For a chemical burn, (A) brush away dry powders, and then (B) flood the area with water. *(Photos courtesy of Michal Heron)*

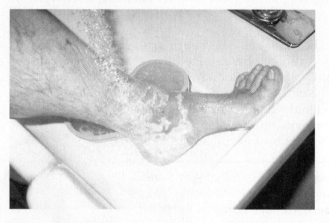

Figure 16-13 Acid burn of the ankle being irrigated.

(Photo courtesy of Roy Alson, MD)

Ideally, all contaminated patients should be decontaminated prior to transport to limit skin damage and prevent contamination of the ambulance or hospital. Remember, removing the patient from the dangerous environment or removing the dangerous environment from the patient is your first priority for patient care. Critical interventions including airway management can be initiated prior to and during the decontamination process. If the patient has not been fully decontaminated prior to transport, notify the receiving hospital as soon as possible, so that they can be prepared to manage the patient.

Irrigation of caustic chemicals in the eye is especially important because irreversible damage will occur in a very short period of time (less than the transport time to get to the hospital). Irrigation of injured eyes may be difficult because of the pain associated with eye opening. However, you must begin irrigation to prevent severe and permanent damage to the corneas (Figure 16-14). Check for contact lenses or foreign bodies and, if present, remove them early during irrigation. A nasal cannula hooked to an IV bag of normal saline and placed over the bridge of the nose makes an excellent bilateral eyewash system during transport. Tap water can be used to irrigate the eyes if saline is not available.

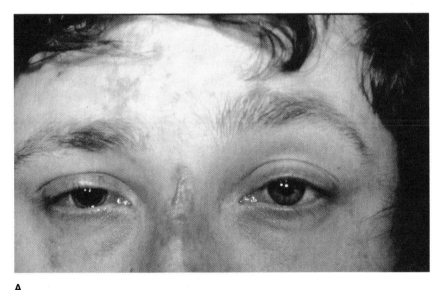

A

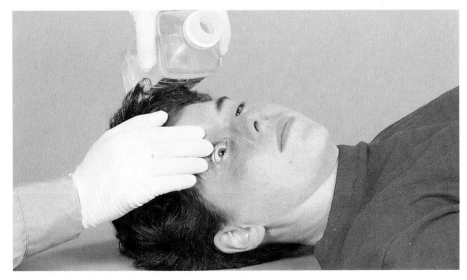

B

Figure 16-14 (A) Chemical burns to the eyes; (B) emergency care of chemical burns to the eye.

Electrical Burns

In cases of electrical burns, damage is caused by electricity entering the body and traveling through the tissues. Injury results from the effects of the electricity on the function of the body organs and from the heat generated by the passage of the current. Extremities are at risk for more significant tissue damage, versus the torso, because their small size results in higher local current density (Figure 16-15). The factors that determine severity of **electrical injury** include the following:

• Type and amount of current (alternating versus direct current and also the voltage)
• Path of the current through the body
• Duration of contact with the current source

The most serious and immediate injury that results from electrical contact is cardiac arrhythmia. Any patient who receives an electric current injury, regardless of how stable he looks, should have a careful immediate evaluation of his cardiac status and continuous monitoring of cardiac activity. The most common life-threatening arrhythmias are premature ventricular contractions, ventricular tachycardia, and ventricular fibrillation.

Aggressive cardiac life support in accordance with AHA/ILCOR guidelines for the management of arrhythmias should be undertaken because these patients are often younger and have normal, healthy hearts. Most of the victims do not have pre-existing cardiovascular disease, and their heart muscle tissue is usually not damaged as a result of the electricity. With good CPR, the chances for resuscitation are excellent. Even under circumstances of prolonged CPR, resuscitation is often possible. Once those efforts at managing cardiac status are complete, provide field care as previously described for thermal burns.

Electrical injuries cause skin burns at the entrance and exit sites because of high temperatures generated by the electric arc 4,500°F (2,500°C) at the skin surface. Additional surface flame burns may result if the patient's clothing is ignited. Fractures and dislocations may be present due to the violent muscle contractions that electrical injuries cause. Often victims are involved in construction and may sustain fractures or other injuries due to falls after an electric shock. Internal injuries usually

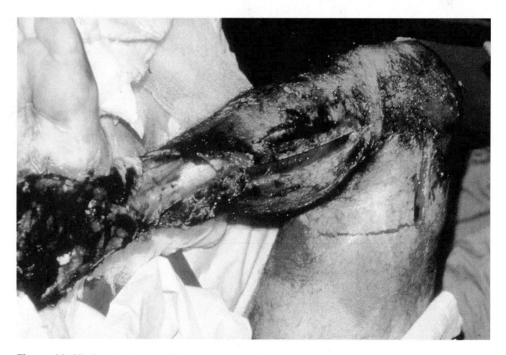

Figure 16-15 Electrical burn of the lower leg and foot. *(Photo courtesy of Roy Alson, MD)*

involve muscle damage, nerve damage, and possible intra-vascular blood coagulation due to electrical current passage. Internal chest or abdominal organ damage due to electrical current is exceedingly rare.

At the scene of an electrical injury, your first priority is scene safety. Determine if the patient is still in contact with the electrical current. If so, you must remove the patient from contact without becoming a victim yourself (Figure 16-16). Handling high-voltage electrical wires is extremely hazardous. Special training and special equipment are needed to deal with downed wires. Never attempt to move wires with makeshift equipment. Tree limbs, pieces of wood, and even manila rope may conduct high-voltage electricity. Even firefighter gloves and boots do not offer adequate protection in this situation. If possible, leave the handling of downed wires to power company personnel or develop a special training program with your local power company to learn how to use the special equipment designed to handle high-voltage lines. If power company personnel are turning off the electricity, be sure they test it to be sure it is off before you approach the scene.

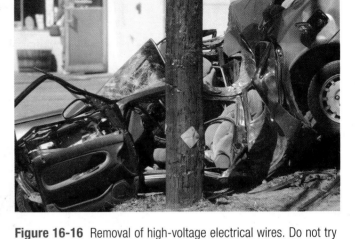

Figure 16-16 Removal of high-voltage electrical wires. Do not try to remove wires with safety equipment (or sticks) unless specially trained. Turn off the electricity at the source or call the power company to remove the wires. *(Photo © Mark C. Ide)*

In the field setting, it is impossible to tell the total extent of the damage in electrical burns because much of the burn injury is deep within the muscle. Therefore, all electrical burn patients should be transported for hospital evaluation. Due to the potential for arrhythmia development, routine IV access should be initiated in the ambulance, along with continuous cardiac monitoring. IV fluid resuscitation should be started during transport in this situation. Because of extensive tissue destruction, the fluid needs during interfacility transport of an electrical burn patient are often higher than for patients with thermal burns.

Electrical burn patients are at risk for developing **rhabdomyolysis**, which is the breakdown of muscle with the release of myoglobin into the circulation and renal failure, as the myoglobin crystals block the kidney tubules. In those cases, the rule of nines is not applicable, and adequate fluid resuscitation is indicated by maintaining a urine output of 0.5 to 1 cc/kg body weight per hour. This level of urine flow also helps to reduce the risk of renal failure from rhabdomyolysis. Also with breakdown of muscle cells, potassium is released into the circulation and can lead to hyperkalemia, which can result in cardiac arrhythmias and death. Tall peaked T-waves on the ECG may be a sign of hyperkalemia. Intravenous calcium (gluconate or chloride) along with intravenous sodium bicarbonate, 50% dextrose, and insulin can temporarily reduce the effects of hyperkalemia on the heart.

rhabdomyolysis: disintegration (lysis) or dissolution of muscle. This releases large amounts of myoglobin into the blood, which can precipitate in the kidneys, causing renal failure.

Lightning Injuries

Lightning kills more persons in North America each year than any other weather-related phenomenon. A **lightning injury** is very different from other electrical injuries in that lightning produces extremely high voltages (> 10,000,000 volts) and currents (> 2,000 amps), but has a very short duration (< 100 msec) of contact.

Lightning produces a flashover phenomenon, in which the current flows around the outside of the victim's body. Consequently, the internal damage from current flow seen with generated electricity is not seen in a lightning strike. Most of the effects from a lightning strike are the result of the massive DC (direct current) shock that is received. Classic lightning-strike burns produce a fernlike or splatter pattern across the skin (Figure 16-17).

The victim does not need to be struck directly to sustain an injury. Lightning can strike an adjacent object or nearby ground and still produce an injury to a victim. Often the victim's skin is wet, from either sweat or rain. This water, when heated by

lightning injury: injury by the multiple effects of very short duration, very high voltage direct current on the body. The most serious effect is cardiac and respiratory arrest.

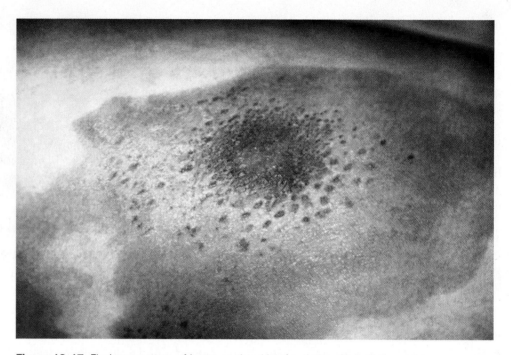

Figure 16-17 Flashover pattern of burns on the skin of a victim of a lightning strike.

the lightning current, is quickly vaporized to steam, producing superficial and partial-thickness burns, and may literally explode the clothing off the victim. Because these burns are superficial, aggressive fluid resuscitation is not required.

The most serious effect of a lightning strike is cardiorespiratory arrest, with the massive current acting like a defibrillator to briefly stop the heart. Cardiac activity often spontaneously resumes within minutes. However, the respiratory drive centers of the brain are depressed by the current discharge and take longer to recover and resume the normal respiratory drive. Consequently, the victim remains in respiratory arrest, which is followed by a second cardiac arrest from hypoxia.

The essential component of the management of the lightning-strike victim is restoration of cardiorespiratory function, while protecting the cervical spine. Follow standard guidelines for CPR and advanced cardiac life support (ACLS). Because lightning strikes can occur at sporting events and other outdoor gatherings, strikes often become multiple-casualty events. It must be stressed that in a multiple-casualty lightning strike, the conventional triage approach of a pulseless or nonbreathing patient equaling a dead patient should not be followed. If a patient is awake or breathing after a lightning strike, he will most likely survive without further intervention. Resuscitative efforts should concentrate on those victims who are in respiratory or cardiac arrest because prompt CPR and ACLS increase the chance that these victims will survive.

Long-term problems have been seen in lightning-strike patients, such as the development of cataracts, or neurologic and/or psychologic difficulties. Perforation of the eardrum is quite common, and rarely long bone or scapular fractures, as seen in the victims of generated high-voltage electrical injuries, may be seen. Those fractures are managed as described in Chapter 14.

There are over 200 reported deaths in North America each year due to lightning strikes. This represents only 30% of lightning-strike victims, so it is possible that you will have to care for such a victim. These events often involve multiple victims, with varying degrees of severity. Prompt CPR greatly improves the chances of survival. When confronted with a naked (or partially unclothed) unconscious or confused patient, with perforated eardrums and a fern-like or splatter burn pattern on his body, think lightning strike.

Radiation Burns

Ionizing radiation damages cells by breaking molecular bonds. Skin burns from radiation look exactly like thermal burns and cannot be differentiated by their appearance alone. However, radiation burns develop slowly over days and so generally do not present as an emergency. Because of the damage to the skin cells, **radiation injury** heals very slowly. The burns can cause fluid loss just as thermal burns do and are even more prone to infection.

Patients with radiation burns are not radioactive unless they are contaminated with radioactive material. If there is any danger that they might be contaminated, you should call for the hazardous materials team to scan them for radiation and perform decontamination if needed. Noncontaminated radiation-burn patients are treated the same as any burn patient. Decontamination of patients contaminated by radioactive material is beyond the scope of this course.

radiation injury: injury to the skin and tissues from the effect of ionizing radiation. The injury is caused by the radiation breaking molecular bonds within the cell and cannot be differentiated from thermal burns by appearance alone.

Circumferential Burns

As mentioned earlier in patient management, circumferential full-thickness burns can lead to neurovascular compromise. Although that is rarely a problem on the fire scene, it may become significant during an interfacility transfer. Full-thickness burns that are circumferential on an extremity can act as a tourniquet as edema progresses. Early on, the patient may complain of loss of sensation and tingling and eventually develop ischemic pain with loss of pulses. Circumferential full-thickness burns on the extremities will require an escharotomy by the physician, especially if long transport times are involved. Circumferential burns of the chest can interfere with chest expansion and thus compromise respirations. Again, escharotomy in this setting can improve ventilatory status.

Be sure to alert the receiving facility if you are transporting a patient with full-thickness circumferential burns.

Secondary Transport

Major burns often do not occur in locations where immediate transport to a burn center is possible. As a result, transport from a primary hospital to a burn center is commonly necessary. After the initial stabilization, prompt transfer to a burn center can improve patient outcome. During this transport, it is important for the emergency care providers to continue resuscitation initiated at the referring facility.

Prior to secondary transport, the transferring physician should have completed the following:

- Stabilization of respiratory and hemodynamic function, which may include intubation and IV access for fluid administration
- Assessment and management of associated injuries
- Review of appropriate lab data (specifically, blood gas analysis)
- Insertion of nasogastric tube in patients having burns covering more than 20% of the body surface area
- Placement of a Foley (urinary) catheter to allow measurement of urine output, which can assist in determining the adequacy of ongoing fluid resuscitation
- Assessment of peripheral circulation and appropriate wound management
- Proper arrangements with the receiving hospital and physician

Parkland formula is a formula to calculate initial fluid resuscitation of the burn patient. The formula is fluid needs for first 24 hours equal 4 cc of Ringer's lactate or normal saline multiplied times the % of burn area multiplied times the body weight in kilograms.

You should specifically discuss the transport with either the referring or the receiving physician to determine what special functions may need monitoring and to determine the appropriate range for fluid administration because burns often require

PEARLS
Secondary Transport

- Plan all secondary transports to burn centers and effectively continue resuscitation during such transports.
- Do not begin a secondary transport of a patient with a possible airway burn without the patient being intubated before transport.

extremely large hourly IV rates for appropriate cardiovascular support. Initial resuscitative fluid needs in a burn patient are calculated using the Parkland formula:

4 cc × % burn area × body weight (kg) = amount of Ringer's lactate or normal saline needed in the first 24 hours

Half of this fluid is given in the first 8 hours and the remainder over the next 16 hours. If large amounts of fluids are to be given, Ringer's lactate is preferred. Normal saline in large amounts can cause hyperchloremic acidosis.

Burn patients will need appropriate IV analgesics during transport.

It is important for you to maintain careful records indicating patient condition and treatment during transport. You should also make an in-depth report to the receiving facility.

Minor Burns

There may be times when an emergency care provider is asked to care for minor burns, such as when providing responder medical support at a major fire. Burn wounds should be cooled with tepid water, not ice. After drying the area, assess for burn depth. Full-thickness burns should be evaluated by a physician, preferably a burn specialist. Partial-thickness burns without blisters can be covered with a sterile dressing. Topical burn agents such as silver sulfadiazine or bacitracin may be applied.

If the patient is going to be seen soon at a medical facility, then do not apply the topical agent because emergency department personnel will remove it upon arrival. Do not use silver containing antibiotic creams on exposed places, such as the face, because they can be photoreactive and darken the skin. Partial-thickness burns with blisters can be debrided, based on local protocol and scope of practice of the emergency care provider. Because they are likely to rupture on their own, large, flimsy blisters (>2 in or >6 cm) can be debrided. Smaller blisters that affect joint movement can also be debrided. Apply dressings along with a topical burn agent or one of the newer membrane dressings.

All these patients should be seen by a burn specialist or surgeon in follow up. Do not forget that burns are painful and the patient will need appropriate analgesics.

Pediatric Burns

Children represent nearly one-half of all patients who seek treatment for burns. Because of their thinner skin, they are at greater risk for severe injury following a burn. Post-burn problems, such as hypothermia, are more likely to occur in children because of their larger surface area to body mass ratio. Because of differences in anatomy, the rule of nines must be modified, because in small children the head represents a larger portion of the body surface. The Lund and Browder chart is better for estimating burn size in children (Table 16-3). The patient's palmar surface (1%) rule applies to children as well as adults.

Sadly, burns in children may be the result of intentional abuse, and in fact, 20% of all abuse cases in the United States involve burns. You should be alert for signs of abuse. They include burns that match shapes of objects such as curling irons, irons, or cigarette burns. Also suspicious for abuse are multiple stories of how the injury occurred or stories of the burn being caused by activities by the child that are inconsistent with the child's development. Burns to the genitalia, perineum, or in a stocking or glove distribution (Figure 16-18) should

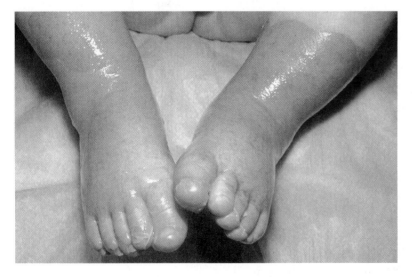

Figure 16-18 Scald burns on a child. This is a typical pattern of child abuse burns. *(Photo courtesy of Roy Alson, MD)*

raise suspicion. If there is a suspicion of abuse, this must be reported to child protective services or law enforcement. Follow your local laws and protocols.

Fire and EMS personnel can help reduce burns in children through community education. Programs to teach parents about limiting the temperature on household water heaters to 120°F (49°C) and programs to teach children about fire safety can make a significant impact on the incidence of pediatric burns in your community. You should be aware that the elderly may also be victims of abuse by burns. (See Chapter 18.)

Case Presentation (continued)

On arrival the fire officer informs you the fire is out and all hazards are controlled. You notice a large number of empty beer bottles around the yard and near the grill. Your triage sweep reveals only two victims, both of whom are ambulatory, talking, and following commands. When you ask what happened, you are told one of the guests threw a cup of gasoline onto the grill to get it to burn faster. He sustained burns to his face, chest, and arms. A second person who was also close to the grill has some burns to the face only.

You direct your partner to check on the person with facial burns, and you go to assess the person with burns to his face, arms, and chest. Your initial assessment reveals the patient has a normal speaking voice and respiration and a strong radial pulse that is slightly fast. No wheezes are heard. A focused exam reveals singeing of his head hair, eyebrows, and nasal hairs. Both forearms show blisters along with charred skin, with burns that appear to be circumferential. There is erythema in his nose, mouth, and pharynx.

Your patient walks to the ambulance and is placed on the cot. At this time it is noted that his voice is becoming husky, and he is complaining of feeling short of breath. An ITLS Ongoing Exam reveals bilateral wheezes, but the pulse oximeter reading is 95% on 15 liters of oxygen by nonrebreather mask. The presence of airway signs should lead you to consider presence of upper airway burns and possibly losing the airway.

Your ambulance has a transcutaneous carbon monoxide monitor, which shows your patient has a carboxyhemoglobin (HbCO) level of 9%. Normally flash burns outdoors do not pose risk of inhalation injury, but given that his clothes ignited, he has sustained more than a flash burn. Your unit does not have DAI capability, and the patient has an active gag reflex and will not tolerate intubation, so you do not attempt one at this time. You do notify the burn center of the potential airway problem, and just in case, remind yourself where the needle cricothyrotomy equipment is located. Your patient is given an albuterol nebulizer treatment and taken to the nearest burn center due to both airway involvement and circumferential arm burns.

The patient undergoes DAI in the emergency department, and a smaller-than-usual size endotracheal tube is placed using a fiberoptic scope. He has bilateral escharotomies of his forearms. His oxygen saturation falls, and he is admitted to the burn ICU, where he develops adult respiratory distress syndrome (ARDS) and has a protracted course. However, because of his youth and general good health, he survives. His upper airway burns resulted from inhalation of the vapor, and the ARDS resulted from probable aspiration.

Assessment of the patient who sustained only facial burns showed his burns are superficial. Your partner has called for a second unit to transport him because the first patient is a load and go, and his patient is refusing transport to the hospital. The firefighters on scene will monitor him until the second unit arrives.

Summary

The mechanisms of burn injuries are potentially deadly for both you and your patient. Remember scene safety! All burns are serious and should be evaluated at the hospital. Do not forget the basics: Half of all burn deaths are from inhalation injuries. Aggressive airway management may be needed. Stop the burning process by quickly irrigating the burn with room-temperature water. A clean sheet is all you need to put on the burn, other than a blanket to cover the patient to prevent hypothermia. In the opposite of load and go, patients with chemical burns must be decontaminated immediately or the burn damage will continue to progress during transport. Electrical burns and lightning injury are commonly associated with cardiac arrest, but rapid evaluation and management are usually life saving. High-voltage electricity is extremely dangerous, so get trained personnel to turn off the current before approaching the patient. Do not begin secondary transfer of a burn patient until the patient has been properly stabilized and the airway protected.

Bibliography

Borron, S. W., F. J. Baud, P. Barriot, M. Imbert, and C. Bismuth. "Prospective Study of Hydroxocobalamin for Acute Cyanide Poisoning in Smoke Inhalation." *Annals of Emergency Medicine* 49, no. 6 (June 2007): 794–801.

Committee on Trauma, American College of Surgeons. "Injuries Due to Burns and Cold." In *Advanced Trauma Life Support*, 9th ed., 230-44. Chicago: American College of Surgeons, 2012.

Danks, R. R. "Burn Management: A Comprehensive Review of the Epidemiology and Treatment of Burn Victims." *Journal of Emergency Medical Services* 28, no. 5 (May 2003): 118–41.

Fortin, J. L., J. P. Giocanti, M. Ruttimann, and J. J. Kowalski. "Prehospital Administration of Hydroxocobalamin for Smoke Inhalation-Associated Cyanide Poisoning: Eight Years of Experience in the Paris Fire Brigade." *Clinical Toxicology* 44, Suppl. 1 (2006): 37–44.

Gausche-Hill, M., K. M. Brown, Z. J. Oliver, C. Sasson, P. S. Dayan, N. M. Eschmann, T. S. Weik, B. J. Lawner, R. Sahni, Y. Falck-Ytter, J. L. Wright, K. Todd, and E. S. Lang. "An Evidence-Based Guideline for Prehospital Analgesia in Trauma." *Prehospital Emergency Care* 18, Suppl. 1 (2014): 25–34.

Jenkins, J. A. "Emergent Management of Thermal Burns." *MedScape* Web page, updated February 10, 2014. Accessed March 2, 2015, at http://emedicine.medscape.com/article/769193-overview.

Leybell, I. "Cyanide Toxicity." *MedScape* Web page, updated July 21, 2014. Accessed January 1, 2015, at http://emedicine.medscape.com/article/814287-overview.

Lloyd, E. C, B. C. Rodgers, M. Michener, and M. S. Williams. "Outpatient Burns: Prevention and Care." *American Family Physician* 85, no. 1 (January 2012): 25–32.

Miller, K., and A. Chang. "Acute Inhalation Injury." *Emergency Medicine Clinics of North America* 21, no. 2 (May 2003): 533–57.

Miller, S., and C. Menckhoff. "Optimizing Outcome in the Adult and Pediatric Burn Patient." *Trauma Reports* 10, no. 2 (March 2009): 1.

Hettiaratchy, S., and R. Papini. "Initial Management of a Major Burn: Overview." *British Medical Journal* 328, no. 7455 (2004): 1555–57.

Get more information about this course by calling
ITLS International at 888-495-4875
(outside the United States call +1-630-495-6442) or visit

www.itrauma.org

17

Pediatric Trauma

Patrick J. Maloney, MD
Ann Marie Dietrich, MD, FACEP, FAAP

Traumi Pediatrici	Traumatismo en Niños	Traumatisme dans les Enfants
Urazy u dzieci	Trauma beim Kind	Ozljede u djece
إصابات الأطفال	trauma dece	Poškodbe otrok
Gyermekkori trauma		

Key Terms

child abuse, *p. 328*
child restraint seat, *p. 345*
consent, *p. 328*
fluid resuscitation, *p. 341*
length-based tape, *p. 328*
SCIWORA, *p. 345*

Objectives

Upon successful completion of this chapter, you should be able to:

1. Describe effective techniques for gaining the confidence of children and their parents.
2. Predict pediatric injuries based on common mechanisms of injury.
3. Describe the ITLS Primary and Secondary Surveys in the pediatric patient.
4. Demonstrate understanding of the need for immediate transport in potentially life-threatening circumstances, regardless of the availability of immediate parental consent.
5. Differentiate the equipment needs of pediatric patients from those of adults.
6. Describe the various ways to perform spinal motion restriction (SMR) on a child and how this differs for an adult.
7. Discuss the need for involvement of EMS personnel in prevention programs for parents and children.

Chapter Overview

Providing appropriate and efficient prehospital care for pediatric patients is challenging. The goal of all prehospital care is to minimize further injury, ensure patient safety, and treat life-threatening conditions. When applying these principles to the pediatric population, you must remember that children are not just little adults. They differ from adults in that they have unique patterns of injuries, frequently have different physical and psychosocial responses to those injuries, require special equipment for assessment and treatment, and can be challenging to assess and communicate with. Doctors as well as emergency care providers are frequently less confident treating children because of these differences and the fact that children are treated less frequently. As a result, providers do not develop as much expertise as they would like. Those with children of their own are further hampered by the intense emotions felt when treating a seriously injured child.

For all these reasons, you should study this chapter carefully. It offers a review of the ITLS Primary Survey, stresses the differences between children and adults, and describes how to manage critical injuries. In addition, the U.S. Emergency Medical Services for Children (EMSC) program promotes pediatric prehospital care and may assist both individual emergency care providers as well as medical directors as a pediatric resource.

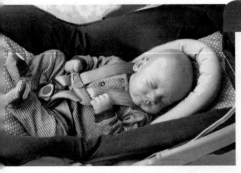

(Photo courtesy of Herjua/Shutterstock)

Case Presentation

Yours is one of several ALS ambulances that have responded to the scene of a multiple-vehicle collision involving a truck. Fire service has controlled the hazards on scene. On arrival the EMS supervisor directs you to the rear of a sedan that was hit on the left side. Two elderly occupants in the front seat are being cared for by other emergency care providers. Your attention is directed to the 10-month old infant still secured in a car seat that was found on the floor between the rear and front seats of the car. The driver (grandfather) states the child has been awake but periodically crying since the collision. You perform an initial assessment of the little girl and find her to be alert, with good skin color and easy respirations.

Before proceeding, consider these questions: Pending arrival of the mother, what steps should you take to reassess and treat the child, and how should the infant be readied for transport? Given the mechanism of injury, should she be removed from her car seat? What form, if any, of spinal motion restriction should be considered, and will her age affect this decision? How does the evaluation of an infant differ from that of an adult? Would awaiting the arrival of the mother facilitate such an evaluation?

Keep these questions in mind as you read through the chapter. Then, at the end of the chapter, find out how the emergency care providers managed this patient.

Communication with the Child and Family

Children are part of a family unit, which is the one constant factor in the child's life, so family-centered care for an injured child is ideal. (Remember that the caregiver of a child will not always be a parent, but for simplicity the generic term *parent* is used in this chapter when referring to the guardian/caregiver of a child.) Following an injury to their child, parents should be involved as much as possible in his or her care. Parents who receive careful instructions and guidance may be helpful to the emergency provider. Explain to them what you are doing and why you are doing it, and then use their trust relationship with the child to enhance your history gathering, physical examination, and care of the patient. Inclusion and respect of the family will improve the performance of all aspects of the stabilization of an injured child.

The best way to gain parental confidence is to demonstrate your competence and compassion in managing the child. Parents are more likely to be cooperative if they see that you are confident, organized, and using equipment that is designed for children. Show the parents you know how important they are by involving them in the care of their child. Whenever possible, keep parents in physical and verbal contact with the child. They can perform simple tasks such as holding a pressure dressing or holding the child's hand. Parents can explain to the child what is going on or sing their favorite songs.

Occasionally, the emotional stress of an ill or injured child may be too much for a parent. When that happens, parents may become visibly anxious, agitated, or even quiet, withdrawn, and "frozen." As the emergency care provider, it is important to recognize the emotional response of the parent. Remember, most children will look to their parents for clues on how to act. If their parent is calm and cooperative, the child will more likely also be composed, but if a parent is panicking and unable to calm down, the child will more likely also be anxious and uncooperative. In situations where the parent is unable to follow your instructions and remain calm, it is sometimes best to ask the parent to step back. It is important to use your best judgment of what is best for the child in these difficult situations. Make sure that the parents receive appropriate care if they were also injured or if they need help dealing with the situation.

When evaluating an injured child, emergency care providers must remember that children of different ages have different cognitive skills and interact with the world in different ways. By making a child-friendly environment and using child-friendly language and gestures, your patient will feel more comfortable and will be more cooperative with your evaluation and treatment.

Remember to speak and act in a way that is understandable and calming to the child and parents. This will not only help console the scared and hurt child, but it also will help you accurately assess the child's condition. A child who can be consoled and interacts normally with a parent likely has a normal mental status. In contrast, a child who cannot be consoled or cannot interact in the usual way may have a head injury, may be in shock, may be hypoxic, or may be in severe pain. Because they are familiar with a child's baseline mental status, the parents are your best resource for detecting subtle changes in the child's behavior. They will notice when the child is "not acting right" before you will. This is especially helpful in dealing with a "special needs" children, who may not respond in a manner typical for a child their age. Record and report your observations just as you would report changes in level of consciousness of an adult.

Children younger than 9 months old like to hear "cooing" sounds or the jingle and sight of keys. Children younger than 1 year of age know many "ah" sounds, like "mama" and "papa." Try to use them. Older children are very literal in their understanding of language. Therefore, always choose your words carefully and explain exactly what you mean in simple terms. For example, when placing an IV in a child, instead of using the word "flush," which will likely make the child think of a toilet, you may describe the saline as "clear water that makes the medicine and blood move."

Whenever possible, try to give a child and parent reasonable options. This will not only give them a sense of participation and control but also will avoid the trap of asking a 2-year-old for permission. Rather than ask, "May I listen to your heart and lung?" which will usually be answered with an emphatic "No!" by a toddler, ask the child if he or she would like you to listen to his or her heart or look in his or her mouth first. When there are no options, such as when placing a cervical collar or transporting a child in an ambulance, clearly tell the child what you are doing in a calm tone and with a smile on your face. When possible, show it does not hurt, perhaps by doing it to a parent or yourself. Never lie to a child.

Always try to tell the child and parents what you are going to do before you do it. Most children do not like surprises when they are scared or uncomfortable. For example, say, "We are going to hold your head still. Mom, this is important in case he has hurt his neck." Speak simply, slowly, and clearly. Be gentle and firm.

Distraction is a great tool. Infants and children younger than 1 year old often can be easily distracted with a simple flashlight. The toddler and young child can benefit from holding a toy or doll. Ask the parent to get one favorite belonging, if easily available, for the ride to the hospital. It will make the trip to and through the hospital easier.

Before you leave the scene with the child, be sure to ask the parent about other children. Sometimes they are so concerned about one that they forget other small children who may be in a high-risk situation, such as alone in the house.

Parental Consent

Many jurisdictions have **consent** laws that exist to protect children. Although consent to treat is necessary for children who are stable and desirable in children who are injured, any critically injured child should not have care delayed while attempting to obtain consent. Prehospital care providers have to assess the situation quickly and decide whether delaying emergency care to obtain parental consent could possibly harm the child. In a situation in which a child needs emergency care (such as a child in a bicycle/motor-vehicle collision and no parent present), you must treat that child immediately. When in doubt, always err on the side of treating and transporting any seriously injured child, regardless of the ability to obtain appropriate consent. Remember to document why you are transporting without permission, and always notify medical direction of this action. As soon as safe and feasible, you should attempt to notify a parent or other caretaker.

If the parents or legal guardians do not want you to transport or treat, try to persuade them. If available, utilize online medical direction for assistance in talking to the parents. Often, if parents are told by a doctor on the phone or radio that their child is potentially very ill or injured, the parents will agree to treatment and transport. If you cannot convince them, document your actions on the written report, and ask the parent or guardian to sign a refusal of care form. If the child has a critical injury and the parents refuse transport, notify law enforcement and the appropriate social services authorities immediately and try to continue care of the child until they arrive. If you suspect **child abuse**, notify authorities at the appropriate time. You should not confront the possible abuser but act in the best interests of the child.

Assessment and Care
Pediatric Equipment

Table 17-1 contains a list of suggested pediatric equipment for the prehospital provider. A more detailed list can be downloaded from the American Academy of Pediatrics website. Keep pediatric equipment separate from your adult equipment so you do not have to search for it when needed urgently. It would be ideal to keep equipment for each size child in separate compartments. However, lack of storage space and high expense make multiple containers and duplicate equipment impractical. Using a **length-based tape** makes it much simpler to determine the appropriate equipment and medication doses for a child.

---

consent: the granting of permission to undergo treatment. In the pediatric patient, it is usually given by the parents or legal guardians but is not required in an emergency situation if neither is present.

PEARLS
Abuse

You are the emergency care provider at the scene of the injury. Be alert to signs of child abuse, such as: the story about how the injury occurred changes, the child was injured while doing something a child of that age cannot physically do, the injury pattern resembles a hand or object, or there are multiple contusions in varied states of healing.

child abuse: physical or emotional violence or neglect toward a person from infancy until age 15.

PEARLS
Equipment

Children require special equipment. Without this equipment, you cannot provide the pediatric patient with adequate care.

length-based tape: a method of estimating the appropriate-size equipment and doses of medications for children. The method is based on the fact that a child's weight is proportional to his length.

Table 17-1: Prehospital Pediatric Equipment and Supplies

BLS Equipment and Supplies

Essential	Desirable
• Infant car seat • Oropharyngeal airways: infant, child, and adult sizes (sizes 00–5) with tongue blades for insertion • Self-inflating resuscitation bag, child and adult sizes • Masks for bag-valve-mask device: neonatal, infant, child, and adult sizes • Oxygen masks; infant, child, and adult sizes • Nonrebreathing mask: pediatric and adult sizes • Stethoscope • Pediatric femur traction splint • Pediatric backboard with head immobilizer • Pediatric cervical collars (rigid) • Blood pressure cuff, infant and child • Portable suction unit with a regulator • Suction catheter: tonsil-tip and 6F–14F • Extremity splints: pediatric size • Bulb syringe • Obstetric pack • Thermal blanket • Water-soluble lubricant	• Nasopharyngeal airways: sizes 18F–34F, or 4.5–8.5 mm • Glasgow Coma Score reference • Small stuffed toy • Finger-stick blood glucose device • Pulse oximeter

ALS Equipment and Supplies

ALS units should carry everything on the BLS list, plus the following items:

Essential	Desirable
• Transport monitor • Blood glucose analysis system • Defibrillator with adult and pediatric paddles • Monitoring electrodes: pediatric sizes • Endotracheal tubes, uncuffed sizes 2.5–6 mm; cuffed sizes 3–8 mm • Endotracheal tube stylets: pediatric and adult sizes • Infant and child laryngoscope straight blades sizes 0–3 and curved blades sizes 2–4 • Nasogastric tubes, sizes 8F–16F • KED (immobilization device) • Magill forceps: pediatric and adult • IO needles, sizes 16, 18, 20 gauge • Butterfly cannulae, 23 and 25 gauge • Over-the-needle catheters, 16–24 gauge • Pediatric armboards • Broselow© (or other length-based) tape • Nebulizer	• Disposable CO_2 detection device • End-tidal CO_2 monitors

Figure 17-1 Use of length-based tape.

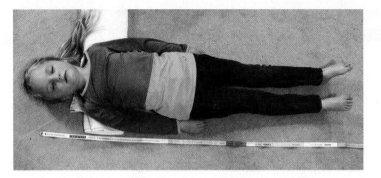

The length-based tape helps you measure the length of a child, estimate the child's weight, appropriately choose equipment of the correct size, and administer precalculated doses of fluid and medications (Figures 17-1 and 17-2). The device allows you to focus on the patient instead of trying to remember the correct equipment size and drug dose. The length-based tape estimates weight and equipment size better than medical professionals. Although there is some controversy about the accuracy of length-based medication dosages because of the increased incidence of childhood obesity, standard length-based resuscitation systems continue to be recommended as safe, rapid, and accurate tools. Trying to calculate medication doses can also lead to medication errors. Besides length-based systems, there are other methods emergency care providers can use to determine appropriate dosages and equipment sizes. Local medical direction should determine which system an organization will use and ensure all providers are trained.

Common Mechanisms of Injury

Children are most commonly injured from falls (either from standing height or higher), motor-vehicle collisions, automobile–pedestrian or bicycle crashes, burns, submersion injuries (drownings), and child abuse. Blunt trauma is much more

Figure 17-2 Standard Pediatric Aid to Resuscitation Card system has color-coded tape and a booklet of precalculated doses of fluids, medications, and equipment. *(Photos courtesy of Kyee Han, MD)*

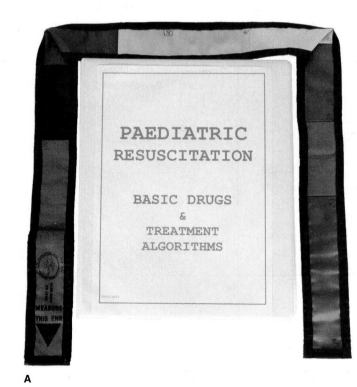

A

Figure 17-2 (continued)

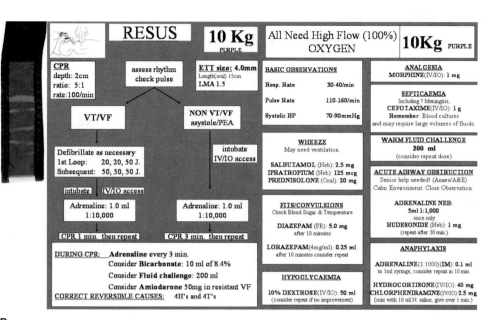

B

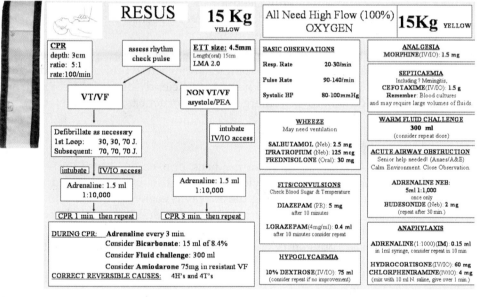

C

common than penetrating injuries in children. Young children who fall from higher than a few feet often land on their heads because the head is disproportionately large and heavy compared to the body of a small child. Fortunately, when children fall from a height of less than three feet, they rarely sustain serious head injuries. One exception to this rule is infants younger than three months of age, who may be seriously injured from seemingly minor falls. Injuries sustained by children riding bicycles, motorcycles, and dirt bikes, especially if they are not wearing a helmet, are often severe. Motor-vehicle collisions, especially if car seats, booster seats, and lap-belt restraints are improperly used, may result in seat-belt syndrome, which can include life-threatening injuries to the liver, spleen, intestines, or lumbar spine.

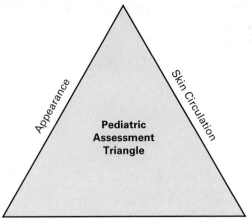

Pediatric
Assessment
Triangle

Appearance

Skin Circulation

Work of Breathing

Figure 17-3 A tool, developed by the American Academy of Pediatrics, to help you efficiently prioritize your care and communicate your findings.

Any situation in which the victim's injury pattern is not consistent with the mechanism may be child abuse, which is also called *nonaccidental trauma (NAT)*. Suspect abuse if the history does not match the injury or if the mechanism of injury is not consistent with the child's developmental status (for example, a two-month-old infant cannot walk and therefore cannot break his or her leg running across the floor). Other warning flags include a delay in seeking care, if the story about the incident frequently changes during your assessment, if stories vary between parents or caregivers, or if you have any other concerns. Remember to report any of these findings to the emergency department team and/or appropriate local authorities. Be familiar with the reporting requirements for your agency.

General Assessment

When arriving at the scene of an injury, it is very important to quickly assess the situation and the injured child. After ensuring your own safety, your next step is to develop a general impression of the injured child, usually from across the room or scene. Before ever touching an injured child, try to decide whether he or she appears to be severely injured or in distress. Make a mental note of the child's initial level of consciousness, work of breathing, and overall circulation as you begin your assessment. Although a preschool child may appear to be sleeping rather than unconscious from an injury, remember that most children will not sleep through the arrival of emergency vehicles. Following a traumatic event, a decreased level of consciousness may suggest hypoxia, shock, head trauma, or seizure.

One tool to help you develop this overall impression of the severity of the child's condition is the Pediatric Assessment Triangle, an objective tool developed by the American Academy of Pediatrics. It will help you efficiently prioritize your care and communicate your findings to the emergency department team. A version of it is shown in Figure 17-3.

Assessment of the Airway

As you begin your assessment, stabilize the neck in a neutral position with your hands. Do not take time to apply a cervical collar until you have finished the ITLS Primary Survey (Figure 17-4). Inspecting the airway is easier in the child than in the adult. It is true that the child's tongue is large, the tissue is soft, and the airway obstructs easily, but other characteristics make it easier to manage the child's airway. For example, neonates are obligatory nose breathers, so clearing the nose with a bulb syringe can be life saving. To use the bulb syringe, first collapse the bulb end of the syringe, and then put the point end in the nose of the child and release the bulb. When you remove the syringe from the nose, squeeze the bulb to empty the mucus, blood, or vomit, and repeat. The bulb syringe can be used to remove secretions from the posterior pharynx of infants as well.

Look for signs of airway obstruction in the child, including apnea, stridor, and "gurgling" respirations. If identified, perform a jaw-thrust maneuver without moving the neck. That will help lift the relatively large tongue out of the way of the airway. Suctioning oral secretions and any vomit from the posterior pharynx also can help. Inserting an oropharyngeal airway may help keep the obstructed airway patent in an unconscious child. (See Chapter 5.) If a tooth is loose, be sure to remove it from the mouth so that the child does not aspirate and choke on it. Also, remember that in small children, the occiput is rather large compared to the torso. When positioned flat on a spinal immobilization board or stretcher, the occiput will often flex the neck and the floppy upper airway. This can result in occlusion of the airway. To prevent this from happening, place a pad underneath the torso of children younger than eight years old to keep the neck in a neutral position. (See Figure 17-5 and Chapter 11.) Hyperextension of the neck also may cause airway occlusion.

ITLS PRIMARY SURVEY

SCENE SIZE-UP
Standard Precautions
Hazards, Number of Patients, Need for additional resources, **Mechanism of Injury**

↓

INITIAL ASSESSMENT
GENERAL IMPRESSION
Age, Sex, Weight, General Appearance, Position, Purposeful Movement, Obvious Injuries, Skin Color
Life-threatening Bleeding

LOC
A-V-P-U
Chief Complaint/Symptoms

AIRWAY (CONSIDER C-SPINE CONTROL)
Snoring, Gurgling, Stridor; Silence

BREATHING
Present? Rate, Depth, Effort

CIRCULATION
Radial/Carotid Present? Rate, Rhythm, Quality
Skin Color, Temperature, Moisture; Capillary Refill
Has bleeding been controlled?

↓

RAPID TRAUMA SURVEY
HEAD and NECK
Wounds?
Neck Vein distention? Tracheal Deviation?

CHEST
Asymmetry (Paradoxical Motion?), Contusions, Penetrations, Tenderness, Instability, Crepitation
Breath Sounds
Present? Equal? (If unequal: percussion)
Heart Tones

ABDOMEN
Contusions, Penetration/Evisceration; Tenderness, Rigidity, Distension

PELVIS
Tenderness, Instability, Crepitation

LOWER/UPPER EXTREMITIES
Obvious Swelling, Deformity
Motor and Sensory

POSTERIOR
Obvious wounds, Tenderness, Deformity

If radial pulse present:
VITAL SIGNS
Measured Pulse, Breathing, Blood Pressure

If altered mental status: Brief Neurological exam
PUPILS
Size? Reactive? **Equal?**

GLASGOW COMA SCALE
Eyes, Voice, Motor

Figure 17-4 Steps in the assessment and management of the trauma patient are the same for both children and adults.

Figure 17-5 Most children require padding under their back and shoulders to keep the C-spine in a neutral position. *(Photo courtesy of Bob Page, MEd, NRP, CCP, NCEE)*

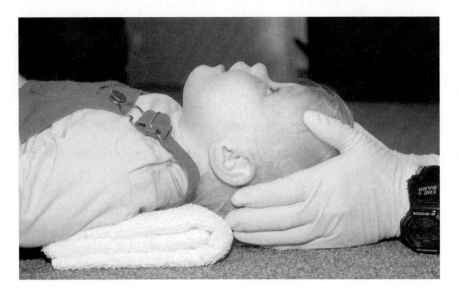

Assessment of Breathing

Assess the child for breathing difficulty and rate. Most children breathe faster than adults normally do. However, children usually breathe even faster when they are having difficulty; and then, when they can no longer compensate, they will have periods of apnea or a very slow respiratory rate. Note whether the child is "working" to breathe, demonstrated by subcostal or suprasternal retractions, nasal flaring, or grunting. Look at the chest rise, listen for air going in and out, and feel the air coming out of the nose. If there is no movement, reposition the jaw to remove any anatomical obstruction. If you still do not sense any air exchange, you must breathe for the child. If you have any doubt that the child is breathing adequately on his or her own, immediately assist the child's breathing. Provide supplemental oxygen to a child with respiratory difficulty.

Artificial Ventilation

The most common cause of cardiac arrest in children, including trauma victims, is hypoxia and respiratory failure. Therefore, the most important skill you must master is artificial ventilation with a bag-valve-mask resuscitation device. Remember, if you can mechanically oxygenate and ventilate a child, you can keep that child alive.

It is crucial that your bag-valve-mask device has a good seal around the face. If the face mask does not fit well, try a different size face mask or try turning the mask upside down for a better seal. Pay attention to your hand placement as well (Figure 17-6). Large adult hands can easily obstruct the airway or injure a child's eyes. Give each breath slowly over one second. Try to use the lowest pressure necessary to see good chest rise with each breath. If the chest is rising, air is getting into the lungs. If you do not see good chest rise, too little air is entering the lungs. Check air entry on both sides of the chest with your stethoscope. If the child is not getting good chest rise with each breath, make sure you have a good mask seal and air entry is not obstructed. If still unsuccessful, you may need to provide more pressure with each rescue breath. Be careful not to provide too much pressure because that can cause a pneumothorax or overinflate the stomach and cause vomiting. Remember that most pediatric resuscitation bags have a pop-off valve. In the prehospital setting, it is usually best to ensure that this valve is turned off.

When providing artificial ventilation, typical rates are 20 per minute for a child younger than one year of age, 15 per minute for older than one year of age, and 10 per minute for an adolescent. Studies have found that rescuers tend to hyperventilate even when consciously trying not to. Always make sure that your bag is

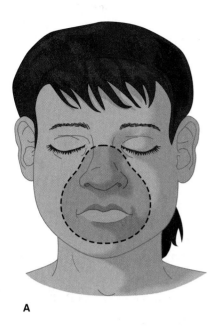

A

Figure 17-6a The mask should fit on the nose and the cleft above the chin.

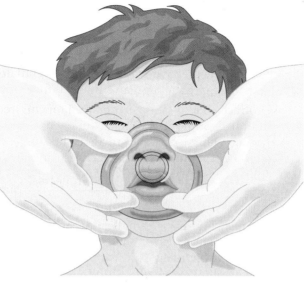

B

Figure 17-6b Two-handed face mask seal.

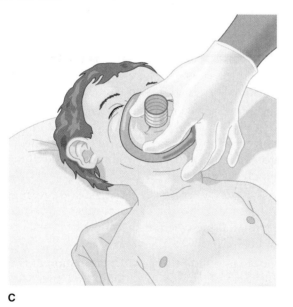

C

Figure 17-6c One-handed face mask seal.

connected to oxygen and that it is flowing (usually 10–15 LPM). Cricoid pressure (Sellick maneuver; see Chapter 4) is not currently recommended in a child because excessive cricoid pressure can easily obstruct a child's airway, and the maneuver has not been shown to prevent aspiration.

Endotracheal Intubation If bag-valve-mask ventilation of the child is effective, then intubation is an elective procedure. Studies have not shown that prehospital intubation improves the outcome of children. It is usually better not to intubate the child in the field if you can ventilate successfully with a bag-valve mask. Rapid and safe transportation to a trauma center, where definitive care is readily available, is one of the most important prognostic factors in trauma patients. Therefore, any unnecessary time spent at the scene should be avoided.

PEARLS
Endotracheal Intubation

The endotracheal tube in a child may become dislodged easily, especially during movement of the child. Frequent reassessment is very important. Constant end-tidal CO_2 monitoring (capnography) is very helpful.

Pediatric intubation is extremely difficult to perform even in an emergency department, so if you must intubate in the field, be prepared. While you set up your equipment, your partner should preoxygenate the child by applying a nonrebreather mask if the child is breathing on his or her own adequately. If the child is not breathing adequately, preoxygenate (not hyperventilate) with five to seven breaths of high-flow oxygen via a bag-valve mask at the normal rate for the age of the child.

Orotracheal intubation is preferred for children. There are several ways to choose the right size for the endotracheal tube. The simplest is to refer to your length-based tape system. Other techniques include choosing a tube that is about the same diameter as the tip of the child's little finger or using the following equation:

$$4 + \frac{\text{age in years}}{4} = \text{size of tube (mm)}$$

In small children the smallest part of the airway is just below the cords. As a result, traditional practice is to use an uncuffed tube in children younger than eight years old. However, most experts now recommend using cuffed endotracheal tubes in all patients. If using a cuffed tube, choose a tube that is 0.5 mm smaller unless using a 3.0 mm tube (in which case you should not downsize at all). In general, you should not inflate the cuff unless directed to do so by your medical direction because a cuff that is overinflated may damage the child's airway.

There is a significant risk of neck movement with any tracheal intubation, so have someone manually stabilize the patient's neck during intubation. Using a straight blade (Miller blade), enter the mouth on the right and gently sweep the tongue to the left. Then place the blade to lift the epiglottis and visualize the larynx. Compared to adults, the small child's larynx is closer to the mouth as well as more anterior (higher up). If you cannot see the cords because of the relatively large and floppy epiglottis, advance the laryngoscope blade to the epiglottis and lift again. The cords should be seen easily.

A common scenario is one in which the laryngoscope is initially advanced beyond the glottis and into the esophagus. If you encounter this clinical situation, gently and slowly withdraw your laryngoscope while visualizing the anatomy. You will likely see the vocal cords "drop down" into your visual field, at which point you may insert your endotracheal tube.

The laryngeal mask (LMA) and the King LT airways are available in pediatric sizes and can be used as rescue airways. They should not be used for airway burns or airway swelling from allergic reactions because they are supraglottic and so do not keep the glottis open.

Pulse oximetry should be used during every intubation. It is a good tool for knowing when you need to stop your intubation attempt to oxygenate the patient again prior to another attempt (usually when the SpO_2 drops below about 90%). Remember, in general, children will desaturate faster than adults. Other ways to make sure that you remember to ventilate include holding your breath when no one is breathing for the child. As soon as you get an urge to breathe, but after no more than 15 seconds, stop trying to intubate, bag the child to reoxygenate, and try again in a few minutes. An alternative effective method is to have the team member who is manually stabilizing the neck count aloud to 15 slowly.

Confirm the endotracheal tube is in the correct place by following the confirmation protocol. (See Chapter 5.) Although a disposable, qualitative end-tidal carbon dioxide detection device can be used to confirm that it is correctly positioned within the airway, capnography is the best way to both confirm the tube is in place and continually monitor its position. Be sure to secure the tube in place. Apply benzoin to the cheek and lip. Firmly tape (or tie with linen tape or plastic oxygen tubing) the tube to the corner of the mouth. Alternatively, a commercial endotracheal tube holder may be used, if available. Beware that simple flexion of the neck can push the tube into the right mainstem bronchus, and extension of the neck can pull the tube out of the trachea. Fortunately, the rigid cervical collar is an easy and practical adjunct to limit any unnecessary head and neck movement in children (collars are not available for infants). Therefore, applying a rigid cervical collar not only protects the trauma patient's cervical spine from potential further injury but also helps reduce the likelihood of endotracheal tube movement and dislodgement in both trauma and nontrauma patients.

Supplemental Oxygen Packaging a child often calls for some improvisation with tape and straps. However, both can restrict chest movement, so assess the child's ventilation frequently en route. Any child with a significant injury should receive supplemental oxygen (as close to 100% oxygen as possible), even if there seems to be no difficulty breathing. Injury, fear, and crying all increase oxygen demands on tissues. Children with any type of injury are likely to vomit, so be prepared. Remember to give ventilation instructions to your teammate before moving to assessment of circulation.

Assessment of Circulation

In a young child, the brachial and femoral pulses are usually easy to feel (so is the dorsalis pedis pulse), whereas the carotid pulse is not. Because tachycardia also occurs with fear and anxiety, the child should then be assessed for signs of poor perfusion, weak peripheral pulses compared to central pulses, cool distant extremities, and delayed capillary refill time. A weak rapid pulse with a rate over 130 is usually a sign of shock in children of all ages except neonates (Table 17-2).

Prolonged capillary refill, cool extremities, and skin mottling may indicate decreased tissue perfusion. Capillary refill may be used along with other methods to assess circulation, but do not depend on it alone to diagnose shock because refill time is prolonged by anything that causes vasoconstriction of the skin, such as cold environment or fear. To test capillary refill time, compress the nail bed, the entire foot, or the skin over the sternum for two seconds. Then release to see how quickly the blood returns and the skin color normalizes. Skin color should return to the precompressed state within two seconds. If it does not, the child has vasoconstriction, which may be a sign of shock.

Control of Bleeding Obvious bleeding sources must be controlled to maintain adequate blood volume and circulation. Remember, the child's blood volume is about 80 to 90 mL/kg, so a 10 kg (22 lb) child has less than one liter of blood. Three or four lacerations can cause a 200 mL blood loss, which is about 20% of the child's total volume. Therefore, pay closer attention to blood loss in a child than you do in an adult. Remember that bleeding may not be immediately evident if the child is fully clothed or lying on an absorbent surface such as carpet or grass. Be sure to expose the child's body and look for bleeding. Posterior scalp lacerations are especially notorious for causing unnoticed bleeding. Use pressure firm enough to control arterial bleeding if necessary. If you ask the parent or a bystander to help hold pressure, monitor them to be sure they are applying enough pressure to stop the bleeding.

One mistake parents as well as emergency medical personnel commonly make is using a large bulky dressing, towel, or piece of clothing to attempt to stop bleeding.

PEARLS
Shock

Because of strong compensatory mechanisms, children can look surprisingly well in early shock. When they deteriorate, however, they often "crash." If you have a long transport time and the mechanism of injury or the assessment suggests the possibility of hemorrhagic shock, be prepared. When you give fluid resuscitation to a child, give 20 mL/kg in each bolus, then reassess. Make sure the total amount of fluid you give is reported to the hospital.

Table 17-2: Ranges for Vital Signs				
Age	Weight (kg)	Respiration (per minute)	Pulse (per minute)	Systolic Blood Pressure (mm Hg)
Newborn	3–4	30–50	120–160	> 60
6 mo–1 yr	8–10	30–40	120–140	70–80
2–4 yr	12–16	20–30	100–110	80–95
5–8 yr	18–26	14–20	90–100	90–100
8–12 yr	26–50	12–20	80–100	100–110
> 12 yr	> 50	12–16	80–100	100–120

Unfortunately, bulky dressings often do not provide enough direct pressure to stop the bleeding. Instead, they simply absorb large amounts of blood and disguise potentially serious bleeding. Your gloved hand and fingers in combination with a 4 × 4 sterile gauze pad is usually your best tool for applying constant firm pressure to the site of bleeding. Once the bleeding is under control, you may attempt to apply a more secure dressing. Be sure to recheck the dressing and wound often to ensure that the bleeding has not recurred.

Hemostatic agents may be used to control hemorrhage in children. In addition, tourniquets are recommended for life-threatening bleeding that cannot be controlled by other means. Their life-saving benefits outweigh the small potential risk of further limb injury and loss. (See Chapters 9 and 14.)

Rapid Trauma Survey or Focused Exam

Perform a rapid head-to-toe exam (rapid trauma survey) for children who have been injured by a generalized mechanism or when you do not know the mechanism of injury. Children who have a focused (isolated) injury or an insignificant injury may have a focused exam of the injured part only. Children with insignificant mechanisms of injury may not require an ITLS Secondary Survey.

Rapid Trauma Survey

The rapid trauma survey is a quick examination of the head, neck, chest, abdomen, pelvis, and extremities. A brief neurological exam also is included if there is altered level of consciousness. Look for life-threatening injuries. By this time, the child should be adequately exposed to assess all the injuries. Parents may be able to assist with this because most children are taught not to allow strangers to disrobe them. You cannot assess what you cannot see. Examine head to toe and front to back, following the sequence of the rapid trauma survey. This will reduce the likelihood that you will miss a critical injury.

Rapidly check the head and neck for signs of injury, such as bruises, abrasions, lacerations, and puncture wounds. Also look for distended neck veins and tracheal deviation. What appears to be minor trauma to the neck can be life threatening because any bleeding or swelling within the neck can compress and obstruct a child's airway very quickly.

Look at, listen to, and feel the chest. Look for deformities, contusions, abrasions, perforations, burns, tenderness, lacerations, and swelling (DCAP-BTLS). Listen to breath sounds on each side, and note any abnormalities. Feel for tenderness, instability, and crepitus (TIC). If not already done, have one of your partners stabilize flail segments, seal open wounds, or decompress a tension pneumothorax.

Gently palpate the abdomen, and note any contusions, abrasions, penetrations, or distention. If there is no complaint of pain in the pelvic area, gently palpate the pelvis noting any TIC. Quickly evaluate the extremities for obvious injury.

After the rapid trauma survey, if indicated, transfer the child to a spinal motion-restriction device. Remember to log roll the child the same way you would an adult. (See Chapter 12.) This is the time to check the child's back carefully for any injuries. If an appropriate size cervical collar is available, place it on the child, securing the body first and then the head to the SMR device. If a rigid cervical collar is unavailable, you may use bulky towel rolls to help immobilize the child's head and neck.

Critical Trauma Situation

If you have found a critical trauma situation, the child needs rapid transport. Once you have the child packaged, you should leave the scene as quickly as possible. Remember to use a pad under the upper torso to align the neck in a neutral position. Pediatric-size rigid cervical collars are useful, especially in children older than one year of age, and can help remind the patient and providers not to move the head. Do not depend on the cervical collar alone, however. Restrict motion of the head with tape and a head motion-restriction device, sandbags, or bulky towel rolls. There are very few procedures that should be done in the field. Minutes count, especially in children. On-scene times of less than five minutes are desirable.

Administer 100% oxygen to all pediatric patients who have potentially serious injuries. There is strong evidence to support the policy that bag-valve-mask ventilation of the critical child is preferable to placing an endotracheal tube, if the transport time to an appropriate emergency department is short.

When considering transportation options, providers should be aware of local and regional resources and policies. This includes deciding on the appropriate destination for a particular patient (the nearest emergency department versus a regional pediatric trauma center) as well as choosing the best transportation mode (BLS versus ALS versus air ambulance). As a general rule, any child with life-threatening injuries or hemodynamic instability should be transported to the nearest facility with the capabilities to stabilize the patient further. See Table 17-3 for a partial list of mechanisms of injury that are criteria for transport to an emergency department approved for pediatrics or a pediatric trauma center.

If a pediatric patient needs a procedure, you must decide whether it is worth the time. You should consider how long it will take to perform, how urgent the procedure is, how difficult it will be at the scene versus in the back of the ambulance or at the hospital, and how much it will delay reaching definitive care. Issues found during the ITLS Primary Survey must be corrected. However, if you can adequately mask ventilate the pediatric patient, then immediate intubation in the field is not necessary. If you have a three-minute procedure (an IV) and a 30-minute transport, the intravenous (IV) line probably should be started en route. If you are awaiting the arrival of a helicopter, you may attempt the procedure, but be sure to have the child packaged and ready when transportation arrives. Some procedures may be best performed in the ambulance while en route to the hospital. Always call ahead so that the emergency department can have the necessary equipment and personnel ready. Perform the ITLS Ongoing Exam and ITLS Secondary Survey en route if there is time.

Table 17-3: Suggested Criteria for Transfer to an Emergency Department Approved for Pediatrics or a Pediatric Trauma Center
Criteria
• Obstructed airway
• Need for an airway intervention
• Respiratory distress
• Shock
• Altered mental status
• Dilated pupil
• Glasgow Coma Scale score < 13
• Pediatric Trauma Score < 8

• Mechanism of injury (less reliable indicators) associated with severe injuries:
  • Fall from a height of 10 feet or more
  • Motor-vehicle collision with fatalities
  • Ejection from an automobile in an MVC
  • In an MVC, significant intrusion into the passenger compartment
  • Hit by a car as a pedestrian or bicyclist
  • Fractures in more than one extremity
  • Significant injury to more than one organ system

Table 17-4: Pediatric Glasgow Coma Scale

		> 1 year	< 1 year	
Eyes Opening	4	Spontaneously	Spontaneously	
	3	To verbal command	To shout	
	2	To pain	To pain	
	1	No response	No response	

		> 1 year	< 1 year	
Best Motor Response	6	Obeys		
	5	Localizes pain	Localizes pain	
	4	Flexion—withdrawal	Flexion—normal	
	3	Flexion—abnormal (decorticate rigidity)	Flexion—abnormal (decorticate rigidity)	
	2	Extension (decerebrate rigidity)	Extension (decerebrate rigidity)	
	1	No response	No response	

		> 5 years	2–5 years	0–23 months
Best Verbal Response	5	Oriented and converses	Appropriate words and phrases	Smiles, coos, cries appropriately
	4	Disoriented and converses	Inappropriate words	Cries
	3	Inappropriate words	Cries and/or screams	Inappropriate crying and/or screaming
	2	Incomprehensible sounds	Grunts	Grunts
	1	No response	No response	No response

If, after completing the ITLS Primary Survey, you find no critical trauma situation, place the child on a stretcher and do a methodical ITLS Secondary Survey.

ITLS Secondary Survey

To perform an ITLS Secondary Survey for pediatric patients, record accurate vital signs, take a SAMPLE history, and perform a complete head-to-toe exam, including a more detailed neurologic exam as you would for an adult. In addition, during your neurologic exam make a notation of the child's behavior and response to the environment (alert and reaching for mom, and so on) and calculate the Glasgow Coma Scale (GCS) score or, if the patient is younger than two years old, the GCS for Infants and Children (Table 17-4). Finish bandaging and splinting, and transport the child while continuously monitoring. Notify medical direction.

Potentially Life-Threatening Injuries
Hemorrhagic Shock

The most common sites of severe internal bleeding in children are the chest, abdomen, pelvis, and long bones (femur fractures). Although intracranial blood loss rarely causes hemorrhagic shock, it may occur in the very young infant. Of course, external bleeding from wounds is also an important source of blood loss. Early shock (often referred to as *compensated shock*) is far more difficult to diagnose in a child than in an adult because of a child's ability to hemodynamically compensate and maintain a normal blood pressure despite life-threatening bleeding. *Persistent tachycardia is the most reliable early indicator of shock in a child.*

Individual variances and environmental factors can make some of the signs of shock normal for a particular child. Tachycardia can occur because of fear or fever. Mottling can be normal in an infant younger than six months of age, especially when exposed to cool environmental temperatures, but it also can be a sign of poor circulation, so note it. Extremities can be cold because of cold exposure or poor perfusion. Capillary refill can be prolonged in a child who is cold. Though all that is true, in general, a child should be carefully evaluated and assumed to have signs of shock if there is persistent tachycardia or signs of poor peripheral perfusion (prolonged capillary refill time, weak peripheral pulses, or cool or mottled extremities).

Low blood pressure is a late sign of shock in children (also called *decompensated shock*). Do not be falsely reassured by a normal blood pressure. A child may still have a serious injury and be compensating to maintain a normal blood pressure. When measuring a children's blood pressure, the rule of thumb for cuff size is to use the largest one that will fit snugly on the patient's upper arm. If there is too much noise, you can perform a blood pressure by palpation. Find the radial pulse, pump up the blood pressure cuff until you no longer feel the pulse, and allow air to leak slowly while observing the dial on the blood pressure cuff. Record the pressure at which you first feel the pulse, and label it "p," for palpation. This will be a systolic blood pressure only and will be slightly lower than a blood pressure that can be ausculated. As a general estimate, the lower limit of normal (fifth percentile) for systolic blood pressure is approximately 60 mm Hg in neonates (<30 days old), 70 mm Hg in infants (one month to one year old), and (70 + [2 × age in years]) mm Hg in children one year and older. (Remember that these are not normal parameters, but rather low values that should prompt you to be very concerned.) A systolic blood pressure below those values should be treated as decompensated shock, which means the child has lost a very significant amount of blood.

fluid resuscitation: the replacement of intravascular volume in a hypovolemic patient by infusing a crystalloid solution.

It is useful to routinely measure blood pressures in all children to enhance your comfort and skill with this procedure so you are able to obtain a blood pressure quickly and efficiently in a frightened or significantly injured child. With repeated practice in healthy children you will be more prepared for the difficult situations.

Fluid Resuscitation

If shock is suspected (compensated with a normal blood pressure or decompensated with a low blood pressure), the child requires **fluid resuscitation**. You should establish vascular access quickly and give a fluid bolus. The initial bolus should be 20 mL/kg of normal saline given as rapidly as possible. If there is no response, another 20 mL/kg may be given. When considering a peripheral IV, try to insert the largest practical catheter available to give the fluid bolus quickly. If the child is in shock, it may be difficult to see or feel a peripheral vein. If you cannot start an IV in two attempts or 90 seconds, you will need to insert an intraosseous (IO) needle. (See Figure 17-7 and Chapter 9 for technique.) There is no scientific data available at this time to suggest that any child in hemorrhagic shock should not be given IV fluids. Remember that cardiac output equals stroke volume multiplied by heart rate. Children cannot increase their stoke volume significantly compared to adults, so when hypovolemic and returning less blood to the heart, they can only maintain perfusion by vasoconstriction and increasing their heart rate. Sometimes children in severe shock develop bradycardia, and this can cause a severe and frequently fatal decrease in perfusion. Treat hypovolemia early.

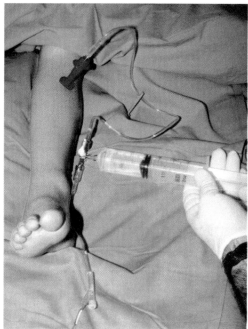

Figure 17-7   An IO needle in a child's proximal tibia being used for venous access. *(Photo courtesy of Bob Page, MEd, NRP, CCP, NCEE)*

Traumatic Brain Injury

Traumatic brain injuries are the most common cause of death in pediatric patients. The head is the primary focus of injury because a child's head is proportionately larger than an adult's. The goal of managing head injuries is twofold. First, it is important to quickly recognize life-threatening intracranial emergencies such as epidural hematomas. In the prehospital setting, this means transporting all children with potentially serious brain injuries to an emergency department equipped to provide definitive care. Second, you should focus on preventing any secondary injury to the brain. Although some of the injury to the brain occurs from the initial impact, further injury to the brain results from preventable causes (secondary brain injury) such as hypoxia and shock. To minimize those risks, you should prioritize three simple principles:

- *Give oxygen.* Brain injury increases brain cell metabolic rate and decreases blood flow in at least part of the brain. So all pediatric patients with a suspected traumatic brain injury should receive 100% oxygen. Similar to adults, children with brain injuries should not be hyperventilated unless they have evidence of cerebral herniation syndrome. (See Chapter 10.) Remember to monitor ventilation with capnography, if available.

- *Ensure adequate cerebral perfusion.* Blood must get to the brain to carry oxygen. It is therefore critical to recognize early signs of shock (tachycardia and poor perfusion) and aggressively correct hypovolemia. Remember, a systolic blood pressure less than 60 mm Hg in a young infant (>1 month of age), 70 mm Hg in a child one month to one year old, and [70 + (2 × age in years)] in children older than one year should be considered hypotension. Hypotension has been shown to be a predictor of poor outcome in traumatic brain injury patients.

- *Be prepared to prevent aspiration.* Head-injury patients frequently vomit. *Be prepared.* Suction should be readily assessable for any child with a head injury.

Changing level of consciousness is the best indicator of traumatic brain injury. A child entering the emergency department with a GCS of 10 that has deteriorated from a GCS of 13 in the field will be approached very differently than a child who has a GCS score of 10 that has improved from a GCS of 7 in the field. Assessments using vague words like semiconscious are not helpful. Instead, note specific points such as whether the child is alert and interactive, asking for parent/crying, reaching for the parent, or reacting to pain or voice, and so on.

Assessment of pupils is as important in a child with altered level of consciousness as in an adult. Note also whether the eyes are moving both left and right or whether they remain in one position. Do *not* move the head to determine this.

A child who is following simple commands has an intact central nervous system and is adequately perfusing the brain. Overall, it may be difficult at the scene to assess the extent of a child's head injury. So, always assume an injured child might have a serious traumatic brain injury. Priorities should be focused on prevention of secondary brain injury and rapid transport to a trauma center equipped to provide definitive care.

Chest Injury

Children with chest injuries generally give visible signs of respiratory distress, such as tachypnea, grunting, nasal flaring, and retractions. Any injured child with any respiratory distress will benefit from supplemental oxygen. Be aware that children's normal respiratory rates are higher than those of adults (Table 17-2, p. 337). As a general rule, a child breathing faster than 40, or an infant faster than 60, usually has respiratory distress.

Other signs of respiratory distress include nasal flaring (the nose moves like a rabbit's nose), and retractions, which are the caving in of the suprasternal, intercostal, or subcostal areas upon inspiration. Grunting is usually abnormal and indicates significant respiratory distress or a severe intra-abdominal injury and indicates a need for ventilatory assistance. Observe the child's breathing pattern as well. Shallow breathing, apnea spells (10–20 seconds of no breathing), or agonal respirations are all signs of respiratory failure and mandate ventilatory assistance.

Children with blunt chest injury are at risk for pneumothorax. Because the chest is small, a difference in breath sounds from side to side may be more subtle than in the adult. You may not be able to tell a difference, even by listening carefully. It is also difficult to diagnose tension pneumothorax in young children, who usually have short, fat necks that mask both neck vein distention and tracheal deviation. If a tension pneumothorax develops, the trachea should eventually shift away from the side of the pneumothorax, although this is a very late finding. Needle thoracostomy can be life saving. (See Chapter 7.)

Children in the preadolescent age group have highly elastic chest walls. Therefore, rib fractures, flail chest, pericardial tamponade, and aortic rupture are seldom seen. However, pulmonary contusion is common. If a child does have rib fractures or a flail chest, he has sustained a significant force to his chest and should be assumed to have serious internal injuries.

Abdominal Injury

The second leading cause of traumatic death in pediatric trauma centers is blunt abdominal trauma resulting in solid organ injury and bleeding. Common mechanisms include motor-vehicle collisions, bicycle crashes, sports-related injuries, and child abuse. In children, the liver and spleen are relatively large and both protrude below the ribs, exposing these organs to blunt trauma.

Abdominal injuries are difficult to diagnose in the field and are frequently missed because the presentation can be subtle. Children may have a difficult time communicating that they have abdominal pain, or the history may be limited secondary to the age of the child or other injuries the child has sustained. Any injured child who complains of abdominal pain should be assumed to have an intra-abdominal injury. The physical exam also may be challenging because of fear, pain, and the age of the child. A child can have a severe abdominal injury with minimal signs of trauma. Findings on examination that suggest significant abdominal injury include tenderness, bruising, and signs of shock. Seat-belt marks and bicycle handlebar marks are also worrisome. Presence of bruising or seat-belt marks on the abdomen should increase suspicion for abdominal injury.

Your assessment should be quick but thorough. If a child with blunt trauma is in shock with no obvious source of bleeding, assume that the patient is bleeding internally, and your decision should be to load and go as quickly as possible. Remember, however, that normal vital signs (heart rate and systolic blood pressure) do not rule out serious intra-abdominal injury.

Life-saving interventions should be made en route to the hospital. If you have a short (5- to 10-minute) transport time to a trauma center, it is not necessary to attempt an IV line. If the child is critical and the transport time is long, you should make no more than two attempts at IV lines before going to an IO needle. Any child who has been crying or suffered an abdominal injury may develop gastric distention and a tendency to vomit, so be prepared.

Spine Injury

Children have short necks, big heads, and loose ligaments. Fortunately, cervical-spine injuries are uncommon before adolescence. When they do occur, children younger than nine years of age usually have upper cervical-spine injuries (C1-C3) in contrast to older children and adults, who usually have lower cervical-spine injuries (C5-C7). There is no proven protocol for "clearing" the spine of a child in the field. A cervical collar is not necessary if the head is properly restricted in a padded device. Again, try to make a game of packaging the child. You can promise you will give him a ride in the ambulance as a reward after you get him all wrapped up and ready.

SCAN 17-1 Stabilizing an Apparently Uninjured Child in a Car Seat

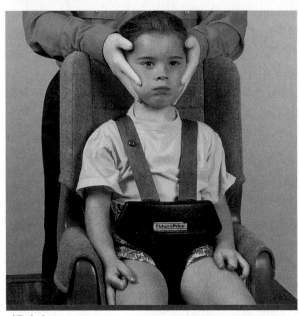

17-1-1 One emergency care provider stabilizes the car seat in an upright position and applies and maintains manual in-line stabilization throughout the SMR process.

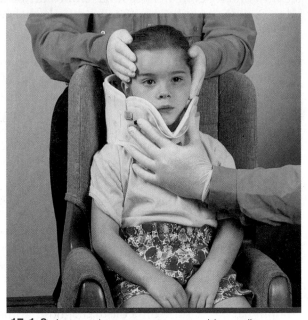

17-1-2 A second emergency care provider applies an appropriate size cervical collar. If one is not available, improvise using a rolled hand towel.

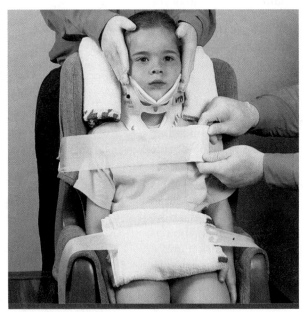

17-1-3 The second emergency care provider places a small blanket or towel on the child's lap, then uses straps or wide tape to secure the chest and pelvic areas to the seat.

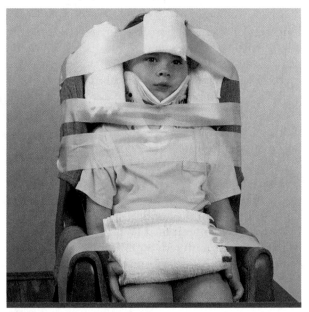

17-1-4 The second emergency care provider places towel rolls on both sides of the child's head to fill the voids between the head and seat. He tapes the head into place, taping across the forehead and the collar, but avoiding taping over the chin, which would put pressure on the neck. The patient and seat can be carried to the ambulance and strapped to the stretcher, with the stretcher head raised.

Have a parent or other familiar person assist, if possible. Be sure your packaging does not restrict chest movement. As mentioned before, children up to about eight years of age will need a pad under the torso to keep the neck in a neutral position.

Spinal-cord injury without radiographic abnormality (**SCIWORA**) refers to spine injuries that are not seen on plain x-rays or a CAT scan. Patients often report early or transient neurologic symptoms such as weakness or numbness. This injury most often involves the cervical spine. Plain x-rays of the spine show no bony abnormalities, and an MRI is required to see the injuries in the spinal cord. Spinal motion restriction (SMR) is indicated in these patients.

SCIWORA: refers to spine injuries that are not identified on plain x-rays or a CAT scan. The letters stand for spinal-cord injury without radiographic abnormality.

Child Restraint Seats

If properly restrained in a **child restraint seat**, a child in a motor-vehicle collision is much less likely to have a serious injury than an unrestrained passenger. Unfortunately, many children are not properly restrained in the car seat or the car seat itself is not correctly anchored to the vehicle. Appropriate use of car seats is an area of injury prevention in which EMS can play a significant role through public education.

If in a car seat that is correctly secured in the vehicle, the child can be transported without being removed from the device. Assess the child as you would any other trauma patient. If no injury is found and the seat's integrity appears to be intact, place padding around the child's head and tape the head directly to the car seat (Scan 17-1). This method of transportation should be used only after a complete assessment has revealed no injury to the child. Be aware of your local protocols regarding this. If the child has evidence of any serious injuries, then remove the child from the car seat and package appropriately based on exam and injuries found.

child restraint seat: a piece of safety equipment in which a child sits and that is designed to protect a child in case of a motor-vehicle collision. It must fit the child, and the child must be properly strapped into the seat for it to be effective.

Case Presentation *(continued)*

You are assessing a 10-month-old child who is in a car seat that was thrown to the floor during a collision and ended up in front of the rear seat. Child has been crying periodically since the accident per the grandfather. With the initial assessment (using the Pediatric Assessment Triangle) normal, the emergency care provider approaches the infant for a more detailed evaluation. Keeping in mind that the child was restrained in the child seat but that the seat was loose in the auto and fell forward onto the rear floor, you are concerned about the possibility of a spine injury.

While the infant remains in the car seat, you begin quietly talking to the child and playing with her feet, with the child smiling when tickled. The responder gently palpates the legs and hips while the child is distracted by a flashlight. Gently palpating the child's abdomen produces more giggling but no distress. You now unzip the child's jump suit and note that the torso is unmarked, though to your chagrin, the diaper is wet. The child's chest and abdomen move easily with breathing, and show no signs of injury. The respiratory rate is about 30. As you attempt to auscultate his chest, the child stops playing with the flashlight and starts grabbing the stethoscope. You note that the child's head moves freely forward and to both sides. Her head is unmarked and tousling her hair reveals no sign of trauma, tenderness, or swelling. The arms move freely and the brachial pulse is about 120 and strong.

You determine that, absent any sign of injury or distress, and with the child seat undamaged, you will transport the child in her child seat with padding placed around her head/neck. You communicate to the child's grandparents, who are being treated by another ambulance crew, that there are no major injuries found and that the child will be transported in the child seat to the hospital. Because you have no diapers on the ambulance, you make a mental note to tell the emergency department staff that the child will need a diaper change.

Summary

To provide good trauma care for children, you must have the proper equipment, know how to interact with frightened parents, know the normal vital signs for various ages (or have them posted in your trauma box), and be familiar with the injuries that are more common in children. Fortunately, the assessment sequence is the same for children as for adults. If you perform your assessment well, you will obtain the information needed to make the right decisions in management. Focusing on assessment and management of the child's airway (with cervical-spine control), breathing, and circulation will result in the best possible outcome.

Although assessment and management of the injured child are life-saving skills, all responders involved in the care of the seriously injured child also should be concerned about prevention. Car seats, bicycle helmets, seat belts, all-terrain vehicle injuries, water safety, scald-burn injuries, firearm safety, and active shooter drills are within the EMS area of concern. Consider volunteering your time to teaching safety (Figure 17-8) and speaking out for laws (infant seat restraints, seat belts, drunk driving) that save lives.

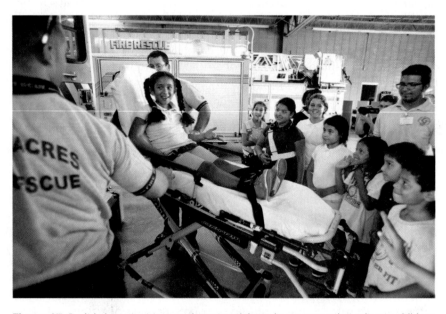

Figure 17-8   It is important to organize or participate in programs that educate children about injury prevention and health care. *(© ZUMA Press, Inc/Alamy)*

Bibliography

American College of Surgeons Committee on Trauma, American College of Emergency Physicians, National Association of EMS Physicians, Pediatric Equipment Guidelines Committee of the EMS for Children Partnership for Children Stakeholder Group, and American Academy of Pediatrics. "Policy Statement—Equipment for Ambulances." *Pediatrics* 124, no. 1 (July 2009): 166–71.

Bliss, D., and M. Silen. "Pediatric Thoracic Trauma." *Critical Care Medicine* 20, Suppl. 11 (November 2002): S409–15.

Dietrich, A., S. Shaner, and J. Campbell. *Pediatric International Trauma Life Support*, 3rd ed. Oakbrook Terrace, IL: International Trauma Life Support, 2009.

DiRusso, S. M., T. Sullivan, D. Risucci, P. Nealson, and M. Slim. "Intubation of Pediatric Trauma Patients in the Field: Prediction of Negative Outcome Despite Risk Stratification." *Journal of Trauma* 59, no. 1 (July 2005): 84–91.

Emergency Medical Services for Children (EMSC) National Resource Center. Accessed January 9, 2014, at http://childrensnational.org/emsc.

Fleicher, G. R., S. Ludwig, and M. Henretig. *Textbook of Pediatric Emergency Medicine,* 6th ed. Philadelphia: Lippincott Williams & Wilkins, 2010.

Gausche, M., R. J. Lewis, S. J. Stratton, B. E. Haynes, C. S. Gunter S. M. Goodrich, P. D. Poore, M. D. McCollough, D. P. Henderson, F. D. Pratt, and J. S. Seidel. "Effect of Out-of-Hospital Pediatric Endotracheal Intubation on Survival and Neurological Outcome: A Controlled Clinical Trial." *Journal of the American Medical Association (JAMA)* 283, no. 6 (February 2000): 783–90.

Holmes, J. F., P. E. Sokolove, W. E. Brant, M. J. Palchak, C. W. Vance, J. T. Owings, and N. Kuppermann. "Identification of Children with Intra-abdominal Injuries After Blunt Trauma." *Annals of Emergency Medicine* 39, no. 5 (May 2002): 500–509.

Holmes, J. F., P. E. Sokolove, W. E. Brant, and N. Kuppermann. "A Clinical Decision Rule for Identifying Children with Thoracic Injuries After Blunt Torso Trauma." *Annals of Emergency Medicine* 39, no. 5 (May 2002): 492–99.

Kokoska, E. R., M. S. Keller, M. C. Rallo, and T. R. Weber. "Characteristics of Pediatric Cervical-Spine Injuries." *Journal of Pediatric Surgery* 36, no. 1 (January 2001): 100–105.

Kuppermann, N., J. F. Holmes, P. S. Dayan, J. D. Hoyle Jr., S. M. Atabaki, R. Holubkov, F. M. Nadel, D. Monroe, R. M. Stanley, D. A. Borgialli, et al. "Identification of Children at Very Low Risk of Clinically-Important Brain Injuries After Head Trauma: A Prospective Cohort Study." *Lancet* 374, no. 9696 (October 3, 2009): 1160–70.

Murray, B. L., and R. J. Cordie. "Pediatric Trauma." In *Rosen's Emergency Medicine,* 8th ed., Edited by J. A. Marx, R. S. Hockberger, and R. M. Walls, 305–23. Philadelphia: Mosby/Elsevier, 2014.

Olufolabi, A. J. G. A. Charlton, and P. M. Spargo. "Effect of Head Posture on Tracheal Tube Position in Children." *Anaesthesia* 59, no. 11 (November 2004): 1069–72.

Pang, D. "Spinal Cord Injury Without Radiographic Abnormality in Children, 2 Decades Later." *Neurosurgery* 55, no. 6 (December 2006): 1325–43.

Rozzelle, C. J., B. Aarabi, S. S. Dhall, D. E. Gelb, R. J. Hurlbert, T. C. Ryken, N. Theodore, B. C. Walters, and M. N. Hadley. "Management of Pediatric Cervical Spine and Spinal Cord Injuries." *Neurosurgery* 72, Suppl. 2 (March 2013): 205–26.

Viccellio, P., H. Simon, B. D. Pressman, M. N. Sha, W. R. Mower, J. R. Hoffman; NEXUS Group. "A Prospective Multicenter Study of Cervical-Spine Injury in Children." *Pediatrics* 108, no. 2 (August 2001): E20.

Vitale, M. G., J. M. Goss, H. Matsumoto, and D. P. Roye, Jr. "Epidemiology of Pediatric Spinal Cord Injury in the United States: Years 1997 and 2000." *Journal of Pediatric Orthopedics* 26, no. 6 (November–December 2006): 745–49.

Walls, R. M., and M. F. Murphy. *Manual of Emergency Airway Management,* 4th ed. Philadelphia: Lippincott Williams & Wilkins, 2012.

Note: Because of increasing demand for further training in management of the injured child, ITLS has developed a one-day course (Pediatric ITLS) that covers this subject in detail.

Get more information about this course by calling ITLS International at 888-495-4875 (outside the United States call +1-630-495-6442) or visit

www.itrauma.org

18

Geriatric Trauma

Leah J. Heimbach, JD, RN, EMT-P
Jonathan G. Newman, MD, MMM, EMT-P, FACEP
Jere F. Baldwin, MD, FACEP, FAAFP

Traumi dell'anziano   Traumatismo en el Adulto Mayor

Traumatisme dans les Personnes âgées   Urazy u osób w podeszłym wieku

Trauma im Alter   Ozljede u osoba starije Životne dobi   إصابات الكبار

trauma starih osoba   Poškodbe pri starostnikih   Időskori trauma

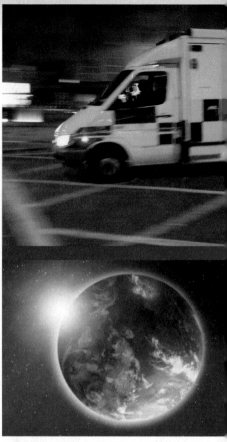

(Photo courtesy of Piccelle/Getty Images)

Key Terms

altered mental status, *p. 351*
compensate, *p. 351*
chronic disease, *p. 353*
kyphotic deformity, *p. 351*
osteoporosis, *p. 351*
pathophysiology of aging, *p. 350*

Objectives

Upon successful completion of this chapter, you should be able to:

1. Describe the changes that occur with aging.
2. Explain how these changes can affect your assessment and management of the geriatric trauma patient.
3. Describe the assessment of the geriatric trauma patient.
4. Describe the management of the geriatric trauma patient.

Chapter Overview

Worldwide, there are more than 500 million people over the age of 65, per the United Nations. Citizens of the United States over the age of 65 comprise over 14% of the U.S. population, and that number is expected to double in the next 25 to 30 years. The age group 85 and older is the fastest-growing segment of the U.S. population. The geriatric population also comprises a significant number of patients being transported by ambulance. In the United States, over 30% of all patients transported by ambulance are over the age of 65.

"Elderly" is often understood as being 65 years or older in the United States because retirement benefits are usually initiated at about this point in life. However, chronological age is not the most reliable definition of "elderly." It is more appropriate to consider the physiologic processes that change with time, such as fewer numbers of neurons, decreased functioning of the kidneys, and decreased elasticity of the skin and tissues.

As a group, elderly (also referred to as geriatric) patients tend to respond to injury poorly compared to younger adults. Geriatric patients who are injured are more likely to experience fatal outcomes, compared to the population at large, even if the injury is of a relatively low severity. According to the U.S. National Safety Council, falls, thermal injury, and motor-vehicle collisions have been identified as common causes of traumatic death in the geriatric population. This is an even greater concern given that, as a whole, the elderly population continues to assume more active lifestyles, making them more prone to injury.

Falls account for the majority of major injuries in the geriatric population, the most common pathology being fractures of the hip or femur and wrist or head injuries. Motor-vehicle collisions account for approximately 25% of geriatric deaths, although the elderly drive fewer miles. The geriatric population has a higher incidence of collision than other age groups, second only to those under the age of 25. Eight percent of geriatric deaths are attributable to thermal injuries, which include inhalation, contact with a heat source resulting in scalding and flame burns, and electrical injury.

Older patients have a worse outcome from trauma compared to similarly injured younger patients, including increased mortality. Research has not pinpointed all the reasons. However, by gaining an understanding of the normal physiologic changes involved in the aging process, you will be prepared to identify subtle and occult injuries, provide optimum care, and select the most appropriate receiving facility for the geriatric trauma victim.

This patient population is one in which EMS can have a significant impact through prevention programs. Unlike many other health-care providers, EMS does enter the homes of patients and has the ability to observe the presence of hazards and other issues that put the patient at risk. Referral to the appropriate agencies to arrange for support for the patient or mitigation of the risk should be part of the care that EMS provides. As the concept of community or primary care paramedicine moves forward in communities, EMS will have more of an opportunity to help prevent traumatic injuries in the elderly patient population.

This chapter addresses aging processes, highlights illnesses to which the geriatric patient is susceptible, and shows how those processes and illnesses make it difficult to predict the physiologic response to trauma in the geriatric patient.

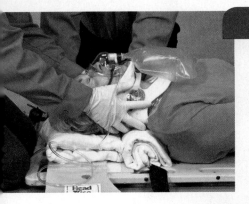

Case Presentation

Your advanced life support (ALS) ambulance has been dispatched to the scene of a motor-vehicle collision with multiple vehicles involved. You are responding at the request of units already on scene. As you arrive on scene, you see an overturned truck and are advised by the fire service that the minor leak has been contained. You are directed to a sedan to take care of a woman sitting in the passenger seat. You note a crack in the windshield on her side of the car. The patient is an 80-year-old woman covered in cornstarch, with seatbelt in place. She is responsive to voice, seems confused, and asks repeatedly, "What happened?" As you approach her, you notice a growing hematoma on the right side of her head.

Before proceeding, consider these questions: What kind of assessment should you perform? Is this patient at increased risk for having occult injuries, more so than a younger person? Should this patient be managed without spinal motion restriction (SMR)? Does this patient require immediate transport? Keep these questions in mind as you read through the chapter. Then, at the end of the chapter, find out how the emergency care providers managed this patient.

Pathophysiology of Aging

pathophysiology of aging: the process of aging that consists of the gradual decline in the normal function of many body systems, which may in part be responsible for greater risk of injury in the elderly population.

The **pathophysiology of aging** is a gradual process whereby changes in bodily functions occur. The changes are in part responsible for the greater risk of injury in the geriatric population.

The Aging Body
Airway
Changes in airway structures of the geriatric patient may include tooth decay, gum disease, and use of a dental prosthesis. Caps, bridges, dentures, and fillings all present potential airway obstructions in the geriatric trauma patient. In addition, arthritic changes may make airway management more challenging, due to decreased movement of the mandible and decreased neck mobility.

Respiratory System
Changes in the respiratory system begin to appear in the early adult years and increase markedly after the age of 60. Circulation to the pulmonary system decreases 30%, reducing the amount of carbon dioxide and oxygen exchanged at the alveolar level. There is a decrease in chest wall movement and in the flexibility of the muscles of the chest wall. The changes cause a decreased inhalation time, resulting in rapid breathing. There is a decrease in vital capacity (the amount of air exchanged per breath) because of an increased residual volume (volume of air remaining in the lungs after deep exhalation). Overall breathing capacity and maximal work rate may decrease. If there is a history of cigarette smoking or a history of working in an area with pollutants, the changes in breathing are even more significant. Rib fractures can result in increased mortality for patients admitted to trauma centers. They may be associated with underlying organ injuries, such as heart, great vessels, liver, spleen, and lungs.

Cardiovascular System
Circulation is reduced in the elderly due to changes in the heart and the blood vessels. Cardiac output and stroke volume may decrease, and the conduction system may degenerate. The ability of the valves of the heart to operate efficiently may decline.

Those changes can predispose the patient to congestive heart failure and pulmonary edema. Arteriosclerosis occurs with increasing frequency in the course of the aging process, resulting in an increased peripheral vascular resistance (and perhaps systolic hypertension). There may be a normally higher blood pressure in the elderly. Thus, a significant change in tissue perfusion may occur in a patient when normal blood pressure of 160 drops to 120 as a result of trauma. All of these changes contribute to older patients having a reduced cardiac output, compared to younger patients.

Neurologic and Sensory Function

Several changes occur in the brain with age. The brain shrinks, and the outermost meningeal layer, the dura mater, remains tightly adherent to the skull. This creates a space or an increased distance between the brain and the skull. Instead of protecting the brain during impact, this space allows an increased incidence of subdural hematoma following even minor trauma. There is also a hardening, narrowing, and loss of elasticity of some arteries in the brain. A deceleration injury may cause blood vessel rupture and potential bleeding inside the skull.

With aging, there is a decline in both visual and auditory function. As a result, elderly patients may not see potential hazards or hear warnings and thus are more likely to sustain an injury. Because of diminished balance and reflexes, elderly patients are at an increased risk for falls. Because of osteoporosis and other aging processes, even a fall from standing can produce significant injury in an older patient.

There is decreased blood flow to the brain. The patient may experience a slowing of sensory responses such as pain perception and decreases in hearing, eyesight, or other sensory perceptions. Many older patients may have a higher pain tolerance from living with conditions such as arthritis or from being on analgesic medications chronically. This can result in their failure to identify areas in which they have been injured. Other signs of decreased cerebral circulation due to the aging process may include confusion, irritability, forgetfulness, altered sleep patterns, and mental dysfunctions such as loss of memory and regressive behavior. There may be a decrease, even an absence, of the ability to **compensate** for shock.

Some elderly patients will develop dementia or a psychiatric illness that can make assessment of their mental status challenging. It is helpful to check with family or caregiver about whether the patient's mental status is altered from their baseline.

Thermoregulation

Mechanisms to maintain normal body temperature may not function properly in the elderly. The patient may not be able to respond to an infection with a fever or may not be able to maintain a normal temperature in the face of injury. The geriatric patient with a broken hip who has been lying on the floor in a room where the temperature is 64°F (18°C) can experience hypothermia.

Renal System

A decrease in the number of functioning nephrons in the kidneys of the geriatric patient can result in a decrease in filtration and a reduced ability to excrete urine and drugs. Older patients may therefore be more sensitive to drugs that cause sedation. It has been recommended that the dosages of these medications be reduced by 20% to 40% to reduce the risk of oversedation.

Musculoskeletal System

The geriatric patient may exhibit signs of changes in posture. There may be a decrease in total height due to the narrowing of the vertebral discs, slight flexion of the knees and hips, and decreased muscle strength. This can result in a **kyphotic deformity** of the spine, resulting in an "S" curvature often seen in the stooped elderly. The geriatric patient also may have advanced **osteoporosis**—a thinning of the bones resulting in a decrease in bone density. This renders the bones more

---

compensate: the body's natural ability to adapt to a range of conditions. In the elderly patient there may be a decrease in the ability, or even an absence of the ability to compensate for shock or other conditions.

PEARLS
Altered Mental Status

Elderly patients with **altered mental status** should always be checked for hypoglycemia, shock, and head trauma, rather than assuming that they are senile.

altered mental status: a diminished level of awareness or consciousness. It can range from mild confusion to coma and indicates effects of medications, damage to the brain, or inadequate delivery of oxygen or nutrients.

kyphotic deformity: a condition caused by narrowing of the vertebral discs and gradual collapse of the osteoporotic thoracic vertebral bodies often seen in the elderly who present in a stooped posture with an "S" shape to the spine.

osteoporosis: a condition frequently seen in the elderly in which there is gradual loss of calcium from the bones with a decrease in bone mass and density, making the bones more easily fractured.

susceptible to fractures. Patients who are older than 65 years of age have an increased risk for cervical-spine fractures after injury. Further, mechanisms of injury alone may be an insufficient predictor of potential for injury because the elderly are at greater risk from lower intensity trauma than the general population.

Frequently in the elderly, diminished subcutaneous tissue decreases protection from falls and blunt trauma. This lack can decrease the person's ability to respond to temperature changes. Also, as skin loses elasticity as well as its natural padding, there is an increased risk of developing pressure sores. Appropriate padding and appropriate removal from hard surfaces, such as a long spineboard, can decrease this risk. Finally, there may be a weakening in the strength of the muscle and bone from a decrease in physical activity. This also will render the geriatric person more susceptible to fractures from only a slight fall.

Gastrointestinal System

Saliva production, esophageal motility, and gastric secretion may decrease as a person ages. This can result in decreased ability to absorb nutrients. Constipation and fecal impactions are common. The liver may be enlarged because of disease processes or may be failing due to disease or malnutrition. This can result in a decreased ability to metabolize medications. Associated poor intake, especially of fluids, can leave older patients dehydrated and thus at increased risk for shock following injury.

Immune System

As the aging process continues, the geriatric patient may be less able to fight off infection. The patient who is in a poor nutritional state will be more susceptible to infection from open wounds, IV access sites, and lung and kidney infections. The geriatric trauma patient who is not otherwise severely injured may die from sepsis due to an impaired immune system.

Other Changes

The total body water and total number of body cells may be decreased in the elderly. An increase in the proportion of the body weight as fat may exist as well. There also may be a loss in the capacity of the body's systems to adjust to illness or injury.

Medications

Many geriatric patients take several medications that can interfere with the ability to compensate after sustaining trauma. Anticoagulants may increase bleeding time. Antihypertensives and peripheral vasodilators can interfere with the body's ability to constrict blood vessels in response to hypovolemia. Beta-blockers can inhibit the heart's ability to increase the rate of contraction, even in hypovolemic shock. Pain medications and medications taken for behavioral problems may depress the level of consciousness, making assessment of head injury challenging.

Antihypertensives, anticoagulants, beta-blockers, sedatives, and hypoglycemic agents may alter the response of the geriatric patient to traumatic injury. Knowledge of the medications the patient is taking can alert you to the fact that the patient's condition may be more unstable than indicated by current signs and symptoms.

Aging and Injury

A number of the aging processes contribute to the increased risk of injury to the geriatric patient. The changes that may increase susceptibility to injury include the following:

- Slower reflexes
- Failing eyesight
- Hearing loss

- Arthritis
- Fragile skin and blood vessels
- Fragile bones

Causative factors related to the aging process have been linked with specific injuries such as tripping over furniture and falling down stairs. Further investigation reveals that those falls are often related as much to a decrease in the function of special senses, such as loss in peripheral vision, as they are to syncope, postural instability, transient impairment of cerebrovascular perfusion, alcohol ingestion, or medication usage. Alterations in perception and delayed response to stressors may contribute to injury in the geriatric patient. When treating the geriatric trauma patient, remember that the priorities are the same as for all trauma patients. However, you must give consideration to three important issues:

- General organ systems may not function as effectively as those in the younger adult, especially the cardiovascular, pulmonary, and renal systems.
- The geriatric patient may have a chronic illness that may complicate the effectiveness of trauma care.
- Bones may fracture more easily with less force. Fractures of major bones such as hips or femurs can be life threatening even with proper care.

Assessment and Management

Geriatric patient assessment, as any assessment, must take into account priorities, interventions, and life-threatening conditions. However, you must be acutely aware that geriatric patients can die from less-severe injuries than younger patients. In addition, it is often difficult to separate the effects of the aging process or of a chronic illness from the consequences of an injury. The chief complaint may seem trivial because the patient may not report truly important symptoms. You must search for important signs or symptoms. In the geriatric patient, it is not uncommon for the patient to suffer from more than one illness or injury at the same time. Remember, the elderly patient may not have the same response to pain, hypoxia, or hypovolemia as a young person. Do not underestimate the severity of the patient's condition.

You may have difficulty communicating with the patient. This could result from the patient's diminished senses, hearing or sight impairment, or depression. The geriatric patient nonetheless should not be approached in a condescending manner. Do not allow others to take over the reporting of events from the patient who is able and willing to communicate reliable information. Unfortunately, the patient may minimize or even deny symptoms out of fear of becoming dependent, bedridden, institutionalized, or even of losing a sense of self-sufficiency. It is important that you explain any actions, including removing any clothing, before initiating the physical assessment.

There are other considerations in assessing the geriatric trauma patient. Peripheral pulses may be difficult to evaluate. Older patients often wear many layers of clothing, which can impede physical assessment. You also must distinguish between signs and symptoms of a **chronic disease** and an acute problem. For instance: A geriatric patient may have nonpathologic rales. Or the loss of skin elasticity and the presence of mouth breathing may not necessarily represent dehydration. Or dependent edema may be secondary to venous insufficiency with varicose veins or inactivity rather than congestive heart failure.

Pay attention to deviation from expected ranges in vital signs and other physical assessment findings in the geriatric patient. An injury that is isolated and uncomplicated in the young adult may be debilitating in the older adult. This may be due to the patient's overall condition, lowered defenses, or inability to keep the effects of an injury localized.

chronic disease: a long-lasting or recurrent illness that may be underlying the acute problem that prompted need for emergency care. Signs and symptoms between the chronic disease and trauma may need to be distinguished. Such diseases may impair the ability of the patient to compensate for injury.

When obtaining the patient's past medical history, it is important to note what medications the patient may be taking. As noted earlier, medications can mask or inhibit responses to injury.

ITLS Primary Survey
Scene Size-up
Size up the scene to decide if it is safe, to determine the number of patients, and to identify the mechanism of injury. Observe the surrounding area for indications that the patient is able to provide his or her own care; for signs of alcohol abuse or ingestion of multiple medications; and for signs of violence, abuse, or neglect. Unfortunately, abuse and neglect of the elderly are common. When your assessment of the patient and surroundings is suspicious for them, notify the proper authorities. Be sure to gather the patient's medications and bring them to the hospital.

Initial Assessment
As with any trauma patient, you must evaluate and provide an adequate airway and maintain spinal motion restriction (SMR) while assessing the initial level of consciousness. It has more significance with elderly patients than with younger patients because subsequent health-care providers may attribute a decreased level of consciousness to a pre-existing condition rather than to the trauma. This is more likely to occur if you have not clearly indicated that the patient was clear, lucid, and cooperative at the scene.

If a patient responds appropriately to initial verbal statements, he or she has an open airway and is conscious. If the patient does not respond, gently open the airway with a modified jaw-thrust maneuver while maintaining the neck in a neutral position. This position may be difficult to determine with certainty because of arthritis and kyphosis of the spine. It is important to recognize this and not to forcibly place the occiput flat on the backboard or ground. You should add padding to the backboard to maintain the patient's usual spinal position. The vacuum backboard is very helpful here.

There is increased potential for the airway to be partially obstructed. Clear the airway, being alert to possible teeth fragments due to decay and gum disease and dental devices such as caps, bridges, dentures, and fillings. Look in the mouth for partially eaten food or regurgitated stomach contents.

Look, listen, and feel for movement of air. Ensure that the rate and volume of air exchange is adequate. The geriatric patient with unresolved airway difficulty or a decreased level of consciousness should be transported immediately. In such a case, frequently monitor the respiratory effort and level of consciousness (remember to check blood glucose). Consider intubation. If drug-assisted intubation is being performed, remember that you might not need as much sedation.

Place your face over the patient's mouth to look at the chest rise, to listen to the quality of the breath sounds from the mouth, and to feel the patient's breath against your ear. If the breathing is so fast that there is inadequate air exchange (more than 20 breaths per minute), or if it is too slow (fewer than 10 breaths per minute), or if the volume of air being exchanged is inadequate, provide assisted ventilation with 100% supplemental oxygen. Capnography is an effective way to monitor the patient's ventilation objectively.

Check the rate and quality of the pulse at the wrist (check at the neck if there is no pulse at the wrist). Evaluate skin color and condition. Scan the patient for bleeding, and control any bleeding with pressure.

Rapid Trauma Survey or Focused Exam
The choice between the rapid trauma survey and the focused exam depends on the mechanism of injury and/or the results of the initial assessment. If there is a dangerous generalized mechanism of injury (auto crash or fall from a height, for instance) or if the

patient is unconscious, you should perform a rapid trauma survey. If there is a dangerous focused mechanism of injury suggesting an isolated injury (such as a bullet wound to the thigh or a stab wound to the chest), you may perform the focused exam, which is limited to the area of injury.

If there is no significant mechanism of injury, and the initial assessment is normal (the patient is alert with no history of loss of consciousness, breathing normally, and a radial pulse less than 100, not complaining of dyspnea or chest, abdominal, or pelvic pain), you may move directly to the focused exam based on the patient's chief complaint. Be aware that elderly patients may not become tachycardic after trauma due to aging processes or medications.

To perform a rapid trauma survey, examine the head, neck, chest, abdomen, pelvis, and extremities. That is, briefly assess the head and neck for injuries and to see if the neck veins are flat or distended and if the trachea is midline. You may apply a rigid extrication collar at this time. Then look, feel, and listen to the chest. Look for both asymmetrical and paradoxical movement. Note if the ribs rise with respiration or if there is only diaphragmatic breathing. Look for signs of blunt trauma or open wounds. Feel for tenderness, instability, or crepitation (TIC). Listen to see if breath sounds are present and equal bilaterally.

Make appropriate interventions for chest injuries. Remember that chest injuries are more likely to cause serious problems in older people with poor pulmonary reserve. Be especially alert to problems in patients with chronic lung disease. Those patients usually have borderline hypoxia even when they are not injured. Briefly notice heart sounds so you will have a baseline for changes such as development of muffled heart sounds. Rapidly expose and look at the abdomen (distention, contusions, penetrating wounds), and gently palpate the abdomen for tenderness, guarding, and rigidity. Check the pelvis and extremities for wounds, deformity, and TIC. Note whether the patient can move fingers and toes before transferring to a backboard.

Critical Transport Decisions

A few procedures may be initiated on scene, but do not delay transport. Examples of critical interventions that may be initiated at the scene are the following:

- Provide airway management.
- Assist ventilation.
- Begin CPR.
- Control major bleeding.
- Seal sucking chest wounds.
- Stabilize flail chest.
- Decompress a tension pneumothorax.
- Stabilize impaled objects.

Consider whether or not the time delay in initiating those procedures outweighs the risks of delaying transportation. The chance of survival decreases with a corresponding increase in the length of scene time. The same indications for immediate transport apply for the elderly as for younger patients. (See Chapter 2.) Remember, you may not have as dramatic a response to injury in the elderly, so you should ensure early transport. If one of the critical conditions is present, immediately transfer the patient to a long backboard (vacuum backboard is recommended) with appropriate padding, apply oxygen, load the patient into the ambulance, and transport rapidly to the nearest appropriate trauma facility.

Packaging and Transport

Package or prepare the elderly patient for transport as quickly and gently as possible. If clinically indicated, take extra care when performing SMR on the geriatric

PEARLS
Chronic Illnesses

Chronic illnesses such as congestive heart failure and COPD should be taken into account as you make judgments about interventions needed to care for the elderly trauma patient.

PEARLS
SMR

- When performing SMR on an elderly patient, steps should be taken to remove him or her from the backboard as soon as is practical. While the patient is on the long spine board, padding should be used to minimize injury to bony prominences. The vacuum backboard is far superior to a hard backboard for use with the elderly patient.
- Extra padding also may be required under the head and shoulders to maintain the cervical spine in its normal alignment.

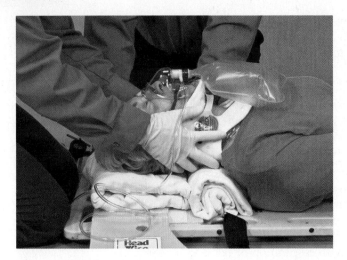

Figure 18-1 Elderly patients with kyphosis require padding under the head and shoulders to maintain the spine in its usual alignment.

trauma patient. This includes padding void areas that may be exaggerated due to the aging process. The elderly patient with kyphosis will require padding under the shoulders and head to maintain the neck in its usual alignment (Figure 18-1). Do not force the neck into a neutral position if it causes pain to do so or if the neck is obviously fused in a forward position. Remember to treat and transport the geriatric trauma patient, as you do all trauma patients, gently and quickly.

ITLS Secondary Survey and Ongoing Exams

Perform an ITLS Secondary Survey on scene if the patient is stable. If there is any question about the patient's condition, you should transport and perform the ITLS Secondary Survey en route. Perform frequent ITLS Ongoing Exams. If IV therapy is to be started, it should be done en route to the hospital. If you start large-bore IV lines en route, monitor the patient's response to IV fluid infusion very closely. Volume infusion may precipitate congestive heart failure in patients with underlying cardiovascular disease. However, do not withhold IV fluids in a patient who is showing signs of hypovolemic shock. Frequently assess the patient's pulmonary status, including lung sounds and cardiac rhythm. All elderly patients should have cardiac monitoring, pulse oximetry, and capnography, if available.

Case Presentation (continued)

You are on the scene of a multiple-vehicle collision. You have been assigned to assess and care for an elderly woman who is the front seat passenger. Her vehicle collided with a motorcyclist who has already been transported. Her husband is in the driver's seat and is being assessed by another crew for his extremity fractures. As you approach your patient, you note she is responding but seems dazed and somewhat confused. You also observe a hematoma on the right side of her head. You find that her airway is open, she is breathing at about 15–20 times per minute, and she keeps asking what happened, over and over. You explain that someone will keep her head from moving too much as an EMT takes manual control of her C-spine. You then check her pulse at the wrist and find it strong, though irregular, with a rate of about 84. In doing so, you note bruising of her right forearm. Otherwise, her skin color and temperature are cool and dry, without pallor or cyanosis.

In response to questioning, the patient says she thinks she may have blacked out.

She admits to pain at the site of the hematoma, but says she does not think she hurts anywhere else. A rapid palpation of the neck, chest, abdomen, pelvis, and extremities reveals no tenderness or crepitation. To allow for better access and extrication of the patient in the rear seat, you decide to rapidly extricate her to a long backboard. Placing a C-collar, you proceed to extricate her onto the stretcher and to transfer her to the ambulance, explaining to her that her husband will be cared for by other emergency care providers.

Once on the ambulance, you carefully remove the backboard from under her by pulling the board from her feet while holding her on the stretcher. She thanks you as you strap her head and torso to the stretcher. You then explain you will perform a rapid head-to-toe examination to discover if she has any other injuries. She agrees. Carefully cutting away her clothes, you note mildly elevated neck veins. She answers that she is treated for high blood pressure, mild congestive heart failure, an irregular heartbeat, and takes a pill for high blood sugar. Her medications are in her purse and include a beta-blocker for hypertension and Coumadin, which she takes for her "irregular heartbeat." While you continue with a rapid trauma survey, noting some bruising at the sternum and anterior iliac crest (seat belt?), your partner prepares to take vital signs and attach a pulse oximeter and cardiac monitor. It is at that moment that the patient becomes suddenly unresponsive and has a brief tonic-clonic seizure.

You repeat the initial assessment and find the patient is now unresponsive, her airway clear, respirations rapid, her pulse about 60, and her blood pressure 164/60. You check her pupils and find the right pupil "blown" (dilated and nonreactive). A neurologic exam reveals that she has no eye opening or verbal response to pain, and withdraws her right arm and leg only. (No movement on the left.) Suspecting a cerebral bleed (possibly epidural, in light of the history of possible initial loss of consciousness, lucid interval, and sudden loss of consciousness), you determine the need to transport immediately to the trauma center.

En route you contact the trauma center to report the situation, place the patient on high-flow oxygen, and prepare to assist ventilation, which has become irregular. With the IV established, you consider endotracheal intubation using rapid sequence intubation (RSI). However, due to short transport time you decide to support the airway with a bag-valve mask. Upon arrival at the hospital, you give a report to the trauma team. A CAT scan of her head reveals an epidural hematoma and subarachnoid hemorrhage. She undergoes an evacuation of the hematoma and after a long hospitalization is discharged to a rehabilitation facility.

Summary

You will be called on to treat and transport an increasing number of geriatric trauma patients. Although the mechanisms of injury may be different from those of younger adults, the prioritized evaluation and treatment is the same. As a general rule, elderly patients have more serious injuries and more complications than younger patients. Some suggest that an age greater than 60 years is sufficient reason to take an injured patient to a level 1 trauma center. The physiologic processes of aging and frequent concurrent illnesses make evaluation and treatment more difficult. You must be aware of the differences to provide optimal care to the patient.

Bibliography

Bergeron, E., A. Lavoie, D. Clas, L. Moore, S. Ratte, S. Tetreault, J. Lemaire, and M. Martin. "Elderly Trauma Patients with Rib Fractures Are at Greater Risk of Death and Pneumonia." *Journal of Trauma* 54, no. 3 (March 2003): 478–85.

Bledsoe, B. E., R. S. Porter, and R. A. Cherry. *Paramedic Care: Principles & Practice*, 4th ed. Vol. 6, Sec. 6: Geriatrics, 175–222. Upper Saddle River, NJ: Pearson Education, 2012.

Centers for Disease Control and Prevention. "Falls Among Older Adults: An Overview." Home and Recreational Safety Web page. Last updated December 30, 2014. Accessed January 19, 2015, http://www.cdc.gov/HomeandRecreationalSafety/Falls/adultfalls.html.

Davidson G. H., C. A. Hamlat, F. P. Rivara, T. D. Koepsell, G. J. Jurkovich, and S. Arbabi. "Long-term Survival of Adult Trauma Patients." *Journal of the American Medical Association* (*JAMA* 305, no. 10 (March 9, 2011): 1001–07.

Diku, M., and K. Newton. "Geriatric Trauma." *Emergency Medicine Clinics of North America* 16, no. 1 (February 1998): 257–74.

Greenbaum, J., N. Walters, and P. D. Levy. "An Evidence-Based Approach to Radiographic Assessment of Cervical Spine Injuries in the Emergency Department." *Journal of Emergency Medicine* 36, no. 1 (January 2009): 64–71.

Jacobs, D. G. "Special Considerations in Geriatric Injury." *Current Opinions in Critical Care* 9, no. 6 (December 2003): 535–39.

Patel, V. I., H. Thadepalli, P. V. Patel, and A. K. Mandal. "Thoracoabdominal Injuries in the Elderly: 25 Years of Experience." *Journal of the National Medical Association* 96, no. 12 (December 2004): 1553–57.

Pudelek, B. "Geriatric Trauma: Special Needs for a Special Population." *AACN Clinical Issues* 13, no. 1 (February 2002): 61–72.

Sasser, S., R. C. Hunt, M. Faul, D. Sugerman, W. S. Pearson, T. Dulski, M. M. Wald, G. J. Jurkovich, C. D. Newgard, E. B. Lerner, et al. "Guidelines for Field Triage of Injured Patients: Recommendations of the National Expert Panel on Field Triage, 2011." *Morbidity and Mortality Weekly Report (MMWR)* 61(RR01): 1–20.

Stevenson, J. "When the Trauma Patient Is Elderly." *Journal of Perianesthesia Nursing* 19, no. 6 (December 2004): 392–400.

Shifflette, V. K., M. Lorenzo, A. J. Mangram, M. S. Truitt, J. D. Amos, and E. L. Dunn. "Should Age Be a Factor to Change from a Level II to a Level I Trauma Activation?" *Journal of Trauma* 69, no. 1 (July 2010): 88–92.

Staudenmayer, K. L., R. Y. Hsia, N. C. Mann, D. A. Spain, and C. D. Newgard. "Triage of Elderly Trauma Patients: A Population-Based Perspective." *Journal of the American College of Surgeons* 217, no. 4 (October 2013): 569–76.

Zarzaur, B. L., M. A. Croce, L. J. Magnotti, and T. C. Fabian. "Identifying Life-Threatening Shock in the Older Injured Patient: An Analysis of the National Trauma Data Bank." *Journal of Trauma* 68, no. 5 (May 2010): 1134–38.

Get more information about this course by calling
ITLS International at 888-495-4875
(outside the United States call +1-630-495-6442) or visit

www.itrauma.org

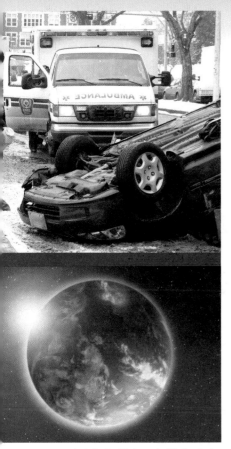

Trauma in Pregnancy

Walter J. Bradley, MD, MBA, FACEP

il trauma nel pregancy   Trauma en el embarazo

Traumatisme de la grossesse   Urazy psychiczne w ciąży

Trauma in Schwangerschaft   traume u trudnoći   صدمة في الحمل

traume u trudnoći   travme v nosečnosti   trauma a terhesség alatt

Jack Dagley Photography/Shutterstock

Key Terms

abruptio placenta, *p. 366*
domestic violence, *p. 366*
physiologic changes, *p. 361*
supine hypotension syndrome, *p. 364*

Objectives

Upon successful completion of this chapter, you should be able to:

1. Understand the dual goals in managing the pregnant trauma patient.
2. Describe the physiologic changes associated with pregnancy.
3. Understand the pregnant trauma patient's response to hypovolemia.
4. Describe the types of injuries most commonly associated with the pregnant trauma patient.
5. Describe the initial assessment and management of the pregnant trauma patient.
6. Discuss trauma prevention in pregnancy.

Chapter Overview

When the crossroads of pregnancy and trauma meet, there are unique challenges. The vulnerability of the pregnant trauma patient and potential injuries to the unborn child serve as reminders of the dual roles of providing care to both mother and fetus. In addition, the pregnant patient is often at risk for a higher incidence of accidental trauma. The increase in fainting spells, hyperventilation, and excess fatigue commonly associated with early pregnancy, as well as the physiologic changes that affect balance and coordination, add to risks.

Trauma is a leading cause of morbidity and mortality in pregnancy. Although maternal mortality due to other causes (such as infection, hemorrhage, hypertension, and thromboembolism) has declined over the years, the number of maternal deaths due to penetrating trauma, suicide, homicide, and motor-vehicle collisions has risen steadily. In the United States approximately 6% to 20% of all pregnant women experience some degree of trauma, not all of which are accidental. Significant trauma occurs in approximately 1 in 12 patients who are injured. Injuries requiring hospital intensive care unit (ICU) admission occur in three to four pregnancies per 100 deliveries. Motor-vehicle collisions account for 65% to 70% of trauma in pregnant patients. Falls, abuse and domestic violence, penetrating injuries, and burns follow. Because minor injuries rarely present problems for emergency care providers, the following discussion focuses on the more severe traumatic injuries to the pregnant patient. Several factors impact trauma in pregnancy and affect fetal morbidity and mortality. They include hypoxia, infection, drug effects, and preterm delivery.

Case Presentation

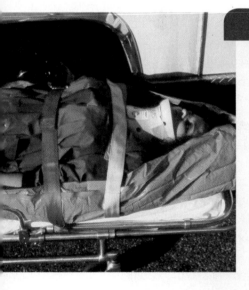

An advanced life support (ALS) ambulance is on the scene of a single-car motor-vehicle collision. The driver of the car swerved to avoid hitting a dog and hit a tree at an approximate speed of 30 miles (50 km) per hour. The patient was restrained, and the airbag deployed from the steering wheel. The scene is safe, and law enforcement is interviewing the driver, who is ambulatory. EMS is asked to evaluate the driver because she is concerned about her unborn baby. She is eight months pregnant. She denies loss of consciousness and head, neck, or back pain. Her only complaint is a tender abdomen. Upon inspection there is a superficial abrasion running horizontally across her abdomen.

Before proceeding, consider these questions: What is likely to have caused this abrasion? Should this patient be transported and evaluated at the emergency department or in the birthing center at the hospital? Might the incident induce premature labor? If she goes into labor, is the fetus old enough to be viable? Could this patient be managed without spinal motion restriction (SMR)? If SMR is indicated for a pregnant patient, are there special precautions to consider?

Keep these questions in mind as you read through the chapter. Then, at the end of the chapter, find out how the emergency care providers managed these patients.

Pregnancy
Fetal Development

The effect of trauma on pregnancy is influenced by the gestational age of the fetus, the type and severity of the trauma, and the extent of disruption of normal uterine and fetal physiology. The fetus is formed during the first three months of pregnancy.

3 Months   **8 Months**

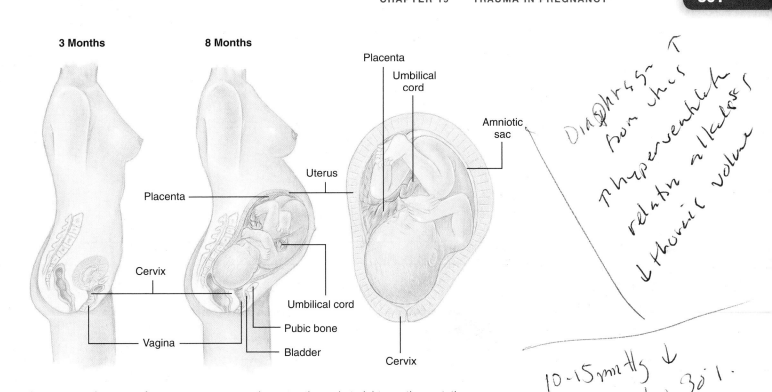

Figure 19-1 Anatomy of pregnancy: uterus at three months and at eight months gestation.

After the third month of gestation, the fully formed fetus and uterus grow rapidly, reaching the umbilicus by the fifth month and the epigastrium by the seventh month (Figure 19-1 and Table 19-1). In countries with well-developed health-care systems, the fetus is considered viable at 24 weeks with over 50% survival reported.

Physiologic Changes During Pregnancy

During pregnancy, dramatic **physiologic changes** occur. These changes, which are unique to the pregnant state, affect and sometimes alter the physiologic response by both the mother and fetus. Changes include blood volume (increases), cardiac output (increases), and blood pressure (decreases; Figure 19-2). The respiratory system also changes significantly due to an enlarging uterus that will elevate the diaphragm and decrease the overall volume of the thoracic cavity. That leads to a relative alkalosis and predisposes the patient to hyperventilation. There is, in addition, an increase in both red blood cells and plasma. With the increase of plasma greater than red

physiologic changes: the normal changes that occur to the body of a woman as she progresses through her pregnancy. These affect blood volume, vital signs, and even response to hypovolemia.

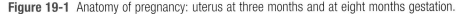

Table 19-1: Assessment of a Pregnancy			
	First Trimester (1–12 weeks)	**Second Trimester (13–24 weeks)**	**Third Trimester (25–40 weeks)**
Viability	Fetus not viable	Potential viability	Fetus viable
Vaginal bleeding	Potential for miscarriage	Potential miscarriage	Potential preterm birth
Fetal heart tones	Not obtainable consistently	120–170 beats per minute	120–160 beats per minute
Height of fundus above symphysis pubis	Difficult to measure	Halfway to umbilicus equals 16 weeks; to the umbilicus equals 20 weeks	1 cm equals 1 week until 37 weeks, then uterus height decreases as the baby settles into the pelvis

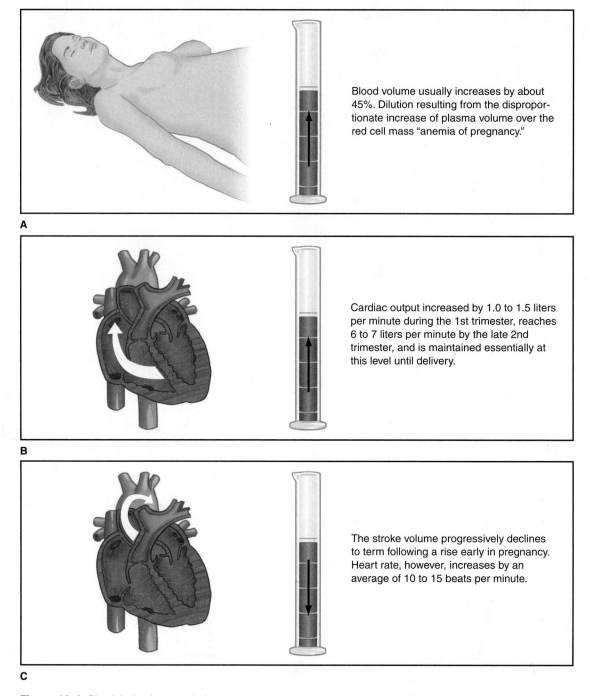

A

Blood volume usually increases by about 45%. Dilution resulting from the disproportionate increase of plasma volume over the red cell mass "anemia of pregnancy."

B

Cardiac output increased by 1.0 to 1.5 liters per minute during the 1st trimester, reaches 6 to 7 liters per minute by the late 2nd trimester, and is maintained essentially at this level until delivery.

C

The stroke volume progressively declines to term following a rise early in pregnancy. Heart rate, however, increases by an average of 10 to 15 beats per minute.

Figure 19-2 Physiologic changes during pregnancy.

blood cells, the patient will appear to be anemic (physiologic anemia of pregnancy). However, many pregnant patients have poor nutritional intake during pregnancy and, because the fetus draws iron stores, may develop an absolute anemia. Gastric motility is also decreased; thus, always assume the stomach of a pregnant patient is full. Always guard against vomiting and aspiration. Table 19-2 illustrates changes during pregnancy.

Responses to Hypovolemia

Acute blood loss results in a decrease in circulating blood volume. The cardiac output decreases as the venous return falls. This hypovolemia causes the arterial blood

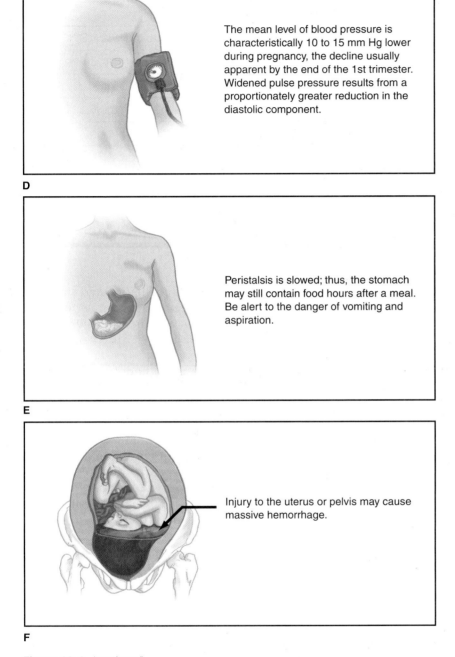

The mean level of blood pressure is characteristically 10 to 15 mm Hg lower during pregnancy, the decline usually apparent by the end of the 1st trimester. Widened pulse pressure results from a proportionately greater reduction in the diastolic component.

D

Peristalsis is slowed; thus, the stomach may still contain food hours after a meal. Be alert to the danger of vomiting and aspiration.

E

Injury to the uterus or pelvis may cause massive hemorrhage.

F

Figure 19-2 (continued)

pressure to fall, resulting in an inhibition of vagal tone and the release of catecholamines. The effect of this response is to produce vasoconstriction and tachycardia.

The vasoconstriction profoundly affects the uterus. Uterine vasoconstriction leads to reduction in uterine blood flow by 20% to 30%. Because of the increased blood volume, the pregnant patient may lose up to 1,500 cc of blood before any detectable change is noted in the blood pressure. The fetus reacts to this hypoperfusion by a drop in the arterial blood pressure and a decrease in heart rate. The fetus then begins to suffer from reduced oxygen concentration in the maternal circulation. Therefore, it is important to give 100% oxygen to the mother to provide sufficient oxygen to the fetus, who can suffer from both oxygen starvation and inadequate blood supply. A shock state in the mother is associated with an 80% fetal mortality rate.

PEARLS
Hypovolemia

- Do not mistake normal vital signs in pregnant patients as signs of shock. The pregnant patient has a normal resting pulse that is 10 to 15 beats faster than usual, and the blood pressure is 10 to 15 mm Hg lower than usual. However, it is also important to realize that a blood loss of 30% to 35% can occur in these patients before there is a significant change in blood pressure. Therefore, be especially alert to all signs of shock, and monitor the vital signs with frequent ITLS Ongoing Exams.

- Cardiac arrest in the pregnant patient is treated the same as for other victims. Defibrillation settings and drug dosages are the same. For hypovolemic arrest, the volume of required fluid increases, and four liters of normal saline should be given as fast as possible during transport.

Table 19-2: Physiologic Changes During Pregnancy

Parameter Monitored	Normal Female	Change
Blood volume	4,000 mL	Increased 40% to 50%
Heart rate	70	Increased 10% to 15%
Blood pressure	110/70	Decreased 5 to 15 mm Hg
Cardiac output	4 to 5 LPM	Increased 20% to 30%
Hematocrit/hemoglobin	13/40	Decreased
PCO$_2$	38	Decreased
Gastric motility	Normal	Decreased

Assessment and Management
Special Considerations

Major goals in caring for the pregnant trauma patient are evaluation and stabilization. The ITLS Primary Survey is the same for the pregnant patient as for other patients. (See Chapter 2.) All prehospital interventions are directed toward optimizing both fetal and maternal outcomes. If the patient is pregnant, there are two patients being treated. *Optimal care for the fetus is appropriate treatment of the mother.* Oxygen administration (100% by nonrebreather mask or by endotracheal intubation) should be rapid. Promptly obtain venous access and begin administration of IV fluids. Monitoring of this patient should be immediate and constant because the anatomic and physiologic changes of pregnancy make the trauma assessment more difficult.

supine hypotension syndrome: the drop in blood pressure seen when a woman who is greater than 20 weeks pregnant is in the supine position. The hypotension is caused by the weight of the pregnant uterus pressing on the inferior vena cava and decreasing the return of blood to the heart by up to 30%.

Called **supine hypotension syndrome**, acute hypotension in the pregnant patient due to decreased venous return requires special mention. It usually occurs when the patient is in a supine position with a 20-week or larger uterus (uterus up to umbilicus). The enlarged uterus compresses the inferior vena cava, leading to decreased venous return and resulting in decreased cardiac output (Figure 19-3). This leads to maternal hypotension, syncope, and fetal bradycardia. Left uterine displacement increases cardiac output by 30% and restores circulation. Uterine displacement must be maintained at all times during resuscitation, transport, and perioperatively for nonobstetric surgery. Therefore, the transport of all pregnant trauma patients, if no contraindication exists, should be by one of the following methods to alleviate vena cava compression:

- Tilt or rotate the backboard 15 to 30 degrees to the patient's left.
- Elevate the right hip four to six inches (10 to 15 centimeters) with a towel, and manually displace the uterus to the left.

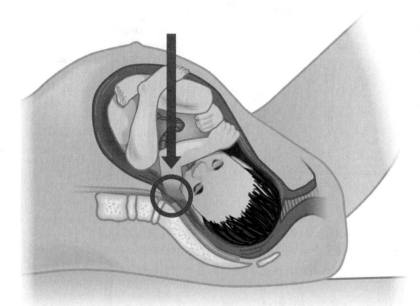

Figure 19-3 Venous return to the maternal heart may be decreased up to 30% because of vena cava compression by the fetus. Transport the patient tilted left side down or manually displace uterus to the left.

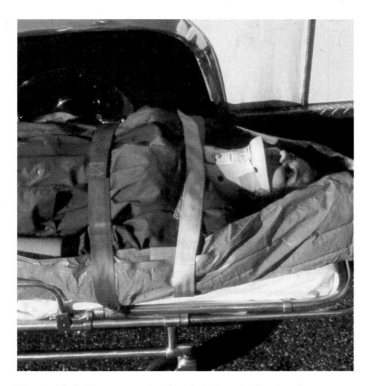

Figure 19-4 The pregnant patient is better stabilized and more comfortable in a vacuum backboard than a hard backboard.

You must be very careful when strapping a third-trimester pregnant patient onto a long backboard. Many patients (and backboards) will roll right over onto the ambulance floor if the tilted backboard is not secured to the stretcher. The vacuum backboard (Figure 19-4) is more comfortable and makes it easier to maintain SMR of the pregnant patient. Table 19-3 illustrates evaluation of uterine size and its effect on management of the pregnant patient.

Types of Trauma
Motor-Vehicle Collisions

Though relatively minor abdominal trauma can cause fetal death, the most common cause of fetal death in trauma is maternal death. Motor-vehicle collisions (MVCs)

PEARLS
Treatment

- You are treating two patients. However, the mortality of the fetus is directly related to the treatment provided to the mother. The goal of prehospital intervention is to maximize the chances of maternal survival, which will provide the fetus with the best chance for survival.
- If the mother dies, continue CPR and notify the hospital to be prepared for immediate cesarean section. Have them bring a sonogram machine to the emergency department for immediate evaluation of the fetus.
- Hypoxemia of the fetus may go unnoticed in the injured pregnant patient. Treatment should include high-flow oxygen.

Table 19-3: ITLS Primary Survey Brief Evaluation of Uterine Size	
Uterine Size < 20 Weeks	**Uterine Size > 20 Weeks**
Uterus Not to Umbilicus	Uterus to Umbilicus or Higher
↓	↓
Pregnancy Management Unchanged	Lateral Displacement of Uterus
↓	↓
Maternal Stabilization	Brief Confirmation of Fetal Heart Activity (if possible)
	↓
	Maternal Stabilization Secondary Fetal Stabilization

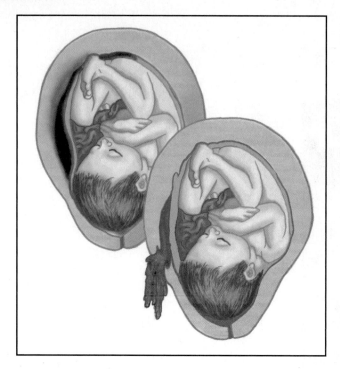

Figure 19-5 Blunt trauma to the uterus may cause separation of the placenta (abruptio placenta) or rupture of the uterus. Massive bleeding may occur, *but there may not be visible vaginal bleeding early.*

abruptio placenta: the separation of the placenta from the wall of the uterus.

PEARLS
Abdominal Trauma

Trauma to the abdominal compartment can cause occult bleeding in either the intrauterine or retroperitoneal area. Keep in mind that gradual stretching of the abdominal wall during pregnancy, along with hormonal changes within the body, make the peritoneal surface less sensitive to irritable stimuli. Therefore, bleeding can occur intraperitoneally, and the signs of rebound, guarding, and rigidity may not be present.

domestic violence: physical or emotional abuse in the home usually from spouse or partner. During the second and third trimesters, it is estimated that 1 in 10 pregnant women experiences physical abuse.

---

account for 65% to 75% of pregnancy-related trauma in North America. Fetal distress, fetal death, **abruptio placenta**, uterine rupture (Figure 19-5), and preterm labor are often seen in pregnant patients who have been in MVCs. A review of the literature indicates that less than 1% of pregnant patients will sustain injury when there is only minor damage to the vehicle.

Head injury is the most common cause of death in pregnant patients involved in MVCs. This is closely followed by uncontrolled hemorrhage. Pregnant victims of MVCs have associated injuries, such as pelvic fractures, that often result in concealed hemorrhage within the retroperitoneal space. The retroperitoneal area, because of its low-pressure venous system, can accommodate the loss of four or more liters (eight or more units) of blood into that area with few clinical signs. Seat-belt use with both a shoulder restraint and lap belt can significantly decrease patient mortality and has not shown any increase in uterine injuries. In late-term pregnancy some women will either not wear seat belts or wear them improperly, due to discomfort caused by the belt over the gravid abdomen. They are at increased risk for injury as a result.

Penetrating Injuries

Gunshot wounds and stabbings are the most common penetrating injuries encountered. If the path of entry is below the fundus, the uterus often offers protection to the mother, absorbing the force of the bullet or knife. Upper abdominal wounds often injure the bowel due to its displacement upward by the uterus. Studies have shown that gunshot wounds to the pregnant abdomen carry a high mortality rate for the fetus (40% to 70%). Mortality rate is lower for the mother (4% to 10%) because the large uterus usually protects vital organs. Stab wounds follow much the same pattern of outcome, with fetal mortality rates of about 40%. Definitive care will depend on several factors, involving degree of shock, associated organ injury, and time of gestation.

Domestic Violence

A large number of pregnant women experience **domestic violence**. The frequency appears to worsen as pregnancy progresses. Through the second and third trimesters, it is estimated that 1 in 10 women experiences abuse during pregnancy. Physical abuse is more likely to be manifest with proximal and midline injuries than the distal injuries of accidental trauma. The face and neck are most common. Domestic abuse has been associated with low birth weight, which leads to problems for the child. The pregnant patient who is under great stress produces hormones (high circulating adrenaline levels, and so on) that negatively affect the pregnancy. The folklore that pregnant patients should be shielded from frightening or disturbing situations may be true. Spouses and boyfriends are the perpetrators of the violence in 70% to 85% of cases.

Falls

The incidence of falls increases with the progression of pregnancy. This is in part due to an alteration in the patient's center of gravity. The incidence of significant injury is proportionate to the force of impact and the specific body part that sustains the impact. Pelvic injuries may result in fetal fractures and *abruptio placentae* (separation of the placenta from the uterine wall causing placental hemorrhage with separation from the uterus leading to fetal hypoxia and often fetal death). Placental abruption is characterized by severe abdominal pain with little or no vaginal bleeding. Emergency department evaluation and monitoring is recommended for even minor abdominal trauma during pregnancy.

Burns

Of the 2.2 million patients that suffer burn injuries in the United States annually, less than 4% are pregnant. The overall mortality and morbidity resulting from thermal injuries to the pregnant patient is not markedly different from the non-pregnant patient. However, it is important to remember that the fluid requirement for the pregnant patient is greater than that of the nonpregnant woman. Fetal mortality increases when the maternal surface burn exceeds 20%. The pregnant patient and the fetus are at significant risk when exposed to carbon monoxide (CO), especially as CO binds preferentially to fetal hemoglobin. Any pregnant woman with CO exposure should receive 100% oxygen by mask, and emergency care providers should consider transport to a center with hyperbaric oxygen capability.

FAST Exam

The use of ultrasound in the assessment and treatment of trauma patients is rapidly becoming a mainstay in the prehospital and hospital settings.

The focused assessment with sonography in trauma, abbreviated "FAST," is a rapid bedside ultrasound examination performed by surgeons, emergency physicians, and trained paramedics as a screening test for blood surrounding the chest and abdominal organs.

The FAST exam assesses four classic areas for free fluid often due to the presence of blood. The four areas are the:

- Perihepatic space
- Perisplenic space
- Pericardium
- Pelvis

This noninvasive exam involves no exposure to radiation, is less costly than a CT scan, and offers a rapid assessment in the hemodynamically unstable patient. Newer technology allows this test to be performed in the field setting. Its use in the care of trauma in pregnancy has been well established. FAST offers an effective means of addressing the double jeopardy concept of two patients, mom and fetus, in the traumatized pregnancy patient.

A newly updated FAST exam, labelled the extended FAST exam or "e FAST," allows for additional evaluation of both the lungs by adding bilateral anterior thoracic ultrasonography. Although an additional adjunct in the assessment of trauma care, it is important for caregivers to recognize the appropriate applications, pitfalls, and technical limitations of its use. There is still an imperfect nature of the exam. Nonetheless, expertise in its use is strongly encouraged.

Trauma Prevention in Pregnancy

Upon reviewing major causes of trauma in pregnancy, it is clear that specific recommendations such as proper seat belt use in motor vehicles, reporting and counseling for domestic violence, as well as education of the multiple physiologic, anatomic, and emotional changes associated with pregnancy will all serve to reduce trauma in pregnancy. Some patients get very little if any prenatal care, and even less prenatal education. If the situation is not critical, you should not hesitate to educate your pregnant patients when you are called to see them.

Case Presentation (continued)

An advanced life support (ALS) ambulance is on scene of a car versus tree collision at 30 miles (48 km) per hour. After assessing the scene for hazards and mechanism, the emergency care providers find that the driver, who is eight months pregnant, was restrained and the airbag deployed from the steering wheel. The patient denies loss of consciousness and head, neck, or back pain. Her only complaint is tenderness beneath a superficial abrasion running horizontally across her abdomen.

Because of the mechanism of injury, the team performs a rapid trauma survey that is normal with the exception of generalized tenderness of the abdomen but no rebound.

The fundus of the uterus is at the xyphoid. The vital signs are normal. It appears the patient had her lap belt across her abdomen instead of her pelvis, and it could have caused uterine or intrauterine injury so the patient is placed on the ambulance stretcher in the semireclining position, with no SMR, and transported nonemergency to the hospital where her obstetrician practices. A sonogram was done in the emergency department, and no abnormality was seen, so a fetal monitor was applied, and the patient was observed overnight. She developed premature labor during the night and delivered a healthy 5-pound, 6-ounce (2.4 kg) boy. She had a normal postpartum course, and she and the baby did well.

Summary

Management of the pregnant trauma patient requires knowledge of the physiologic changes that occur during pregnancy. Pregnant patients require rapid evaluation and also rapid interventions for stabilization, including aggressive oxygen administration and fluid resuscitation. They require special techniques in packaging and transport to prevent the vena cava compression syndrome. Because of the difficulty in early diagnosis, you should have a low threshold for load and go, if there is any danger of the development of hemorrhagic shock. Pregnant patients with serious injuries should be directly transported to a facility (trauma center) capable of managing these complex patients. Optional fetal care is dependent on optimal care of the mother.

Bibliography

Chang, J., C. J. Berg, L. E. Saltzman, and J. Herndon. "Homicide: A Leading Cause of Injury Deaths Among Pregnant and Postpartum Women in the United States, 1991–1999." *American Journal of Public Health* 95, no. 3 (March 2005): 471–77.

Coker, A. L., M. Sanderson, and B. Dong. "Partner Violence During Pregnancy and Risk of Adverse Pregnancy Outcomes." *Paediatric and Perinatal Epidemiology* 18, no. 4 (July 2004): 260–69.

El-Kady, D., W. M. Gilbert, J. Anderson, B. Danielsen, D. Towner, and L. H. Smith. "Trauma During Pregnancy: An Analysis of Maternal and Fetal Outcomes in a Large Population." *American Journal of Obstetrics and Gynecology* 190, no. 6 (June 2004): 1661–68.

Esposito, T. J. "Trauma During Pregnancy." *Emergency Medicine Clinics of North America* 12, no. 1 (February 1994): 167–99.

Fildes J., L. Reed, N. Jones, M. Martin, and J. Barrett. "Trauma: The Leading Cause of Maternal Death." *The Journal of Trauma* 32, no. 5 (March 1992): 643–45.

Hill, D. A., and J. J. Lense. "Abdominal Trauma in the Pregnant Patient." *American Family Physician* 53, no. 4 (March 1996): 1269–74.

Lewiss, R. E., T. Saul, and M. Del Rios. "Focus On: EFAST—Extended Focused Assessment with Sonography for Trauma." American College of Emergency Physicians website, *ACEP News*, January 2009. Accessed January 2, 2015, at http://www.acep.org/Clinical---Practice-Management/Focus-On--EFAST---Extended-Focused-Assessment-With-Sonography-for-Trauma/

Maghsoudi, H., R. Samnia, A. Garadaghi, and H. Kianvar. "Burns in Pregnancy." *Burns: Journal of the International Society for Burn Injuries* 32, no. 2 (March 2006): 246–50.

Pons, P. T. "Prehospital Considerations in the Pregnant Patient." *Emergency Medical Clinics of North America* 12, no. 1 (February 1994): 1–7.

Vaizey, C. J., M. J. Jacobson, and F. W. Cross. "Trauma in Pregnancy." *British Journal of Surgery* 81, no. 10 (October 1994): 1406–15.

Weiss, H. B., T. Songer, and A. Fabio. "Fetal Deaths Related to Maternal Injury." *Journal of the American Medical Association* 286, no. 15 (October 17, 2001): 1863–68.

Mendez-Fiqueroa, H., J. D. Dahlke, R. A. Vrees, and D. J. Rouse. "Trauma in Pregnancy: An Updated Systematic Review." *American Journal of Obstetrics and Gynecology* 209, no. 1 (July 2013): 1–10.

Get more information about this course by calling
ITLS International at 888-495-4875
(outside the United States call +1-630-495-6442) or visit

www.itrauma.org

20

The Impaired Patient

Jonathan G. Newman, MD, MMM, FACEP, EMT-P

Paziente Intossicato da Alcool o Droghe   Pacientes Intoxicados por alcohol o drogas

Les Patients sous l'influence d'alcool ou de drogues

Pacjent pod wpływem alkoholu lub narkotyków

Patienten unter dem Einfluss von Alkohol oder Drogen

Ozljeđenici pod utjecajem alkohola ili droga   المخدر مريض تحت تأثير الكحول أو

pacijent pod uticajem alkohola ili droga   Pacienti pod vplivom alkohola ali drog

Ittas vagy kábítószer hatása alatt lévő sérült

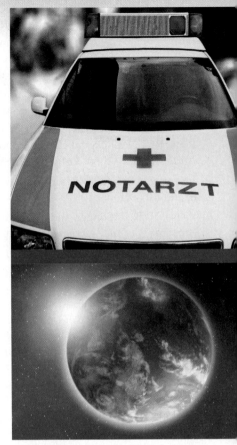

(Ambulance photo courtesy of Alexander Ivanov, Shutterstock.com)

Key Terms

capacity, *p. 375*
closed-ended questions, *p. 374*
excited delirium, *p. 374*
interactive style, *p. 373*
patient restraint, *p. 374*
uncooperative patient, *p. 374*

Objectives

Upon successful completion of this chapter, you should be able to:

1. List signs and symptoms of patients under the influence of alcohol and/or drugs.
2. Describe some strategies you would use to help ensure cooperation during assessment and management of a patient under the influence of alcohol and/or drugs.
3. Define excited delirium.
4. List the special considerations for assessment and management of patients in whom substance abuse is suspected.

Chapter Overview

The relationship between alcohol and trauma is well documented. For instance, it is reported that car crashes involving alcohol result in injuries to about 500,000 people a year. Studies of individuals who are substance abusers note that those persons are at greater risk of suffering an injury than the general population, and they are more likely to have repeated injuries.

Abuse of drugs and alcohol is a worldwide problem. Substance abuse includes individuals who have abused alcohol, drugs, or both. It has been associated with a number of traumatic events, often resulting from accidents, car crashes, suicides, homicides, and other violent crimes. Further, a study reported in the *Journal of the American College of Surgeons* found a high rate of alcohol and illicit drug use in patients who die from trauma. Therefore, it would not be surprising to find that a number of seriously injured trauma patients are under the influence of alcohol or some other substance. This group of trauma patients often presents with unique challenges that can require some special patient management techniques along with good ITLS care.

Case Presentation

This case is a continuation of the case from Chapter 16: You are the senior emergency care provider in an advanced life support team called as a second response unit to the scene of a burn injury. The first patient was critical, and the first ambulance had to make an emergency transport. Fire personnel have been monitoring the second patient while waiting for your arrival. The scene is safe. You have one patient. He has redness to his face, and his eyebrows are singed. He is slurring his speech and is unsteady on his feet. He admits to "drinking a few beers." When you begin to examine him, he becomes confrontational and tells you to leave him alone.

Before proceeding, consider these questions: How would you approach this patient? What critical signs are you looking for? Could some effects of alcohol intoxication mimic trauma-related signs and symptoms? Is this a load-and-go patient? Could the scene dynamics change and become unsafe? Keep these questions in mind as you read through the chapter. Then, at the end of the chapter, find out how the emergency care providers managed this patient.

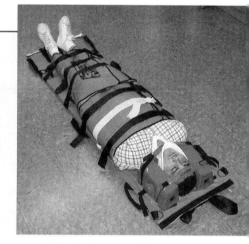

Substance Abuse

A high index of suspicion combined with the results of the physical exam, the history obtained from the patient or bystanders, and evidence at the scene can clue you in to whether your patient is under the influence of alcohol or drugs. Table 20-1 includes commonly abused drugs, along with signs and symptoms of their use.

Prescription medications are carefully formulated to contain the drug in the amount listed on the label, but street drugs are not. They are often mixed or "cut" with other active drugs or inactive fillers. The drugs that are used to cut the main substance will change the effect the drug has and may alter the signs and symptoms the patient experiences. The fillers used change the amount of the primary drug contained in each dose. Therefore, the patient's report of how much was used is a helpful but not 100% reliable indication of what symptoms to expect.

For example, methamphetamines may be mixed with bath salts, resulting in an increase in the variety of signs and symptoms seen. Heroin is often cut with inactive and sometimes active materials, such as fentanyl. Occasionally it is cut less than

Table 20-1: Commonly Abused Drugs with Their Associated Signs and Symptoms

Drug Category	Common Names	Signs and Symptoms of Use or Abuse
Alcohol	Beer, whiskey, wine, mouthwash	Altered mental function, confusion, polyuria, slurred speech, coma, hypertension, hyperthermia
Amphetamines/ methamphetamines	Bennies, ice, speed, uppers, dexies, Ecstasy, MDMA, Adderall, bath salts, crystal	Excitement, hyperactivity, dilated pupils, hypertension, tachycardia, tremors, seizures, fever, paranoia, psychosis
Cocaine	Coke, crack, blow, rock	Same as amphetamines plus chest pain; lethal dysrhythmias
Hallucinogens	Acid, LSD, PCP, peyote, mushrooms	Hallucinations, dizziness, dilated pupils, nausea, rambling speech, psychosis, anxiety, panic
Marijuana	Grass, hash, pot, tea, weed, K2, and Spice (contain synthetic marijuana compounds)	Euphoria, sleepiness, dilated pupils, dry mouth, increased appetite
Narcotics/opiates	Heroin, horse, big H, Darvon, codeine, stuff, morphine, smack, fentanyl, Percocet, opana	Altered mental status, constricted pupils, bradycardia, hypotension, respiratory depression, hypothermia
Sedatives and psychoactive medications	GHB; barbiturates; benzodiazepines (e.g., Librium, Valium, Xanax, Ativan, Rohypnol) Antidepressants: Elavil, Prozac, Sinequan, Effexor Antipsychotics: Thorazine; Zyprexa, Abilify	Altered mental status, dilated pupils, cardiac dysrhythmias, hypotension, respiratory depression, hypothermia

usual. When patients use their usual amount of such drugs, more extreme signs and symptoms are experienced, and an increased number of deaths occur.

New or emerging drugs, such as "Krokodil," which is desomorphine, also may be expected. Desomorphine has been used in Russia since the early 2000s. Its use in the United States was first reported in 2013. It has an effect similar to heroin but lasts for a shorter period of time. Its use is associated with tissue damage and can result in skin ulcers and gangrene. Amputations are sometimes necessary.

"N-bomb" includes a group of designer drugs called 25B-NBOMe, 25C-NBOMe, and 25I-NBOMe. These drugs target the serotonin receptor and cause hallucinations. Patients will have signs and symptoms similar to the hallucinogens listed in Table 20-1. However, small amounts of these drugs have caused seizures, cardiac and respiratory arrest, and death.

Salvia is a hallucinogen. It is found in southern Mexico. It can produce an altered perception of the external reality that results in a patient becoming unable to interact properly in his or her surroundings. Users may have dizziness, trouble walking, and slurred speech.

Assessment and Management

Your ITLS Primary and Secondary Surveys should follow the ITLS guidelines already described in this book. (See Chapter 2.) However, there are some particular aspects to be aware of when conducting an exam on a patient for whom you suspect substance abuse. Pay particular attention to mental status, pupils, speech, and respiration, and note any needle marks you may discover. An altered mental status can be seen in every form of substance abuse. However, remember that an altered level of consciousness is always due to a head injury, shock, or hypoglycemia until proven otherwise. Also remember that all patients have an emergency medical condition until proven otherwise.

Pupils often are constricted in patients who have abused opiates. Dilated pupils are common in patients exposed to amphetamines, cocaine, hallucinogens, and marijuana. Patients who use barbiturates will have pupils that are constricted early on. However, if high doses have been consumed, the pupils can eventually become fixed and dilated. Speech can be slurred when patients use alcohol or sedatives, and patients who are under the influence of hallucinogens may seem to ramble when they talk. Respiration can be significantly depressed with opiates and sedatives. Stimulant agents, such as cocaine, can produce tachycardia and hypertension, which may make identifying occult blood loss more difficult. Also many drugs of abuse lessen the patient's perception and response to pain, making your assessment more challenging.

The history supplied by the patient or bystanders can help to establish whether substance abuse is involved. Try to find out what was used, when it was taken, and how much was taken. If you know the name of the drug taken, you may need to check with your local poison control center because the number of prescription medications that are abused is in the hundreds, and many have serious toxic effects.

However, be aware that patients often deny that they have used or abused any substance. If possible, inspect the patient's surroundings for clues that drugs or alcohol may have been used. Note any alcoholic beverage bottles, pill containers, injection equipment, smoking or snorting paraphernalia, or unusual odors.

Trauma patients under the influence of alcohol or drugs can challenge the provider not only by their traumatic injuries but also by their attitudes. The way in which you interact with patients who have abused substances can determine if the patient will be cooperative or uncooperative. How you speak to them can be as important as what you are doing for them. Your interaction style, if offensive, can make patients uncooperative and force you both to lose precious minutes of the Golden Period. If your **interactive style** is positive and nonjudgmental, the patient is more likely to be cooperative and allow all the appropriate medical interventions, thus decreasing on-scene time. As noted before, all the substances that are abused can cause an altered mental state. When interacting with patients, you must be prepared to deal with euphoria, psychosis, paranoia, or confusion and disorientation.

interactive style: your speech and body language as you interact with a patient. A positive, nonjudgmental interactive style facilitates assessment and interventions while decreasing scene time.

Some interaction strategies that can help you gain your patient's cooperation are as follows:

- Identify yourself to patients and orient them to the surroundings. Tell them your name and your title (for example, "Paramedic"). Ask for their names and how they would like to be addressed. Avoid using generic names like "Bub" or "Honey." With this patient population, it may be necessary to orient patients to place, date, and what is going on multiple times. Repetitive questions by the patient may be a sign of a head injury, rather than intoxication.

- Treat patients in a respectful manner and avoid being judgmental. Often a lack of respect can be heard in the tone of your voice or how you say things, not just in what you say. Never forget that you are there to save lives. This includes all patients. You are not a police officer, and you are not there to pass judgment on a patient's worth to society. Also take care not to destroy evidence.

- Acknowledge the concerns and feelings of patients. Those who are scared or confused may be more comfortable with what is taking place if you recognize and address those feelings. Be gentle but firm. Explain all treatment interventions before they are performed. Be honest; backboards and extrication collars are uncomfortable, and IV lines hurt.

closed-ended questions:
questions that can be answered with a "yes" or "no." This is often the best approach with patients under the influence of alcohol or drugs due to their limited ability to concentrate.

patient restraint: methods of limiting the motion and mobility of patients to prevent them from becoming a danger to themselves or others.

uncooperative patients: patients who behave inappropriately and do not respond to reasonable requests and limits placed on them for their own safety and that of caregivers. Based on jurisdiction, a range of options are available for restraining patients against their will when warranted for patient safety, assessment, and care. A variety of physical and chemical restraints can be implemented.

excited delirium: a syndrome characterized by sympathetic nervous system excitation with tachycardia, hyperthermia, and hypertension. These patients often hallucinate and are very agitated. They are at risk for cardiac dysrhythmias and death.

- Let patients know what will be required of them. For instance, they may be confused and not realize that they need to hold still while responders are trying to stabilize them.
- Ask **closed-ended questions** when getting a history from patients. Closed-ended questions can be answered with a yes or no. Patients may only be able to concentrate for short periods of time, and they may ramble when asked open-ended questions that require a full answer. Consider getting as much of the history as you can from relatives, friends, or bystanders. This might help improve the reliability of what you discover. Get as much relevant history as you can, but do not delay transport.

The Uncooperative Patient

A small percentage of your patients may be uncooperative. You must be firm with them. Set limits to their behavior, and let them know when their behavior is inappropriate. Consider physical **patient restraint** or chemical restraint only if you are not able to secure enough cooperation to provide adequate care. Often being direct without being confrontational may be enough to convince an **uncooperative patient** to allow medical care to be provided. Respond to aggressive statements without adopting aggressive speech or posture yourself. Do not argue because it can increase the tension. With intoxicated patients you often have to redirect them back toward what you want them to do.

Other things EMS can do to prevent escalation is to avoid yelling at the patient, respect the patient's personal space, and avoid talking to the patient in a condescending manner. Acknowledge the patient's concerns, and try to maintain eye contact.

You should watch for clues regarding physical violence, such as verbal threats, aggressive posture by the patient, rapidly shifting eye movements, and fist clenching. If the situation becomes physical, you should back out to safety and allow law enforcement officers to perform their job. Given that many traumatic events involve motor-vehicle collisions or violent acts such as assault, it is a good policy to have law enforcement on the scene. The actual dispatch of law enforcement is governed by local protocol, but do not hesitate to request their support if you feel it is needed.

Excited Delirium

Excited delirium (EXD) is a syndrome characterized by agitation and aggressive behavior. The syndrome often results in death of patients, especially when restrained. The patient exhibits tachycardia, hyperthermia, and hyperactivity and often hallucinates. These patients are often difficult to handle because they can display incredible strength. Deaths have been attributed to the patient being placed into prone restraint with hands behind the back and legs bent forward ("hog tie position"), resulting in positional asphyxia. However, it is now believed that the effects of stimulants (cocaine, methamphetamine, others) lead to cardiac dysrhythmias, and their signs reflect sympathetic nervous system overstimulation. Often to safely subdue these patients, less-than-lethal weapons, such as pepper spray or a Taser®, will be used by law enforcement. Decontaminate the patient if he or she has been pepper sprayed. Cardiac monitoring should be applied due to the tachycardia, though the diaphoresis may make it difficult for pads to stick.

Management of these patients can be challenging. Preventing injury to yourself and other responders is important, along with protecting the patient from further injury. Rapidly sedating the patient is the most effective way to control the situation. IM benzodiazepines and haloperidol have been used effectively. Recent studies have shown good results with IM ketamine. Local protocol will determine which agents can be used. Take care to avoid a needlestick injury when dealing with the struggling patient.

Plan for these types of patient encounters. First, check with your local jurisdiction to determine what protocol you must use when restraining patients against their will. Many jurisdictions allow police officers to place people in custody if they are a threat to themselves or others. Severely injured trauma patients who refuse or will not cooperate with care may be considered a threat to themselves.

The decision on whether patients can refuse care is based on a patient's **capacity** to refuse. This varies with jurisdictions. For emergency care providers to treat, patients must consent to care. In many places unresponsive patients are able to be treated based on the concept of implied consent. These are situations in which it is assumed a reasonable person would want care when not receiving care carries significant risk to the patient. For patients to refuse, they must display the capacity to do so. This means patients have no alteration of mental status, such as a head injury, intoxication, hypoxia, or hypoglycemia, and that they understand the risks and possible detrimental outcomes (up to and including death) if they refuse care.

capacity: the ability of patients to understand their situation and to make an informed decision about their care.

This is a very difficult situation for emergency care providers because they are there to help. The decision of whether the patient has the capacity to refuse care should be documented.

Once the decision has been made to restrain the patient, it must be carried out with care. The actual process of physically restraining the patient is beyond the scope of this course, and the emergency care providers should receive this training from the agency for which they work. At the simplest level, securely strapping a patient to a backboard with use of a cervical collar and head motion-restriction device can serve to restrain most patients. Caution must be taken not to worsen any current injuries or to inflict any new ones.

There is often no good solution to this predicament. Restrained patients could struggle so hard that spinal motion restriction (SMR) is rendered ineffective. The Reeves sleeve is one of the few pieces of equipment that can be effective both in providing spinal motion restriction and in restraining patients. Note that it may be very difficult to place an agitated and combative patient into the Reeves sleeve (Figure 20-1).

Restrained patients must always have a provider who can manage the airway, should the patient vomit. If SMR is not needed, the patient can be restrained on the ambulance stretcher with head elevated. Be sure to check extremities distal to restraints for pulse, motor function, and sensation as part of your ITLS Ongoing Exam.

Crews should plan and practice procedures for restraining patients, ideally in cooperation with local law enforcement. The trauma scene is not the place to learn new skills. Reassess restrained patients often. Restrained patients must have an emergency care provider with them during the entire time they are under EMS care. They also should be attached to the appropriate monitor. Intoxicated patients, especially those on stimulants are at risk for death during transport.

The standard ITLS approach to patient care will work well, even with patients under the influence of alcohol or drugs. Ensure that the scene is safe, determine the number of injured, and discover the mechanism of injury. Use standard precautions. Many patients who are dependent on drugs and/or alcohol are at increased risk for infection with hepatitis B, hepatitis C, and HIV. Follow the ITLS

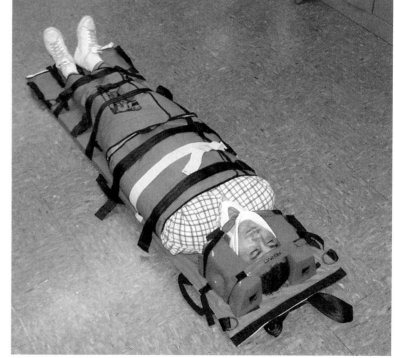

Figure 20-1 Reeves sleeve.

Table 20-2: Drug Categories and Specific Treatments to Consider or Areas to Assess Closely

Drug Category	Specific Treatments and Areas to Assess
Alcohol	Administer IV thiamine and glucose; use D50W if indicated; watch for hypothermia.
Amphetamines/ methamphetamine	Monitor for seizures and dysrhythmias; treat seizures with diazepam or lorazepam.
Cocaine	Monitor for seizures and dysrhythmia; treat rhythm disorders. Avoid beta-blockers, as these may increase myocardial ischemia. Benzodiazepines may be helpful for agitation
Hallucinogens	Provide reassurance. Benzodiazepines may be helpful for agitation
Marijuana	Provide reassurance. Benzodiazepines may be helpful for agitation
Narcotics/opiates	Try naloxone*, watch for hypothermia, hypotension, and respiratory depression (CO_2 monitor).
Sedatives	Try naloxone* and consider flumazenil**, watch for hypothermia, hypotension, and respiratory depression (end-tidal CO_2 monitor).

*Naloxone should be titrated to the patient's respirations. Repeated doses may be indicated because the narcotic may last longer than the effects of the naloxone.

**Flumazenil use is controversial. It can precipitate seizures in patients dependent on benzodiazepines. Further, flumazenil use may cause seizures in those who have been using benzodiazepines to prevent seizures and in those patients who have overdosed on tricyclic antidepressants. Flumazenil should be given only on direct order of medical direction.

PEARLS
Management

- Check finger-stick glucose and provide ECG monitoring on every patient with altered mental status.
- In this population, hypothermia, hypotension, and respiratory depression are common and must be treated aggressively. Involve the poison control center early if the person has taken a drug with which you are not familiar.

Primary and Secondary Surveys as recorded in Chapter 2. Remember to note any mental status changes that might be associated with substance abuse.

When performing the ITLS Secondary Survey, be sure to include the specific areas that can provide clues to substance abuse. As with all trauma patients, treatment includes the consideration of oxygen, an IV line, cardiac monitoring, and O_2 saturation or expired CO_2 monitoring. Check blood sugar in all patients with altered mental status.

Table 20-2 lists drug categories and associated specific treatments or areas requiring close attention when substance abuse is suspected. A survey of American teenagers by the National Institute on Drug Abuse (NIDA), published in 2014, shows that overall drug use continues to decline in that age group. However, they reported that the perception of 3, 4-Methylenedioxymethamphetamine (MDMA or Ecstasy) as harmful is going down, and this might be a precursor to an increase in the use of this drug. The NIDA also expressed concern about the nonmedical use of the narcotics Vicodin (hydrocodone) and OxyContin (oxycodone).

Case Presentation *(continued)*

The ITLS Primary Survey is intact because the patient is ambulatory and speaking with no distress. However, he is acting clinically intoxicated. The singeing of facial hair and superficial facial burns are concerning for possible inhalation injury. He keeps stating that he is fine and he wants to stay at the party. He becomes loud and abusive toward EMS personnel. You attempt to convince him of the need to be assessed. You firmly and repeatedly tell him about the need to be evaluated. Despite your calm demeanor, he becomes agitated. Because he had treated the fire personnel the same way, the Fire Officer had called for police to respond. A police officer now tells the patient he can go with the ambulance or he can go in the police car, but he is too intoxicated to refuse care. The patient reluctantly agrees to be evaluated and transported. The ITLS Secondary Survey shows only superficial facial burns and no wheezes, stridor, or other signs of respiratory compromise. The patient does try to get off the stretcher several times during transport, but each time sits down when politely but firmly told to do so.

He is evaluated in the hospital emergency department, treated for his superficial burns, and allowed to "sleep off" his intoxication. A urine drug screen also shows presence of cannabis but no other drugs. The emergency department staff gives him information about alcohol and substance abuse and treatment options because this is not his first visit to the hospital due to being intoxicated. The patient is discharged in the care of his father, who is unhappy about having to pick him up in the middle of the night.

Summary

Knowing the signs and symptoms of alcohol and drug abuse will allow you to recognize the patient who may be impaired. Assessing the patient for signs and symptoms outlined in this chapter can help you confirm your suspicions. Determining that your patient has abused some substance will allow you to pay attention to specific areas for critical changes as well as provide life-saving interventions that may be indicated for individual substances. The five interaction strategies for improving patient cooperation are very important when dealing with the patient under the influence of alcohol or drugs, but those strategies also should be used with all patients. Remember that the patient's safety is a primary concern. If you must restrain a patient for his or her safety, do so in a planned manner that is most sensitive to your patient's needs.

Bibliography

Bledsoe, B., R. Porter, and R. Cherry. *Paramedic Care: Principles and Practice*, 3rd Edition, Vol. 3, 499–507, and Vol. 5, 206–207. Upper Saddle River, NJ: Prentice Hall, 2009.

"Commonly Abused Drugs Chart." National Institute of Drug Abuse website, revised March, 2011. Accessed January 3, 2015, at http://www.drugabuse.gov/drugs-abuse/commonly-abused-drugs-charts/commonly-abused-drugs-chart

"Commonly Abused Prescription Drugs Chart." National Institute of Drug Abuse website, revised October, 2011. Accessed January 3, 2015, at http://www.drugabuse.gov/drugs-abuse/commonly-abused-drugs-charts/commonly-abused-prescription-drugs-chart

Demetriades D., G. Gkiokas, G. C. Velmahos, C. Brown, J. Murray, and T. Noguchi. "Alcohol and Illicit Drugs in Traumatic Deaths: Prevalence and Association with Type and Severity of Injuries." *Journal of the American College of Surgeons* 199, no. 5 (November 2004): 687–92.

"Drug Facts: Nationwide Trends." National Institute on Drug Abuse website, last updated/revised January, 2014. Accessed January 3, 2015, at http://www.drugabuse.gov/infofacts/nationtrends.html

Elling, B., K. M. Elling, and the American Academy of Orthopedic Surgeons. "Toxicology and Behavioral Emergencies." In *Paramedic: Pharmacology Applications*, 274–278. Sudbury, MA: Jones & Bartlett Learning, 2009.

"Emerging Trends: Krokodil." National Institute on Drug Abuse website, last updated/revised November, 2014. Accessed January 3, 2015, at http://www.drugabuse.gov/drugs-abuse/emerging-trends

Miller, T. R., D. C. Lestina, and G. S. Smith. "Injury Risk Among Medically Identified Alcohol and Drug Abusers." *Alcoholism, Clinical and Experimental Research* 25, no. 1 (January 2001): 54–59.

"Salvia Divinorum and Salvinorin A." Drug Enforcement Administration webpage, October 2013. Accessed January 3, 2015, at http://www.deadiversion.usdoj.gov/drug_chem_info/salvia_d.pdf

Su, H. K., M. Baker, and L. J. Baraff. "Design Drug 25B-NBOMe Use Likely to Land Overdose Cases in Your Emergency Department." American College of Emergency Physicians, *ACEP Now* website, November 19, 2014. Accessed January 3, 2015, at http://www.acepnow.com/article/designer-drug-25b-nbome-use-likely-land-overdose-cases-emergency-department/

Takeuchi, A., T. L. Ahern, and S. O. Henderson. "Excited Delirium." *West Journal of Emergency Medicine* 12, no. 1 (January 2012): 77–83.

"251-NBOMe, 25C-NBOMe, and 25B-NBOMe." Drug Enforcement Administration webpage, November 2013. Accessed January 3, 2015, at http://www.deadiversion.usdoj.gov/drug_chem_info/nbome.pdf

Vike, G. M., M. L. DeBard, et al. "Excited Delirium Syndrome (ExDS): Defining Based on a Review of the Literature." *Journal of Emergency Medicine* 47, no. 5 (November 2012): 897–905.

Get more information about this course by calling
ITLS International at 888-495-4875
(outside the United States call +1-630-495-6442) or visit

www.itrauma.org

Trauma Arrest

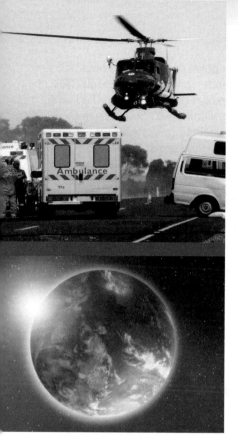

Ray Fowler, MD, FACEP
Ahamed Idris, MD
Jeremy Brywczynski, MD

Arresto CardioRespiratorio Post Traumatico   Paro Cardiopulmonar Traumático

Arrêt Cardiorespiratoire   Zatrzymanie krążenia u chorego po urazie

Herz- Kreislaufstillstand nach Trauma   Zastoj srca i disanja u traumi

إصابات توقف القلب والرئة   kardiorespiratorni zastoj usled traume

Kardiopulmonalni zastoj zaradi poškodbe

Traumás eredetű keringés-légzésleállás

(Ambulance photo courtesy of David Hancock, Shutterstock.com)

Key Terms

foreign body airway obstruction
    (FBAO), *p. 385*
traumatic cardiopulmonary arrest
    (TCPA), *p. 380*
unsalvageable patient, *p. 380*
withholding or termination of
    resuscitation, *p. 381*

Objectives

Upon successful completion of this chapter, you should be able to:

1. Identify treatable causes of traumatic cardiopulmonary arrest.
2. Describe the proper evaluation and management of the patient in traumatic cardiopulmonary arrest.
3. Identify patients in traumatic cardiac arrest for whom you should withhold resuscitation attempts.

Chapter Overview

You will encounter trauma patients who are found either pulseless or apneic on scene or who deteriorate rapidly and develop those signs while under your care. Although CPR in traumatic arrest is considered futile, there are several causes of traumatic cardiac arrest that are correctable, and prompt recognition and intervention could be life saving. This chapter will discuss guidelines for when to attempt resuscitation and when it would be futile. You also will review the causes of the traumatic cardiac arrest and the best plan of action to rapidly identify the cause and match your response to that cause.

Case Presentation

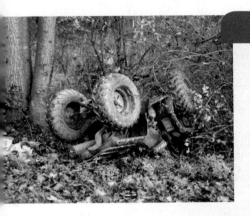

A basic life support (BLS) ambulance arrives at scene of an all-terrain vehicle crash in a very rural area. The closest hospital is 15 miles away, and the closest level 2 trauma hospital is 45 miles away. In this EMS system, advanced life support (ALS) is only dispatched on request of the BLS ambulance on scene. The scene size-up reveals a safe scene with one patient (approximately 20 years old) from an all-terrain vehicle that appears to have failed to negotiate a curve in the dirt road. The all-terrain vehicle and helmetless driver left the roadway and struck a tree.

The patient is unresponsive, not breathing, and pulseless. There is an obvious deformity to the skull, multiple rib fractures, and deformity to the left femur. There were no witnesses to the crash, and it is difficult to determine when the crash occurred. An AED is applied, and it indicates, "No shock advised."

Before proceeding, consider these questions: Should CPR be initiated? Should the BLS ambulance request an ALS response? If ALS does respond, should they respond with "lights and sirens"? What are likely causes of this cardiac arrest? Keep these questions in mind as you read through the chapter. Then, at the end of the chapter, find out how the emergency care providers managed this patient.

The Unsalvageable Patient

traumatic cardiopulmonary arrest (TCPA): a grouping of conditions defined by the common precipitating factor of trauma as the origin for the cardiac arrest.

unsalvageable patient: one who does not have a reasonable expectation for resuscitation and survival based on defined clinical indicators and parameters. It is acceptable to withhold resuscitation under those conditions.

Attempting to resuscitate the patient in **traumatic cardiopulmonary arrest (TCPA)** can put you and the public in danger. Research has shown that emergency lights-and-sirens traffic can be hazardous to both prehospital providers and to the safety of the public. Do not attempt resuscitation unless there is some chance of the patient's survival. One review of 195 trauma patients who presented unconscious, without palpable pulse or spontaneous respiration, found that patients with sinus rhythm and nondilated (< 4 mm) reactive pupils had a good chance of survival. However, in those patients with asystole, agonal rhythm, ventricular fibrillation, or ventricular tachycardia (**unsalvageable patients**), there were no survivors. The National Association of EMS Physicians and the American College of Surgeons Committee on Trauma have jointly developed guidelines for **withholding or termination of resuscitation** in prehospital traumatic cardiopulmonary arrest (Table 21-1). You also should be familiar with your local protocols that relate to traumatic cardiac arrest.

Advanced cardiac life support (ACLS) has always been directed toward dealing with a cardiac cause for the pulseless patient. In trauma cases, however, cardiopulmonary arrest is usually not due to primary cardiac disease, such as coronary atherosclerosis with acute myocardial infarction. You must direct your treatment by identifying the

Table 21-1: Guidelines for Withholding or Terminating Resuscitation of Prehospital Traumatic Cardiopulmonary Arrest*

1. Resuscitation should be withheld in cases of:

   a. Blunt trauma with no breathing, pulse, or organized rhythm on ECG on EMS arrival at the scene.

   b. Penetrating trauma with no breathing, pulse, pupillary reflexes, spontaneous movement, or organized ECG activity.

   c. Any trauma with injuries obviously incompatible with life (such as, decapitation).

   d. Any trauma with evidence of significant time lapse since pulselessness, including dependent lividity, rigor mortis, etc.

2. Cardiopulmonary arrest patients in whom the mechanism of injury does not correlate with the clinical condition, suggesting a nontraumatic cause of the arrest, should have standard resuscitation initiated.

3. Termination of resuscitation efforts should be considered (consult medical direction):

   a. With EMS-witnessed cardiopulmonary arrest and 20 minutes of unsuccessful resuscitation and the patient remains in a "nonshockable" rhythm or PEA at a rate less than 40 beats per minute.

   b. When transport time to the hospital emergency department is more than 15 minutes and the preceding condition exists.

4. Special consideration should be given to victims of near drowning, lightning strike, and hypothermia.

**Joint Position Statement of the National Association of EMS Physicians and the American College of Surgeons Committee on Trauma (Revised 2012).*

withholding or termination of resuscitation: based on research and published guidelines, attempting to resuscitate the patient in cardiac arrest may be withheld or terminated in certain instances.

underlying cause of the arrest, or you will almost never be successful in resuscitation. Use the ITLS Primary Survey to determine both the cause of the arrest and to identify those patients for whom you should attempt resuscitation.

Airway and Breathing Problems

Hypoxemia is the most common cause of traumatic cardiopulmonary arrest. Acute airway obstruction or ineffective breathing will be clinically manifested as hypoxemia. Carbon dioxide accumulation from inadequate breathing contributes to the unsuccessful resuscitation of such patients. Airway problems such as those listed in Table 21-2 lead to hypoxemia by preventing the flow of oxygen to the lungs. Drugs and alcohol, often in conjunction with minor head trauma, can result in airway obstruction by the tongue as well as by respiratory depression.

Careful monitoring of the intoxicated patient may prevent respiratory or cardiac arrest. The same is true of the patient who is unconscious from a head injury. The lax muscles in the pharynx allow the tongue to fall back and obstruct the airway. Obtaining and maintaining an open airway by use of the modified jaw-thrust maneuver along with an oro- or nasopharyngeal airway is vital for patients with no gag reflex. You may use a blind insertion supraglottic airway device (King Airway™, LMA™, and others) if tolerated by the patient and if there is no airway injury distal to the epiglottis. The role of endotracheal intubation (ETI) in the major trauma patient is an area of wide debate and ongoing study. Theoretically, management of the airway should be simpler with ETI, but studies have questioned its benefit and any role in improving survival. In any case, the provider should use all efforts available to prevent aspiration, including having an effective suction device readily available.

Patients with TCPA caused by airway obstruction may respond to advanced life support if the anoxic period was not prolonged.

Patients with hypoxia secondary to a breathing problem have an adequate airway, but they are unable to oxygenate their blood because they cannot get oxygen and

PEARLS
Cardiac Arrest

Cardiac arrest following trauma is usually not due to cardiac disease.

Table 21-2: Causes of Prehospital Traumatic Cardiopulmonary Arrest

1. Airway Problems
   a. Foreign body
   b. Tongue prolapse
   c. Swelling
   d. Tracheal damage
   e. Hemorrhage into the airway
   f. Misplaced advanced airway

2. Breathing Problems
   a. Tension pneumothorax
   b. Open pneumothorax (sucking chest wound)
   c. Flail chest
   d. Diaphragmatic injury
   e. High spinal-cord injury
   f. Carbon monoxide inhalation
   g. Smoke inhalation
   h. Aspiration
   i. Near-drowning
   j. Central nervous system depression from drugs/alcohol
   k. Apnea secondary to electric shock or lightning strike

3. Circulatory Problems
   a. Hemorrhagic shock (empty heart syndrome) from any cause, including traumatic aortic dissection and other vascular injuries
   b. Tension pneumothorax
   c. Pericardial tamponade
   d. Myocardial contusion
   e. Acute myocardial infarction
   f. Cardiac arrest secondary to electric shock

blood together at the alveolar-capillary membrane of the lungs. This could be from one or more of the following:

- Inability to ventilate, as in a tension pneumothorax, open pneumothorax, flail chest, pulmonary contusion, or high spinal-cord (C-3 or above) injury

- Lung tissue filled with fluid, as in the patient with aspiration of blood or vomitus or adult respiratory distress syndrome (ARDS, also known as noncardiogenic pulmonary edema). Near-drowning patients have hypoxemia early from lack of oxygen, and later their lungs develop ARDS.

- Lungs filled with gas (smoke inhalation) that does not contain the appropriate amount of oxygen but instead contains harmful gases such as carbon monoxide or cyanide. In addition, the hot vapor can result in pulmonary edema, further preventing oxygenation by increasing the distance (by alveolar capillary membrane swelling) between the red blood cells and oxygen.

- Hypoventilation caused by head injury, lightning strike, or drugs and alcohol.

Patients with breathing problems should have aggressive appropriate airway management and assisted ventilation with high-flow oxygen. Many of these patients will respond quickly if they have not been anoxic for too long. It is important for you to remember that the patient in shock is very sensitive to positive pressure ventilation (also known as "assisted" ventilation). Positive pressure ventilation will diminish venous return to the heart. This lowers cardiac output and hence blood pressure, worsening the shock state. This will be covered in more detail later in this chapter.

Circulatory Problems

The causes of TCPA due to circulatory failure are found in Table 21-2. Hypovolemic shock (shock due to blood loss) is the most common circulatory cause of TCPA. Blood loss may be external, internal, or both, and it may be classified as controlled or uncontrolled. Massive internal bleeding causing cardiac arrest is usually fatal and can display any of the cardiac arrest ECG rhythms on the monitor.

Massive external bleeding causing TCPA often can be controlled in such conditions as amputations, and tourniquets may be life saving in such cases. Prompt intravenous (IV) fluid replacement—especially with blood and blood products—presents an opportunity for salvage in this group of patients.

Massive internal bleeding that produces cardiac arrest is due to a transected blood vessel, injury to an internal organ (such as liver and spleen), or both. TCPA in these patients is usually fatal. Arrival at a trauma center with some cardiac electrical activity presents slight hope for successful resuscitation with prompt care by the trauma team.

Traumatic tension pneumothorax reduces venous return due to increased intrathoracic pressure in the affected pleural space, accompanied by pressure against the mediastinum late in its course. Decreased venous return reduces cardiac output, and shock occurs. Jugular venous distention, tachycardia, and cyanosis occur, appearing similar to pericardial tamponade, and the patient's trachea may deviate away from the affected side with increasing pressure against the mediastinum late in the course of the condition. The latter clinical finding may be difficult to identify.

It is vital to diagnose tension pneumothorax if it is present during TCPA. This is one potentially correctable cause of TCPA, and needle decompression of the pleural space on the affected side may be life saving.

Traumatic pericardial tamponade (another form of "mechanical" or obstructive shock) producing TCPA is quickly fatal. This condition is usually encountered in a patient with penetrating trauma to the chest wall. The heart is squeezed by blood and clots in the pericardial sac and less able to fill with blood during each beat. The pressure within the pericardial sac is transmitted to the chambers of the heart, preventing them from filling during diastole. That reduces venous return to the heart, and cardiac arrest and shock occur. Because of poor lung perfusion, cyanosis usually develops.

These patients often show Beck's triad, which is a "quiet heart" (muffled heart tones because the heart is nearly empty), evidence of blood not getting into the heart (jugular venous distention), and hypotension (due to low cardiac output) in the setting of equal bilateral breath sounds (unless a lung injury is also present).

Peripheral pulses diminish as hypotension worsens, and indeed, cardiac output may be so low that you cannot feel a pulse. Tachycardia is usually present on the monitor until cardiac arrest is imminent. The peripheral pulses may decrease or disappear with inspiration (termed *pulsus paradoxus*), which is an exaggeration of the slight (less than 10 mm Hg) decrease in systolic blood pressure that occurs during normal inspiration.

Importantly, the multiple-trauma victim may have massive hemorrhage in addition to cardiac tamponade (or tension pneumothorax), reducing the distention of neck veins and making the tamponade (or tension pneumothorax) more difficult to detect. The critical take-home point here is that the patient who is bleeding to death may not have enough blood within the vascular space to show distended neck veins in a tension pneumothorax or cardiac tamponade.

Patients with pericardial tamponade may appear to be in pulseless electrical activity (PEA) and commonly will not respond to ACLS protocols. Emergency care providers

PEARLS
ACLS Protocols

Do not rely on advanced cardiac life support (ACLS) protocols alone. TCPA protocols should include rapid and adequate volume replacement, as well as chest decompression when indicated. Also, if the patient has had a chest seal applied to an open chest wound and experiences a TCPA, remove the seal to help decompress a possible tension pneumothorax that may have developed.

can try administering IV fluids to increase "pre-load" and improve venous return. If allowed by protocol or by virtue of licensure and training, an emergency care provider can perform a pericardiocentesis. Removal of as little as 10 cc of blood can result in return of spontaneous circulation (ROSC).

Acute myocardial infarction and myocardial contusion can produce inadequate blood flow (circulation) by either one or a combination of three mechanisms. Those mechanisms are dysrhythmia, acute pump failure, and pericardial tamponade. The patient with a myocardial contusion has usually been in a deceleration collision resulting in trauma to the chest. In such an incident there may be a chest wall or sternal contusion.

Ventricular fibrillation (VF) triggered by a blow to the anterior chest wall during cardiac repolarization is most commonly seen in teenage boys who are engaged in sporting activities (such as being hit in the chest with a helmet while being tackled playing football) or from compression of the chest against a steering wheel. This condition is known as *commotio cordis*. Prompt recognition that the VF may have been caused by a blow to the chest is critical, and rapid defibrillation is often life saving. The placement of automated external defibrillators at sporting events that might result in such chest trauma is an important public health consideration.

TCPA from an electrical shock usually presents as ventricular fibrillation. It may respond to ACLS protocols if you are able to initiate resuscitation early enough following TCPA. Electrical shock from alternating current usually induces ventricular fibrillation. Thus standard ACLS, especially early defibrillation can be life saving. The cardiac arrest seen following a lightning strike is frequently due to the prolonged apnea that may follow the lightning strike. The victim of an electrical shock has suffered severe muscle spasm and respiratory muscle paralysis and may well have been thrown down or fallen a great distance. Thus the same systematic approach to this patient as to any other is required to identify all associated injuries and to give the patient the best chance for a good outcome. However, it should be remembered that patients in TCPA after electrical or lightning injury have a higher rate of survival than arrest from other causes, and full resuscitation should always be attempted when they are encountered. Be sure the patient is no longer in contact with the electricity source. Do not become a victim yourself!

It should be noted that in a lightning strike with multiple victims, emergency care providers should begin resuscitating those victims who are pulseless and/or apneic. This is an exception to the classic triage rule of not resuscitating pulseless patients in a mass-casualty event. A patient who has a pulse after a lightning strike has a greater than 98% chance of surviving.

In summary, patients with cardiopulmonary arrest related to inadequate circulation have either one of the following clinical conditions:

- Inadequate return of blood to the heart because of
  —Increased pressure in the chest causing decreased venous return to the heart, as in tension pneumothorax or pericardial tamponade
  —Hemorrhagic shock with inadequate circulating blood volume because of blood loss
- Inadequate pumping of the heart because of
  —Cardiac rhythm disturbances as in myocardial contusion, acute myocardial infarction, *commotio cordis*, or electrical shock
  —Acute heart failure with failure of the cardiac pumping mechanism as in large myocardial contusion or acute myocardial infarction, which may be complicated by pulmonary edema

Approach to Trauma Patients in Cardiac Arrest

TCPA patients are a special group. Many are young and do not have pre-existing cardiac conditions or coronary disease. Ensuring a complete scene size-up is important because many cases involve criminal activity (stabbings, shootings), so carefully record your observations of the scene after the EMS call is completed. Some TPCA patients may be resuscitated if you arrive soon enough and if you pay attention to the differences from the usual medical cardiac arrest.

The extremely poor resuscitation rate for TCPA patients is probably due to the fact that many of them have been hypoxic for a prolonged period of time before the arrest occurred. Prolonged hypoxia causes such severe acidosis that the patient may not respond to attempted resuscitation. One study concluded that of 138 patients requiring prehospital CPR at the scene or during transport because of the absence of blood pressure, pulse, and respirations, none of the patients survived, whether the victim of blunt or penetrating trauma. In addition, there has been no survival benefit noted in traumatic cardiac arrest patients transported by ground or air EMS services.

Patients who suffer TCPA from isolated head injury usually do not survive. However, they should be aggressively resuscitated because the extent of injury cannot always be determined in the field, and therefore, you cannot predict the outcome for the individual patient. Also, these patients are potential organ donors. With suspected head-injured patients, it is important to avoid hyperventilation because it decreases oxygen supply to the already injured brain tissue through constricting arterial circulatory flow to the brain. Patients who are found in asystole after massive blunt trauma are dead; their resuscitation may be terminated in the field.

Children are a special case. Although some reports show the same dismal results for resuscitation of children in cardiac arrest in the field as for adults, one review of over 700 cases of children who received CPR in the field found that 25% survived to discharge. This may be in part because sometimes the pulse is difficult to find in a child. In any case, you should be especially aggressive in attempting to resuscitate children with no palpable pulse. Limit pulse check to 10 seconds. If no pulse has been found after 10 seconds, begin CPR.

General Plan of Action

As you approach the patient, note obvious injuries. The patient in cardiac arrest will have no active bleeding, but if he or she is in a pool of blood, you have strong evidence of an arrest from exsanguination. After determining unresponsiveness and breathlessness (or only gasping), restrict the motion of the cervical spine. Take no longer than 10 seconds to check for a pulse, and then begin chest compressions immediately, at a compression rate of 110 to 120 compressions per minute. For one emergency care provider the ratio of chest compressions to breaths is 30:2. For two emergency care providers, the ratio is 15:2 compressions to breaths with compression rate of 100 to 110 per minute. Pauses in compressions should be limited to less than 10 seconds.

A significant number of childhood deaths are from foreign body aspiration, which is most frequent in children under five years of age. Two-thirds of foreign body aspiration deaths occur in infants. The management of a **foreign body airway obstruction (FBAO)**, for which the airway is blocked and there is no coughing, in a victim who is responsive or unresponsive is as follows.

FBAO Responsive Patient

For the child or adult, start with subdiaphragmatic abdominal thrusts. For an infant, start with five back blows followed by five chest compressions until the object is expelled.

PEARLS
Pregnant Patients

Cardiac arrest in the pregnant patient is treated the same as in other patients. Defibrillation settings and drug dosages are exactly the same. For hypovolemic arrest, the volume of fluid needed increases, and four liters of normal saline (or other electrolyte solution approved by medical direction) should be given as fast as possible during transport.

PEARLS
Children in Cardiac Arrest

Because children who are in traumatic cardiac arrest are more likely to respond to resuscitation than adults, they are treated aggressively unless obviously unsalvageable.

PEARLS
Proper Response

An adequate number of emergency care providers are required to handle this situation well: one to drive the ambulance, one to ventilate, one to do chest compressions, and one to diagnose and treat the cause of the arrest.

foreign body airway obstruction (FBAO): any foreign body (vomitus, blood, food, and so on) that obstructs the airway.

FBAO Unresponsive Patient

If the cause of the collapse is known to be FBAO, start CPR with chest compressions. (Do not perform pulse check.) After 30 compressions, check the airway. (Do not perform blind finger sweeps.) Ventilate two times.

Open the airway with the modified jaw-thrust maneuver. You will need assistance to maintain cervical motion restriction. The patient must be on a firm, flat surface because there is a chance of injuring the spine if there is an associated vertebral injury, but this is of less concern if the patient is dying of an airway obstruction. If still unsuccessful, you may attempt cricothyroidotomy or translaryngeal jet ventilation if you are trained in the procedures and if your protocols permit you to perform them.

If the airway is not obstructed, give two full breaths and then check the pulse. If no pulse is palpable, you must begin chest compressions immediately. Prepare for immediate transport, if you are not planning to terminate resuscitation. Allow two other emergency care providers to do the cardiopulmonary resuscitation while you get the monitor. Perform at least two minutes of continuous chest compressions, and then check the cardiac rhythm. If either ventricular fibrillation or pulseless ventricular tachycardia (VF/pVT) is present, continue compressions while charging the defibrillator. Defibrillate with the energy recommended in your treatment guidelines. Evidence suggests that higher energy settings may have some benefit. Resume compressions for two minutes after defibrillation before reanalyzing the rhythm.

If either asystole or PEA is present or if VF/pVT persists after the shock, you should evaluate the patient for the cause of the arrest, while continuing CPR. If the patient is a victim of blunt trauma and systole is present, consider termination of resuscitation. If the patient has penetrating trauma, quickly check the pupils. If the pupils are dilated and nonreactive, consider termination of resuscitation unless VF/pVT are present. As mentioned earlier in this situation, it may be beneficial to attempt bilateral needle decompression in the second intercostal space anteriorly (or fourth intercostal space laterally) because tension pneumothorax is one reversible cause of traumatic cardiac arrest. Resuscitation efforts should not be initiated for patients with either injuries incompatible with life or for those who have evidence of prolonged time since the arrest and are in asystole (Table 21-1). If resuscitation attempts have already begun on these patients, it is appropriate to follow the resuscitation policy as directed by your local medical direction, which may permit termination of resuscitation.

For patients with an organized rhythm on ECG, you must quickly evaluate and treat for the cause of the arrest. This should be done in the ambulance during transport, if possible. Use the ITLS Primary Survey that you follow for every trauma patient to try to determine the cause of the TCPA.

PEARLS
Asystole

Patients found in asystole after massive blunt trauma are dead. There is no reasonable expectation of achieving successful resuscitation in these patients.

PEARLS
Transport

Rapid transport to a surgical facility is necessary. Perform procedures in the ambulance during transport. Do not waste valuable time. It is important to recognize that it is very difficult to perform effective CPR in a moving ambulance.

Procedure

Initial Assessment and Critical Actions

1. Establish and control the airway using the appropriate airway adjunct according to your treatment guidelines. Ventilate with 100% oxygen. While the other emergency care providers are ventilating and performing chest compressions, you must systematically look for reversible causes of the arrest.

2. Look for breathing problems as a cause of the arrest. Answering the following questions may

allow you to identify any breathing problems that may be the cause or a contributing factor:

a. *Look at the neck.* Are the neck veins flat or distended? Is the trachea midline? Is there evidence of soft-tissue trauma to the neck?

b. *Look at the chest.* Does the chest rise symmetrically each time you ventilate? Are there chest injuries (penetrations, bruising, flail segment)? If there is spontaneous respiration, is there any paradoxical motion noted?

c. *Feel the chest.* Is there any instability or asymmetry? Is there any crepitation? Is there any subcutaneous emphysema?

d. *Listen to the chest.* Are breath sounds present on both sides? Are the breath sounds equal?

If breath sounds are not equal, percuss the chest. Is the side with the absent or decreased breath sounds hyperresonant or dull? If the patient has been intubated, is the endotracheal tube inserted too far?

If there are distended neck veins, decreased breath sounds on one side of the chest, with the trachea deviated away from the side of the injury, and hyperresonance to percussion of the chest on the affected side, then the patient may have a tension pneumothorax. An improperly positioned endotracheal tube can cause unequal breath sounds and may be harmful to the patient because only one lung is being ventilated. You should always recheck the position of the endotracheal tube before you make a diagnosis of tension pneumothorax because it is much more common to have a poorly positioned endotracheal tube (such as in a mainstem bronchus) than to have a tension pneumothorax. A tension pneumothorax requires needle decompression of the affected side of the chest, if you are trained in the procedure and your protocols allow for this. If required, call medical direction immediately for permission to decompress. Continue ventilation with 100% oxygen.

Do not discontinue chest compressions until either there is a palpable pulse or resuscitation is terminated. Even though you have found a cause, there may be other causes for the patient's arrest. Other breathing problems (sucking chest wound, flail chest, simple pneumothorax) will be adequately treated by airway control and ventilation with high-flow oxygen. Once you have established an airway and are applying positive pressure ventilation to the TCPA patient, you no longer have to seal sucking chest wounds or apply external stabilization to flails. Remember, though, that positive pressure ventilation can convert a simple pneumothorax to a tension pneumothorax.

Once the patient has both adequate airway management and is being appropriately ventilated, you may concentrate on the circulatory system. As soon as IV access is obtained, rapidly give two liters of normal saline or other resuscitation fluid approved by medical direction. Once again, do not delay at the scene. In the traumatic cardiac arrest patient, all treatment past establishing the airway should be done during transport, if the decision has been made to continue resuscitation.

Hemorrhagic shock is the most common circulatory cause of traumatic cardiopulmonary arrest. If there is a large amount of blood on or around the patient, you should note the source of the bleeding because this must be controlled if you resuscitate the patient. If there is no external bleeding, the patient must be carefully examined for evidence of internal bleeding. Reexamine the neck veins. Flat neck veins in the presence of sinus tachycardia on the monitor favor the presence of hypovolemic shock. Attempt to start two large-bore IV lines while en route. Intraosseous (IO) lines are acceptable alternatives to IV lines, though the flow rate of the IO needle may not always approach that of large-bore IV catheters. A 10 cc flush of normal saline into the IO needle after placement into the bone often improves flow rate.

PEARLS
ITLS Primary Survey

The pulseless trauma patient requires careful attention during the ITLS Primary Survey to identify treatable problems in the proper priority.

Decreased breath sounds on one side with percussion dullness on the same side suggests a hemothorax of such degree that shock will be present, though dullness to percussion may also suggest a ruptured diaphragm. Obvious bleeding, distended abdomen, multiple fractures, or an unstable pelvis also suggest that hemorrhagic shock is the cause of the TCPA. Transport rapidly while rapidly infusing two liters of normal saline.

Penetrating wounds of the chest or upper abdomen, or contusions of the anterior chest, are associated with pericardial tamponade and/or myocardial contusion. If the neck veins are distended, the trachea is midline, and breath sounds are equal, you should suspect pericardial tamponade. Attempt to start two large-bore IV lines while proceeding with all possible haste to the emergency department.

Electrical shock creates a special situation. It usually presents as ventricular fibrillation. Severe acidosis can develop rapidly, making resuscitation more difficult. TCPA secondary to electric shock may respond readily to ACLS protocols if you arrive before the acidosis is too severe. Do not forget to follow spinal motion-restriction protocols. A victim of high-voltage electrical shock may have fallen from a power line or have been thrown several feet by the violent muscle spasm associated with the shock. Be sure the patient is no longer in contact with the electrical source. Do not become a victim!

Considerations in Traumatic Cardiac Arrest Management

Research continues into how to optimize patient evaluation and management in TCPA patients. These patients present many challenges, requiring the ITLS provider to maintain current understanding in the care of these critically ill trauma victims.

Airway Management

It is unclear what the optimal airway is for the patient in TCPA. Prolonged periods of hypoxia have been demonstrated for patients on whom ETI is attempted in the prehospital phase of care. Excessive manipulation of the airway during ETI has been associated with increased risk of aspiration. A recent study has revealed no difference in survival to hospital discharge in cardiac arrest patients when comparing the use of ETI to Combitube® placement in the prehospital phase of care.

What is apparent is the airway needed in managing a TCPA patient is that which can adequately do the job. If a bag-valve-mask ventilation is adequate, then use that. Laryngeal fracture from blunt trauma or severe vocal cord edema due to inhaling burning gases may require cricothyrotomy. "One size fits all" does not apply in airway management of the patient in TCPA.

If the trauma patient had previously been intubated and then develops a cardiac arrest, assess the airway using the DOPE algorithm: D—displacement of the endotracheal tube, O—obstruction of the endotracheal tube, P—pneumothorax development, or E—equipment problems (ventilator failure, loss of oxygen supply), correcting the problems as they are identified.

Ventilation

We now know that positive pressure ventilations reduce venous return, whether via bag-valve mask, ETI, or supraglottic airways. You must attempt to provide adequate air exchange while avoiding overventilation. In the TCPA patient it is reasonable to begin with an assisted ventilation rate of one breath every eight seconds with a tidal volume of 750 cc, which is about eight times per minute using roughly a one-hand squeeze on a standard bag. This should provide good chest rise and provides a minute ventilation of about five liters per minute. The patient should be reassessed continuously during the resuscitation to determine if this rate of assisted ventilation is appropriate, too high, or too low.

Ultrasound

Over the last few years there has been an increasing use of portable ultrasound machines in the prehospital setting. Although still expensive and most often used by physicians or critical care transport programs, an ultrasound can help identify presence of cardiac tamponade, identify pneumothoraces, and even assess the level of cardiac activity in a rhythm suspected of being PEA.

Capnography

Oxygen is supplied to cells by the lungs and vascular system. The oxygen is transported to the cells of the body, where energy substrate (such as carbohydrate) is enzymatically burned in the cells, producing energy, water, and carbon dioxide (CO_2). CO_2 is produced proportionally to the supply of O_2 to the cells by the lungs and vascular system. The CO_2 is returned to the lungs to be exhaled. CO_2 can be measured at the airway through a technique called "waveform capnography" (literally: graphing the wave of exhaled CO_2). Thus waveform capnography provides a glimpse of the actual metabolism of the body, and the normal level measured at the airway is approximately 40 mm Hg during exhalation. A low measured level of CO_2 at the airway in TCPA patients is an indication that O_2 supply to the cells is low and the patient is in a shock state. Rising CO_2 levels during resuscitation of TCPA patients is an indication of improving circulation, though caution should be taken to make sure that the respiratory circuit is working appropriately.

Overventilation of the TCPA patient can reduce cardiac output by decreasing venous return to the heart. This lowers O_2 delivery to the tissues, reducing CO_2 production and measured capnography. Thus, measuring capnography at the airway is a useful guide to establishing the correct ventilation rate and tidal volume (literally, minute ventilation) in the TCPA patient, allowing the emergency care provider to adjust the ventilation rates downward if capnography measures under 10 mm Hg. Specific guidelines to ventilation rate and capnography measurements should come from your local medical direction.

Case Presentation (continued)

A BLS ambulance is on the scene of an all-terrain vehicle versus tree, unwitnessed and time of impact undetermined. The closest hospital is 15 miles away; level 2 trauma hospital, 45 miles away. The scene is safe with one patient (approximately 20 years old) who is helmetless, unresponsive, breathless, and pulseless. There is an obvious deformity to the skull, multiple rib fractures, and deformity to the left femur. An AED is applied, and it indicates, "No shock advised."

Because the cardiac rhythm could not be determined by the AED, CPR is initiated, and an ALS unit is requested to respond. ALS arrives within 5 minutes of being sum-moned. The ALS team assesses the patient and finds him unresponsive, no spontaneous respirations, and no pulses (with or without CPR). The heart monitor is applied, and the ECG reveals asystole in two leads. The ALS team contacts medical direction to request the termination of resuscitative efforts. Medical direction approves the request, and resuscitative efforts are stopped.

The autopsy of the victim revealed massive cerebral trauma, rib fractures, pulmonary contusion, a lacerated liver, and pelvic and left femur fractures. Cause of death was cited as accidental traumatic brain injury and exsanguination.

Summary

The trauma patient in cardiopulmonary arrest is usually suffering from a breathing or circulatory problem. If you are to save this patient, you must identify the cause of the arrest with the ITLS Primary Survey and then rapidly transport the patient while performing those procedures that specifically address the cause of the arrest. Although it is very rare to successfully resuscitate a patient suffering from a trauma arrest secondary to hemorrhagic shock, attention to detail will allow you the best chance to "bring one back from the dead," which is one of the greatest challenges and greatest satisfactions in EMS.

Bibliography

American Heart Association. "Guidelines for Cardiopulmonary Care Resuscitation (CPR) and Emergency Cardiovascular Care Science." *Circulation* 122, no. 18, Suppl. 3 (November 2, 2010): S640–S920.

Cera, S. M., G. Mostafa, R. F. Sing, J. L. Sarafin, B. D. Matthews, and B. T. Heniford. "Physiologic Predictors of Survival in Post-Traumatic Arrest." *The American Surgeon* 69, no. 2 (February 2003): 140–44.

Davis, D. P., D. Hoyt, M. Ochs, D. Fortlage, T. Holbrook, L. K. Marshall, and P. Rosen. "The Effect of Paramedic Rapid Sequence Intubation on Outcome in Patients with Severe Traumatic Brain Injury." *Journal of Trauma, Injury, Infection, and Critical Care* 54, no. 3 (March 2003): 444–53.

Di Bartolomeo, S., G. Sanson, G. Nardi, V. Michelutto, and F. Scian. "HEMS vs. Ground-BLS Care in Traumatic Cardiac Arrest." *Prehospital Emergency Care* 9, no. 1 (January–March 2005): 79–84.

Fontanarosa P. B. "Electric Shock and Lightning Strike." *Annals of Emergency Medicine* 22, no. 2 Pt 2 (February 1993): 378–87.

Hopson, L. R., E. Hirsh, J. Delgado, R. M. Domeier, N. E. McSwain, and J. Krohmer. "Guidelines for Withholding or Termination of Resuscitation in Prehospital Traumatic Cardiopulmonary Arrest: Joint Position Statement of the National Association of EMS Physicians and the American College of Surgeons Committee on Trauma." *Journal of the American College of Surgeons* 196, no. 1 (January 2003): 106–12.

National Association of EMS Physicians and American College of Surgeons Committee on Trauma. "Withholding of Resuscitation for Adult Traumatic Cardiopulmonary Arrest." *Prehospital Emergency Care* 17, no. 2 (April–June 2013): 291.

Perron, A. D., R. F. Sing, C. C. Branas, and T. Huynh. "Predicting Survival in Pediatric Trauma Patients Receiving Cardiopulmonary Resuscitation in the Prehospital Setting." *Prehospital Emergency Care* 5, no. 1 (January–March 2001): 6–9.

Rosemurgy A. S., P. Norris, S. M. Olson, J. M. Hurst, and M. H. Albrink. "Prehospital Traumatic Cardiac Arrest: The Cost of Futility." *Journal of Trauma* 35, no. 3 (September 1993): 468–74.

Saunders C. E., and C. Heye. "Ambulance Collisions in an Urban Environment." *Prehospital and Disaster Medicine* 9, no. 2 (April–June 1994): 118–24.

Wang H. E., and D. M. Yealy. "How Many Attempts Are Required to Accomplish Out-of-Hospital Endotracheal Intubation?" *Academic Emergency Medicine* 13, no. 4 (April 2006): 372–77.

Warner K. J., J. Cuschieri, M. Copass, G. J. Jurkovich, and E. M. Bulger. "The Impact of Prehospital Ventilation on Outcome After Severe Traumatic Brain Injury." *Journal of Trauma* 62, no. 6 (June 2007): 1330–38.

Get more information about this course by calling
ITLS International at 888-495-4875
(outside the United States call +1-630-495-6442) or visit

www.itrauma.org

Standard Precautions and Transmission-Based Precautions

Katherine West, BSN, MSEd, CIC
Howard Werman, MD, FACEP
Richard N. Nelson, MD, FACEP

Precauzioni Standard   Precauciones Estándar   Précautions standard

Środki ostrożności   Eigenschutz   Standardne mjere zaštite

الاحتياطات الواجب اتباعها   standarne mere opreza

Standardni varnostni ukrepi   Általános óvintézkedés

CandyBox Images/Shutterstock

Key Terms

airborne precautions, *p. 403*
bacille de Calmette et Guérin (BCG), *p. 397*
blood and OPIM, *p. 393*
contact precautions, *p. 402*
droplet precautions, *p. 402*
hepatitis B virus (HBV), *p. 393*
hepatitis C virus (HCV), *p. 394*
human immunodeficiency virus (HIV), *p. 395*
post-exposure prophylaxis (PEP), *p. 396*
standard precautions, *p. 395*

Objectives

Upon successful completion of this chapter, you should be able to:

1. Discuss the three most common bloodborne viral illnesses to which emergency care providers are likely to be exposed in the provision of patient care.
2. Discuss the signs and symptoms of airborne and droplet-transmitted diseases, and describe protective measures to reduce possible exposure to them.
3. Describe precautions emergency care providers can take to prevent exposure to blood and other potentially infectious materials (cerebrospinal fluid, synovial fluid, amniotic fluid, pericardial fluid, pleural fluid, or any fluid with gross visible blood).
4. Describe procedures for emergency care providers to follow if they are accidentally exposed.
5. Discuss multidrug-resistant organisms, and describe precautions for care of patients with multidrug-resistant illnesses and airborne/droplet diseases.
6. Be able to identify those situations in which a higher level of personal protective equipment is needed, beyond the basic equipment used in daily patient care.
7. List vaccines and immunizations recommended for EMS personnel.

Chapter Overview

All occupations carry some risk. For EMS, risks have included highway hazards, fires, downed electrical wires, toxic substances, and scene security problems. The provision of patient care may pose the additional possibility of exposure to bloodborne and other diseases. Fortunately, there are precautions that can be taken to markedly reduce those risks. In addition, if personal protective equipment could not be used or failed, medical post-exposure treatment is available to reduce the chances of acquiring disease following an exposure event. And of course, there are vaccines and immunizations that protect personnel from many diseases to which they may be exposed. Exposure does not mean infection. Exposure can be treated or prevented.

A discussion of the entire spectrum of diseases to which you are potentially exposed is beyond the scope of this chapter. However, the three most common types of viral bloodborne infections are appropriate to discuss in conjunction with trauma management because their modes of spread are primarily by contaminated blood and other potentially infectious materials (OPIM). They are hepatitis B (HBV), hepatitis C (HBC), and HIV infection.

It is a common misconception that all body fluids are potentially infectious. Body fluids that do not pose a risk for HBV, HCV, and HIV are tears, sweat, saliva, urine, stool, vomitus, nasal secretions, and sputum unless they *contain visible blood contamination*. It is also important to note that vaginal secretions and semen are only a risk through sexual contact.

This chapter offers a review of the three most common types of viral bloodborne infections plus a brief review of the airborne- and droplet-transmitted diseases that can pose a risk to emergency care providers. These airborne and droplet diseases include tuberculosis, measles, mumps, rubella, chickenpox, and influenza. Recently, there has been an increase in cases of these diseases in more developed countries, despite successful prevention programs directed toward them. This rise is attributed to a decline in vaccination rates. Last, a brief overview of infections caused by multidrug-resistant organisms is included to increase emergency care provider awareness of the risk such infections present.

Case Presentation

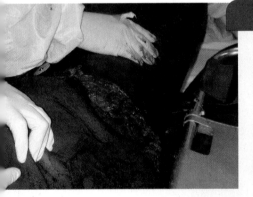

An advanced life support (ALS) tactical medical team is on scene with law enforcement's Special Response Team (SRT). The team is preparing to enter a dwelling where there is known crack/cocaine and methamphetamine sales and usage. Just prior to entry, a noise, flash, diversionary device (NFDD) is detonated inside the dwelling. Entry is made, and the scene is secured. However, during the initial commotion, one of the occupants of the dwelling tried to escape by jumping through a large glass window. The suspect is taken into custody, and tactical emergency care providers are cleared to assess him.

The nearly naked male patient is approximately 25 years old and has multiple lacerations on his face, neck, and arms. There is severe, active bleeding from the lateral aspect of the patient's right thigh. It is believed an artery has been lacerated. The patient is still conscious and is physically and verbally abusive.

Before proceeding, consider these questions: How should the "bleeder" be managed? Is a tourniquet indicated? Are the emergency care providers and others at risk of being exposed to blood or other potential infectious material (OPIM)? Does the patient's lifestyle (suspected drug user) make him at high risk for having infectious diseases? What personal protective equipment (PPE) should the emergency care providers don? Keep these questions in mind as you read the chapter. Then, at the end of the chapter, find out how the emergency care providers managed this patient.

Diseases of Concern

Bloodborne Diseases

Hepatitis B

The term *viral hepatitis* is used to describe a group of viral infections involving the liver. At least five types of hepatitis virus have been described: hepatitis A, B, C, D, and E. Hepatitis A and E are spread primarily through contact with contaminated fecal material and are not bloodborne. They are most prevalent in Africa. Hepatitis D is transmitted through blood and body-fluid exposure to patients already infected with hepatitis B. Because of their frequent contact with blood and needles, health-care workers are considered at risk of becoming infected with the **hepatitis B virus**. Fortunately, hepatitis B is the one form of hepatitis for which there is an effective preventive vaccine. Today, in the United States there is universal vaccination. Similar programs exist in many other countries. Health-care providers have been receiving vaccine since 1982, all newborns since 1990, and all middle school, high school, and college students since 2000. As a result, there has been a 95% reduction in occupationally acquired hepatitis B infection and a decrease in all cases in the United States.

Hepatitis B virus is an infectious virus usually spread by exposure to infected blood. It is the major cause of acute and chronic hepatitis, cirrhosis, and liver cancer. There are three effective vaccines available to prevent infection: Heptavax, Recombivax-B, and Engerix-B. Following an acute infection, 3% to 5% of hepatitis B patients become chronic carriers of the virus and remain potentially infectious.

In 2011, the U.S. Centers for Disease Control (CDC) reported that hepatitis B infection in health-care workers acquired through occupational exposure is an infrequent or rare event. HBV is spread by contact with contaminated blood or OPIM, sexual transmission, and direct contact with a contaminated item and nonintact skin. Infection usually occurs from contaminated needlesticks or through sexual contact. The risk for acquiring HBV infection by occupational exposure is only an issue for personnel who have not been vaccinated and who do not report an exposure. In those situations there is an estimated 6% to 30% risk for contracting HBV infection, if the source patient is positive for active disease. If the nonvaccinated EMS provider reports the exposure, he or she can be treated. There is also a special treatment protocol for those who did not previously mount an antibody response to the vaccine and have an exposure.

Besides vaccination, other steps can be taken to decrease risk for emergency care providers. Use of devices to minimize needlestick as mandated by the Needlestick Safety and Prevention Act of 2000 requires the use of needle-safe or needleless devices (Figure 22-1). The use of devices designed to comply with this legislation has cut the number of sharps injuries by more than half since its implementation. Infection also can occur by contact of bloody secretions with open skin lesions or mucosal surfaces, so use of standard precautions is key. Routine testing of donor blood for HBV makes transmission from blood transfusions very rare.

In the United States, the Occupational Safety and Health Administration (OSHA) mandated in 1991 that all employers of health-care workers offer HBV vaccine to any health-care worker at risk of occupational exposure to **blood and OPIM**. This must occur within 10 days of being hired and before the health-care worker performs at risk tasks. The HB vaccine offers lifelong protection. Vaccines available today are recombinant; they contain no human components, thus eliminating the possibility of the person being vaccinated from contacting HBV. A titer (blood test) is performed one to two months after completion of the vaccine series to document response to the vaccine. If positive, no further titer testing is needed or recommended. The vaccine is safe and produces immunity in over 90% of people vaccinated.

Another form of protection is hepatitis B immunoglobulin (HBIG). This preparation contains antibodies to HBV and provides temporary, passive protection against it.

PEARLS
An EMS Standard

All patients are potential carriers of infectious disease. That is why standard precautions are the EMS standard for practice.

hepatitis B virus (HBV): virus responsible for hepatitis B, transmitted through contact with blood or body fluids.

PEARLS
HBV Immunization

Complete all three doses for full lifelong coverage! Be prepared! Stay up to date on all your immunizations.

PEARLS
OPIM

The abbreviation "OPIM" refers to other (than blood) potentially infectious materials. Those materials include:

- Cerebrospinal fluid (CSF)
- Synovial fluid
- Amniotic fluid
- Pericardial fluid
- Pleural fluid
- Any fluid with gross visible blood

blood and OPIM: blood or other body fluids or tissues that can carry infectious organisms

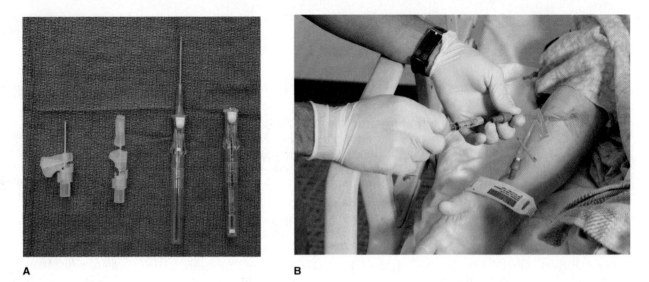

A   **B**

Figure 22-1 (A) Safety needles and (B) needleless medication administration system. *(Photos courtesy of Stanley Cooper, EMT-P)*

HBIG is only 70% effective and, when effective, provides protection for only four to six months. HBIG is used only when there has been a significant exposure to HBV in an unimmunized person and should be given in conjunction with vaccine to offer full coverage post exposure. There are five protocols for medical follow-up for exposure to HBV based on the vaccine status of the medical provider. Thus, it is important for the EMS agency's designated officer for infection control to have easy access to medical records 24/7 should an exposure occur.

Hepatitis C

hepatitis C virus (HCV): virus that causes hepatitis C.

The hepatitis C virus (HCV) is an infectious virus primarily spread by exposure to infected blood. The hepatitis C virus (HCV) was identified in 1988–1989 and was previously called non-A, non-B hepatitis. The incubation period is six to seven weeks. HCV infection tends to be less severe than HBV during the initial infection. However, there appears to be a greater likelihood of becoming a chronic carrier of HCV following infection. Liver failure and cirrhosis occur in 20% to 80% of chronic HCV carriers.

The incidence rate for occupational transmission is low and usually related to a contaminated needlestick injury. Health-care workers can acquire infection through hollow-bore needlesticks with contaminated needles. Fortunately, the use of needle-safe devices has led to a significant decrease in contaminated sharps injuries. The risk rate for developing HCV after a needlestick is about 1.5%, if the source is positive for HCV.

In 2012, there were over 1,700 cases of HCV reported in the United States. Note that a number of those cases were patients who were infected by health-care workers who had the disease but who did not follow infection control protocols properly or at all. Prior to 1992, HCV was the leading cause of hepatitis resulting from blood transfusions. Today, as a result of better testing of donated blood, HCV is no longer transmitted via this route. The virus also appears to be spread by sharing of intravenous needles, sexual contact, tattooing, and body piercing, much like HBV.

There is currently no vaccine available to protect against HCV infection. Evidence suggests that there is no protective effect provided by administering immune globulin following exposure to HCV. Now, rapid HCV testing can be performed on the source patient. If the source is positive, the exposed provider will undergo close monitoring and repeat testing for the virus.

Treatments are available for people who acquire HCV, which have resulted in a cure in most of those who receive treatment. It also appears that with early treatment, chronic infection with HCV can be prevented.

Human Immunodeficiency Virus Infection

HIV infection is caused by the **human immunodeficiency virus (HIV)**. Patients with HIV infection have difficulty fighting certain infections due to a compromised immune system. This predisposes the HIV-infected patient to a variety of unusual infections not generally seen in healthy patients of similar age. They are called "opportunistic infections" and pose a risk to the patient but not to the care provider. An example is *Pneumocystis jirovecii* (formerly known as *P. carinii*) pneumonia (PCP). Most individuals have this yeast-like fungus in their lungs, but it does not cause illness because a healthy immune system prevents it from causing infection. PCP is not transmissible from an infected patient to care providers with intact immune systems. Other examples of opportunistic infections in HIV patients are those caused by atypical mycobacteria. This is a medical issue for the patient but does not pose a risk to the healthy health-care worker.

Patients infected with HIV can present with a wide spectrum of clinical manifestations. Early symptoms, like many viral illnesses, resemble the flu. Many patients with HIV infection are asymptomatic. Other patients will test positive for HIV because they had an exposure at some time but did not develop the disease and thus cannot transmit the disease to others. HIV patients being treated with current drugs may be free of virus circulating in their blood and, as such, pose only a minute risk. Current studies show that after 48 weeks of treatment, 96% of those treated HIV patients have no circulating virus in their blood. Knowing that a patient is HIV positive may not be enough information to assess risk for infection. Testing the source patient's blood for viral load may be needed to determine risk for transmission following an exposure.

HIV appears to be transmitted in a manner similar to HBV. Although the virus has been cultured from a variety of body fluids, only blood has been implicated in the transmission of the virus in the workplace. This is because other body fluids do not carry enough virus particles to transmit the disease. Semen and vaginal secretions have been shown to transmit the virus during sexual activity only. There is no evidence to suggest that HIV is transmitted by casual contact.

Transmission to health-care workers has been documented only after accidental parenteral exposure (needlestick) or exposure of mucous membranes and open wounds to large amounts of infected blood. Measurable risk data for occupational exposure is 0.3% for needlestick injuries and 0.09% for mucous membrane exposure. There is one documented case of transmission from infected blood on nonintact skin. This case was reported in 2002 and involved a health-care worker with extensive dermatitis who did not always use gloves appropriately when caring for a patient coinfected with HIV and HCV.

HIV appears to be different from the hepatitis B virus in two ways: First, it does not survive outside the body. Routine germicidal cleaning agents are effective. Second, it is transmitted far less efficiently than HBV.

Several groups have been identified as having a high risk of HIV infection. They include men who have sex with men (MSM), intravenous drug abusers, patients who have received blood transfusions or pooled-plasma products prior to 1992 (such as hemophiliacs), and heterosexual contacts of HIV-positive persons. However, because of the difficulty in identifying HIV-infected patients, all contacts with blood and OPIM should be considered a potential HIV exposure. This concept (all patient blood/OPIM except sweat is potentially infective) is why **standard precautions** are "universally" applied.

There is currently no available vaccine to protect against HIV infection. Antiretroviral drug regimens, though not a cure, have been shown to prolong the lives of HIV/AIDS

PEARLS
TB

If your patient has a persistent cough plus other symptoms suggestive of TB, place a surgical mask on the patient, not on yourself. You should also wear a mask especially if the patient requires oxygen and cannot wear a mask. The appropriate mask for emergency care providers is an N-95 respirator.

human immunodeficiency virus (HIV): a virus that weakens the immune system, predisposing a patient to a wide range of unusual infections.

standard precautions: steps each health-care worker takes to protect themselves and their patient from exposure to infectious agents; includes treating each patient and himself as if they were infectious.

patients. Life expectancy is now believed to be 50 years post diagnosis. This would make HIV-infection today a chronic disease. Some studies have suggested that antiretroviral agents may reduce the risk of HIV transmission in health-care workers if administered within hours following a significant exposure to HIV-infected blood and OPIM. The decision to administer such agents should be based on the nature of the exposure, the likelihood that the patient is infected with HIV, the duration of time following exposure, and consultation with the exposed health-care worker. In general, large-gauge hollow-needle exposures are more significant than solid instruments (such as a scalpel).

post-exposure prophylaxis (PEP): the administration of medications to prevent infection from the agent to which the person was exposed.

If the exposure meets the CDC criteria for **post-exposure prophylaxis (PEP)**, and it is planned to offer drugs post exposure to the health-care worker, PEP should be administered within hours but not days of the exposure. Recommendations are for early post-exposure treatment to reduce the risk of acquiring the disease. Exposed personnel need to be counseled about the side effects and other issues involving the use of these drugs before they are started. Baseline lab work also needs to be drawn. By performing rapid HIV testing on the source patient, an emergency care provider may be able to avoid being placed on medications unnecessarily while awaiting results of additional blood work on the source.

Rapid HIV testing is recommended as part of the post-exposure workup. The cost is low, and testing takes about 10 to 20 minutes. If PEP drugs are to be offered in the emergency department, the treating physician (in North America) should call the toll-free PEP Hotline at 1-888-448-4911 for a second opinion. In other areas of the world, treating physicians should follow facility protocols before the drugs are prescribed. Remember, all post-exposure medical follow-up begins with testing the source patient, not the exposed emergency care provider.

An important and encouraging finding in the past few years is that persons who have been under treatment for HIV for over 48 weeks and whose viral levels are nondetectable (no circulating HIV virus in the blood) are not infectious. This may reduce the need for PEP, if this type of patient is a source. It is the responsibility of the physician treating the exposed emergency care provider to assess the risk of transmission and to provide guidance to the exposed emergency care provider. Emergency care providers often do not know all the details about the status of the patient's HIV disease and must assume all blood is potentially infectious.

Airborne Transmissible Diseases

Tuberculosis

From 1985 to 1993, the incidence of active tuberculosis increased significantly to over 25,000 cases in the United States. It was the result of an increase in cases among people infected with HIV and an increase in immigration of people from areas where tuberculosis infection is endemic (Asia, Latin America, the Caribbean, Africa). Because of better public health measures, tuberculosis has been declining in the past several years. Cases decreased by over 84% from 1997 to 2009. In fact, the number of cases in 2012 was the lowest ever reported in the United States.

PEARLS
Notification of Exposed Emergency Care Providers

The Ryan White Comprehensive AIDS Resources Emergency Act, U.S. Public Law 101-381, required inclusion of all emergency response employees—firefighters, emergency medical technicians, paramedics, law enforcement officers, and volunteers—in the post-exposure medical notification process in the event of an exposure to a bloodborne or airborne transmissible disease.

Risk factors for tuberculosis include homelessness, certain immigrant populations (Asia, Africa), patients at risk for HIV infection, and people who live in congregate settings (correction facilities, nursing homes, homeless shelters). On a global perspective, there is an effort to eliminate the disease by 2015.

Tuberculosis is caused by a bacterium, Mycobacterium tuberculosis, which is spread from an infected person to susceptible people through the air, especially by coughing or sneezing. This is not a highly communicable disease. Contracting tuberculosis requires prolonged direct contact, as in a family living situation. Only persons with active infection of the lung or throat spread tuberculosis.

Clinical manifestations of the disease become apparent only when the patient's immune system fails to keep the bacteria in check. The bacteria then begins to infect the lungs and may spread to other portions of the body, particularly the kidneys, spine, or brain. Infections outside the lung are called *extrapulmonary* and are not communicable to the care provider. Signs and symptoms of active tuberculosis are most prominent in the lungs and include a productive cough that lasts longer than three weeks in conjunction with two or more of the following: pain in the chest, coughing up bloody sputum, weakness or fatigue, unexplained weight loss, loss of appetite, fever, chills, night sweats, or hoarseness.

Treatment of tuberculosis includes antibiotic agents. A positive TB skin test (PPD) means the person is infected with TB (TB infection), but it does not necessarily indicate active disease. *TB disease* is the term for the active disease. If there is a positive skin test but no indication of active TB, isoniazid (INH) or rifampin may be given for a short course of treatment, usually once a week for 12 weeks. More extensive and prolonged antibiotic therapy is necessary if active TB is confirmed. Multidrug-resistant TB is a more serious form of the disease and means that the organism has become resistant to two of the first-line antibiotics. Additional drugs are available to treat both conventional and multidrug-resistant TB.

Since 1995, the CDC has recommended placing a surgical mask on any patient suspected of having TB. The CDC recommends that when treating patients with active TB or suspected TB, emergency care providers should wear an N-95 mask. Health-care workers should receive tuberculin skin testing prior to employment and periodically thereafter, depending on the TB risk assessment in their work area, to ensure that tuberculosis has not been acquired. This is in keeping with the CDC guidelines published on December 30, 2005, which OSHA is enforcing. Annual TB skin testing is only continued if more than three active untreated TB patients were transported by an EMS service in the previous 12 months. It should be noted that to continue annual testing in low-risk areas leads to false-positive tests. The International Association of Fire Fighters (IAFF) and the National Fire Protection Association's NFPA 1581 Infection Control Standard defer to the CDC guidelines.

Outside the United States, **bacille de Calmette et Guérin (BCG)** is a vaccine used to prevent TB. In portions of Europe and Asia universal vaccination with BCG is the standard. The protection offered by the vaccine is not lifelong, and the reported efficacy in preventing TB infection has varied. It should be noted that if vaccinated with BCG, a person will always test positive if given a PPD test. Even if vaccinated with BCG, an emergency care provider should utilize appropriate PPE and isolation techniques when caring for a suspected TB patient.

bacille de Calmette et Guérin (BCG): vaccine against tuberculosis prepared from a strain of bovine tuberculosis that has been weakened; not commonly used in the United States.

Chickenpox—Varicella Zoster

Chickenpox is considered to be a highly communicable disease. It is transmitted from one person to another by inhalation of aerosols or by touching drainage from the lesions. The incubation period is between 10 and 21 days after the exposure event. An infected person may be able to transmit the disease one to two days before the rash appears. A person with chickenpox is considered to be communicable until all the lesions become crusted and dried.

Signs and symptoms of chickenpox include fever and a rash that progresses to a plump lesion or lesions, and photosensitivity (the patient wants to be in the dark). The rash usually begins on the covered areas of the body.

The primary prevention measure for chickenpox is vaccination if the person is not immune. Immunity is documented by written diagnosis, a titer or documentation of vaccination with two doses of vaccine given one month apart. Protection from acquiring chickenpox helps reduce the chance of a person developing shingles (Zoster). Shingles is caused by latent chickenpox virus. A person who is not protected against chickenpox and cares for a patient with shingles is at risk for developing chickenpox.

The chickenpox vaccine is given in two doses one month apart. Women of childbearing age are to be counseled not to become pregnant for four weeks after each dose of vaccine, which needs to be documented.

Rubeola (Red Measles/Hard Measles)

Rubeola is a virus primarily transmitted by the airborne route. Health care personnel are considered a higher risk for becoming infected than members of the general public. This disease has been preventable since measles vaccination programs started in 1963. Cases of measles have increased due to a decline in the vaccination rate over concerns that the vaccine for measles, mumps, and rubella (MMR) is associated with autism. This concern has not been supported by any clinical evidence.

All health-care workers should receive measles vaccinations. Immunity is documented by evidence per written documentation showing the person has received two doses of live measles vaccine, a titer showing immunity, or written documentation of disease. Lacking immunity verification, give the MMR vaccine. Of special note: Persons who were vaccinated between 1963 and 1967, need to be revaccinated with live-measles vaccine because the killed-virus vaccine that was used previously has been shown not to be protective.

Signs and symptoms of measles include rash, fever, coryza and conjunctivitis, and Koplik spots (whitish/gray spots on the buccal mucosa). The incubation period is 7 to 18 days following an exposure event.

Droplet Diseases

Pertussis—Whooping Cough

Pertussis is caused by the bacterium and is a highly contagious disease. As this text goes to press, increasing numbers of cases are being reported, with several significant outbreaks in the United States.

Pertussis is characterized by uncontrollable, violent coughing spells that often make it difficult to breathe. After a coughing attack, someone with pertussis often needs to take deep breaths, which makes the whooping sound from which the disease gets its name. This may be followed by vomiting.

Pertussis more commonly affects infants and young children whose smaller airways are at risk for compromise. Most adults and health-care workers have not been vaccinated against pertussis since they were 11 to 14 years of age. In 2005, and again in 2011, the CDC recommended that all health-care workers should receive a booster dose of Tdap (tetanus, diphtheria, and pertussis).

If pertussis is contracted or a provider exposed, the person can be treated with antibiotics. Persons with suspected or active pertussis should wear a surgical mask. Providers should wear surgical masks and above all, be vaccinated.

Mumps

Mumps is childhood disease caused by a viral infection. Signs and symptoms of this disease include fever and swelling and inflammation of the salivary glands. Dehydration often follows due to poor fluid intake, especially in young children.

Since MMR vaccine programs began in 1963, cases of mumps in the United States decreased dramatically. However, outbreaks began occurring again in 2008–2009 and continue. This resurgence of the mumps is related to the drop in vaccinations because of unfounded concerns about the safety of the MMR vaccine.

Primary prevention is vaccination. Care providers should make sure they have received two doses of mumps vaccine if they have not had the mumps. Vaccine is 80% to 85% protective after one dose of vaccine. After two doses of vaccine, the protection level is 79% to 95%. This is a live virus vaccine, so women of childbearing age need to be counseled not to become pregnant for four weeks after each dose of vaccine.

PEARLS

Preventing Droplet-Transmitted Diseases

The first prevention method for many droplet-transmitted diseases is vaccination using the MMR vaccine. The secondary prevention method is placing a surgical mask on the suspect patient, or, health-care workers should wear a surgical *mask*.

It is important to document immunity for all health-care workers. The mumps vaccine is not effective if given post exposure. If a worker is not already protected, vaccination is the best prevention method. If not immune and need to transport a suspect patient, put a surgical mask on the patient.

Rubella—German Measles

Rubella is also known as the three-day measles. This illness is viral and is the third disease covered in the MMR vaccine. This is generally referred to as a benign disease. However, this illness in pregnant women can lead to birth defects in the fetus, including blindness, deafness, mental retardation, and congenital heart defects. The incubation period for rubella is 12 to 23 days. A person is considered contagious from the onset of the rash. The signs and symptoms of rubella include fever, rash, and swollen lymph glands.

Rubella was declared eliminated from in the United States in 2005. Again with a decline in vaccinations, cases of rubella are again being seen. The MMR vaccine is effective, and its protection is long lasting. All health-care workers should have immunity to rubella. Primary protection is afforded by vaccination in the absence of history of the disease.

Meningitis, Viral or Bacterial

Meningitis is a disease caused by the inflammation of the protective membranes (the meninges) covering the brain and spinal cord. There are two types of meningitis—viral and bacterial. Viral meningitis accounts for over 90% of U.S. cases and is not communicable. In contrast, bacterial meningitis, or meningococcal meningitis, is communicable by direct contact with the infected patient's oral secretions or through respiratory droplets. The CDC defines exposure to bacterial meningitis as close contacts with a patient who has meningococcal disease. Such close contacts include household members, child-care center contacts, college dormitory roommates, and persons directly exposed to the patient's oral secretions (kissing, mouth-to-mouth resuscitation, endotracheal intubation, or endotracheal tube management). Those who have had significant exposure to a patient with meningococcal meningitis need to be treated with a short course of antibiotics. Vaccination against bacterial meningitis is now recommended by the CDC for all, beginning at age 13.

Meningitis infections are characterized by a sudden onset of fever, headache, and stiff neck. It is often accompanied by other symptoms, such as nausea, vomiting (projectile), photophobia (sensitivity to light), altered mental status, sudden onset severe headache, and neck stiffness.

Influenza

Influenza (flu) is a communicable respiratory illness caused by influenza viruses (Type A or Type B viruses). Influenza causes mild to severe illness and at times can lead to death. Worldwide, influenza kills over 200,000 people each year, more than any of the other diseases discussed in this chapter. The elderly, young children, pregnant women, and people with lowered immune systems are at high risk for serious flu complications. Flu complications can include bacterial pneumonia, ear infections, sinus infections, and dehydration. Flu can also exacerbate chronic medical conditions such as congestive heart failure, asthma, and diabetes. People who have the flu often feel some or all of the following symptoms: fever or feeling feverish/chills, cough, sore throat, headache, body aches (myalgias), fatigue, and runny nose.

Flu viruses spread mainly by droplets made when people with the flu cough or sneeze. A person might get flu by touching a surface or object that has flu virus on it and then touching his or her own mouth, eyes, or nose. Annual vaccinations are the best way to prevent contracting the flu. By taking flu vaccine each year, protection builds up in a person's immune system against more of the different strains of seasonal flu viruses. This also serves to decrease illness and workers' absenteeism.

PEARLS
Preventing Meningitis Transmission

Placing a surgical mask on a suspect patient blocks transmission. If the patient cannot be masked, health-care workers should wear surgical masks. In the field it is not possible to differentiate between viral and bacterial meningitis, therefore use appropriate PPE on *all* suspected meningitis cases.

PEARLS
Influenza Transmissions

Annual flu vaccinations are the first line of defense for preventing influenza. Placing a surgical mask on a suspected flu patient blocks transmission. If the patient cannot be masked, health-care workers should wear surgical masks.

Follow the CDC's work restriction guidelines if personnel come to work ill with the flu. The importance of work restriction was stressed during the H1N1 flu outbreak in 2009 and 2010. Flu vaccine is viewed not only as emergency care provider protection but as patient protection as well. There are new influenza vaccines available that do not contain mercury or antibiotics and are not egg based. So, many more providers can participate in the program. It is a problem that EMS is one of the lowest groups for compliance with annual vaccination campaigns.

Multidrug-Resistant Organisms (MDROs)

Since the early 1960s the number of multidrug-resistant organisms has been increasing. First reported in the hospital care setting, such infections are now also in the general population. Hospital-associated infections (HAIs) are now a leading cause of extended hospital stay and increased costs. Many health-care systems are actively trying to lower HAIs.

Methicillin-resistant *Staphylococcus aureus* (MRSA) is perhaps the most prevalent HAI. There now is a community acquired (CA-MRSA) strain that is more common and more easily transmissible than the HA form. The new CA strain is called USA 300 or USA 400. It is transmitted by close personal contact with nonintact skin, close contact sports (wrestling, football), and poor personal hygiene. Household pets have also been identified as a source for transmission. These infections are often is misdiagnosed as a "spider bite."

Referring to MRSA as methicillin resistant is a bit misleading. MRSA strains are currently resistant to several different antibiotics, including penicillin, oxacillin, and amoxicillin. HA-MRSA is often also resistant to tetracycline and erythromycin. Generally, it presents as a localized soft-tissue infection (abscess) and is easily treated by incision and drainage. However, the organism can affect organs and joints. Complications of MRSA infection may include endocarditis, necrotizing fasciitis, osteomyelitis, sepsis, and death.

Prehospital care personnel are not at high risk for contracting MRSA when performing job tasks. Gloves, good hand washing, and clean surfaces and equipment are important for protection of patients and care providers. EMS agencies also should have cleaning routines established for exercise equipment and enforce work-restriction guidelines for personnel who have nonintact skin that is not able to be covered with a dressing. There is no post-exposure treatment for exposure to MRSA recommended.

Vancomycin-Resistant Enterococci (VRE)

Vancomycin-resistant enterococci (VRE) is primarily a hospital-acquired infection commonly found in urinary tract and bloodstream infections. Enterococci are common bacteria of the gastrointestinal and urinary tracts and sometimes cause infection. Vancomycin is the primary drug used to treat this infection. In some cases, enterococci have become resistant to this drug and are called vancomycin-resistant enterococci (VRE). VRE has also been found in livestock stool, uncooked chicken, and persons who work at farms or processing plants. VRE can live on surfaces for long periods of time, so cleaning is important after patient delivery. VRE is transmitted by direct contact with contaminated surfaces or equipment or by direct contact with a patient's wound drainage. A health-care worker must have an open cut or sore to allow the organism entry.

Prevention against VRE includes using standard precautions, including gloves and good hand washing when in contact with wound drainage, urine, or stool. A cover gown is only needed if there will be contact wound drainage with an emergency care provider's uniform. Following transport, it is important to clean any ambulance surface or equipment that came in contact with the suspected VRE patient. Focus on high-touch items. Standard surface disinfectants will adequately clean surfaces contaminated with VRE.

VRE is treated using newer synthetic antibiotics. People in good health are not at risk of infection. However, health-care workers may play a role in transmitting the

PEARLS
Artificial Ventilation

Be prepared! Have appropriate barrier devices with you so you are not required to do mouth-to-mouth breathing. However, you have an obligation to perform mouth-to-mouth resuscitation if your patient needs it and you forgot your equipment.

PEARLS
VRE Exposure

If you sustain direct contact with an open wound and VRE body fluids, notify your infection control officer and complete a report. No medical treatment post exposure is indicated.

organism if they do not practice careful hand washing and other infection control precautions. Methods for VRE transmission are direct contact with hands, environmental surfaces, or medical equipment contaminated by the feces of an infected person. There is no recommended medical follow-up for exposure to VRE.

Clostridium Difficile (C-diff)

Clostridium difficile (C-diff) is not a multidrug-resistant organism, but it is treated as if it were. It results from prolonged antibiotic treatment and is generally related to a patient's hospital stay. C-diff replaces "good" bacteria in the intestines and leads to watery, green, and foul-smelling diarrhea, fever, nausea, loss of appetite, and abdominal tenderness/pain. It is an issue also for patients who find themselves in the long-term care (LTC) setting. LTC personnel should advise an EMS crew what precautions are to be used for transport.

Generally, this illness resolves in two to three days after discontinuing antibiotics. Complications that result from *C. diff* infection include pseudomembranous colitis, sepsis, and perforations of the colon. Glove use, good hand washing with warm water and soap, and cleaning contaminated surfaces with an appropriate cleaning agent is important for reducing transmission risks. Alcohol-based hand cleaners do not kill *C. diff*. Use soap and warm water to wash hands.

Health-care workers should report and document contamination of open skin areas. No medical follow-up is recommended.

Multidrug-resistant organisms will continue to be an issue until several key influencing factors are addressed. They include good hand washing practice, cleaning of vehicles and equipment, education regarding the nonuse of antibiotics when not needed, removal of antibiotics from animal foods, and altering prescription habits. With the advent of new and emerging resistant organisms, obtaining a travel history on all patients is important.

> **PEARLS**
> **C. Difficile Cleaning**
>
> Alcohol-based products are *not* effective for decontaminating surfaces that have been exposed to C-diff. C-diff is a spore-forming agent so a chlorine-based cleaning solution is required.

Precautions for Prevention of Transmission of Infectious Agents

Standard precautions refer to treating everyone (including you) as if they are infectious. Your goal is to prevent the spread of infection from you to the patient and from the patient to you. In today's environment, you must use appropriate precautions based on each and every patient's care needs. Consider the use of personal protection based on the task being performed (Table 22-1).

> **contact precaution:** steps health-care workers can take to protect themselves and patients from contracting diseases transmitted through direct contact with infected patients or materials.
>
> **droplet precautions:** steps health-care workers can take to protect themselves and patients from contracting diseases transmitted through droplets of fluid, such as nasal or respiratory secretions; includes use of mask, gown, and googles.
>
> **airborne precautions:** steps health-care workers can take to protect themselves and patients from contracting diseases transmitted through inhalation, including use of N-95 respirator.

Table 22-1: Infectious Diseases and Route of Transmission

Bloodborne *(includes body fluids)*	Airborne	Droplet
HIV	Chickenpox	Influenza
Hepatitis B	Measles	Pertussis
Hepatitis C	Tuberculosis	Rubella
Rabies		Mumps
Cutaneous anthrax		N. meningitis (bacterial meningitis
Viral hemorrhagic fevers (Ebola)		SARS
		Diphtheria
		Novel influenza virus (H1N1)

Procedure

General Considerations

1. Be knowledgeable about infection from hepatitis B, hepatitis C, and HIV. Understand their etiologies, signs and symptoms, routes of transmission, and epidemiology (relationships of the various factors determining the frequency and distribution of a disease).

2. If you have on your own body open or weeping lesions, take special precautions to prevent exposure of those areas to blood and OPIM. Lesions should be covered with a bandage. If the lesions cannot be adequately protected, get placed on work restriction. Avoid invasive procedures, other direct patient care activities, and handling of equipment used for patient care.

3. Perform routine hand washing before and after all patient contact. Wash hands as soon as possible following exposure to blood or OPIM. Wash hands after glove removal. Alcohol-based foam or gel is best for in-field use. Emergency care providers should not have artificial nails or extensions because they can be hard to clean and can trap potentially infectious materials.

4. Become immunized against the hepatitis B virus, chickenpox, measles, mumps, and rubella if you are not protected by acquired immunity. Get your Tdap booster.

5. Report any exposure event to your designated infection control officer (DICO).

Procedure

Transmission-Based Precautions

When the way in which a disease is transmitted is identified, there are specific methods to prevent that transmission. Those methods are called *transmission-based precautions*. There are three categories of transmission precautions—contact, droplet, and airborne precautions. Note that these are *always* used in conjunction with standard precautions

Contact Precautions

Contact precautions are meant to reduce the risk of transmission of organisms spread by direct or indirect contact, including GI illnesses (Norovirus), multidrug-resistant organisms, skin and wound infections, and head lice. In addition to standard precautions, contact precautions are as follows:

1. Wear gloves.
2. Wear gown when in contact with the individual, surfaces, or objects within the immediate environment.

3. Clean and disinfect all reusable items, such as blood pressure cuff and stethoscope.
4. Follow surface cleaning protocol for the vehicle and stretcher, using appropriate viricidal or germicidal agents.

Droplet Precautions

Certain diseases can be transmitted by droplets, such as influenza, pertussis, and meningococcal disease. So, in addition to standard precautions use the following **droplet precautions**:

- Wear a surgical mask when within three feet (one meter) (for smallpox six feet or two meters) of persons known or suspected of having diseases spread by droplets.
- If large droplets are produced with coughing or sneezing, place a surgical mask on the patient for transport. If you are unable to do so, then don a surgical mask yourself.

- If you are ill, practice cough and sneeze etiquette yourself.

Airborne Precautions

With individuals known or suspected of having diseases spread by fine particles dispersed by air currents, such as tuberculosis, measles, and chickenpox, use **airborne precautions** such as wearing goggles or a face shield during *all* contact with the individual, not just when splashes or sprays are anticipated. All persons should wear an N-95 respirator.

Procedure

Handling and Cleaning of Items Exposed to Blood or OPIM

- Prevent sharps injuries by using needle-safe or needleless devices. It is the law in the United States and in your best interest.
- Any disposable equipment such as masks, gowns, gloves, mouthpieces, and airways that have been contaminated by blood or OPIM should be collected in an impervious plastic bag. The plastic bags should then be disposed of according to governmental definitions of medical waste in proper waste containers available in hospital emergency departments or other health-care locations. Nondisposable gowns should be laundered at the hospital or EMS facility. There should be linen bags or containers designated for contaminated gowns, and so on.
- Use a low-sudsing detergent with a neutral pH to wash any surface spills on nondisposable equipment that does not usually come in contact with skin or mucous membranes. The equipment should then be wet down or soaked in a 1:100 dilution of household bleach (or 70% isopropyl alcohol). In this concentration, bleach will not cause corrosion of metal objects.
- Using a low-sudsing detergent with a neutral pH, wash nondisposable medical devices that will frequently contact skin or mucous membranes. Check manufacturer's recommendations for disinfection so the warranty is not voided. If appropriate after washing, soak equipment for 30 to 40 minutes or more in 2% alkaline glutaraldehyde (such as Cidex®) or similar solution in a well-ventilated area, rinse in sterile water, and package until reuse.

Procedure

Personal Protection During Patient Exposures

Follow standard precautions and use transmission-based precautions. (See Table 22-2.)

- Wear gloves if exposure to blood or OPIM is anticipated. Always take this precaution when performing an invasive procedure or handling any item soiled with blood or body fluids. Almost all trauma patients are risks for exposure to blood or body fluids.
- Disposable gowns, masks, and eye coverings are necessary when extensive contact with blood or body fluids is anticipated. Those precautions are advised when airborne spread of blood or body

(continued)

Procedure (*continued*)

Table 22-2: Recommended Personal Protective Equipment for Worker Protection Against HIV and HBV Transmission in Prehospital Settings*

Task or Activity	Disposable Gloves	Gown	Mask	Protective Eyewear
Bleeding control with spurting blood	Yes	Yes	Yes	Yes
Bleeding control with minimal bleeding	Yes	No	No	No
Emergency childbirth	Yes	Yes	Yes	Yes
Blood drawing	Yes	No	No	No
Starting IV line	Yes	No	No	No
ET intubation or use of BIAD	Yes	No	No, unless splashing is likely	No, unless splashing is likely
Oral/nasal suctioning, manually cleaning airway	Yes	No	No, unless splashing is likely	No, unless splashing is likely
Handling and cleaning instruments with microbial contamination	Yes	No, unless soiling is likely	No	No
Measuring blood pressure	No	No	No	No
Measuring temperature	No	No	No	No
Giving an injection	Yes	No	No	No

*From CDC Guidelines for Public Safety Personnel & U.S. OSHA Guidelines.

fluids is likely, such as with endotracheal intubation, blind insertion airway device, vaginal deliveries, and major trauma.

- When treating any patient with respiratory complaints, mask the patient with a surgical mask or nonrebreather oxygen mask. It is also important to get a travel history.

- Direct mouth-to-mouth ventilation of patients during CPR is discouraged. Use disposable mouthpieces when artificial ventilation is performed.

Procedure

Reporting Accidental Exposure to Blood or OPIM

- Thoroughly wash or irrigate the exposed area immediately following an exposure to blood or contaminated body fluids. In the United States, you must contact your designated infection control officer (DICO), which all employers of HCWs must have. The DICO will deal with the incident and the medical facility from this point, including contacting the DICO from the hospital emergency department where you delivered the patient.

- The DICO will make the first determination regarding whether or not an exposure occurred and will notify the receiving facility of the possible exposure at the time of the incident. The DICO will ask the facility to cooperate in determining the serologic status of the source. Know your local rules, laws, and responsibilities.

- Write a report of the incident as soon as possible. The minimum information that should be recorded on the report is included in Figure 22-2.

REPORT OF EXPOSURE TO BLOOD OR OPIM

NAME OF EMS PERSONNEL _____

NAME OF EMS SERVICE _____

SSI _____

ADDRESS OF EMS SERVICE _____

PHONE NUMBER (HOME)_____ (WORK) _____

DATE OF EXPOSURE _____TIME OF EXPOSURE _____

NAME OF PATIENT_____

HOSPITAL ID NUMBER _____

PATIENT ADDRESS_____

PHONE NUMBER (WORK) _____ (HOME) _____

ROUTE OF EXPOSURE: _____

( ) Parenteral exposure (needlestick or sharp instrument)

( ) Mucous membrane

( ) Open skin

( ) Intact skin

( ) Other_____

TYPE OF FLUID:

( ) blood   ( ) emesis   ( ) saliva

( ) stool   ( ) urine   ( ) other_____

SOURCE OF EXPOSURE:

HIV:	( ) Yes	( ) No	( ) Unknown	
Hepatitis B:	( ) No	( ) Acute	( ) Chronic Carrier	( ) Unknown
Hepatitis C:	( ) No	( ) Acute	( ) Chronic Carrier	( ) Unknown
Tuberculosis:	( ) No	( ) Yes		

RISK FACTORS:

( ) Homosexual   ( ) IV Drug Abuser

( ) Hemophilia   ( ) Dialysis Patient

( ) Sexual Contact of the Above

( ) Other_____

HIV Test: ( ) Pos.   ( ) Neg.   ( ) Unknown

Date of HIV Test: _____

HBsAg: ( ) Pos.   ( ) Neg.   ( ) Unknown

Date of HBsAg Test _____

Description of Circumstances Surrounding the Exposure, Including Measures Taken After Exposure:

_____

_____

_____

INSTITUTION NOTIFIED: _____

PHYSICIAN OR RESPONSIBLE PERSON: _____

DATE OF NOTIFICATION: _____TIME OF NOTIFICATION: _____

NAME OF EXPOSED PERSONNEL _____ DATE _____

SIGNATURE _____

Figure 22-2 Sample report form.

(*continued*)

Procedure (*continued*)

The written ambulance report may be used to supplement, but not replace, the exposure report. In many systems, you will be required to fill out a confidential exposure report form, which only the exposed emergency care provider, the DICO, and the treating physician are allowed to see and be involved in the communication process. An exposed emergency care provider has become a patient and has a right to privacy.

- Blood tests (if any) to be done on the exposed emergency care provider depend on reports of testing of the source patient. If the results of rapid HIV testing and rapid HCV are negative, then no further testing of the emergency care provider is needed.

  If the source patient is positive for HIV, then the exposed employee should undergo HIV serology determination close to the time of the incident. Repeat testing should be done at six weeks and four months. The four-month test should be done using rapid testing. If the source patient is HCV

positive, the exposed emergency care provider can be tested for HCV-RNA in two weeks following the exposure. If the source patient is HBV positive and the exposed emergency care provider has not already been immunized, hepatitis B vaccine should be administered.

The administration of HBIG should be determined by the serologic testing of both the source (where possible) and the exposed health-care provider, as well as by the assessment of the risk of the exposure. If the care provider has a positive titer report in his or her chart, no treatment is indicated.

- Exposure plans must include a mechanism for information exchange between the DICO and medical facility. In addition to EMS reporting of exposures by emergency care providers, this mechanism should include the notification of the DICO when the medical facility identifies, after the fact, that an emergency care provider may have been exposed to an infectious disease from a patient he or she transported.

Case Presentation (*continued*)

An ALS tactical medical team is on scene with law enforcement's Special Response Team (SRT). The team has entered a dwelling where there is known crack/cocaine and methamphetamine sales and usage. During the entry by law enforcement, one of the occupants tried to escape by jumping through a large glass window. As a result, the 25-year-old male has multiple lacerations on his face, neck, leg, and arms. There is severe, active bleeding from the lateral aspect of the right thigh, likely caused by a lacerated artery. The patient is conscious and physically and verbally abusive. He is quickly restrained by the law enforcement officers.

Both emergency care providers and law enforcement officers don supplemental personal protective equipment (face shields and gowns). The ITLS Primary Survey reveals the patient is conscious and combative, verbally abusive, and spitting. Attempts to control the patient's

bleeding with direct pressure are unsuccessful. A commercially made tourniquet is applied proximal to the bleeding site, and the hemorrhage is controlled. Although being manually and mechanically restrained, the patient continues to resist.

Respiratory rate is 30, pulse rate is 120, and breath sounds are clear and equal. Minor lacerations, with minimal bleeding, are noted on the chest, forearms, and lower legs. The patient is immediately transported. No useful additional information is gathered during the ITLS Secondary Survey. Due to combativeness a blood pressure is not obtained, but skin color is good, capillary refill is normal, and peripheral pulses, although rapid, are present and weak. An IV is established, with 4 mg of lorazepam and a 20 mL/kg bolus of normal saline administered. During transport the receiving hospital is notified of the incoming patient status and the suspicions of drug use and excited delirium syndrome. His excited delirium is finally controlled with ketamine in the emergency department.

The patient is admitted to the hospital and undergoes repairs of his multiple lacera-tions. He is also treated for polydrug abuse and hepatitis C virus infection. Because of the proper use of personal protective equip-ment, none of the EMS or law enforcement personnel sustained an exposure.

Summary

Like most HCWs, you are at risk of exposure to many contagious diseases. Because of the presence of blood and contaminated secretions in many trauma victims, you must take extra precautions to avoid exposure to the viruses that cause hepatitis B, hepatitis C, and HIV and to the bacteria that cause tuberculosis. Knowledge of the modes of exposure, as well as adherence to barrier precautions, or post-exposure medical follow-up will reduce your risk of contracting any of those infections. In the United States, the government standards released make adherence to precautions mandatory for HCWs at risk for exposure to contaminated blood or OPIM with the exception of not delaying care if personal protective equipment is not readily avail-able. Taking recommended vaccines and immunizations also lowers risk for expo-sure to vaccine-preventable diseases.

Bibliography

Coll, W. E., and K. West. "Emergency and Other Pre-Hospital Medical Services." In *APIC Text of Infection Control and Epidemiology*, 4th ed., clinical editor P. Grotta. An online text from the Association for Professionals in Infection Control and Epidemiology, Inc., last updated June 6, 2014. Accessed December, 2014, at http://text.apic.org/item-55/chapter-54-emergency-and-other-pre-hospital-medical-services

"Bloodborne Infectious Diseases: HIV/AIDS, Hepatitis B, Hepatitis C: Management and Treatment Guidelines." CDC Web page, last updated July 21, 2014. Accessed December 16, 2014, at http://www.cdc.gov/niosh/topics/bbp/guidelines.html

Chapman, L. E., E. E. Sullivent, L. A. Grohskopf, E. M. Beltrami, J. F. Perz, K. Kretsinger, J. F. Perz, K. Kretsinger, A. L. Panlilio, et al. "Recommendations for Postexposure Interventions to Prevent Infection with Hepatitis B Virus, Hepatitis C Virus, or Human Immunodeficiency Virus, and Tetanus in Persons Wounded During Bombings and Other Mass-Casualty Events—United States, 2008: Recommendations of the Centers for Disease Control and Prevention." *MMWR Recommendations and Reports* 57, no. RR-6 (August 1, 2008): 1–19.

Clinical Consultation Center. "Post-Exposure Prophylaxis (PEP)." University of California, San Francisco, Web page © 2015. Accessed January, 2015, at http://nccc.ucsf.edu/clinician-consultation/post-exposure-prophylaxis-pep/

"Hand Hygiene in Health Care Settings." CDC Web page, last updated January 8, 2015. Accessed February 5, 2015, at http://www.cdc.gov/handhygiene/

Jensen, P. A., L. A. Lambert, M. F. Iademarco, and R. Ridzon. "Guidelines for Preventing the Transmission of Mycobacterium Tuberculosis in Health-Care Settings. *MMWR Recommendations and Reports* 54, no. RR-17 (December 30, 2005): 1–141.

Kuhar, D. T., D. K. Henderson, K. A. Struble, W. Heneine, V. Thomas, L. W. Cheever, A. Gomaa, A. L. Panlilio; U.S. Public Health Service Working Group. "Updated U.S. Public Health Service Guidelines for the Management of Occupational Exposures to Human Immunodeficiency Virus and Recommendations for Postexposure Prophylaxis." *Infection Control and Hospital Epidemiology* 34, no. 9 (September 2013): 875–92.

PEARLS
Reporting an Exposure

Any possible exposure to dis-eased blood or OPIM should be immediately reported to your designated infection control offi-cer. (Know who the DICO is and how to contact him or her 24/7.) The medical facility is required under the new Ryan White dis-ease list to inform the DICO if a crew has transported a patient suspected for or diagnosed with an airborne or droplet transmitted disease.

PEARLS
Mandatory Reporting

Reporting of exposure to HBV, HBC, HIV, as well as airborne and droplet disease exposures is man-datory in the United States and has significantly reduced the inci-dence and spread of infection in health-care providers in the last 15 years.

Needlestick Safety and Prevention Act, Public Law 106–430. *U.S. Federal Register* 66, no. 12 (2001): 5318–24.

NFPA 1581: Standard on Fire Department Infection Control Program. (Quincy, MA: National Fire Protection Association, 2015). Accessed January, 2015, at http://www.nfpa.org/codes-and-standards/document-information-pages?mode=code&code=1581

"Occupational Latex Allergies." NIOSH Web page, Workplace Safety and Health Topics, last updated July 10, 2010. Accessed February 5, 2015, at http://www.cdc.gov/niosh/topics/latex/.

Ryan White Comprehensive AIDS Resources Emergency Act; Emergency Response Employees; Notice, Centers for Disease Control, Department of Health and Human Services, Federal Register, March 21, 1994—Reauthorized September 30, 2009, Part G. *U.S. Federal Register,* 76, no. 212 (Wednesday, November 2, 2011). Disease Listing for Ryan White Law. Accessed March 4, 2015, at http://www.gpo.gov/fdsys/pkg/FR-2011-11-02/pdf/2011-28234.pdf

Shefer, A., W. Atkinson, C. Friedman, D. T. Kuhar, G. Mootrey, S. R. Bialek, A. Cohn, A. Fiore, L. Grohskopf, J. L. Liang, et al. "Immunization of Health-Care Personnel: Recommendations of the Advisory Committee on Immunization Practices (ACIP)." *MMWR Recommendations and Reports* 60, no. RR-7 (November 25, 2011): 1–45.

"Testing for HCV Infection: An Update for Guidance for Clinicians and Laboratorians." *MMWR Recommendations and Reports* 62, no. 18 (May 7, 2013): 362–65.

Weiner, H. R. "Community-Associated Methicillin-Resistant *Staphylococcus Aureus*: Diagnosis and Treatment." *Comprehensive Therapy* 34, no. 3-4 (2008): 143–46.

Get more information about this course by calling
ITLS International at 888-495-4875
(outside the United States call +1-630-495-6442) or visit

www.itrauma.org

Index

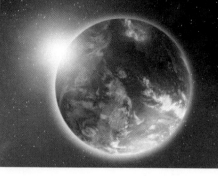